MEDICAL COMPLICATIONS OF TYPE 2 DIABETES

Edited by **Colleen Croniger**

Medical Complications of Type 2 Diabetes
Edited by Colleen Croniger

Published by InTech
Janeza Trdine 9, 51000 Rijeka, Croatia

Publishing Process Manager Mirna Cvijic

Technical Editor Teodora Smiljanic

Cover Designer InTech Design Team

Additional hard copies can be obtained from orders@intechopen.com

Medical Complications of Type 2 Diabetes, Edited by Colleen Croniger
p. cm.
978-953-307-363-7

For EU product safety concerns:
IN TECH d.o.o., Prolaz Marije Krucifikse Kozulić 3, 51000 Rijeka, Croatia,
info@intechopen.com or visit our website at intechopen.com.

Meet the editor

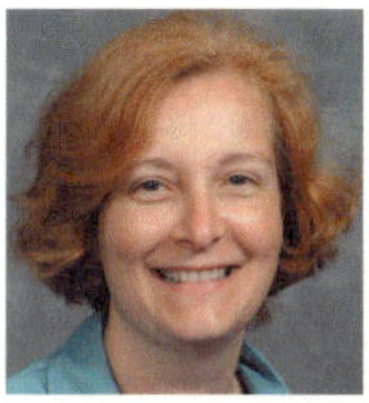

Dr. Colleen Croniger received her graduate degree in Molecular Biology from Case Western Reserve University in Cleveland, Ohio. After completing her graduate studies, she studied and learned metabolism from her post-doctoral mentor, Dr. Richard Hanson at Case Western Reserve. In 2002, Dr. Croniger joined the faculty of the Nutrition Department at Case Western Reserve as an Siistant Professor. Her research is focused on obesity, diabetes, nonalcoholic steatohepatitis (NASH) and alcoholic steatohepatitis (ASH) using genetically modified mouse models. She also teaches graduate and medical students nutrition and metabolism. Dr. Croniger has received Scholarship in Teaching award for her teaching, and for the design and implementation of the current medical school curriculum. In addition Dr. Croniger is a member of American Diabetes Association (ADA) and American Society for Biochemistry and Molecular Biology (ASBMB). Finally Dr. Croniger is the Metabolic Core director for the Case Western Reserve University Mouse Metabolic Phenotyping Core (MMPC). The Case MMPC is one of six centers that are NIH-NIDDK funded.

Contents

Preface

Obesity and type 2 diabetes are increasing worldwide problems. In this book we reviewed insulin secretion in both healthy individuals and in patients with type 2 diabetes. Because of the risk associated with progression from insulin resistance to diabetes and cardiovascular complications increases along a continuum, we included several chapters on the damage of endothelial cells in type 2 diabetes and genetic influences on endothelial cell dysfunction. Cardiovascular complications occur at a much lower glucose levels, thus a review on the oral glucose tolerance test compared to other methods was included. The medical conditions associated with type 2 diabetes such as pancreatic cancer, sarcopenia and sleep disordered breathing with diabetes were also discussed. The book concludes with several chapters on the treatments for this disease offering us hope in prevention and successful alleviation of the co-morbidities associated with obesity and type 2 diabetes.

Colleen Croniger
Department of Nutrition, Case Western Reserve University,
School of Medicine, Cleveland,Ohio
US

Part 1

Insulin Resistance

1

Insulin Secretion and Actions

Sarawut Jitrapakdee[1] and Briony E. Forbes[2]
[1]*Deparment of Biochemistry, Faculty of Science, Mahidol University, Bangkok,*
[2]*School of Molecular and Biomedical Science, University of Adelaide, Adelaide,*
[1]*Thailand*
[2]*Australia*

1. Introduction

1.1 Insulin biosynthesis

The islets of langerhans are the clusters of the endocrine tissue that scatter among the exocrine cells in the pancreas. The islets occupy approximately 1-2% of the total pancreatic tissue. Approximately, 1 million islets are scattered in the 25 cm long human pancreas. The insulin-producing cells make up 80% of each islet, while the remaining includes glucagon-producing α-cells, somatostatin-producing δ-cells and the pancreatic polypeptide (PP) F-cells (Unger et al., 1978). Insulin is first synthesized as a 110-amino acid polypeptide chain known as pre-proinsulin. This precursor form contains a hydrophobic 24-amino acid at its N-terminus known as the signal peptide. This signal peptide is removed during translocation from the cytoplasm to the endoplasmic reticulum, producing the proinsulin which comprises of chains A, B and C with three disulfide bonds. Further proteolysis of proinsulin in the secretory vesicles by the prohormone convertases (PC1 and PC2) and the carboxypeptidase E, removes the C-peptide from the rest of the molecule while still retains three disulfide bonds. This remaining part or mature insulin contains 21 amino acids on chain A and 30 amino acids on chain B (Steiner, 1969).

1.2 Biphasic insulin secretion and insulin exocytosis

The mature insulin is stored in the secretory granules which can be divided into two distinct pools, i.e. the reserve pool (RP) and the readily releasable pool (RRP) (Barg et al., 2002; Bratanova-Tochkova et al., 2002). The RRP is located close to the plasma membrane and is a rather small pool of insulin, comprising only 1-10% of total insulin in the cell. In contrast, the RP is located intracellularly and is a largest insulin pool. Once insulin granules in the RRP are released, the RP moves close to the plasma membrane to replenish the RRP (Barg et al., 2002; Bratanova-Tochkova et al., 2002).

Unlike other endocrine cells in the pancreas, β-cells secrete insulin. This occurs not only under low glucose conditions (non-stimulatory conditions) (3-5 mM glucose) but also when the glucose concentration in plasma is high during the postprandial period (10-25 mM glucose) when β-cells secrete much larger amounts of insulin into the circulation. Although several nutrients including glucose, some amino acids and non-esterified fatty acids can stimulate insulin secretion, glucose appears to be the most potent insulin secretagogue. The mechanism of glucose-induced insulin secretion (GSIS) is the most extensively studied. Secretion of insulin in response to the elevated levels of glucose in plasma is rapid and occurs in a two-step process known as *biphasic insulin secretion* (Straub and Sharp, 2002; Straub and Sharp, 2004). The first phase occurs very rapidly within a first few minutes upon stimulation. At this stage, the insulin granules in the RRP are fused very rapidly with the plasma membrane, resulting in a sharp release of insulin in the blood circulation. The first phase lasts only for a few minutes before the second phase begins and is sustained to the peak at 30-40 min or longer, depending on whether the concentration of plasma glucose is still high. The amount of insulin released during the second phase is much higher than the first phase. It is estimated that 99% of total insulin is secreted in this second phase, with an approximate release rate of 5-40 granules/cell/minute (Barg et al., 2002; Straub and Sharp, 2004). Therefore the second phase of insulin secretion is more physiologically important. Not unexpectedly, this biphasic insulin secretion appears to be impaired in the patients with type 2 diabetes. The translocation of the insulin granules in the RP to become the RRP, as well as the docking of secretory vesicles to the plasma membrane are dynamic processes, requiring the rearrangement of cytoskeleton proteins inside the β-cell (Wang and Thurmond, 2009). During basal conditions, the F-actin filaments are polymerized as a dense network below the plasma membrane. This web structure of filamentous F-actin not only blocks the access of insulin granules in the reserved pool to the plasma membrane but also prevents the interaction of the v-SNARE protein, VAMP2, in the insulin granule vesicles with the t-SNARE proteins (syntaxin 1 and 4) on the plasma membrane. This process is a prerequisite for granule exocytosis. Under glucose stimulation conditions, F-actin filaments are depolymerized and there is an increased microtubule polymerization rate, allowing the RP of insulin granules to translocate to the plasma membrane where the interaction of vSNAREs and tSNAREs are maximized (Farshori and Goode, 1994; Howell and Tyhurst, 1979; Thurmond et al., 2003).

2. Biochemical basis of glucose-induced insulin secretion

2.1 K_{ATP}-dependent GSIS: Roles of glycolysis, mitochondrial metabolism and ATP-sensitive potassium channels

Unlike other ligands, glucose does not require a cellular receptor to mediate signal transduction to stimulate insulin secretion in β-cells. This signal transduction is initiated by the rapid uptake of glucose through the glucose transporter 2 (GLUT2) in rodents (Chen et al., 1990) or glucose transporter 1 (GLUT1) in humans (De Vos et al., 1995) located on the plasma membrane of β-cells. GLUT2 transporters allow the high-capacity and low affinity transport needed to equilibrate glucose concentrations across the plasma membrane and to support the β-cell's very high metabolic rate. Glucose then undergoes phosphorylation by a glucokinase which possesses a high K_m for glucose, allowing the elevated levels of plasma glucose present during the postprandial period to enter β-cells for glycolysis (Matschinsky, 1990). As glucokinase has low binding affinity for glucose, this means that the glycolytic rate is never saturated during the postprandial period. Because the β-cell contains very low activity of lactate dehydrogenase, most glycolysis-derived pyruvate enters the mitochondria and is oxidized to acetyl-CoA by the pyruvate dehydrogenease complex. Acetyl-CoA is then oxidized in the TCA cycle, concomitant with the production of the reducing equivalents, NADH. In contrast to other cell types, β-cells possess very high mitochondrial glycerol-3-phosphate dehydrogenase activity, which is a key enzyme in the mitochondrial-3-phosphate dehydrogenase shuttle (MacDonald, 1981). This allows NADH formed during glycolysis to be transported to the mitochondria for oxidative phosphorylation. The reducing equivalents obtained from glycolysis and TCA cycle are subsequently oxidized through the electron transport chain to produce cellular ATP. The key component that links the metabolic signal and the insulin granule exocytosis is the ATP-sensitive potassium channel (K_{ATP}). This channel is an octamer comprising four pore forming subunits of Kir6.2 and four subunits of the sulfonylurea receptor (SUR1) (Aguilar-Bryan et al., 1995). Under unstimulated conditions, K_{ATP} channels are opened, allowing the diffusion of K^+ across plasma membrane of β-cells near equilibrium. However, when the ratio of ATP:ADP ratio is high due to a high rate of glucose oxidation, ATP binds to the Kir6.2 component of the K_{ATP} channel, causing the channel to close. The depolarization of the membrane caused by the closure of the K_{ATP} channel opens the voltage-gated Ca^{2+} channel, causing Ca^{2+} influx into the cells (Ashcroft et al., 1984). This electrophysiological cascade results in the exocytosis of the insulin granues in the RRP. The increase of intracellular Ca^{2+} also stimulates the calmodulin-dependent protein kinase II which can phosphorylate several targets including the myosin light chain kinase that controls the cytoskeletal or secretory vesicle proteins (Easom, 1999). The insulin release triggered by the K_{ATP}-dependent mechanism corresponds to the first phase of the biphasic insulin secretion (Straub and Sharp, 2004).

2.2 K_{ATP}-independent GSIS: Anaplerosis and coupling factors

Although the K_{ATP} channel appears to control the GSIS, several lines of evidence suggest that GSIS can be operated independently of K_{ATP} channel. Treating β-cells with a K_{ATP} channel opener, diazoxide, does not completely eliminate GSIS (Gembal et al., 1992). Furthermore, mice lacking Kir6.2 or the SUR1 component of K_{ATP} are still capable of secreting insulin in response to glucose albeit not as robust as the wild type mice (Seghers et al., 2000; Shiota et al., 2002). It has now become clear that GSIS requires "coupling factors" or "metabolic factors" that act as the amplifying signal of insulin secretion. Those coupling factors include NADPH, GTP, long chain acyl-CoA and glutamate. The biochemical pathways or cycles that lead to production of the coupling factors are described below.

NADPH: The pentose phosphate pathway is the major pathway that produces NADPH, however the β-cell does not possess glucose-6-phosphate dehydrogenase to produce this reducing equivalent. Instead, β-cells possess a very high activity of pyruvate carboxylase and pyruvate dehydrogenase (MacDonald, 1993). Although equal proportions of the glycolysis-derived pyruvate enters mitochondria is carboxylated by PC and decarboxylated by pyruvate dehydrogenase, only the flux via the carboxylation reaction is correlated with GSIS (Lu et al., 2002). In β-cells, there is a high rate of the export of TCA cycle intermediates, i.e. citrate and malate from mitochondria to cytoplasm which is known as cataplerosis (MacDonald, 2003). The exported citrate and malate are then recycled back to the mitochondria as pyruvate known as pyruvate cycling as shown in Figure 1. This pyruvate cycling can be shuttled to the pyruvate via pyruvate/malate, pyruvate/isocitrate or pyruvate citrate cycles (MacDonald et al., 2005). As noted in Figure 1, NADPH is a common reducing equivalent produced by malate dehydrogenase, malic enzyme and isocitrate dehydrogenase in the above three cycles, respectively. Pyruvate then re-enters the mitochondria and is carboxylated by pyruvate carboxylase, which is as highly abundant as in the gluconeogenic tissue. Deficiencies in pyruvate carboxylase, cytosolic malic enzyme and cytosolic isocitrate dehydrogenase result in impaired GSIS, indicating the importance of pyruvate cycling in β-cells (Jitrapakdee et al., 2010). Glucose sharply increases the NADPH:NADP ratio proportion to the level of insulin secretion. The mechanism by which NADPH acts on insulin secretion is thought to be mediated through the glutaredoxin and thioredoxin redox pairs. The maintenance of the extra-mitochondria redox state via glutaredoxin and thioredoxin is required to support insulin granule exocytosis. Furthermore, NADPH is also associated with the voltage-dependent potassium channel (K_v) which works in an opposite way to the K_{ATP} channel. This channel functions as K^+ efflux, causing the repolarization of the β-cell plasma membrane for the next cycle of GSIS. Binding of NADPH to the Kv causes the conformational change of its regulatory subunit, reducing the efficacy of this channel for repolarization of the β-cell plasma membrane and enhancing the action of K_{ATP} channel [reviewed by Jitrapakdee et al., 2010].

Long chain acyl-CoA: Long chain acyl-CoA is another coupling factor thought to be required for GSIS (Brun et al., 1996; Corkey et al., 1989; Prentki et al., 1992). Evidence for this is derived from the following observations. Acute exposure of β-cells to glucose sharply increases intracellular levels of malonyl-CoA and long chain acyl-CoA. In supporting this observation, exposure of permeabilized β-cells to long chain acyl-CoA or non-esterified fatty acids also stimulates Ca^{2+}-evoked insulin exocytosis. This is accompanied by elevated levels of acetyl-CoA carboxylase 1 (ACC1), a rate-limiting enzyme of *de novo* fatty acid synthesis. ACC condenses two molecules of acetyl-CoA to malonyl CoA and this enzyme is rapidly induced by high concentrations of glucose in β-cells. Because malonyl-CoA is a potent inhibitor of the carnitine palmitoyl transerase I (CPT-1), the rapid increase of malonyl-CoA level by ACC1 would inhibit β-oxidation of fatty acids, resulting in the elevated levels of long chain acyl-CoA in β-cells (Brun et al., 1996; Corkey et al., 1989; Prentki et al., 1992). This long chain acyl-CoA can be used as the precursor for synthesizing diacyl glycerol and phospholipids. Consistent with this idea, acute exposure of β-cells to glucose also modifies the concentrations of phospholipids and cholesteryl esters. These modifications could affect membrane fluidity and exocytosis of the secretory vesicles. Furthermore diacyl glycerol can also activate protein kinase C which in turn phosphorylates its downstream targets including ion channels.

Although inhibition of ACC1 and fatty acid synthetase activities result in a marked reduction of GSIS, suppression of ATP-citrate lyase expression does not appear to affect GSIS, suggesting the presence of another pathway that can supply acetyl-groups for *de novo* fatty acid synthesis in β-cells [reviewed by Jitrapakdee et al., 2010]]. An alternate pathway that provides acetyl-groups for long chain acyl-CoA synthesis lies within the acetoacetate production catalyzed by acetoacetyl-CoA synthetase. This was demonstrated by the knockdown experiment in which suppression of this enzyme expression impairs GSIS in β-cells (MacDonald et al., 2005). Acute exposure of β-cells to glucose not only stimulates rapid lipogenesis but also alters phospholipid and cholesteryl ester contents in the plasma membrane which in turn affects insulin granule exocytosis and β-cell plasma membrane fluidity (MacDonald et al., 2008).

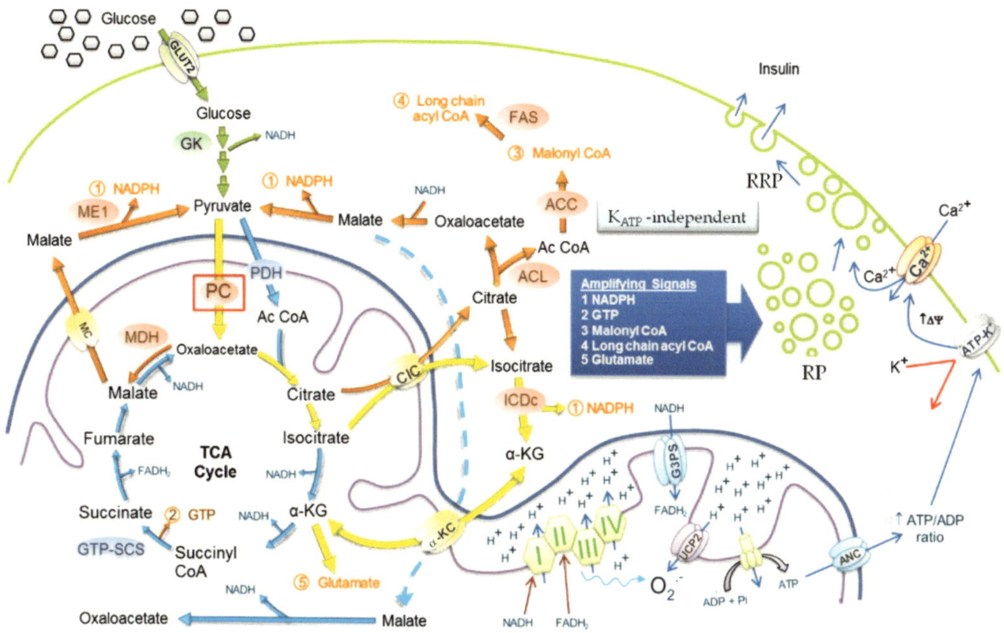

Fig. 1. Biochemical basis of glucose-induced insulin secretion (GSIS). Glucose enters β-cells through GLUT2 transporter and is metabolized to pyruvate by glycolysis. Pyruvate enters the mitochondria where it is oxidized in the TCA cycle. The NADH produced by both glycolysis and TCA cycle are oxidized to produce the cellular ATP. The increased level of ATP:ADP triggers the closure of ATP-sensitive potassium channels resulting in membrane depolarization. This in turn opens the voltage gate-dependent Ca^{2+} channels, causing the influx of Ca^{2+} which triggers the immediate exocytosis of insulin granules in the readily releasable pool, corresponding to the 1st phase of biphasic insulin secretion. Some components of the TCA cycle, i.e. malate, citrate and isocitrate are also exported from the mitochondria to cytoplasm (cataplerosis) where these exported products are converted back to pyruvate (pyruvate cycling) concomitantly with the production of NADPH via pyruvate-malate, pyruvate-citrate and pyruvate-isocitrate shuttles, respectively. PC replenishes OAA in the TCA cycle when malate, citrate and isocitrate are removed for the pyruvate cycling. The exported citrate is converted to oxaloacetate and acetyl-CoA. ACC1 converts acetyl-CoA to malonyl-CoA which is subsequently converted to long chain acyl-CoA by FAS. The NADPH malonyl-CoA, long chain acyl-CoA together with the mitochondrial GTP produced by succinyl-CoA synthetase and glutamate produced by glutamate dehydrogenase serve as "amplifying signals" that correspond to the 2nd phase of biphasic insulin secretion. ACC, acetyl-CoA carboxylase; ACL, ATP-citrate lyase; cICD, cytolsolic isocitrate dehydrogenase; CIC, citrate/isocitrate carrier; GTP-SC, GTP-succinate dehydrogenase; FAS, fatty acid synthase, MDH, malate dehydrogenase; ME, malic enzyme, PC, pyruvate carboxylase; PDH, pyruvate dehydrogenase complex; RP, reserve pool; RRP, readily releasable pool.

Other coupling factors: Acute exposure of β-cells to glucose causes a sharp increase in the level of glutamate, suggesting that glutamate might be a second messenger that promotes insulin secretion (Maechler and Wollheim, 1999). This intracellular source of glutamate is derived from the conversion of α-ketoglutarate by the glutamate dehydrogenase. Although there is a strong correlation between the rapid increase of an intracellular level of glutamate upon an acute stimulation by glucose, there is no direct evidence indicating that the rise of glutamate level results in the insulin secretion (MacDonald and Fahien, 2000). Incubation of β-cells with glutamine, a precursor of glutamate production does not increase GSIS. Furthermore the GDH ablated mice showed only 30-40% loss of GSIS indicating that glutamate may not be the second messenger for insulin secretion (Carobbio et al., 2009).

The level of mitochondrial GTP may be one of the coupling factors that regulate GSIS. The succinyl-CoA synthetase catalyzes the conversion of succinyl-CoA to succinate, concomitant with the production of GTP. Suppression of the succinyl-CoA synthetase expression results in impaired GSIS in β-cells, indicating the importance role of mitochondrial GTP in GSIS (Kibbey et al., 2007).

Incubation of β-cells with high concentrations of glucose not only stimulates ATP production via electron transport system but also triggers the production of the reactive oxygen species in the mitochondria. There is evidence that the reactive oxygen species may be an obligatory signal for insulin secretion (Leloup et al., 2009; Pi et al., 2007). Incubation of β-cells with certain reactive oxygen species stimulates insulin secretion. Because these reactive oxygen species are toxic to the cells and they are removed very quickly by the antioxidant enzymes in the β-cells the question remains whether this transient increase of reactive oxygen species is a bona fide coupling factor for GSIS.

3. Other insulin secretagogues

Although glucose is the most potent insulin secretagogue, certain amino acids including leucine and glutamine can also stimulate insulin secretion (Fahien et al., 1988; Malaisse-Lagae et al., 1982). Leucine stimulates insulin secretion because its acts as an allosteric activator of the glutamate dehydrogenase, an anaplerotic enzyme that converts glutamate to α-ketoglutarate in the TCA cycle. Glutamine by itself cannot stimulate insulin secretion, however combination of glutamine and leucine stimulates insulin secretion as robustly as glucose because glutamine can be converted to glutamate, and leucine acts as allosteric activator of glutamate dehydrogenase in the presence of excess glutamate substrate. Unlike leucine, arginine can stimulate only the 1st phase but not the amplifying phase of insulin secretion. The reason for this is because arginine is not metabolized in the mitochondria in the glycolysis or TCA cycle.

Free fatty acids by themselves cannot stimulate insulin secretion but low concentrations of them augment glucose-induced insulin secretion (Deeney et al., 2000; Poitout, 2003). Free fatty acids can be metabolized to long chain fatty acyl-CoA which is one of the coupling factors as described earlier. However, chronic exposure of β-cells to high concentration of fatty acids promotes β-cell apoptosis via the formation of ceramides or other reactive lipids (Giacca et al., 2011; Poitout and Robertson, 2002).

Apart from the nutrient secretagogues, some hormones can stimulate insulin secretion. The well known insulinotropic peptide hormones include the glucagon-like-peptide-1 (GLP-1) and gastic-inhibitory peptide (GIP) (Holst, 2007). GLP-1 is secreted from the enteroglucagonproducing cells (L-cells) in the lower intestine, while GIP is secreted from K-cells in the upper gastrointestinal tract. These two peptides are secreted in response to the ingestion of glucose. GLP-1 acts to increase insulin secretion via the circulation acting directly on pancreatic β cells and also via the sensory afferent neurons acting on the central nervous system (Holst et al. 2007). In the brain GLP-1 acts a neuropeptide to promote neuroendocrine actions on the autonomic nervous system including regulation of food intake, satiety and pancreatic secretions. GLP-1 is controlled by the dipeptidyl protease 4 (DPP4). DPP4 cleavage renders GLP-1 unable to bind to its target receptor, the glucagon-like peptide-1 receptor (GLP-1R) and thus tightly controls the levels of GLP-1 in the intestine and the circulation. GLP-1 also promotes metabolic control by inhibiting glucagon secretion.

4. Insulin oscillation

In humans, mouse and rat the majority of insulin (>70%) is released in a pulsatile manner with a periodicity of 3-5 min (Matveyenko et al., 2008; Porksen et al., 1997; Song et al., 2000). This pattern is observed both before and after meals, however the amplitude of oscillation is higher during the postprandial period. The oscillation of insulin secretion is believed to be a mechanism to prevent down-regulation of insulin receptors in the target tissues. The pulsatile insulin secretion is most obviously detected in the portal vein and can also be detected in the isolated islets. Remarkably, the oscillations of insulin secretion are also synchronized among one million islets. These tightly synchronized oscillations require the complex factors including the soluble factor, gap junction and intra-pancreatic nerves. However, this pulsatile pattern becomes less obvious in the peripheral blood (Tengholm and Gylfe, 2009). These oscillations are intrinsic to the islets, and are regulated by the concentrations in individual β-cells of cytoplasmic Ca^{2+}, intracellular cAMP and plasma membrane phosphoinositide lipids, as well as the activity of phospholipase C (Tengholm and Gylfe, 2009). The oscillations of insulin secretion from pancreatic islets correlate very well with the oscillation of intracellular Ca^{2+} concentration (Bergsten et al., 1994; Bergsten and Hellman, 1993). Although it is widely accepted that the insulin oscillation is the result of intracellular Ca^{2+} oscillation, it is unclear whether the oscillation of Ca^{2+} levels results from the oscillations of glycolytic and/or mitochondrial intermediates. The oscillation of phosphofructokinase (PFK) activity is well known to produce the oscillation of its product, fructose-1,6-bisphosphate which may in turn regulate oscillation of intracellular Ca^{2+} concentrations (Tornheim, 1997). However, suppression of PFK activity in β-cells did not affect the oscillation of intracellular Ca^{2+} concentration, suggesting that oscillation of PFK activity may not control the pulsatile manner of insulin secretion. However, recent reports reports have shown that there are oscillations of key metabolic products in the mitochondria including citrate, ATP, NAD(P)H, and O_2 consumption (Bertram et al., 2007; Tengholm and Gylfe, 2009). Notably, the oscillations of these metabolic products are also in the same range as that of intracellular Ca^{2+} oscillation. Although the oscillations of key products of mitochondrial metabolism are likely to regulate the oscillations of intracellular Ca^{2+}, Ca^{2+} by itself may feedback inhibit or stimulate the mitochondrial metabolism, resulting in the decrease or increase insulin secretion. The intracellular Ca^{2+} raised upon glucose-induced insulin secretion can enter mitochondria via the uniporter and depolarize the electrochemical potential in the inner membrane of the mitochondria thereby reducing mitochondrial ATP production (Bertram et al., 2007; Tengholm and Gylfe, 2009). However, the intra-mitochondrial Ca^{2+} can also stimulate the activities of several mitochondrial enzymes including the pyruvate dehydrogenase complex, isocitrate dehydrogenase and α-ketoglutarate dehydrogenase (Bertram et al., 2007; Tengholm and Gylfe, 2009). These synchronous oscillations of products of mitochondrial metabolism are believed to orchestrate the oscillation of insulin secretion.

Normoglycaemia is more efficiently maintained when insulin is delivered in a pulsatile fashion, most probably because of enhanced expression on the target tissues of insulin receptors that have a similar recycling periodicity. Significantly, this pulsatile delivery of insulin is lost or severely diminished in type 2 diabetes. This contributes to insulin resistance and the requirement for compensatory hypersecretion by the islets, potentially leading to their exhaustion (Bertram et al., 2007; Tengholm and Gylfe, 2009).

5. Insulin signaling

Insulin signaling controls metabolism as well as growth and survival in many mammalian tissues. It also plays a vital role in controlling lifespan (Longo et al., 2008). In humans, perturbation of insulin signaling results in diabetes but is also implicated in neoplasia (Pollak, 2008). Signaling via the insulin receptor (IR) results in activation of two main signalling pathways: the phosphoinositide 3-kinase/Akt (PI3K/Akt) and the mitogen activated protein kinase (MAPK) pathways. Both mitogenic and metabolic signalling outcomes are activated via the IR and the response arising depends on expression levels of the receptor and downstream signaling molecules by the cells within the target tissues.

The IR exists in two isoforms arising from alternative splicing (Belfiore et al., 2009; Denley et al., 2003). The exon 11+ (IR-B) isoform is expressed in insulin sensitive tissues and primarily in the liver. This receptor is responsible for the metabolic control processes classically associated with insulin's action. The exon 11- (IR-A) isoform, which lacks the 12 amino acids normally encoded by exon 11, is expressed mainly in fetal tissues including liver, kidney and muscle. Interestingly, both insulin and insulin-like growth factor-II (a structurally related mitogenic growth factor) can bind to the IR-A with high affinity to promote cell proliferation and survival. The foetal co-expression of IGF-II and IR-A suggests both may act together to play an important role in foetal growth. Interestingly, expression of both IGF-II and the IR-A is often upregulated in cancer and this represents an additional mechanism by which cancer cells grow and survive (Avnet et al., 2009; Denley et al., 2003).

5.1 Insulin receptor structure

The IR is a transmembrane glycoprotein with tyrosine kinase activity. It is a homodimer with each subunit consisting of an extracellular α subunit and a transmembrane spanning β subunit (see Figure 2) (De Meyts and Whittaker, 2002; Ward and Lawrence, 2009). The receptor is produced from a single proreceptor protein that is glycosylated, dimerised and proteolytically processed into separate α (~135kDa) and β chains (95kDa, mature receptor ~460kDa). The ligand binding region is located in the extracellular α subunits and the tyrosine kinase domain is located in the cytoplasmic region of the β subunits. The stoichiometry of ligand binding is 1:1. A recent crystal structure of the extracellular portion of the IR revealed a folded over conformation with two potential ligand binding pockets (McKern et al., 2006; Smith et al., 2010). The residues important for ligand binding have been identified by a series of detailed site-directed mutagenesis studies, with the use of IR:IGF-1R chimeras and using antibody competition for ligand binding (De Meyts and Whittaker, 2002). Within a single binding pocket ligand contacts the receptor at two sites. Site 1 is made up of residues within the L1 domain (large domain 1 leucine rich region) and ID (insert domain), with each derived from opposite receptor monomers. Site 2 is located within the Fn-III-1 and Fn-III-2 domains (derived from the same monomer as the ID of site 1).

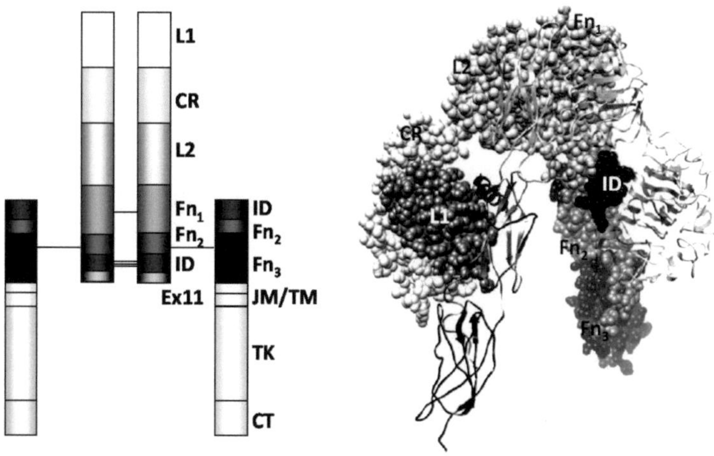

Fig. 2. The IR structure. The IR consists of 2 α and intracellular β subunits made up of the following domains (labelled on one receptor monomer, Left): L1 and L2, large domains 1 and 2 (leucine-rich repeats); CR, Cys-rich domain; Fn1, Fn2, Fn3, fibronectin type III domains 1-3 (also referred in the text as FnIII-1, FnIII-2, FnIII-3); ID, insert domain; Ex11, 12 residues encoded by exon11 (IR-B only); TM, transmembrane; JM, juxtamembrane; TK, tyrosine kinase; CT, C-terminal domains (adapted from Denley et al., 2003). The ligand binding regions are found in the L1, Fn1 and Fn2 (also referred in the text as FnIII-1 and -2) and the ID. (Right) The folded over conformation of the receptor is revealed in the IR ectodomain crystal structure (McKern et al., 2006), pdb 3LOH). The two binding pockets evident in the folded over structure include residues from each receptor monomer. One monomer is depicted in ribbon mode and the other is in surface filled mode.

While there is currently no structure of insulin bound to the intact IR, chemical cross-linking data and the structure of the IR ectodomain have allowed the development of a structural model of the interaction (Lou et al., 2006). Ligand binding cross-links the two receptor monomers leading to a structural change in the ectodomain and precluding binding of a second ligand molecule in the unoccupied binding pocket (as described in the mathematical model by Kiselyov et al., (Kiselyov et al., 2009).

The receptor structural change is transduced across the transmembrane region to the intracellular domain leading to activation of the intracellular tyrosine kinase domain. Crystal structures of the inactive and activated forms of the IR tyrosine kinase domain reveal that the first step in the activation process is the movement of an inhibitory arm reaching from the juxta membrane region that maintains the tyrosine kinase domain in a basal, low activity state. Removal of juxtamembrane domain Tyr984 from its contacts with the amino terminal kinase lobe allows coordination of ATP and subsequent trans autophosphorylation of Tyr1146, Tyr1150 and Tyr1151 within the activation loop of the tyrosine kinase domain (Hubbard, 2004).

5.2 Insulin signaling components

Following tyrosine kinase domain activation several other residues are phosphorylated and these act as docking sites for downstream signaling molecules (Siddle, 2011; Taniguchi et al., 2006). In fact at least 7 tyrosine residues, 12 serine residues and a single threonine have been shown to be phosphorylated in response to insulin (Kohanski, 1993; Lewis et al., 1990; Tavare and Denton, 1988; Tornqvist et al., 1987). Initial autophosphorylation of Tyr960 within a NPXY motif of the transmembrane domain provides an important docking site for insulin receptor substrate 1 and 2 (IRS-1 and IRS-2) and Shc (both substrates for the IR tyrosine kinase). The Grb2-associated binder 1 (Gab 1) and Cas-Br-M (murine) ecotropic retroviral transforming sequence homologue (Cbl) proteins also are substrates of the IR tyrosine kinase and play a role in glucose uptake (see section 6.1). IRS-1 and IRS-2 contain a phosphotyrosine-binding domain and a plekstrin-homology domain which facilitate the interaction with activated IR via phosphoTyr960. IRS and Shc proteins are phosphorylated on multiple sites by the IR and these phosphotyrosines then act as docking sites for different SH2 containing signaling molecules including PI3K and growth receptor binding protein-2 (Grb2). These proteins are the first molecules of the two main insulin stimulated signaling cascades: the PI3K-AKT/protein kinase B (PKB) pathway, which leads to protein translation, metabolic control, cell cycling and cell survival, and the Ras-mitogen-activated protein kinase (MAPK) pathway, which controls cell growth and differentiation.

There are six IRS proteins with IRS-1 and IRS-2 being the most widely expressed (Taniguchi et al., 2006). Knockdown studies *in vivo* and *in vitro* indicate that IRS-1 and IRS-2 play different roles of in insulin signaling. For example, *in vivo* knockdown of hepatic IRS-1 expression is associated with increased gluconeogenesis whereas down-regulation of hepatic IRS-2 is associated with expression of genes involved in lipogenesis. IRS-1 knockout mice are small and insulin resistant with normal glucose homeostasis due to compensatory insulin secretion. IRS-2 knockout mice are normal in size but develop diabetes and are insulin resistant due to reduced β-cell mass (reviewed in (Taguchi and White, 2008)). Although they do recruit many of the same binding partners the signalling differences of the two IRS isoforms may be explained by their differing abilities to bind certain downstream signalling molecules. Subcellular localisation or activation kinetics may also play a role. IRS signalling is controlled by feedback mechanisms predominantly involving serine phosphorylation of the IRS proteins by downstream kinases including Akt, S6K1 and GSK3, and leading to IRS inactivation (Taniguchi et al., 2006).

Several proteins regulate signaling via the IR (Taniguchi et al., 2006). SOCS-3 (suppressor of cytokine signalling-3), induced by cytokine signaling, regulates IR signaling by competing for binding with IRS proteins to phosphorylated Tyr960, thereby down-regulating insulin's action. SOCS proteins have attracted significant interest as they are up-regulated in cases of insulin resistance. Growth factor receptor bound proteins (Grb10/Grb14) act as pseudo substrates for the tyrosine kinase domain of activated IR and thereby inhibit further phosphorylation of downstream signaling molecules including IRS-1. They also protect the phosphotyrosines in the tyrosine kinase domain from dephosphorylation by phosphatases, thus potentially prolonging receptor activation (Holt and Siddle, 2005). One such phosphatase is PTP1B, which directly interacts with the IR tyrosine kinase domain thereby reducing IR signalling activity (Yip et al., 2010). Grb10 also promotes receptor downregulation via its interaction with the ubiquitin ligase NEDD4 (Ramos et al., 2006; Vecchione et al., 2003). Simultaneous knockout of Grb10 and Grb14 improved glucose homeostasis due to enhanced IR signalling (Holt et al., 2009; Holt and Siddle, 2005).

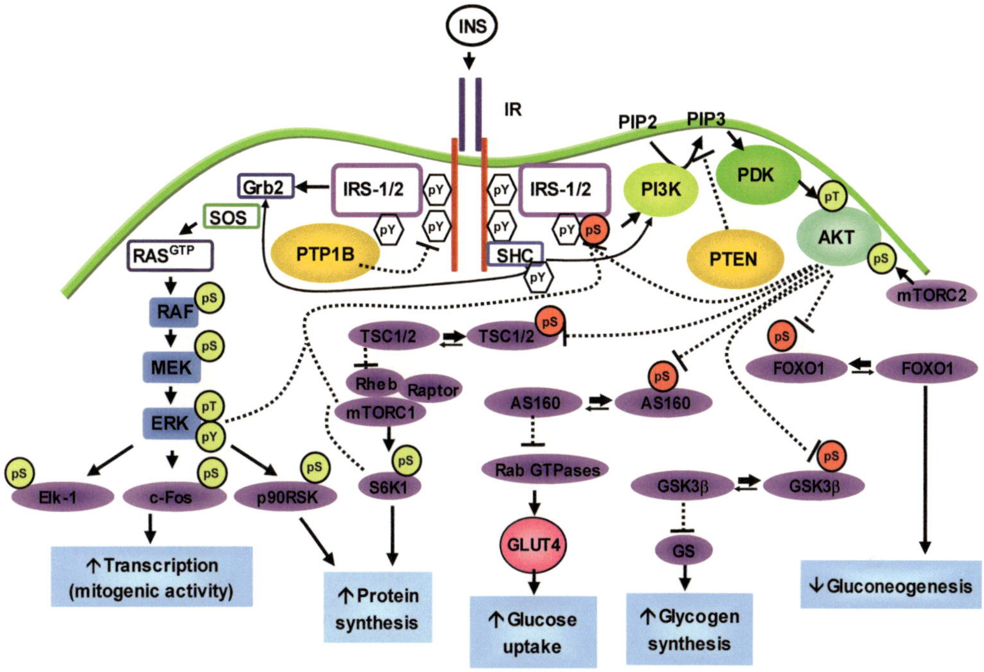

Fig. 3. The canonical insulin receptor signalling pathways (PI3K/AKT and MAPK pathways). Binding of insulin (INS) to the insulin receptor (IR) leads to activation of the intracellular receptor tyrosine kinase. Subsequent autophosphorylation leads to recruitment of IRS-1/2 and Shc. Activated PI3K then converts phosphotidyl inositol (4,5) bisphosphate (PIP2) to phosphotidyl inositol (3,4,5) trisphosphate which then recruits PDK and AKT to the membrane. AKT is phosphorylated on Thr308 by PDK and Ser473 by mTORC2. There are many target substrates of the serine kinase AKT including TSC1/2, which when phosphorylated by AKT becomes inactive and thereby promotes activation of the mTORC1 complex and subsequent protein synthesis. Inactivation of the GTPase activating protein AS160 by AKT relieves the inhibition of RAB GTPase to promote GLUT4 translocation and glucose uptake. Glycogen synthase promotes glycogen synthesis when AKT inactivates GSK3β and phosphorylation of FOXO1 prevents its translocation to the nucleus and thus inhibits gluconeogenesis. AKT signalling is switched off by the phosphatases PTEN (converts PIP3 to PIP2) and PTP1B (direct action on the IR). Mitogenic signalling involves recruitment of Grb2 by activated IRS-1/2 and Shc. SOS bound to Grb2 acts as a guanine exchange factor promoting the formation of active RAS GTP. Activation of RAF and the downstream MAPK signalling cascade follows leading to activation of p90RSK and protein synthesis as well as the transcription factors Elk-1 and c-FOS. IRS proteins are negatively regulated upon serine phosphorylation by AKT, mTORC1, pS6K and activated ERK1/2. Activation is indicated by a solid line and inhibition by a dashed line. IRS, insulin receptor substrate; PI3K, phosphotidylinositol 3-kinase; PDK, protein dependent kinase; mTORC, mammalian target of rapamycin complex; PTEN, phosphatase and tensin homologue; FOXO1, forkhead box O1; GSK3β, glycogen synthase kinase 3β; GS glycogen synthase; AS160, AKT substrate of 160kDa; TSC1/2, tuberous sclerosis complex-1 and -2; Rheb, Ras homologue enriched in brain; Raptor, regulatory associated protein of mTOR; PTP1B, protein tyrosine phosphatase 1B; Grb2, growth receptor binding protein 2; SOS, son-of-sevenless; MEK, MAPK kinase; ERK, extracellular signal-regulated kinase 1 and 2; p90RSK, p90 ribosomal protein S6 kinase; pY, phosphotyrosine; pS, phosphoserine; pT, phosphothreonine.

Activation of the IR by insulin also leads to internalization of the ligand:receptor complex and results in endosomal breakdown of insulin. Internalised receptor is either degraded or recycled back to the membrane for further signaling events (Foti et al., 2004). Interestingly, rapid receptor recycling is linked to sustained Akt signalling (Romanelli et al., 2007), whereas there is evidence that receptor internalization plays a role in prolonged signalling associated with the MAPK pathway and mitogenic activity (Jensen et al., 2007).

6. Insulin actions

6.1 Mitogenic effects

Insulin receptor signaling via the MAPK pathway leads predominantly to mitogenic biological effects such as cell growth, survival and differentiation (Belfiore et al., 2009; Siddle, 2011). Binding and activation of IRS proteins leads to recruitment of Grb2 and the guanyl nucleotide exchange factor SOS (son-of-sevenless). SOS then activates the small GTPase Ras which in turn activates Raf and the MAPK, MEK and Erk1/2 signaling cascade. Activated Erk1/2 phosphorylates a series of targets including p90 ribosomal protein S6 kinase (p90RSK), which promotes protein synthesis, and the transcription factors Elk-1 and c-Fos (Figure 3) (Shaul and Seger, 2007). Erk1 and Erk2 have both overlapping and unique functions. Erk1 knockout mice develop normally and are born a normal size probably due to compensation by Erk2. However, Erk1 knockouts do have deficient thymocyte maturation and some neurological defects. In contrast knockout of Erk2 is embryonic lethal. In relation to metabolism, Erk1 appears to play specific roles in adipogenesis (Taniguchi et al., 2006).

While insulin stimulates mitogenic effects such as promoting pancreatic β cell health through signalling via the IR (Belfiore et al., 2009), it is also able to activate mitogenic pathways upon binding to the highly similar type 1 IGF receptor (IGF-1R) (Pollak and Russell-Jones, 2010). IGFs promote cell proliferation, survival and migration upon activation of the IGF-1R. IGFs are essential for normal growth and development and also promote cancer cell proliferation and survival. Elevated circulating IGF-I levels have been associated with an increased risk of cancer and up-regulation of IGF-I, IGF-II and the IGF-1R is commonly seen in many types of cancer (Pollak, 2008). The affinity of insulin for the IGF-1R is at least 100-fold lower than the affinity of IGF-I for its receptor. Therefore activation of the IGF-1R by insulin only occurs in situations of high insulin concentrations. For this reason there is growing concern that hyperinsulinemia associated with Type 2 diabetes leads to an elevated risk of cancer, highlighting the need for tight glucose control in these patients. Furthermore the potential increased cancer risk is being assessed for patients currently treated with long acting insulin mimetics such as glargine which have increased IGF-1R binding affinities (Pollak and Russell-Jones, 2010).

6.2 Metabolic effects

Insulin exerts its metabolic effects in three major tissues including liver, skeletal muscle and adipose tissues. Those effects include the stimulation of glucose transport, glycolysis, lipogenesis and protein synthesis while inhibiting gluconeogenesis, glycogenolysis, lipolysis and protein breakdown (see Figure 4).

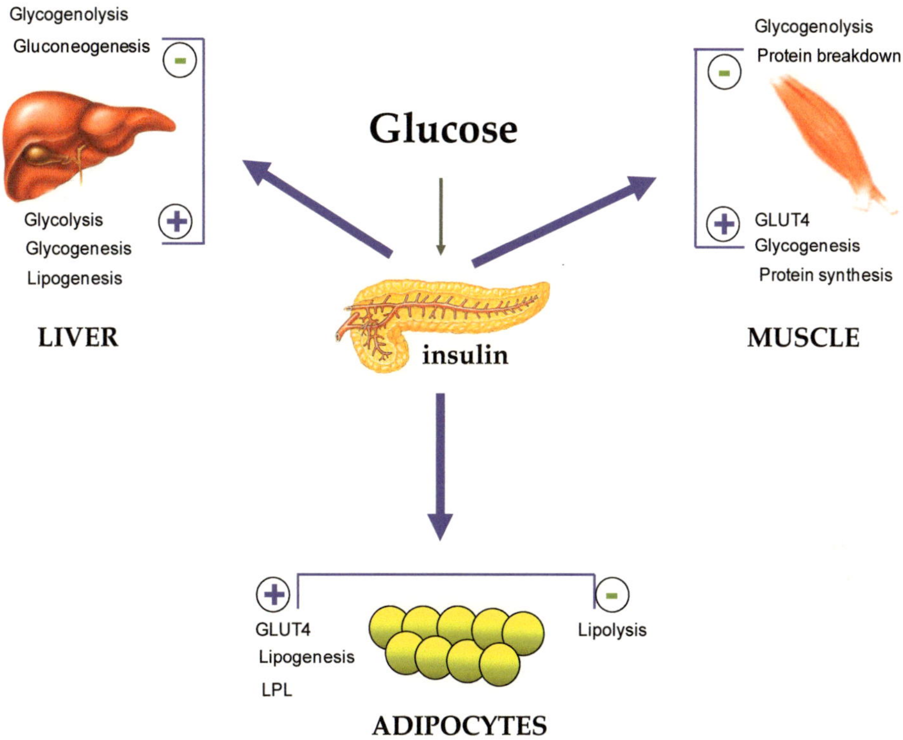

Fig. 4. Metabolic effects of insulin in liver, adipose tissue and skeletal muscle. In liver, insulin stimulates glycogenesis, glycolysis and lipogenesis (*de novo* fatty acid synthesis) but inhibits glycogenolysis and gluconeogenesis. In muscle, insulin stimulates glucose uptake via GLUT4 transporter, glycogenesis and protein synthesis but inhibits protein breakdown and glycogenolysis. In adipose tissue, insulin stimulates glucose uptake via GLUT4, lipogenesis (de novo fatty acid synthesis), and triglyceride synthesis by stimulating LPL activity. -, inhibition; +, stimulation.

6.2.1 Glucose transport

Glucose transporter 4 (GLUT4) is the most abundant transporter isoform in adipocytes and myocytes and is the only isoform that is regulated by insulin (Bryant et al., 2002). GLUT4 acts as the gate that allows extracellular glucose to enter the cells. During nutrient restriction or unstimulated conditions, 5-10% of GLUT4 is located on the plasma membrane while 90-95% is sequestered in an intracellular vesicle-bound form. However, when the concentration of extracellular glucose becomes high and the insulin is released, GLUT4 is translocated from intracellular sites to the plasma membrane (Holman and Cushman, 1994). The molecular mechanism by which insulin promotes the translocation of GLUT4 depends upon phosphorylation of downstream kinases including PI3K and Akt. The production of phosphoinositol(3,4,5) triphosphate by PI3K facilitates the release of the vesicle-bound GLUT4 and allows trafficking to the cell surface. The increased phosphoinositol (3,4,5)-triphosphate also promotes actin polymerization, resulting in the mobilization of the vesicle-bound GLUT4 near the plasma membrane. The other signal that promotes translocation of GLUT4 involves phosphorylation of Cbl that is associated with an adaptor protein, CAP. The CAP-phosphorylated Cbl complex is then translocated to the lipid raft on the plasma membrane where this complex further interacts with three more adaptor proteins, namely Crk, C3G and TC10. Here, TC10 functions as the second signal independent of PI3K activation, facilitating the trafficking of GLUT4 to the plasma membrane. Furthermore, fusion of the vesicle bound GLUT4 to the plasma membrane also requires the interaction between SNARE on the GLUT4 vesicles and the plasma membrane (Huang and Czech, 2007; Ishiki and Klip, 2005; Shisheva, 2008). The translocation of GLUT4 to the plasma membrane occurs within a few minutes after insulin stimulation and this allows rapid uptake of extracellular glucose to the muscle cells. In fact 75% of insulin-dependent glucose disposal occurs through GLUT4-mediated transport into muscle cells.

6.2.2 Glycogen synthesis

Glycogenesis is an important means to store excess glucose in liver and skeletal muscle (Pagliassotti and Cherrington, 1992). Insulin stimulates glycogen synthesis in liver and skeletal muscle through the glycogen synthase kinase 3 (GSK3). There are two isoforms of GSK3, i.e. GSK3α (51 kDa) and GSK3β (47 kDa), both of which share over 98% sequence identity in their kinase domains but different in their N-termini (Forde and Dale, 2007). Both isoforms are capable of phosphorylating glycogen synthase. During starvation when glucose is low, glycogen synthase is phosphorylated by casein kinase II at Ser657. Phosphorylation at this residue of glycogen synthase primes GSK3 to phosphorylate three more serine residues namely, Ser641, Ser645 and Ser649, making glycogen synthase becomes catalytically inactive (Forde and Dale, 2007). However, when insulin is released in response to hyperglycemic conditions, this leads to the activation of the Akt/PKB signaling cascade as mentioned earlier. Akt/PKB in turn phosphorylates Ser21 residue of GSKα or Ser9 residue of GSK3β, causing them become catalytically inactive, and no longer able to phosphorylate glycogen synthase (Sutherland et al., 1993). The non-phosphorylated glycogen synthase can now convert the UDP-glucose into glycogen in muscle and hepatocytes. Insulin also stimulates the activity of protein phosphates 1 (PP1) specifically localized near the glycogen granules (Brady and Saltiel, 2001; Ragolia and Begum, 1998). This enzyme removes a phosphate group from glycogen synthase, rendering it catalytically active.

Insulin not only stimulates glycogen synthesis but also inhibits the process of glycogen breakdown known as glycogenolysis which is important for the supply of glucose during short term starvation. Glycogen phosphorylase releases one unit of glucose in the form of glucose-1-phosphate from the glycogen chain. During starvation when the level of glucagon is high, binding of glucagon to its G-protein couple receptor activates adenylyl cyclase activity to convert ATP to cAMP. cAMP in turn stimulates PKA activity to phosphorylate an inactive form of glycogen phosphorylase (known as the phosphorlyase b form), transforming it to become an active form (glycogen phosphorylase a form) (Johnson, 1992). However, during postprandial period when the level of insulin is high, insulin activates phosphodiesterase which subsequently converts cAMP to AMP. As the level of cAMP is low, PKA is no longer activated, the glycogen phosphorylase remains in an inactive form. Furthermore, insulin activates protein phosphatase-1 to remove phosphate from phosphorylase a, transforming it to an inactive form and results in the inactivation of glycogenolysis (Brady and Saltiel, 2001; Ragolia and Begum, 1998).

6.2.3 Gluconeogenesis

Gluconeogenesis is the pathway that converts non-carbohydrate precursors including glycerol (product from triglyceride hydrolysis), lactate (end product from anaerobic glycolysis in skeletal muscle) and alanine (from protein breakdown in muscle) to glucose through the combined reverse reactions of glycolysis and the four additional reactions catalyzed by pyruvate carboxylase, phosphoenolpyruvate carboxykinase, fructose-1,6-bisphosphatase and glucose-6-phosphatase, respectively (Pilkis and Granner, 1992). Gluconeogenesis is absolutely essential for survival during prolonged fasting because red blood cells and the brain primarily rely on glucose as fuel. The genes encoding these four enzymes are regulated by two transcription factors, i.e. the forkhead transcription factor box O (FoxO) and the cAMP-responsive element binding protein (CREB). During prolonged starvation, glucagon triggers the production of cAMP which in turn stimulates PKA to phosphorylate Ser133 of CREB (Altarejos and Montminy, 2011; Mayr and Montminy, 2001; Montminy, 1997). This phosphorylated CREB together with its coactivator, the transcriptional coactivator of regulated CREB activity 2 (TORC2) (Koo et al., 2005) then binds to the cAMP-responsive element (CRE) in the promoters of PC, PEPCK and G6Pase genes and stimulate their transcription.

Under fasting conditions, FoxO also binds to its responsive element known as the insulin-responsive element (IRE) [(T/C)(G/A)AAACAA] in the promoters of PEPCK and G6Pase genes and stimulate their expression (Barthel et al., 2005; Nakae et al., 2008). Combined actions of CREB and FoxO result in the robust stimulation of gluconeogenic pathway. However, when the level of extracellular glucose is high and the level of insulin is high, the gluconeogenic rate is inhibited. As the result of insulin signaling, Akt phosphorylates FoxO protein at Thr24, Ser256 and Ser319 residues (Barthel et al., 2005; Nakae et al., 2008), preventing its entry to the nucleus thus inhibiting transcription of PEPCK and G6Pase genes (Zhang et al., 2006). Furthermore Akt also phosphorylates TORC2 via another kinase, SIK2, at Ser 171 residue, inhibiting its entry to the nucleus (Dentin et al., 2007; Koo et al., 2005). This in turn prevents transcriptional activation of PC, PEPCK and G6Pase genes. In summary insulin inhibits hepatic gluconeogenesis by inhibiting the entry of FoxO and TORC2 to the nucleus, thereby preventing transcriptional activation of gluconeogenic enzyme genes.

6.2.4 Coordinate control of glycolysis and fatty acid synthesis

Excess glucose is not only stored as glycogen in the liver but is also stored as fat through the *de novo* fatty acid synthesis. Insulin stimulates this effect by stimulating the glycolytic pathway through the increased expression of some glycolytic enzymes including glucokinase and L (liver)-type pyruvate kinase. This allows the production of acetyl-CoA which subsequently enters TCA cycle. A high rate of acetyl-CoA oxidation in the mitochondria accelerates the export of citrate from mitochondria to cytoplasm where it is oxidatively decarboxylated back to oxaloacetate and acetyl-CoA by an ATP-citrate lyase. Acetyl-CoA is converted to malonyl-CoA by the first rate-limiting step enzyme of lipogenesis, namely the acetyl-CoA carboxylase (ACC). Malonyl-CoA formed by the activity of ACC are condensed together to form fatty acyl-CoA in the cytoplasm. Insulin is able to increase both glycolysis and *de novo* fatty acid synthesis by stimulating the expression of two transcription factors, namely the sterol regulatory element binding protein 1c (SREBP1c) and the carbohydrate responsive element binding protein (ChREBP) (Dentin et al., 2005;

Desvergne et al., 2006). SREBP1c binds to the promoters of glucokinase, acetyl-CoA carboxylase and fatty acid synthase genes while ChREBP binds to the promoters of L-type pyruvate kinase, ATP-citrate lyase, acetyl-CoA carboxylase and fatty acid synthase genes (Postic et al., 2007; Towle et al., 1997). The coordinate regulation of glycolysis, citrate export and *de novo* fatty acid synthesis by insulin through the use of ChREBP and SREBP1c transcription factors allows fuel partitioning toward fat storage in hepatocytes.

Insulin can also stimulate glycolysis through the stimulation of one of glycolytic enzymes, i.e. phosphofructokinase 1 (PFK1) activity. PFK1 phosphorylates glucose-6-phosphate to fructose-1,6-bisphosphate thus increasing the level of this intermediate for the glycolytic pathway. Fructose-2,6-bisphosphate is an allosteric activator of PFK1 while it is an inhibitor of FBPaseI (Okar et al., 2001; Pilkis et al., 1995). This fructose-2,6-bisphosphate intermediate is produced by the bifunctional enzyme, phosphofructokinase 2/fructose bisphosphatase 2 (PFK2/FBPase2). PFK2 converts fructose-6-phosphate to fructose-2,6-bisphosphate while FBPase2 converts fructose-2,6-bisphosphate back to fructose-6-phosphate. Glucagon acting via cAMP-dependent protein kinase phosphorylates PFK2, converting it to an inactive form, allowing FBPase2 to convert fructose-2,6-bisphosphate to fructose-6-phosphate. The lower level of fructose-2,6-bisphosphate de-represses the FBPase1 activity, promoting gluconeogenesis. In contrast, insulin stimulates PFK2 activity of this bifunctional enzyme through phosphoprotein phosphatase, dephosphorylating PFK2, converting it into a catalytically active form. This results in the rise of fructose-2,6-bisphosphate level which stimulates PFK1, promoting glycolysis (Okar et al., 2001; Pilkis et al., 1995).

6.2.5 Triglyceride synthesis

Similar to liver, insulin also stimulates expression of some key enzymes in glycolytic pathway and *de novo* fatty acid synthesis, resulting in the increase in the synthesis of fatty acids in adipose tissue.

The dietary fat transported with chylomicrons as well as the *de novo* fat that is synthesized from liver and transported with very low density lipoprotein are taken up in adipose tissue. Because triglycerides cannot be readily transported to adipocytes, they must be first hydrolyzed to free fatty acids and glycerol by the lipoprotein lipase (LPL). The LPL is synthesized by adipocytes and is secreted in the circulation where it is associated with the extracellular matrix on the endothelial cells. After the hydrolysis of triglycerides by LPL, free fatty acids can now be transported across the plasma membrane of endothelial cells to adipocytes. Here, the monoacylglycerol acyltransferase and diacylglycerol acyltransferase re-esterify free fatty acids with glycerol back to triglycerides (Jin et al., 2002). Insulin promotes fat storage by stimulating adipocyte LPL activity, resulting in the uptake of dietary fat and *de novo* fat from liver to adipose tissue. The molecular mechanism by which insulin regulates LPL activity in adipocyte is not well defined, although there is clear evidence that insulin does not stimulate transcription of LPL gene (Raynolds et al., 1990; Semenkovich et al., 1989) but rather enhances the secretion of LPL from adipocytes to the extracellular matrix where the enzyme becomes active (Camps et al., 1990; Chan et al., 1988; Knutson, 2000; Nielsen et al., 1997). It is noted that insulin does not stimulate LPL activity in other tissues such as muscle and myocardium which possesses different LPL. This explains why the fat deposition rate is high in adipose tissue during fed period. In addition to stimulating the LPL activity, insulin inhibits the activity of another lipase called the hormone sensitive lipase (Watt and Steinberg, 2008). Hormone sensitive lipase is inhibited when the level of insulin is high. However, when the level of insulin is low, which is counterbalanced by the high level of glucagon, hormone sensitive lipase becomes active and it hydrolyzes triglycerides to free fatty acids which are released to the blood circulation during prolonged starvation.

6.2.6 Protein synthesis

Another metabolic effect of insulin is protein synthesis in muscle cells. Insulin promotes this anabolic process through the activity of mammalian target of rapamycin (mTOR) which is activated by Akt. Activation of mTOR in turn regulates different steps in the protein synthesis including translation initiation, elongation and ribosome biogenesis (Proud, 2004; Proud, 2006). The initiation factor 4 (eIF4E) functions as the protein that recognizes the CAP structure at the 5'-end of eukaryotic mRNA thus allowing translation to occur in a CAP-dependent manner. During non-stimulated conditions, eIF4E is bound to its inhibitor protein, PHAS1 or 4E-binding protein, resulting in the suppression of translation initiation. However when the level of insulin is high, PHAS1 is phosphorylated by mTOR, causing the dissociation of eIF4E from PHAS1. This results in the initiation of protein synthesis in a CAP-dependent manner (Lin et al., 1994; Wang et al., 2005). Insulin also regulates the recognition of the methionyl tRNA ($tRNA^{Met}$) to the initiation codon through the initiation factor, eIF2. In general, the GTP-bound eIF2 carries the $tRNA^{Met}$ to the initiation codon where the engagement between first codon and $tRNA^{Met}$ occurs, concomitant with the release of the GDP-eIF2. The GDP-eIF2 is then converted back to GTP-eIF2 by another initiation factor, eIF2B. During unstimulated conditions, GSK3 phosphorylates eIF2B, inhibiting its activity to convert GDP-eIF2 to GTP-eIF2, resulting in translational inhibition. However, when the level of insulin is high, GSK3 is phosphorylated by Akt/PKB resulting in the loss of its activity. This causes the de-repression of eIF2B activity, enabling it to activate eIF2B (Cohen and Frame, 2001). Insulin can also regulate the elongation step of protein synthesis by modulating the activity of elongation factor, eEF2 (Proud, 2006; Redpath et al., 1996). In general eEF2 facilitates the translocation of ribosome along the mRNA so that the next codon can be engaged by the corresponding aminoacyl tRNA. This translocation process is regulated by the eEF2 kinase which phosphorylates Thr56 residue of eEF2, inhibiting its activity to translocate the ribosome to the next site. When the level of insulin is high, mTOR phosphorylates eEF2 kinase, allowing eEF2 to regain its activity. Insulin also promotes the dephosphorylation of eEF2, leading to the stimulation of polypeptide chain elongation.

In addition to promoting initiation and elongation steps in the protein synthesis, insulin again stimulates ribosome biosynthesis through mTOR. mTOR phosphorylates p70 ribosomal S6 kinase (p70) and PHAS1 as mentioned earlier. p70 subsequently phosphorylates S6 ribosomal protein in the 40s subunit of the ribosome, resulting in the biosynthesis of active ribosomes (Proud, 2004; Proud, 2006).

Insulin has long been known to inhibit cellular protein breakdown. This is important when considering muscle loss in association with the increased proteolytic activity has been seen in the type 2 diabetic patients. Administration of insulin to the patients can reverse the muscle loss. Insulin inhibits protein breakdown through the inhibition of the non-ubiquitin and ubiquitin-mediated proteolytic activity in the proteasome (Bennett et al., 2000; Duckworth et al., 1994; Hamel et al., 1997). Although an insulin-degrading enzyme has been proposed to be involved in this action, the exact mechanism by which this enzyme mediates the anti proteolytic activity of insulin remains unclear. Signaling through the Akt phosphorylation is also a critical step to control the ubiqutin-mediated proteolytic activity (Faridi et al., 2003). In muscle, two isoforms of ubiqution ligase (E3) namely the atrogin-1 (also known as MAFbx), MuRF-1 are transcriptionally regulated by insulin via FoxO (Sandri et al., 2004). As mentioned earlier, insulin stimulates phosphorylation of FoxO, inhibiting its entry to the nucleus and results in the transcriptional repression of artogin-1 and MuRF-1 genes. As such, the abundance of these two proteins is low, limiting the availability of ubiqutin-mediated proteolytic machinery. Furthermore insulin also inhibits the lysosomal-mediated proteolytic activity (autophagy) through the activation of mTOR protein (Meijer, 2008).

7. References

Aguilar-Bryan, L.et al. (1995). Cloning of the beta cell high-affinity sulfonylurea receptor: a regulator of insulin secretion. *Science,* Vol. 268, No. 5209, pp. 423-426

Altarejos, J.Y. & Montminy, M. (2011). CREB and the CRTC co-activators: sensors for hormonal and metabolic signals. *Nature Reviews Molecular Cell Biology,* Vol. 12, No. 3, pp. 141-151

Ashcroft, F.M.et al. (1984). Glucose induces closure of single potassium channels in isolated rat pancreatic -cells. *Nature,* Vol. 312, No. 5993, pp. 446-448

Avnet, S.et al. (2009). Insulin receptor isoform A and insulin-like growth factor II as additional treatment targets in human osteosarcoma. *Cancer Res,* Vol. 69, No. 6, pp. 2443-2452

Barg, S.et al. (2002). A subset of 50 secretory granules in close contact with L-type Ca2+ channels accounts for first-phase insulin secretion in mouse beta-cells. *Diabetes,* Vol. 51 Suppl 1, No. pp. S74-82

Barthel, A.et al. (2005). FoxO proteins in insulin action and metabolism. *Trends Endocrinol Metab,* Vol. 16, No. 4, pp. 183-189

Belfiore, A.et al. (2009). Insulin receptor isoforms and insulin receptor/insulin-like growth factor receptor hybrids in physiology and disease. *Endocr Rev,* Vol. 30, No. 6, pp. 586-623

Bennett, R.G.et al. (2000). Insulin inhibits the ubiquitin-dependent degrading activity of the 26S proteasome. *Endocrinology,* Vol. 141, No. 7, pp. 2508

Bergsten, P.et al. (1994). Synchronous oscillations of cytoplasmic Ca2+ and insulin release in glucose-stimulated pancreatic islets. *Journal of Biological Chemistry,* Vol. 269, No. 12, pp. 8749

Bergsten, P. & Hellman, B. (1993). Glucose-induced amplitude regulation of pulsatile insulin secretion from individual pancreatic islets. *Diabetes,* Vol. 42, No. 5, pp. 670

Bertram, R.et al. (2007). Metabolic and electrical oscillations: partners in controlling pulsatile insulin secretion. *American Journal of Physiology-Endocrinology And Metabolism,* Vol. 293, No. 4, pp. E890

Brady, M.J. & Saltiel, A.R. (2001). The role of protein phosphatase-1 in insulin action. *Recent Progress in Hormone Research,* Vol. 56, No. 1, pp. 157

Bratanova-Tochkova, T.K.et al. (2002). Triggering and augmentation mechanisms, granule pools, and biphasic insulin secretion. *Diabetes,* Vol. 51, No. suppl 1, pp. S83

Brun, T.et al. (1996). Evidence for an anaplerotic/malonyl-CoA pathway in pancreatic beta-cell nutrient signaling. *Diabetes,* Vol. 45, No. 2, pp. 190

Bryant, N.J.et al. (2002). Regulated transport of the glucose transporter GLUT4. *Nature Reviews Molecular Cell Biology,* Vol. 3, No. 4, pp. 267-277

Camps, L.et al. (1990). Lipoprotein lipase: cellular origin and functional distribution. *American Journal of Physiology-Cell Physiology,* Vol. 258, No. 4, pp. C673

Carobbio, S.et al. (2009). Deletion of glutamate dehydrogenase in beta-cells abolishes part of the insulin secretory response not required for glucose homeostasis. *J Biol Chem,* Vol. 284, No. 2, pp. 921-929

Chan, B.L.et al. (1988). Insulin-stimulated release of lipoprotein lipase by metabolism of its phosphatidylinositol anchor. *Science,* Vol. 241, No. 4873, pp. 1670-1672

Chen, L.et al. (1990). Regulation of beta-cell glucose transporter gene expression. *Proceedings of the National Academy of Sciences,* Vol. 87, No. 11, pp. 4088

Cohen, P. & Frame, S. (2001). The renaissance of GSK3. *Nature Reviews Molecular Cell Biology,* Vol. 2, No. 10, pp. 769-776

Corkey, B.E.et al. (1989). A role for malonyl-CoA in glucose-stimulated insulin secretion from clonal pancreatic beta-cells. *Journal of Biological Chemistry,* Vol. 264, No. 36, pp. 21608

De Meyts, P. & Whittaker, J. (2002). Structural biology of insulin and IGF1 receptors: implications for drug design. *Nat Rev Drug Discov,* Vol. 1, No. 10, pp. 769-783

De Vos, A.et al. (1995). Human and rat beta cells differ in glucose transporter but not in glucokinase gene expression. *Journal of Clinical Investigation,* Vol. 96, No. 5, pp. 2489

Deeney, J.T.et al. (2000). Acute stimulation with long chain acyl-CoA enhances exocytosis in insulin-secreting cells (HIT T-15 and NMRI -cells). *Journal of Biological Chemistry,* Vol. 275, No. 13, pp. 9363

Denley, A.et al. (2003). The Insulin Receptor Isoform Exon 11- (IR-A) in Cancer and other Diseases: A Review. *Horm Metab Res,* Vol. 35, No. (11-12), pp. 778-785

Dentin, R.et al. (2005). Carbohydrate responsive element binding protein (ChREBP) and sterol regulatory element binding protein-1c (SREBP-1c): two key regulators of glucose metabolism and lipid synthesis in liver. *Biochimie,* Vol. 87, No. 1, pp. 81-86

Dentin, R.et al. (2007). Insulin modulates gluconeogenesis by inhibition of the coactivator TORC2. *Nature,* Vol. 449, No. 7160, pp. 366-369

Desvergne, B.et al. (2006). Transcriptional regulation of metabolism. *Physiological Reviews,* Vol. 86, No. 2, pp. 465

Duckworth, W.C.et al. (1994). A direct inhibitory effect of insulin on a cytosolic proteolytic complex containing insulin-degrading enzyme and multicatalytic proteinase. *Journal of Biological Chemistry,* Vol. 269, No. 40, pp. 24575

Easom, R.A. (1999). CaM kinase II: a protein kinase with extraordinary talents germane to insulin exocytosis. *Diabetes,* Vol. 48, No. 4, pp. 675

Fahien, L.A.et al. (1988). Regulation of insulin release by factors that also modify glutamate dehydrogenase. *Journal of Biological Chemistry,* Vol. 263, No. 27, pp. 13610

Faridi, J.et al. (2003). Akt promotes increased mammalian cell size by stimulating protein synthesis and inhibiting protein degradation. *American Journal of Physiology-Endocrinology And Metabolism,* Vol. 285, No. 5, pp. E964

Farshori, P.Q. & Goode, D. (1994). Effects of the microtubule depolymerizing and stabilizing agents Nocodazole and taxol on glucose-induced insulin secretion from hamster islet tumor (HIT) cells. *J Submicrosc Cytol Pathol,* Vol. 26, No. 2, pp. 137-146

Forde, J.E. & Dale, T.C. (2007). Glycogen synthase kinase 3: a key regulator of cellular fate. *Cellular and molecular life sciences,* Vol. 64, No. 15, pp. 1930-1944

Foti, M.et al. (2004). Insulin and IGF-1 receptor trafficking and signalling. *Novartis Found Symp,* Vol. 262, No. pp. 125-141; discussion 141-127, 265-128

Gembal, M.et al. (1992). Evidence that glucose can control insulin release independently from its action on ATP-sensitive K+ channels in mouse B cells. *Journal of Clinical Investigation,* Vol. 89, No. 4, pp. 1288

Giacca, A.et al. (2011). Lipid-induced pancreatic -cell dysfunction: focus on in vivo studies. *American Journal of Physiology-Endocrinology And Metabolism,* Vol. 300, No. 2, pp. E255

Hamel, F.G.et al. (1997). Insulin Inhibition of Proteasome Activity in Intact Cells* 1. *Biochemical and Biophysical Research Communications,* Vol. 234, No. 3, pp. 671-674

Holman, G.D. & Cushman, S.W. (1994). Subcellular localization and trafficking of the GLUT4 glucose transporter isoform in insulin responsive cells. *Bioessays,* Vol. 16, No. 10, pp. 753-759

Holst, J.J. (2007). The physiology of glucagon-like peptide 1. *Physiological Reviews,* Vol. 87, No. 4, pp. 1409

Holt, L.J.et al. (2009). Dual ablation of Grb10 and Grb14 in mice reveals their combined role in regulation of insulin signaling and glucose homeostasis. *Mol Endocrinol,* Vol. 23, No. 9, pp. 1406-1414

Holt, L.J. & Siddle, K. (2005). Grb10 and Grb14: enigmatic regulators of insulin action--and more? *Biochem J,* Vol. 388, No. Pt 2, pp. 393-406

Howell, S.L. & Tyhurst, M. (1979). Interaction between insulin-storage granules and F-actin in vitro. *Biochemical Journal,* Vol. 178, No. 2, pp. 367

Huang, S. & Czech, M.P. (2007). The GLUT4 glucose transporter. *Cell Metabolism,* Vol. 5, No. 4, pp. 237-252

Hubbard, S.R. (2004). Juxtamembrane autoinhibition in receptor tyrosine kinases. *Nat Rev Mol Cell Biol,* Vol. 5, No. 6, pp. 464-471

Ishiki, M. & Klip, A. (2005). Minireview: recent developments in the regulation of glucose transporter-4 traffic: new signals, locations, and partners. *Endocrinology,* Vol. 146, No. 12, pp. 5071

Jensen, M.et al. (2007). Activation of the insulin receptor by insulin and a synthetic peptide leads to divergent metabolic and mitogenic signaling and responses. *J Biol Chem,* Vol. 282, No. 48, pp. 35179-35186

Jin, W.et al. (2002). Lipases and HDL metabolism. *Trends in endocrinology and metabolism,* Vol. 13, No. 4, pp. 174-178

Jitrapakdee, S.et al. (2010). Regulation of insulin secretion: role of mitochondrial signalling. *Diabetologia,* Vol. 53, No. 6, pp. 1019-1032

Johnson, L.N. (1992). Glycogen phosphorylase: Control by phosphorylation and allosteric effectors. *The FASEB journal,* Vol. 6, No. 6, pp. 2274

Kibbey, R.G.et al. (2007). Mitochondrial GTP regulates glucose-stimulated insulin secretion. *Cell Metabolism,* Vol. 5, No. 4, pp. 253-264

Kiselyov, V.V.et al. (2009). Harmonic oscillator model of the insulin and IGF1 receptors' allosteric binding and activation. *Mol Syst Biol,* Vol. 5, No. 243, pp. 1-12

Knutson, V.P. (2000). The release of lipoprotein lipase from 3T3-L1 adipocytes is regulated by microvessel endothelial cells in an insulin-dependent manner. *Endocrinology,* Vol. 141, No. 2, pp. 693

Kohanski, R.A. (1993). Insulin receptor autophosphorylation. II. Determination of autophosphorylation sites by chemical sequence analysis and identification of the juxtamembrane sites. *Biochemistry,* Vol. 32, No. 22, pp. 5773-5780

Koo, S.H.et al. (2005). The CREB coactivator TORC2 is a key regulator of fasting glucose metabolism. *Nature,* Vol. 437, No. 7062, pp. 1109-1111

Leloup, C.et al. (2009). Mitochondrial reactive oxygen species are obligatory signals for glucose-induced insulin secretion. *Diabetes,* Vol. 58, No. 3, pp. 673

Lewis, R.E.et al. (1990). Insulin-sensitive phosphorylation of serine 1293/1294 on the human insulin receptor by a tightly associated serine kinase. *J Biol Chem,* Vol. 265, No. 2, pp. 947-954

Lin, T.A.et al. (1994). PHAS-I as a link between mitogen-activated protein kinase and translation initiation. *Science,* Vol. 266, No. 5185, pp. 653

Longo, V.D.et al. (2008). Turning anti-ageing genes against cancer. *Nat Rev Mol Cell Biol,* Vol. 9, No. 11, pp. 903-910

Lou, M.et al. (2006). The first three domains of the insulin receptor differ structurally from the insulin-like growth factor 1 receptor in the regions governing ligand specificity. *Proc Natl Acad Sci U S A,* Vol. 103, No. 33, pp. 12429-12434

Lu, D.et al. (2002). 13C NMR isotopomer analysis reveals a connection between pyruvate cycling and glucose-stimulated insulin secretion (GSIS). *Proceedings of the National Academy of Sciences of the United States of America,* Vol. 99, No. 5, pp. 2708

MacDonald, M.J. (1981). High content of mitochondrial glycerol-3-phosphate dehydrogenase in pancreatic islets and its inhibition by diazoxide. *Journal of Biological Chemistry,* Vol. 256, No. 16, pp. 8287

MacDonald, M.J. (1993). Estimates of glycolysis, pyruvate (de) carboxylation, pentose phosphate pathway, and methyl succinate metabolism in incapacitated pancreatic islets. *Archives of biochemistry and biophysics,* Vol. 305, No. 2, pp. 205-214

MacDonald, M.J. (2003). The export of metabolites from mitochondria and anaplerosis in insulin secretion. *Biochimica et Biophysica Acta (BBA)-General Subjects,* Vol. 1619, No. 1, pp. 77-88

MacDonald, M.J.et al. (2008). The role of rapid lipogenesis in insulin secretion: Insulin secretagogues acutely alter lipid composition of INS-1 832/13 cells. *Arch Biochem Biophys,* Vol. 470, No. 2, pp. 153-162

MacDonald, M.J. & Fahien, L.A. (2000). Glutamate is not a messenger in insulin secretion. *Journal of Biological Chemistry,* Vol. 275, No. 44, pp. 34025

MacDonald, M.J.et al. (2005). Perspective: emerging evidence for signaling roles of mitochondrial anaplerotic products in insulin secretion. *Am J Physiol Endocrinol Metab,* Vol. 288, No. 1, pp. E1-15

Maechler, P. & Wollheim, C.B. (1999). Mitochondrial glutamate acts as a messenger in glucose-induced insulin exocytosis. *Nature,* Vol. 402, No. 6762, pp. 685-689

Malaisse-Lagae, F.et al. (1982). The stimulus-secretion coupling of amino acid-induced insulin release. Influence of a nonmetabolized analog of leucine on the metabolism of glutamine in pancreatic islets. *J Biol Chem,* Vol. 257, No. 7, pp. 3754-3758

Matschinsky, F.M. (1990). Glucokinase as glucose sensor and metabolic signal generator in pancreatic beta-cells and hepatocytes. *Diabetes,* Vol. 39, No. 6, pp. 647

Matveyenko, A.V.et al. (2008). Measurement of pulsatile insulin secretion in the rat: direct sampling from the hepatic portal vein. *American Journal of Physiology-Endocrinology And Metabolism,* Vol. 295, No. 3, pp. E569

Mayr, B. & Montminy, M. (2001). Transcriptional regulation by the phosphorylation-dependent factor CREB. *Nature Reviews Molecular Cell Biology,* Vol. 2, No. 8, pp. 599-609

McKern, N.M.et al. (2006). Structure of the insulin receptor ectodomain reveals a folded-over conformation. *Nature,* Vol. 443, No. 7108, pp. 218-221

Meijer, A.J. (2008). Amino acid regulation of autophagosome formation. *METHODS IN MOLECULAR BIOLOGY-CLIFTON THEN TOTOWA-,* Vol. 445, No. pp. 89

Montminy, M. (1997). Transcriptional regulation by cyclic AMP. *Annual review of biochemistry,* Vol. 66, No. 1, pp. 807-822

Nakae, J.et al. (2008). The FoxO transcription factors and metabolic regulation. *FEBS letters,* Vol. 582, No. 1, pp. 54-67

Nielsen, M.S.et al. (1997). Segments in the C-terminal folding domain of lipoprotein lipase important for binding to the low density lipoprotein receptor-related protein and to heparan sulfate proteoglycans. *Journal of Biological Chemistry,* Vol. 272, No. 9, pp. 5821

Okar, D.A.et al. (2001). PFK-2/FBPase-2: maker and breaker of the essential biofactor fructose-2, 6-bisphosphate. *Trends in Biochemical Sciences,* Vol. 26, No. 1, pp. 30-35

Pagliassotti, M.J. & Cherrington, A.D. (1992). Regulation of net hepatic glucose uptake in vivo. *Annual review of physiology,* Vol. 54, No. 1, pp. 847-860

Pi, J.et al. (2007). Reactive oxygen species as a signal in glucose-stimulated insulin secretion. *Diabetes,* Vol. 56, No. 7, pp. 1783

Pilkis, S.J.et al. (1995). 6-Phosphofructo-2-kinase/fructose-2, 6-bisphosphatase: a metabolic signaling enzyme. *Annual review of biochemistry,* Vol. 64, No. 1, pp. 799-835

Pilkis, S.J. & Granner, D.K. (1992). Molecular physiology of the regulation of hepatic gluconeogenesis and glycolysis. *Annual review of physiology,* Vol. 54, No. 1, pp. 885-909

Poitout, V. (2003). The ins and outs of fatty acids on the pancreatic [beta] cell. *Trends in endocrinology and metabolism,* Vol. 14, No. 5, pp. 201-203

Poitout, V. & Robertson, R.P. (2002). Minireview: Secondary {beta}-Cell Failure in Type 2 Diabetes--A Convergence of Glucotoxicity and Lipotoxicity. *Endocrinology,* Vol. 143, No. 2, pp. 339

Pollak, M. (2008). Insulin and insulin-like growth factor signalling in neoplasia. *Nat Rev Cancer,* Vol. 8, No. 12, pp. 915-928

Pollak, M. & Russell-Jones, D. (2010). Insulin analogues and cancer risk: cause for concern or cause celebre? *Int J Clin Pract,* No. pp.

Porksen, N.et al. (1997). In humans at least 75% of insulin secretion arises from punctuated insulin secretory bursts. *Am J Physiol,* Vol. 273, No. 5 Pt 1, pp. E908-914

Postic, C.et al. (2007). ChREBP, a transcriptional regulator of glucose and lipid metabolism. *Annu. Rev. Nutr.,* Vol. 27, No. pp. 179-192

Prentki, M.et al. (1992). Malonyl-CoA and long chain acyl-CoA esters as metabolic coupling factors in nutrient-induced insulin secretion. *Journal of Biological Chemistry,* Vol. 267, No. 9, pp. 5802

Proud, C.G. (2004). mTOR-mediated regulation of translation factors by amino acids. *Biochemical and Biophysical Research Communications,* Vol. 313, No. 2, pp. 429-436

Proud, C.G. (2006). Regulation of protein synthesis by insulin. *Biochemical Society Transactions,* Vol. 34, No. 2, pp. 213-216

Ragolia, L. & Begum, N. (1998). Protein phosphatase-1 and insulin action. *Molecular and cellular biochemistry,* Vol. 182, No. 1, pp. 49-58

Ramos, F.J.et al. (2006). Grb10 mediates insulin-stimulated degradation of the insulin receptor: a mechanism of negative regulation. *Am J Physiol Endocrinol Metab,* Vol. 290, No. 6, pp. E1262-1266

Raynolds, M.V.et al. (1990). Lipoprotein lipase gene expression in rat adipocytes is regulated by isoproterenol and insulin through different mechanisms. *Molecular Endocrinology,* Vol. 4, No. 9, pp. 1416

Redpath, N.T.et al. (1996). Regulation of translation elongation factor-2 by insulin via a rapamycin-sensitive signalling pathway. *The EMBO Journal,* Vol. 15, No. 9, pp. 2291

Romanelli, R.J.et al. (2007). Insulin-like growth factor type-I receptor internalization and recycling mediate the sustained phosphorylation of Akt. *J Biol Chem,* Vol. 282, No. 31, pp. 22513-22524

Sandri, M.et al. (2004). Foxo transcription factors induce the atrophy-related ubiquitin ligase atrogin-1 and cause skeletal muscle atrophy. *Cell,* Vol. 117, No. 3, pp. 399-412

Seghers, V.et al. (2000). Sur1 knockout mice. A model for K(ATP) channel-independent regulation of insulin secretion. *J Biol Chem,* Vol. 275, No. 13, pp. 9270-9277

Semenkovich, C.F.et al. (1989). Insulin regulation of lipoprotein lipase activity in 3T3-L1 adipocytes is mediated at posttranscriptional and posttranslational levels. *Journal of Biological Chemistry,* Vol. 264, No. 15, pp. 9030

Shaul, Y.D. & Seger, R. (2007). The MEK/ERK cascade: from signaling specificity to diverse functions. *Biochim Biophys Acta,* Vol. 1773, No. 8, pp. 1213-1226

Shiota, C.et al. (2002). Sulfonylurea receptor type 1 knock-out mice have intact feeding-stimulated insulin secretion despite marked impairment in their response to glucose. *Journal of Biological Chemistry,* Vol. 277, No. 40, pp. 37176

Shisheva, A. (2008). Phosphoinositides in insulin action on GLUT4 dynamics: not just PtdIns (3, 4, 5) P3. *American Journal of Physiology-Endocrinology And Metabolism,* Vol. 295, No. 3, pp. E536

Siddle, K. (2011). Signalling by insulin and IGF receptors: supporting acts and new players. *J Mol Endocrinol,*Vol. 47, No. 1, pp.R1-R10

Smith, B.J.et al. (2010). Structural resolution of a tandem hormone-binding element in the insulin receptor and its implications for design of peptide agonists. *Proc Natl Acad Sci U S A,* Vol. 107, No. 15, pp. 6771-6776

Song, S.H.et al. (2000). Direct measurement of pulsatile insulin secretion from the portal vein in human subjects. *Journal of Clinical Endocrinology & Metabolism,* Vol. 85, No. 12, pp. 4491

Steiner, D.F. (1969). Proinsulin and the biosynthesis of insulin. *The New England journal of medicine,* Vol. 280, No. 20, pp. 1106

Straub, S.G. & Sharp, G.W. (2002). Glucose-stimulated signaling pathways in biphasic insulin secretion. *Diabetes Metab Res Rev,* Vol. 18, No. 6, pp. 451-463

Straub, S.G. & Sharp, G.W. (2004). Hypothesis: one rate-limiting step controls the magnitude of both phases of glucose-stimulated insulin secretion. *Am J Physiol Cell Physiol,* Vol. 287, No. 3, pp. C565-571

Sutherland, C.et al. (1993). Inactivation of glycogen synthase kinase-3 beta by phosphorylation: new kinase connections in insulin and growth-factor signalling. *Biochemical Journal,* Vol. 296, No. Pt 1, pp. 15

Taguchi, A. & White, M.F. (2008). Insulin-like signaling, nutrient homeostasis, and life span. *Annu Rev Physiol,* Vol. 70, No. pp. 191-212

Taniguchi, C.M.et al. (2006). Critical nodes in signalling pathways: insights into insulin action. *Nat Rev Mol Cell Biol,* Vol. 7, No. 2, pp. 85-96

Tavare, J.M. & Denton, R.M. (1988). Studies on the autophosphorylation of the insulin receptor from human placenta. Analysis of the sites phosphorylated by two-dimensional peptide mapping. *Biochem J,* Vol. 252, No. 2, pp. 607-615

Tengholm, A. & Gylfe, E. (2009). Oscillatory control of insulin secretion. *Molecular and cellular endocrinology,* Vol. 297, No. 1-2, pp. 58-72

Thurmond, D.C.et al. (2003). Glucose-stimulated insulin secretion is coupled to the interaction of actin with the t-SNARE (target membrane soluble N-ethylmaleimide-sensitive factor attachment protein receptor protein) complex. *Molecular Endocrinology,* Vol. 17, No. 4, pp. 732

Tornheim, K. (1997). Are metabolic oscillations responsible for normal oscillatory insulin secretion? *Diabetes,* Vol. 46, No. 9, pp. 1375

Tornqvist, H.E.et al. (1987). Identification of insulin receptor tyrosine residues autophosphorylated in vitro. *J Biol Chem,* Vol. 262, No. 21, pp. 10212-10219

Towle, H.C.et al. (1997). Regulation of the expression of lipogenic enzyme genes by carbohydrate. *Annual Review of Nutrition,* Vol. 17, No. 1, pp. 405-433

Unger, R.H.et al. (1978). Insulin, glucagon, and somatostatin secretion in the regulation of metabolism. *Annual review of physiology,* Vol. 40, No. 1, pp. 307-343

Vecchione, A.et al. (2003). The Grb10/Nedd4 complex regulates ligand-induced ubiquitination and stability of the insulin-like growth factor I receptor. *Mol Cell Biol,* Vol. 23, No. 9, pp. 3363-3372

Wang, X.et al. (2005). Distinct signaling events downstream of mTOR cooperate to mediate the effects of amino acids and insulin on initiation factor 4E-binding proteins. *Molecular and cellular biology,* Vol. 25, No. 7, pp. 2558

Wang, Z. & Thurmond, D.C. (2009). Mechanisms of biphasic insulin-granule exocytosis–roles of the cytoskeleton, small GTPases and SNARE proteins. *Journal of cell science,* Vol. 122, No. 7, pp. 893

Ward, C.W. & Lawrence, M.C. (2009). Ligand-induced activation of the insulin receptor: a multi-step process involving structural changes in both the ligand and the receptor. *Bioessays,* Vol. 31, No. 4, pp. 422-434

Watt, M. & Steinberg, G. (2008). Regulation and function of triacylglycerol lipases in cellular metabolism. *Biochem. J,* Vol. 414, No. pp. 313-325

Yip, S.C.et al. (2010). PTP1B: a double agent in metabolism and oncogenesis. *Trends Biochem Sci,* Vol. 35, No. 8, pp. 442-449

Zhang, W.et al. (2006). FoxO1 regulates multiple metabolic pathways in the liver. *Journal of Biological Chemistry,* Vol. 281, No. 15, pp. 10105

2

The Oral Glucose Tolerance Test: An Old but Irreplaceable Test to Evaluate Glucose Metabolism and Cardiovascular Risk

Gian Paolo Fra, Ettore Bartoli and Gian Piero Carnevale Schianca
Internal Medicine, Department of Internal and Experimental Medicine, East Piedmont "Amedeo Avogadro" University
Italy

1. Introduction

The International Diabetes Federation estimates that near 285 million people have known type 2 diabetes: their number will probably double within 20 years (Shaw et al., 2010). Furthermore, worldwide, the number of persons with prediabetes, defined as impaired fasting glucose (IFG) or impaired glucose tolerance (IGT) (Genut et al., 2003), is estimated to be 314 million and is expected to be 418 million in 2025 (Garber et al., 2008). This scenario, amplified by the fact that several subjects do not know they have diabetes (Garber et al., 2008), has a predictable consequence: as the prevalence and progression to type 2 diabetes continues to increase and the afflicted population's age rises, the associated complications of diabetes inevitably will emerge as a major public health care issue. In 2007, for example, the direct and indirect costs related to diabetes, diabetes complications and general medical care amounted to $ 174 billions in the United States (American Diabetes Association [ADA], 2008). Thus, the advantage not only to diagnose, but also to recognize as soon as possible subjects at high risk to develop type 2 diabetes, is evident. If, on one hand, the magnitude of morbidity and early mortality attributable to diabetes has been clearly shown (ADA, 2008), on the other hand a growing body of evidence indicates that earlier detection and consequent earlier treatment of hyperglycaemia and related metabolic abnormalities may be beneficial (DREAM Trial Investigators, 2006; Knowler et al., 2002). In fact, early detection and treatment of subjects with prediabetes has the potential of reducing or delaying the progression to diabetes (DREAM Trial Investigators, 2006; Gillies et al., 2007; Knowler et al., 2002) and related cardiovascular disease (Chiasson et al., 2003; Ratner et al., 2005).

The risk associated with progression to diabetes and cardiovascular complications increases along a continuum, rather than being threshold-dependent, and occurs at much lower glucose levels than those required to diagnose diabetes. Consequently, relying exclusively on diabetic glucose level may delay treatment (Bergman, 2010), as we need to maximize our efforts in diabetes prevention and early disease management.

How can we identify not only unknown diabetics but, above all, those subjects with glucose levels not yet in the diabetic range, who do instead mostly need preventive interventions?

Although the increase in diabetes risk already starts at fasting plasma glucose (FPG) levels still within the normal range (Schulze et al., 2010; Tirosh et al., 2005), it follows that the FPG alone conveys inadequate information.

Recently the American Diabetes Association (ADA) proposed the measurement of glycosylated haemoglobin (A1c) to stratify glucose tolerance (International Expert Committee, 2009). Although A1c represents an easy screening test, and it is not influenced by fasting, drinking a glucose solution, or waiting hours for blood drawing, we believe that it cannot substitute for the information obtained derived from the oral glucose tolerance test (OGTT). In fact the contributions of FPG and post-prandial glucose to A1c levels are not linear: elevated FPG is mostly responsible for higher A1c levels. Instead, borderline A1c values, just above the upper limits of normal, strongly depend upon post-prandial glucose (Monnier et al., 2003). In support of these considerations, the results of well-designed studies (Fajans et al., 2011; Kramer et al., 2010) substantially indicate the insufficient sensitivity of A1c in detecting early diabetes.

Actually the OGTT, based on FPG and 2 h plasma glucose (2hPG) after ingestion of 75 g of glucose (Genut et al., 2003), is currently considered the gold standard to establish whether a subject has normal glucose tolerance (NGT) or altered glucose homeostasis.

In this report, we will discuss the OGTT. In our opinion, this old test, judged obsolete and inaccurate to the point of being considered optional according to ADA recommendations, should be instead reconsidered because of its irreplaceable clinical utility. Moreover, it could provide clear-cut metabolic information capable of recognizing subjects endowed with a metabolic profile prone to a progressive derangement in glucose homeostasis, suggestive of a high risk to develop diabetes.

2. The history of the OGTT

The OGTT is an old test used to diagnose alterations in glucose metabolism; its actual design is the result of a continuous reshaping that has lasted decades.

The notions that fasting hyperglycemia is too late a criterion for the early diagnosis of type 2 diabetes and that many subjects had obvious diabetes when their glucose was measured after a meal, led to the development, by the 1960s, of at least six different procedures for standardized OGTT. This debate involved the glucose load, ranging from 50 to 100 g, several time-points and, especially, the choice of the diagnostic cut-off of glycemic values (Herman, 2007; Valleron et al., 1975).

Based upon the analysis on the bimodal plasma glucose distribution firstly observed in Pima Indians, in 1979 the National Diabetes Data Group (National Diabetes Data Group, 1979) and, subsequently, in 1997 the ADA (ADA, 1997), established the correct procedure and interpretation of OGTT. In particular:

1. The standard glucose load was set at 75 g p.o.
2. Two stages of glucose intolerance, intermediate between NGT and diabetes, were recognized from FPG and 2hPG: IGT was defined by a 2hPG of 140-199 mg/dl in 1979 and confirmed in 1997, and the IFG defined by a FPG of 110-125 mg/dl in 1997.
3. In 1997, the FPG cut-off value to diagnose diabetes was lowered from 140 to 126 mg/dl.

It was evident that the rationale for lowering the cut-off FPG levels (126 mg/dl for diabetes and 110 mg/dl for IFG) was to make the OGTT, just developed and standardized, unnecessary. The ADA was predicting that FPG alone could stratify the different alterations of glucose metabolism, proceeding from NGT to diabetes with an intermediate glucose

intolerance step constituted by IFG. The hope was that, by eliminating the OGTT, considered time consuming, poorly reproducible and not well accepted by patients, a larger number of subjects could be efficiently screened, diagnosed and treated using FPG alone.
Unfortunately, FPG and 2hPG are not equivalent: the first measurement, becomes altered mainly by an impairment in the insulin-induced stimulation of hepatic glucose uptake, whereas postprandial glycemia (i.e.2hPG) rises because of delayed insulin secretion in combination with marked insulin resistance (Rizza, 2010). Thus, IFG and IGT are dependent upon different metabolic pathways. Our group did in fact supply evidence on the diversity of these pre-diabetic stages: we reported a relevant impairment of insulin secretion in IFG and an exquisite faltering in insulin sensitivity in IGT (Carnevale Schianca et al., 2003). Thus, it seems that prediabetes may represent a heterogeneous entity, which does not only entail an increased risk of diabetes, but also of cardiovascular disease (Garber et al., 2008). The attempt to screen glucose tolerance using FPG alone has been disavowed by several epidemiological observations. At variance with one single study involving three ethnic groups in the United Kingdom (Unwin et al., 1998), reporting a better prediction for diabetes from FPG with respect to 2hPG, FPG alone was shown to underestimate the diabetes prevalence when compared to 2hPG (Cheng et al., 2006; Harris et al., 1997). To ameliorate the diagnostic power of FPG, in 2003 the ADA lowered from 110 to 100 mg/dl its cut-off to define prediabetes (Genut et al., 2003). This did not meet the predicted expectations. As an example, a revealing study involving young African-American subjects compared FPG to OGTT to diagnose glucose intolerance. FPG (110 mg/dl) detected only 27.4% of cases, OGTT 87,1%; when the 2003 ADA criteria were applied, the FPG threshold of 100 mg/dl did not perform any better, identifying only 28.9% of glucose intolerance cases (Cheng et al., 2006). Furthermore, beside the evidence that FPG cannot be equated to 2hPG (Carnevale Schianca et al., 2003; Rizza, 2010), it has been demonstrated that 2hPG more efficiently predicts the risk of heart disease than FPG (DECODE Study Group, 1998).
Moreover, although substituting FPG for 2PG seems attractive and convenient both on epidemiological and clinical grounds, it does not yield any metabolically relevant information. The point is that it is misleading to try to assess glucose homeostasis and, at the same time, to stratify cardiovascular risk, without informations derived from post-prandial glucose metabolism. To compare the relative importance of FPG vs 2hPG in detecting diabetes, we studied different FPG cut-off values in detecting glucose intolerance separately identified by OGTT (Sainaghi et al., 2007). Out of 202 subjects with FPG ≥ 100 mg/dl, 121 (60%) had 2hPG < 140 mg/dl; conversely, out of 452 subjects with FPG < 100 mg/dl, 61 (14%) had a 2hPG ≥ 140 mg/dl. Choosing arbitrarily a FPG cut-off of 90 mg/dl, 33 out 266 subjects (12%) still had abnormal 2hPG. These data clearly demonstrate that any reduction of FPG threshold produces a progressive rise in sensitivity coupled to a progressive fall in specificity in detecting high-risk subjects for diabetes. Only the simultaneous information obtained from 2hPG (i.e. OGTT) allows the screening to become effective.
The next point will be explicative of the clinical utility of OGTT.

3. The OGTT in "action"

Despite various attempts to lower the cut-off of FPG to avoid the necessity of executing OGTT, there are extensive data showing that OGTT is more sensitive than FPG alone for diagnosing diabetes or prediabetes (Cheng et al., 2006; Harris et al., 1997; Meigs et al., 2003).

To illustrate the considerable clinical information obtained from the routine execution of OGTT, we will show the results gathered in a cohort of asymptomatic subjects attending a metabolic patient facility.

A series of consecutive 1665 patients with unknown diabetes, underwent an OGTT because of the presence of risk factors such as obesity, hypertension, diabetes inheritability, or dyslipidaemia. In agreement with the 2003 ADA criteria (Genut et al., 2003), as shown in Fig. 1 section A, relying on FPG alone, 1023 subjects (61.4%) were NGT (FPG <100 mg/dl) (group 1), while 642 were affected by glucose intolerance. Of these, 561 had IFG (group 2), 81 diabetes (group 3). As a consequence 4.9% of subjects (group 3) could start the necessary treatments, including pharmacotherapy, while 33.7% (group 2), classified as prediabetics, should be trained to follow appropriate lifestyle changes. Obviously, the remaining 61.4% (group 1), considered "normal", should perhaps be invited to follow scheduled FPG controls.

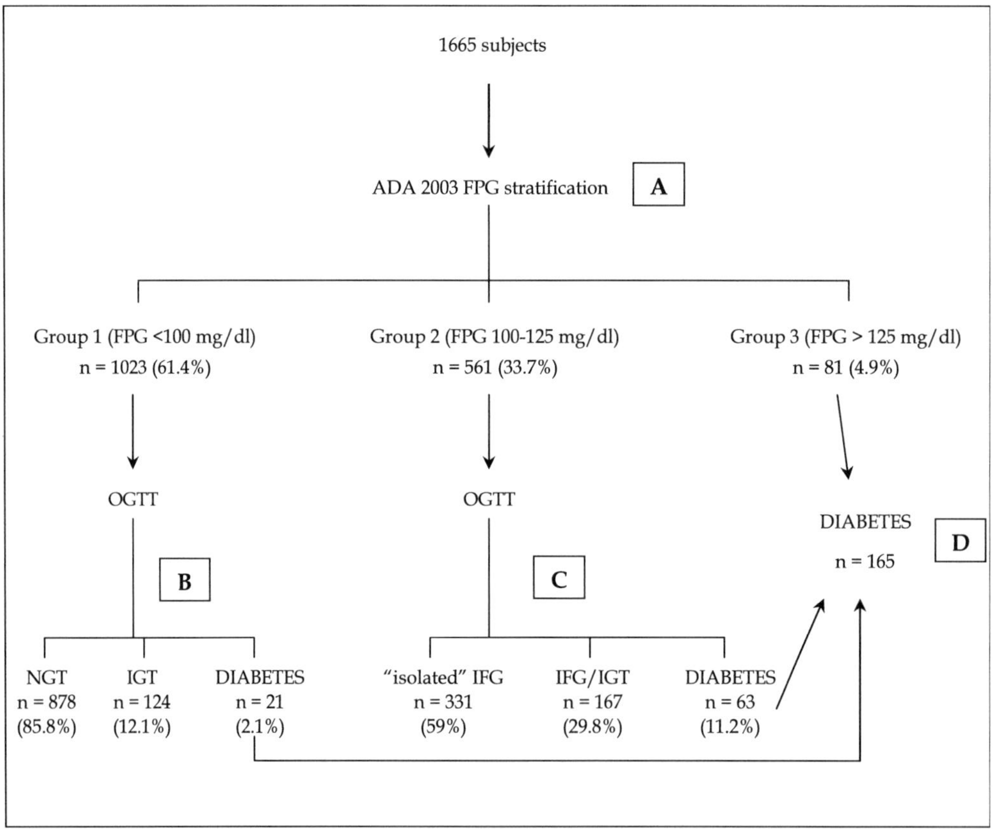

Fig. 1. The stratifications of FPG and OGTT in a cohort of 1665 subjects.
In section A it is shown the ADA 2003 FPG stratification; in section B the OGTT stratification in Group 1 and, in section C, in Group 2. In section D the contributions of both FPG and OGTT to detect subjects with diabetes are shown.

Probably this would be the scenario if FPG were the only test executed for diabetes screening. Using, in addition, criteria for the metabolic syndrome or A1c would not substantially increase the detection power of such a procedure (Expert Panel on detection, evaluation, and treatment of high blood cholesterol in adults, 2001 Fajans et al., 2011; Garber et al., 2008; Kramer et al., 2010).

Will the OGTT add importantly to the previous screening? If we consider group 1 (i.e. subjects with FPG < 100 mg/dl), we note, as shown in Fig. 1 section B, that OGTT gives surprising results. A considerable proportion of these subjects (14.2%) shows abnormal glucose tolerance, such that 124 subjects were affected by IGT and 21 by diabetes! From these data, we can formulate at least two considerations. Firstly, FPG, despite the decision to lower its threshold to more efficiently screen glucose abnormalities (Genut et al., 2003), continues to exhibit low specificity; secondly, OGTT is the only way to formally diagnose IGT, which constitutes the basic pathophysiologic alteration of type 2 diabetes. The identification of IGT is a crucial step in preventive cardiovascular strategies. The progression to diabetes is 6% to 10% per year for patients with IGT (Garber et al., 2008) and, similarly, a higher cardiovascular risk with elevated 2hPG has been reported even in the presence of normal FPG (DECODE Study Group, 1998). Thus, using FPG alone would deceitfully reassure a large proportion of individuals as being NGT and who will not be warned on the benefits of preventive treatments.

Let us now consider group 2, as shown in Fig. 1 (i.e. subjects with FPG 100-125 mg/dl). This large proportion of subjects should be labelled as affected by prediabetes and potentially susceptible of preventive therapies. In 2003, the ADA lowered FPG from 110 to 100 mg/dl to optimize sensitivity and specificity in detecting future diabetes (Genut et al., 2003). Nevertheless, this decision did not yield the expected results, as the development of diabetes in IFG varied widely (Davidson et al., 2003; Garber et al., 2008): for example, in our cohort of 1665 subjects, the percentage of IFG subjects ranged from 13.9% to 33.7%, depending on whether we considered a FPG cut-off value of 110 (ADA, 1997), or of 100 mg/dl (Genut et al., 2003). The weakness of relying on FPG as the only mean to stratify glucose metabolism is then readily apparent. Moreover, the 561 IFG subjects (group 2) are far from being homogeneous as demonstrated by OGTT data of Fig. 1 section C: the majority of these subjects (n=331, 59%) has normal 2hPG, such that they should be classified as "isolated" IFG, whereas 29.8% (n = 167) have 2hPG 140-199 mg/dl, which indicates that are affected by combined IFG and IGT (IFG/IGT). Only 63 (11.2%) had real type 2 diabetes.

It does not seem tenable to abandon OGTT in view of these data, which stress the usefulness of this test to correctly pinpoint, among subjects with similar IFG, those in need of a more accurate screening: they will be warned them about their risk of progression to diabetes, as well as their cardiovascular risk. Re-examining our OGTT data, these 63 subjects correctly identified as affected by diabetes would be promptly treated (DREAM Trail Investigators, 2006; Knowler et al., 2002), the 167 with IFG/IGT would be considered at high cardiovascular risk and, also, more liable to future diabetes (Garber et al., 2008): appropriate preventive strategies would be undertaken. Finally, the 331 subjects correctly identified as affected by "isolated" IFG by virtue of their 2hPG < 140 mg/dl, are probably at lower risk than those whose 2hPG was ≥ 140 mg/dl (Garber et al., 2008), suggesting only lifestyle changes and strict follow-up as initial preventive options. The crucial conclusion is that only OGTT permits this differentiation.

Fig. 1 section D shows the differential contributions of FPG versus OGTT in detecting subjects affected by diabetes: FPG individuated 49.1% of 165 subjects affected by diabetes, while OGTT allowed pinpointing an additional 50.9%. In fact, 11.2% of 561 subjects with

FPG 100-125 and the 2.1% of the 1023 subjects with FPG < 100 mg/dl were truly affected by diabetes. This striking result emphasises the diagnostic weight of OGTT.
As a whole, the evidence of these data demonstrates that, without OGTT, the correct clinical management of a devastating metabolic disease becomes inefficient.

4. The "expansion" of OGTT

The worldwide pandemic of diabetes entails the early detection of high risk subjects to provide with appropriate treatment. Unfortunately, the diabetic risk starts already when FPG values are still within the normal range (Tirosh et al., 2005). It seems, however, unreasonable to classify the vast majority of the population as at risk, as these subjects are presently thought to progress along a continuum similar to that of other chronic diseases, like hypercholesterolemia and hypertension. Thus, using the "raw" OGTT alone, although of crucial clinical importance, may not be sufficient. Epidemiological observations reported that ~ 40% of subjects who will develop diabetes exhibit NGT at baseline blood glucose testing, indicating that there is a large number of NGT subjects who constitute the largest reservoir of diabetes (Unwin et al., 2002). Moreover, the actual definition of prediabetes cannot provide an adequate solution of this dilemma, as not all subjects with IFG, IGT, or both, progress to diabetes; only 30 to 40% of IGT subjects do, in fact, ultimately convert to diabetes (Gerstein et al., 2007; Meigs et al., 2003). Thus, two questions arise: how to recognize normal subjects who will really develop diabetes in their future, and how to recognize prediabetic subjects who, in all likelihood, will never become diabetics.
The present "conventional" interpretation of OGTT, as well as methods using non-OGTT data (Expert Panel on detection, evaluation, and treatment of high blood cholesterol in adults, 2001; Kolberg et al., 2009; Stern et al., 2002), do not answer this question. Independent from the method used, all diabetes screening programmes do not reach the desired sensitivity and specificity. Consequently, a large number of subjects could inappropriately undergo prevention or, to the contrary, be excluded from beneficial interventions.
Recently, the relationship between FPG and 2hPG has been examined in a series of observations aimed at identifying NGT subjects at high risk for progression to diabetes (Abdul-Ghani et al., 2006; Abdul-Ghani et al., 2007; Abdul-Ghani et al., 2009). FPG and 2hPG closely correlate with β-cell function (Carnevale Schianca et al., 2003), the principal factor responsible for the development of diabetes (Gastaldelli et al., 2004). Changes in β-cell function also influence the shape of plasma glucose concentration profile during OGTT (Abdul-Ghani et al.; 2010 Tscritter et al., 2003). It has been reported that NGT subjects whose plasma glucose values fall faster to FPG levels during OGTT, have greater insulin sensitivity and better β-cell function compared to NGT subjects whose plasma glucose values fall more slowly (Abdul-Ghani et al., 2006; Abdul-Ghani et al., 2010; Carnevale Schianca et al., 2010). In agreement with the concept that the faster postload glucose drops towards FPG, or the lower postload glucose rises, the more efficient is β-cell function, we recently introduced a new dynamic appraisal of standard OGTT by computing the percentage increment of 2hPG with respect to FPG (PG%), by using the formula [(2hPG - FPG) / FPG] x 100 (Bartoli et al., 2011; Carnevale Schianca et al., 2010; Carnevale Schianca et al., 2011). Since FPG and 2hPG, that are not interchangeable (Unwin et al., 1998), as they convey different information (Carnevale Schianca et al., 2003;

Gastaldelli et al., 2004), PG% could reflects the fine tuning between insulin secretion and sensitivity. We tested PG% in relation to some estimated indexes of insulin sensitivity and insulin secretion derived from OGTT-data (Carnevale Schianca et al., 2010; Carnevale Schianca et al., 2011). Adding to glycemic measurements the simultaneous determinations of plasma insulin, Stumvoll et al. proposed, based on simple statistical methods using stepwise linear regression analysis and conceived for different sets of OGTT's time points, a series of formulas to calculate estimated indexes of insulin sensitivity and secretion (Stumvoll et al., 2001a). All these estimated indexes were validated by the clamp technique, the "gold" standard to evaluate the β-cell function (DeFronzo et al., 1979). Nevertheless, the evaluation of β-cell function using gold-standard method, is not practically feasible for epidemiological and clinical strategies (Stumvoll et al., 2001b). Among all indexes proposed by Stumvoll et al. we selected those that use FPG, 2hPG and the corresponding plasma insulin values. So with a single test, *i.e.* the OGTT with simultaneous determination of plasma insulin, it is possible to define not only the glucose tolerance and the PG%, but also calculate insulin sensitivity and secretion. We reported that in each glucose tolerance group, the larger is PG%, the lower is insulin sensitivity (Carnevale Schianca et al. 2011). Since insulin sensitivity is negatively related to insulin secretion through a hyperbolic function (Khan, 2003), glucose metabolism is thought to deteriorate when the fall in insulin sensitivity is not compensated by a sufficient increase of secretion. We demonstrated, for example, that NGT subjects with 2hPG near to or below FPG value (i.e., low PG%), are more sensitive to insulin; they do not need, then, the enhanced insulin secretion that, on the contrary, is necessary for NGT subjects with high PG%, a condition where there is a fall in insulin sensitivity (Carnevale Schianca et al., 2010). This is, in all likelihood, attended by an elevation of 2hPG, although still remaining within the "normal" range: probably the 2hPG will remain "normal" until a compensatory insulin secretion is maintained. When this compensation fails, a derangement of glucose tolerance, probably heralded by a rise in PG%, is unavoidable. The PG% could therefore identify, within the NGT range, a distinct phenotype that may predispose to a worsening of glucose tolerance. As previously described in the San Antonio Metabolism study, subjects with 2hPG ranging from 121 to 139 mg/dl had a 60% reduction in β-cell function when compared to subjects with 2hPG < 120 mg/dl (Gastaldelli et al., 2004); this, and our data, demonstrate that β-cell function begins to deteriorate long before we can conventionally identify prediabetes.

The PG% seems also useful when applied to subjects with glycaemic values within the IFG range. In 1997 the ADA proposed to diagnose IFG by FPG ranging from 110 to 125 mg/dl (American Diabetes Association, 1997) and, in 2003, widened this range by lowering the inferior limit of FPG to 100 mg/dl, in the attempt to better predict the development of diabetes (Genut et al., 2003). However, this change increased the overall prevalence of IFG approximately three to fourfold, without any reliable advantage in diabetes prevention (Davidson et al., 2003; Garber et al., 2008; Unwin et al., 2002).

Fig.1 section A shows that the use of FPG alone allows to diagnose IFG in 561 out of 1665 subjects (33.7%). Section C shows the improved stratification of IFG subjects obtained by OGTT: 59% (n=331) of these, with 2hPG < 140 mg/dl, were really affected by "isolated" IFG. This is an example of the utility of standard OGTT to correctly differentiate subjects with similar FPG. Will all these 331 subjects with isolated IFG exhibit the same risk to progress to diabetes? Unfortunately, the standard OGTT, although useful in correctly stratify all subjects with FPG between 100 and 125 mg/dl, does not help us any further. Instead, the calculation of PG% could offer a possibility to recognize, even in the "isolated" IFG range, subjects with abnormalities in β-cell function predisposing to worsening glucose homeostasis.

As an example, we will consider the case of a subject whose OGTT yielded FPG = 107 and 2hPG = 110 mg/dl, and then compare him with another subject whose OGTT gave FPG = 104 and 2hPG = 136 mg/dl. Both subjects suffer, by definition, from isolated IFG. Are they truly similar?

Recently, we demonstrated that the simple calculation of PG% can differentiate subjects with isolated IFG into two different phenotypes, as the higher the PG% the more dysfunctional is the β-cell (Carnevale Schianca et al., 2011). Likewise, even in the NGT and IFG/IGT ranges, we noted a progressive and meaningful worsening of insulin sensitivity proceeding from lower to higher PG% values, while there were no changes in insulin secretion. Only within the NGT range was insulin secretion significantly higher in the upper PG% values. We speculated that this increment, probably secondary to the derangement in insulin sensitivity, is the prerequisite to maintain a subject within the NGT range (Carnevale Schianca et al., 2010).

With this simple calculation of PG%, we add to our diagnostic tools the possibility to detect the pathophysiologic difference between the two IFG subjects of the above example: the first patient has PG% = 2.8%, the second one = 30.8%. Probably, this latter subject has an important deterioration of β-cell function, very likely attended, in the future, by metabolic consequences which could be amenable to preventive treatments. The actual definition of the IFG range forces us to define as prediabetes a large section of the population; the application of PG% can better define the real metabolic risk. As an example, considering the 331 subjects with "isolated" IFG shown in Fig. 1 section C, 156 (47.1%) had a PG% ≤ 0%: their 2hPG values suggest a metabolic efficiency hardly suggestive of a risk of future diabetes.

Unlike IFG, the recognition of IGT is exclusively based on OGTT, which can yield additional critical information if implemented by the computation of PG%. We reported that, within the IGT range, a major increment of PG% indicates subjects probably more liable to develop diabetes (Carnevale Schianca et al., 2010). Although no significant differences in insulin sensitivity and secretion could be disclosed considering a large spectrum of PG%, when the insulin secretion was corrected by insulin sensitivity to estimate β-cell function (Utzschneider et al., 2009), it was significantly impaired in IGT subjects with higher PG%. Since not all IGT subjects progress to diabetes (Gerstein et al., 2007; Meigs et al., 2003), and the decline in β-cell function favours this evolution (Festa et al., 2006), PG% can identify, when elevated, a high-risk subgroup to which a more aggressive preventive treatment could be applied.

5. Conclusions

In conclusion, the PG% can expand the clinical weight of OGTT by simply implementing a more powerful and informative calculation that discloses the efficiency of β-cell function. When high, probably the PG% pinpoints a higher risk of worsening glucose homeostasis. Although prospective studies designed to test the utility of PG% are needed, this computation has the advantage of being simple, feasible and of being obtained by the standard OGTT. This old test, conceived to investigate glucose tolerance and perhaps hurriedly considered obsolete and unsuitable, seems, on the contrary, irreplaceable.

6. References

Abdul-Ghani, M.A.; Williams, K.; DeFronzo, R. & Stern, M. (2006). Risk of progression to type 2 diabetes based on relationship between postload plasma glucose and fasting plasma glucose. *Diabetes Care,* Vol.29, NO.7, (July 2006), pp. 1613-1618, ISSN: 0149-5992

Abdul-Ghani, M.A.; Williams, K.; DeFronzo, R. & Stern, M. (2007). What is the best predictor of future type 2 diabetes? *Diabetes Care* , Vol.30, No.6, (July 2007), pp. 1544-1548, Epub 2007 Mar 23, ISSN: 0149-5992

Abdul-Ghani, M.A.; Lyssenko, V.; Tuomi, T.; DeFronzo R. & Groop, L. (2009). Fasting versus postload plasma glucose concentration and the risk for future type 2 diabetes: results from the Botnia study. *Diabetes Care,* Vol.32, No.2, (February 2009), pp. 281-286, Epub 2008 Nov 18, ISSN: 0149-5992

Abdul-Ghani, M.A.; Lyssenko, V.; Tuomi, T.; DeFronzo, R.A. & Groop, L. (2010). The shape of plasma glucose concentration curve during OGTT predicts future risk of type 2 diabetes. *Diabetes/Metabolism Research and Reviews,* Vol.26, No.4, (May 2010), pp. 280-286, ISSN: 1520-7552

American Diabetes Association. (1997). Report of the Expert Committee on the diagnosis and Classification of Diabetes Mellitus. *Diabetes Care,* Vol. 20, No.7, (July 1997), pp. 1183-1197, ISSN: 0149-5992

American Diabetes Association. (2008). Economics costs of diabetes in the U.S. in 2007. *Diabetes Care,* Vol.31, No.3, (March 2008), pp. 596-615, ISSN: 0149-5992

Bartoli, E.; Fra, G.P. & Carnevale Schianca, G.P. (2011). The oral glucose tolerance test (OGTT) revisited. *European Journal of Internal Medicine,* Vol.22, No.1, (February 2011), pp. 8-12, Epub 2010 Aug 17, ISSN: 0953-6205

Bergman, M. (2010). Inadequacies of absolute threshold levels for diagnosing prediabetes. *Diabetes/Metabolism Research and Reviews,* Vol.26, No.1, (January 2010), pp. 3-6, ISSN: 1520-7552

Carnevale Schianca, G.P.; Rossi, A.; Sainaghi, P.P.; Maduli, E. & Bartoli, E. (2003) The significance of impaired fasting glucose versus impaired glucose tolerance. Importance of insulin secretion and resistance. *Diabetes Care,* Vol.26, No.5, (May 2003), pp. 1333-1337, ISSN: 0149-5992

Carnevale Schianca, G.P.; Colli, E.; Onolfo, S.; Pedrazzoli, R.; Fra, G.P. & Bartoli, E. (2010). Individuation of different metabolic phenotypes in normal glucose tolerance test. *Acta Diabetol Acta Diabetologica,* Vol.47, No.2, (June 2010) pp. 167-172, Epub 2009 Nov 21, ISSN: 0940- 5429

Carnevale Schianca, G.P., Mella, R.; Bigliocca, M.; Colli, E.; Fra, G.P. & Bartoli, E. (2011). Expanding the clinical use of standard OGTT: the percentage increment of 2h with respect to fasting glucose as an index of β-cell dysfunction. *Diabetes/Metabolism Research and Reviews,* Vol.27, No.3, (March 2011), pp. 262-268, doi: 10.1002/dmrr.1166, ISSN: 1520-7552

Cheng, C.; Kushner, H., & Falkner, B.E. (2006). The utility of fasting glucose for detection of prediabetes. *Metabolism Clinical and Experimental,* Vol.55, No.4, (April 2006), pp. 434-438, ISSN: 0026-0495

Chiasson, J.L. ; Josse, R.G. ; Gomis, R.; Hanefeld, M. ; Karasik, A. & Laakso, M.; STOP-NIDDM Trial Research Group. (2003). Acarbose treatment and the risk of cardiovascular disease and hypertension in patients with impaired glucose tolerance: The STOP-NIDDM trial. *Journal of the American Medical Association*, Vol.290, No.4, (July 2003), pp. 486-494, ISSN: 0098-7484

Davidson, M.B.; Landsman, P.B. & Alexander, C.M. (2003). Lowering the criterion for impaired fasting glucose will not provide clinical benefit. *Diabetes Care*, Vol.26, No.12, (December 2003), pp. 3329-3332, ISSN: 0149-5992

DECODE Study Group, on behalf of the European Diabetes Epidemiology Study Group. (1998). Will new diagnostic criteria for diabetes mellitus change phenotype of patients with diabetes? Reanalysis of European epidemiological data. *British Medical Journal*, Vol.317, No.7155, (August 1998), 371-375, ISSN 0959-8138

DeFronzo, R.A.; Tobin, J.D. & Andres, R. (1979). Glucose clamp technique: a method for quantifying insulin secretion and resistance. *American Journal of Physiology: Endocrinology and Metabolism*, Vol.237, No.3, (September 1979), E214-E223, ISSN 0193-1849

DREAM (Diabetes REduction Assessment with ramipril and rosiglitazone Medication) Trial Investigators, Gerstein, H.C.; Yusuf, S.; Bosch, J.; Poque, J.; Sheridan, P.; Dinccag, N.; Hanefeld, M.; Hoogwerf, B.; Laasko, M.; Mohan, V.; Shaw, J.; Zinman, B. & Holman, R.R. (2006). Effect of rosiglitazone on the frequency of diabetes in patients with impaired glucose tolerance or impaired fasting glucose: a randomised controlled trial. *Lancet*, Vol.368, No.9541, (September 2006), pp. 1096-1105, ISSN 0140-6736

Expert Panel on Detection, Evaluation, and Treatment of High Blood Cholesterol in Adults. (2001). Executive summary of the third report of the National Cholesterol Education Program (NCEP) on detection, evaluation, and treatment of high blood cholesterol in adults (Adult Treatment Panel III). *Journal of the American Medical Association*, Vol.290, No.19, (May 2001), pp. 2486-2497, ISSN: 0098-7484

Fajans, S.S.; Herman, W.H. & Oral, E.A. (2011). Insufficient sensitivity of hemoglobin (1C) determination in diagnosis or screening of early diabetic states. *Metabolism Clinical and Experimental*, Vol.60, No.1, (January 2011), pp. 86-91, Epub 2010 August 17, ISSN: 0026-0425

Festa, A.; Williams, K.; D'Agostino, R.; Wagenknecht, L.E. & Haffner, S.M. (2006). The natural course of β-cell function in non-diabetic individuals. The insulin resistance atherosclerotic study. *Diabetes*, Vol.55, No.4, (April 2006), pp. 114-120, ISSN: 0012-1797

Garber, A.J.; Handelsman, Y.; Einhorn, D.; Bergman, D.A.; Bloomgarden, Z.T.; Fonseca, V.; Garvey, T.; Gavin, J.R.3rd; Grunberger, G.; Horton, E.S.; Jellinger, P.S.; Jones, K.L.; Lebovitz, H.; Levy, P.; McGuire, D.K.; Moghissi, E.S. & Nesto, R.W. (2008). Diagnosis and management of prediabetes in the continuum of hyperglycemia: when the risk of diabetes begin? A consensus statement from the American College of Endocrinology and the American Association of Clinical Endocrinologists. *Endocrine Practice*, Vol.14, No.7, (October 2008), pp. 933-946, ISSN: 1530-891X

Gastadelli, A.; Ferrannini, E.; Miyazaki, Y.; Matsuda, M. & DeFronzo, R.A.; San Antonio metabolism study. (2004). Beta-cell dysfunction and glucose intolerance: results from the San Antonio Metabolism (SAM) study. *Diabetologia*, Vol.47, No.1, (January 2004), pp. 31-39, Epub 2003 Dec 10, ISSN: 0012-186X

Genut, S.; Alberti, K.G.; Bennett, P.; Buse J.; DeFronzo, R.; Kahn, R.; Kitzmiller, J.; Knowler, W.C.; Lebovitz; H.; Lenmark, A.; Nathan, D.; Palmer, J.; Rizza, R.; Saudek, C.; Shaw, J.; Steffes, M.; Tuomilehto, J. & Zimmet, P.; Expert Committee on the Diagnosis and Classification of Diabetes Mellitus (2003). Follow-up report on the diagnosis of diabetes mellitus. *Diabetes Care,* Vol.26, No.11, (November 2003), pp. 3160-3167, ISSN: 0149-5992

Gerstein, H.C.; Santaguida, P.; Raina, P.; Morrison, K.M.; Ballion, C.; Hunt, D.; Yazdi, H. & Booker, L. (2007). Annual incidence and relative risk of diabetes in people with various categories of dyslglycemia: a systematic overview and meta-analysis of prospective studies. *Diabetes Research and Clinical Practice,* Vol.78, No.3, (December 2007), pp. 305-312, Epub 2007 Jun 29, *ISSN*: 0168-8227

Gillies, C.L.; Abrams, K.R.; Lambert, P.C.; Cooper, N.J., Sutton, A.J., Hsu, R.T. & Khunti, K. (2007). Pharmacological and lifestyle interventions to prevent or delay type 2 diabetes in people with impaired glucose tolerance: systematic review and meta-analysis. *British Medical Journal,* Vol.334, No.7588, (February 2007), pp. 229, Epub 2007 Jan 19, ISSN: 0959-8138

Harris, M.I.; Eastman, R.C.; Cowie, C.C.; Flegal, K.M. & Eberhardt, M.S. (1997). Comparison of diabetes diagnosis categories in the US population according to 1997 American diabetes Association and 1980-1985 World Health Organization diagnostic criteria. *Diabetes Care,* Vol.20, No.12, (December 1997), pp. 1859-1862, ISSN: 0149-5992

Herman, W.H. (2007). Diabetes epidemiology: guiding clinical and public health practice. The Kelly West Award Lecture, 2006. *Diabetes Care,* Vol.30, No. 7, (July 2007), pp. 1912-1919, Epub 2007 May 11, ISSN: 0149-5992

International Expert Committee. (2009). International Expert Committee Report on the role of the A1C assay in the diagnosis of diabetes. *Diabetes Care,* Vol.32, No.7, (July 2009), pp. 1327-1334, Epub 2009 Jun 5, ISSN: 0149-5992

Kahn, S.E. (2003). The relative contributions of insulin resistance and beta-cell dysfunction to the pathophysiology of type 2 diabetes. *Diabetologia,* Vol.46, No.1, (January 2003), pp. 3-19, Epub 2003 Jan 11, ISSN: 0012-186X

Knowler, W.C.; Barret-Connor, E.; Fowler, S.E.; Hamman, R.F.; Lachin, J.M.; Walker, E.A. & Nathan, D.M. Diabetes Prevention Program Research Group. (2002). Reduction in the incidence of type 2 diabetes with lifestyle intervention or metformin. *N Engl J Med,* Vol.346, No.6, (February 2002), pp. 393-403, *ISSN: 0028-4793*

Kolberg, J.A.; Jørgensen, T.; Gerwiev, R.W.; Hamren, S.; McKenna, M.P.; Moler, E.; Rowe, MW; Urdea, M.S.; Xu, X.M.; Hansen, T.; Pedersen, O. & Borch-Johnsen, K. (2009). Development of a type 2 diabetes risk model from a panel of serum biomarkers from the Inter99 cohort. *Diabetes Care,* Vol.32, No.7, (July 2009), pp. 1207-1212, ISSN: 0149-5992

Kramer C.K., Araneta M.R.G., & Barret-Connor, E. (2010). A1C and diabetes diagnosis: The Rancho Bernardo Study. *Diabetes Care,* Vol.33, No.1, (January 2010), pp. 101-103, Epub 2009 Oct 16, ISSN: 0149-5992

Meigs, J.B.; Muller, D.C.; Nathan, D.M.; Blake, D.R. & Andres, R. (2003). The natural history of progression from normal glucose tolerance to type 2 diabetes in the Baltimore Longitudinal Study of Aging. *Diabetes,* Vol.52, No.6, (June 2003), pp. 1475-1484, ISSN: 0012-1797

Monnier, I.; Lapinski, H. & Colette, C. (2003). Contributions of fasting and postprandial plasma glucose increments to the overall diurnal hyperglycemia of type 2 diabetic patients: variations with increasing levels of HbA(1c). *Diabetes Care,* Vol.26, No.3, (March 2003), pp. 881-885, ISSN: 0149-5992

National Diabetes Data Group. (1979). Classification and diagnosis of diabetes mellitus and other categories of glucose intolerance. *Diabetes,* Vol.28, No.12, (December 1979), pp. 1039-1052, ISSN: 0012-1797

Ratner, R.; Goldberg, R.; Haffner, S.; Marcovina, S.; Orchard, T.; Fowler, S. & Temprosa, M. Diabetes Prevention Program Research Group. (2005). Impact of intensive lifestyle and metformin therapy on cardiovascular disease risk factors in the diabetes prevention program. *Diabetes Care,* Vol.28, No.4, (April 2005), pp. 888-94, ISSN: 0149-5992

Rizza, R.A. Pathogenesis of fasting and postprandial hyperglycemia in type 2 diabetes: implications for therapy. (2010). *Diabetes,* Vol.59, No.11, (November 2010), pp. 2697-2707, Epub 2010 Aug 12, ISSN: 0012-1797 59

Sainaghi, P.P.; Castello, L.; Limoncini, A.M.; Bergamasco, L.; Bartoli, E. & Schianca, G.P.C. (2007). Poor specificity of fasting plasma glucose cut-off values in ruling out glucose intolerance: the complementary usefulness of OGTT. *Experimental and Clinical Endocrinology & Diabetes,* Vol.115, No.2, (February 2007) pp. 112-7, ISSN 0947-7349

Schulze, M.B.; Fritsche, A.; Boeing, H. & Joost, H.G. Fasting plasma glucose and type 2 diabetes risk: a non-linear relationship. (2010) *Diabetic Medicine,* Vol.27, No.4, (April 2010), pp. 473-476, ISSN: 0742-3071

Shaw, J.E.; Sicree, R.A. & Zimmet, P.Z. Global estimates of the prevalence of diabetes for 2010 and 2030. (2010) *Diabetes Research and Clinical Practice,* Vol.87, No.1, (January 2010), pp. 4-14, Epub 2009 Nov 6, ISSN: 0168-8227

Stern, M.P.; Williams, K. & Haffner, S.M. Identification of persons at high for type 2 diabetes mellitus: do we need the oral glucose tolerance test? (2002). *Ann Intern Med Annals of Internal Medicine,* Vol.136, No.8, (April 2002), pp. 575-81, ISSN: 0003-4819

Stumvoll, M.; Van Haeften, T.; Fritsche, A. & Gerich, J. Oral glucose tolerance test indexes for insulin sensitivity and secretion based on various availabilities of sampling times. (2001a) *Diabetes Care,* Vol.24, No4, (April 2001), pp. 796-797, ISSN: 0149-5992

Stumvoll, M.; Fritsche, A. & Häring, H. The OGTT as test for beta cell function? (2001b) European Journal of Clinical Investigation, Vol.31, No.5 (May 2001), pp. 380-381, ISSN: 0014-2972

Tirosh, A.; Shai, I.; Tekes-Manova, D.; Israeli, E.; Pereg, D.; Shochat, T.; Kochba, I., & Rudich, A.; Israeli Diabetes Research Group. (2005). Normal fasting plasma glucose levels and type 2 diabetes in young men. *N Engl J Med,* Vol.353, No.14, (October 2005), pp. 1454-1462, *ISSN: 0028-4793*

Tschritter, O.; Fritsche, A.; Shirkavand, F.; Machicao, F.; Haring, H. & Stumvoll, M. (2003). Assessing the shape of the glucose curve during an oral glucose tolerance test. *Diabetes Care,* Vol.26, No.4, (April 2003), pp. 1026-1033, ISSN: 0149-5992

Unwin, N.; Alberti, K.G.; Bhopal, R.; Harland, J.; Watson, W., & White, M. (1998). Comparison of the current WHO and new criteria for the diagnosis of diabetes mellitus in three ethnic groups in the UK. *Diabetic Medicine,* Vol.15, No.7, (July) pp. 554-557, ISSN: 0742-3071

Unwin, N.; Shaw, J.; Zimmet, P. & Alberti, K.G. (2002). Impaired glucose tolerance and impaired fasting glycaemia: the current status on definition and intervention. *Diabetic Medicine,* Vol.19, No.9, (September 2002), pp. 708-723, ISSN: 0742-3071

Utzschneider, K.M.; Prigeon, R.L.; Faulenbach, M.V.; Tong, J.; Carr, D.B.; Boyko, E.J.; Leonetti, D.L.; McNeely, M.J.; Fujimoto, W.Y. & Kahn, S.E. (2009). Oral disposition index predicts the development of future diabetes above and beyond fasting and 2-h glucose levels. *Diabetes Care* , Vol.32, No.2, (February 2009), pp. 335-341, Epub 2008 Oct 28, ISSN: 0149-5992

Valleron, A.J.; Eschwège, E.; Papoz, L., & Rosselin, G.E. (1975). Agreement and discrepancy in the evaluation of normal and diabetic oral glucose tolerance test. *Diabetes,* Vol.24, No.6, (June 1975), pp. 585-593, ISSN: 0012-1797

3

The Role of Parathyroid Hormone-Related Protein (PTHRP) in the Pathophysiology of Diabetes Mellitus

Ioannis Legakis
Department of Endocrinology, Henry Dunant Hospital, Athens Greece

1. Introduction

Blood glucose homeostasis is controlled by the endocrine cells of **the pancreas, located** in the islets of Langerhans. The islet cells monitor the concentration of glucose in the blood and secrete hormones with opposite effects. When after a meal the blood glucose concentration is increasing, the beta cells, which are the most numerous islet cells, secrete the hormone insulin to reduce blood glucose. Insulin stimulates the uptake of glucose by cells of the body and stimulates the conversion of glucose to glycogen in the liver. If the glucose level falls too far, islet alpha cells secrete the hormone glucagon, which stimulates the breakdown of glycogen to glucose in the liver and therefore increases blood glucose between meals. Optimal control of blood glucose levels depends on delicate changes in insulin production and secretion by the pancreatic beta cells and on their capacity for a large increase of secretion after meals, requiring large stores of insulin [1]. Very important is the need for the beta-cell mass to be closely regulated by glucose and hormonal effects on beta-cell replication, size, apoptotic elimination and, under certain conditions, neogenesis from progenitor cells. Failure to adapt to changes in body mass, pregnancy, insulin sensitivity of peripheral tissues, or tissue injury may lead to the development of chronically elevated blood glucose, or diabetes [2]. The increasing global prevalence of diabetes has stimulated efforts to develop new therapeutic strategies like beta-cell replacement or regenerative medicine. The existing therapies with exogenous insulin or hypoglycemic agents for type 1 and type 2 diabetes are unsatisfactory, since they do not offer a cure and are mostly insufficient for preventing the secondary complications associated with diabetes [3].

Despite an enormous increase in our understanding of islet differentiation and development, there is sparse information regarding the factors and pathways that regulate growth, survival, and death of islet cells. The number of islet beta cells present at birth is mainly generated by the proliferation and differentiation of pancreatic progenitor cells, a process called neogenesis. Shortly after birth, beta-cell neogenesis stops and a small proportion of cycling beta cells can still expand the cell number to compensate for increased insulin demands, albeit at a slow rate. The low capacity for self-replication in the adult is too limited to result in a significant regeneration following extensive tissue injury. Likewise, chronically increased metabolic demands can lead to beta-cell failure to compensate. Neogenesis from progenitor cells inside or outside islets represents a more potent mechanism leading to robust expansion of the beta-cell mass, but it may require external stimuli. For therapeutic purposes, advantage could be taken from the surprising differentiation plasticity of adult pancreatic cells and possibly also from stem cells. **Recently a large number of factors controlling the differentiation of beta-cells has been identified**. They are classified into the following main categories: growth factors, cytokine and inflammatory factors, and hormones such as PTHrP and GLP-1**[4,5]**. In general , treatment with these external stimuli can restore a functional beta-cell mass in diabetic animals, but further studies are required before it can be applied to humans.

2. Parathyroid hormone-related peptide

PTH-related peptide (PTHrP) was first discovered as the most frequent cause of the syndrome of humoral hypercalcemia of malignancy [6-10]. However, PTHrP mRNA is widely expressed under normal conditions, and gene ablation experiments have established that this peptide plays an essential role in normal skeletal development [11]. Human PTHrP can be produced as a 141-amino acid peptide or, through alternative mRNA splicing, as a protein comprising either 139 or 173 amino acids. PTHrP binds to the same receptor as PTH, and the biological responses elicited by either ligand through this common PTH1R-receptor are largely indistinguishable, at least with regard to mineral ion homeostasis [12-15]. For these actions of PTH and PTHrP, the amino-terminal (1–34) peptide fragments are sufficient, as PTH-(1–34) and PTHrP-(1–34) display both high-affinity receptor binding and efficient receptor activation. There is a growing body of evidence, however, suggesting that the midregional and/or carboxy-terminal fragments of either peptide, derived through posttranslational processing mechanisms, also have biological activity [16-18]. However, the observed activities of midregional and COOH-terminal fragments of PTH and PTHrP are unlikely to be related to adult mineral ion homeostasis and are probably mediated through receptors that are distinct from the PTH1R, although these receptors have not yet been identified.

3. Structure-activity relations in PTH and PTHRP

PTH and PTHrP show significant sequence homology within the first 13 amino acid residues (Fig1), and this sequence conservation reflects the functional importance of the amino-terminal residues in receptor signaling [19- 21]. Between PTH and PTHrP, sequence homology decreases markedly in the 14–34 region, where only three amino acids are identical, and beyond residue 34 there is no recognizable similarity.

For both PTH and PTHrP, the 15–34 region functions as the principal PTH1R binding domain, and these portions of the two peptides probably interact with overlapping regions of the receptor, as the two fragments compete equally for binding with radiolabeled PTH-(1–34) or PTHrP-(1–36) to the PTH1R [22,23].These findings also suggest that the two divergent receptor binding domains of PTH and PTHrP **adapt** similar conformations.

The three-dimensional crystal structures of PTH or PTHrP are not known, but the peptides have been analyzed extensively by nuclear magnetic resonance (NMR) spectroscopic methods. In general, these studies indicate that, under certain solvent conditions, PTH-(1–34) and PTHrP-(1–36) analogs contain defined segments of secondary structure, including a relatively stable a-helix in the carboxy-terminal receptor-binding domain, a shorter less stable helix near the aminoterminal activation domain, and a flexible hinge or bend region connecting the two domains [24-26].

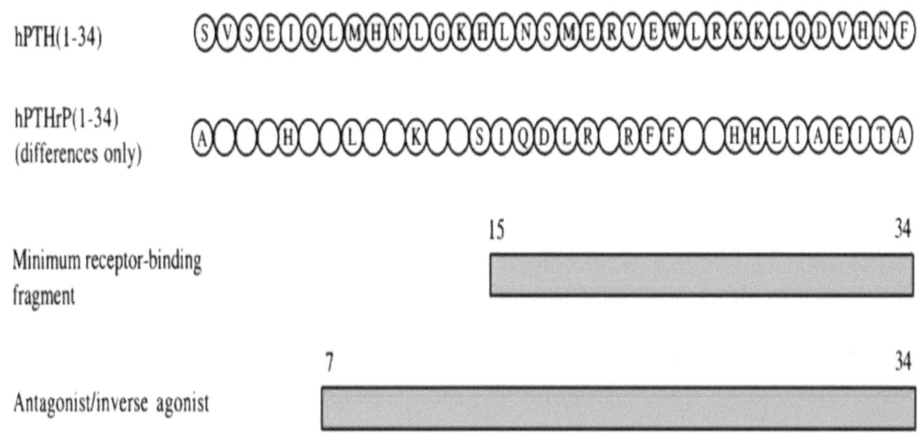

Fig. 1. Parathyroid hormone (PTH) and PTH-related peptide (PTHrP) and analogs: functional domains and receptor selectivity determinants. A: amino acid sequences of the bioactive (1–34) regions of native human PTH and human PTHrP. In the schematic of human PTHrP, only residues that differ from human PTH are provided, and amino acids that are identical to the corresponding residues of PTH are represented by open circles. Bars represent peptide fragments that exhibit weak receptor binding (15–34) or antagonist and inverse agonist properties (7–34)

Although most NMR solution studies find evidence for peptide flexibility, the question of whether the conformations of PTH and PTHrP recognized by the receptor are folded with tertiary interactions, as suggested by some studies [27-29], or extended, as suggested by other analyses , remains unanswered.

4. Receptors for PTH and PTHRP

As indicated above, PTH and PTHrP mediate their actions primarily through the PTH1R PTH/PTHrP receptor, a G protein-coupled receptor (GPCR) with seven membrane-spanning **helices**[30]. The PTH1R forms, along with the receptors for secretin, calcitonin, glucagon, and several other peptide hormones, a distinct family of GPCRs that exhibit none of the amino acid sequence motifs found in the other subgroups of the superfamily of heptahelical receptors [31-32]. These peptide hormone receptors, called class II or family B receptors [31], can be distinguished from other GPCRs by their large, **(150** amino acid) amino-terminal extracellular domain containing six conserved cysteine residues, as well as by several other conserved amino acids that are dispersed throughout the NH2-terminal domain, the membrane-embedded helixes, and the connecting loops.

Significant progress has been made in understanding the role of the common PTH/PTHrP receptor, the PTH1R, in mammalian biology, particularly with regard to its normal role in chondrocyte growth and development, and its pathological role in two rare genetic disorders in humans. Amino acid residues in the PTH1R and PTH2R that are likely to be

important for ligand-receptor interaction and for signal transduction have been identified through mutagenesis methods and through photoaffinity cross-linking techniques.
Although these studies have provided new insights into the mode of ligand-receptor interaction, there is still much that needs to be learned about this complex process.

5. Pancreas development

The pancreas originates from the foregut endoderm as ventral and dorsal buds, beginning at embryonic day (e) 9.5 in the mouse, and the two buds later fuse at approximately e12.5 [33]. The endodermal epithelium proliferates in response to various fibroblast growth factors (FGFs) produced by the adjacent mesenchyme [34], undergoes branching morphogenesis, and differentiates into ductal, exocrine, and endocrine cells. Evagination and development of the ventral pancreatic bud is slightly delayed compared with that of the dorsal bud, and the ventral bud gives rise to fewer endocrine cells than does the dorsal bud [35]. The ventral and dorsal buds also differ with regard to the signals they require for development.

5.1 Dynamic changes in an organism's ß-cell mass

In addition to maintaining ß-cell mass under normal circumstances, as just discussed, an organism must also be able to alter its ß-cell mass in accordance with its requirements for insulin. In states of insulin resistance, such as pregnancy and obesity, ß-cell mass is known to increase [45]. Such ß-cell mass expansion is accomplished primarily by increasing ß-cell proliferation, although neogenesis may also contribute. However, when compensatory ß-cell mass expansion is inadequate, diabetes ensues - gestational diabetes in the case of pregnancy, and type II diabetes in the case of obesity. Although the majority of humans do not become diabetic in these circumstances, a significant portion of the population is predisposed to ß-cell failure, for currently unknown reasons. It is likely that factors that regulate ß-cell proliferation may play a role, although whether the factors that regulate ß-cell mass expansion are the same as those that regulate ß-cell mass maintenance is unclear.

5.2 Regulatory factors of b-cell mass expansion and maintenance

During pregnancy, rats exhibit a greater than 50% increase in ß-cell mass, which is accomplished primarily through an approximate threefold increase in ß-cell proliferation [46]. The chief stimuli of ß-cell proliferation during pregnancy are placental lactogens (PLs), although prolactin (Prl) and growth hormone (GH) also have similar effects on ß-cells and are also elevated during pregnancy. After delivery, ß-cell mass returns to normal levels within 10 days through increased ß-cell apoptosis, decreased ß-cell proliferation, and ß-cell atrophy.
Diet-induced obesity results in insulin resistance and ß-cell mass expansion in humans and mice. The C57Bl/6 mouse strain is notoriously susceptible to these effects, exhibiting a 2.2-fold increase in ß-cell mass and proliferation after 4 months on a high-fat diet versus a control diet [51]. However, these mice eventually become diabetic and lose their ß-cell mass due to increased ß-cell apoptosis and reduced ß-cell proliferation.
In genetic models of obesity and insulin resistance, there is also a compensatory expansion of ß-cell mass. For example, *db/db* mice, which lack a functional leptin receptor, exhibit a twofold increase in ß-cell mass by 8 weeks of age [52]. This timepoint correlates with the onset of diabetes, which progresses from glucose intolerance that is first observed between 4

and 6 weeks of age. A similar rat model, the Zucker diabetic fatty (ZDF) rat (*fa/fa*), also has a homozygous mutation in the gene encoding the leptin receptor. ZDF rats exhibit increased ß-cell mass and increased ß-cell proliferation prior to the onset of diabetes, but increased ß-cell apoptosis prevents them from adequately expanding their ß-cell mass after the onset of diabetes, despite continued high rates of ß-cell proliferation [53]. This phenotype contrasts with what is observed in non-diabetic Zucker fatty (ZF) rats, which possess the same mutation as ZDF rats and also become obese and insulin resistant but do not develop diabetes due to sufficient ß-cell mass expansion through increased ß-cell proliferation, neogenesis, and hypertrophy [53].

Another model of insufficient ß-cell mass expansion is the insulin receptor substrate two null mouse [*Irs2*$^{-/-}$; 54]. Global inactivation of Irs2 results in severe insulin resistance, both centrally in the brain causing obesity, and peripherally, for which ß-cell mass expansion should be able to compensate. However, because ß-cells require Irs2 for proper proliferation and function, *Irs2*$^{-/-}$-mice are unable to expand their ß-cell mass, and they develop diabetes by 10 weeks of age. This phenotype is not observed in *Irs1*$^{-/-}$-mice, despite the fact that these mice exhibit similar insulin resistance, because Irs1 is not required for ß-cell mass expansion. These experiments provide additional evidence that Irs2 is required for ß-cell mass expansion in response to insulin resistance. Furthermore, overexpression of Irs2 in ß-cells (*Rip-Irs2*) is sufficient to prevent ß-cell failure in diet-induced obesity and streptozotocin-induced diabetic models [55].

6. The role of PTHrP in diabetes

PTHrP was discovered in the early 1980s as the factor responsible for humoral hypercalcemia of malignancy. Subsequent studies found PTHrP expression to be widespread in almost all tissues and organs of the body. One such tissue is the islet of Langerhans, in which all four endocrine cell types **(α, ß, γ and δ pancreatic polypeptide cells**) produce PTHrP. Not only is the peptide made in islets, but receptors for PTHrP also seem to be present on ß cells. To begin to evaluate the possible role of PTHrP in pancreatic islets, transgenic mice overexpressing PTHrP in the ß cells of islets were **developed** using the rat insulin II promoter (RIP). These RIP-PTHrP mice displayed islet cell hyperplasia, significant hypoglycemia under both fasting and nonfasting conditions, as well as inappropriate hyperinsulinemia. Insulin expression was shown to be up-regulated both at the messenger RNA and protein level in whole pancreas of RIP-PTHrP mice. [58]

PTHrP is a prohormone that is posttranslationally endoproteolytically cleaved to yield a family of mature secretory peptides [58-60] . These include an amino-terminal secretory form, which binds to and activates the recently cloned parathyroid hormone receptor [10] , as well as several other mid-region, and carboxyl-terminal secretory forms of the peptide. Since the full-length PTHrP(1-141) cDNA was used to construct the transgene, these experiments do not provide information regarding which of the several secretory forms is (or are) responsible for the hyperinsulinemia and islet hyperplasia observed.

The phenotype does not seem to result from a developmental effect of PTHrP on the pancreas, because transgenic mice at 1 week of age were normoglycemic and displayed normal islet mass despite expression of the PTHrP transgene. In contrast, a visible increase in islet mass (2-fold) was observed in RIP-PTHrP mice by 12 weeks of age, and increased further (3- to 4-fold) by 1 yr of age. Both an increase in the number of ß cells per islet as well as an increase in total islet number contribute to the enhancement of islet mass in these mice.

The increase in islet mass in RIP-PTHrP transgenic mice does not seem to be a result of an increase in the proliferation rates of preexisting ß cells of the islet. Thus, the increased islet mass in RIP-PTHrP mice most likely results from a decrease in the normal rate of ß-cell turnover or apoptosis and/or enhanced neogenesis(62). In other cell types like chondrocytes, neuronal cells, and prostate carcinoma cells, PTHrP has been shown to have an antiapoptotic or protective effect against cell death. In line with this, ß cells of the RIP-PTHrP mice have also been shown to be more resistant to the cytotoxic effects of high doses of the diabetogenic agent streptozotocin (STZ): RIP-PTHrP transgenic mice remain relatively euglycemic unlike their normal littermates, which become severely diabetic following STZ injection. Histologically, the resistance to the diabetogenic effects of STZ seems to result, at least partially, from PTHrP-induced resistance to STZ-mediated ß-cell death (63).

Another surprising feature of the RIP-PTHrP mouse is that despite impressive overproduction of PTHrP, systemic hypersecretion of PTHrP does not occur and hypercalcemia does not develop. This is surprising because PTHrP is clearly sorted into the regulated secretory pathway [64-67], and is copackaged with insulin in islet cells [66], and is secreted in response to insulin secretagogues [66]. This may reflect clearance of PTHrP by the liver after it is secreted into the portal circulation.

These findings suggest that PTHrP may have potential in therapeutic strategies designed to increase ß-cell mass and function. Specifically, this peptide could prove to be valuable in improving islet transplant survival in type 1 diabetes.

Recently, the discovery of a family of islet homeobox genes including PDX1/STF1/IPF1/IDX1, ISL1, PAX-4, PAX-6, NeuroD/ß-2 and others [74-77] and putative islet growth factors such as GH, PRL, placental lactogen, hepatocyte growth factor, the reg family of proteins, and the recently identified protein, INGAP [78-80] has focused attention on the mechanisms responsible for pancreatic and islet development and on the mechanisms whereby islet neogenesis occurs in states of islet injury, subtotal pancreatectomy, or pregnancy, and whereby normal islet mass is sustained throughout life. If PTHrP does not have an obvious role in islet cell proliferation or in apoptosis of existing islets but is nevertheless very potent in increasing islet mass, it is possible that PTHrP may play a role in normal islet neogenesis or in differentiation from uncommitted precursor cells, such as ductular epithelial cells. In this regard, it has been reported that PTHrP is indeed expressed in pancreatic ductular cells [81].

For attaining a well-functioning ß-cell mass, PTHrP is a very promising candidate among insulinotropic peptides including hepatocyte growth factor, GLP-1, and exendin-4 [82]. Indeed, rat insulin gene–promoted overexpression of PTHrP in mouse islets presented a twofold increase in total islet number and total islet mass, as well as in insulin content [83]. In contrast, transgenic mice expressing exendin-4, a long-acting GLP-1–like peptide, presented no remarkable change in total islet number and total islet mass [84]. Thus, PTHrP seems to be potent in upholding a well-functioning ß-cell mass.

7. Preleminary clinical observations

As had been the case in so many other tissues, the observation of physiological and pathophysiological responses to PTH was documented in the islet and in insulin target tissues long before the discovery of PTHrP. The significance of these observations was difficult to fathom at the time, since no obvious physiological link between calcium homeostasis and glucose metabolism readily suggested itself. For example, it had long been observed that glucose intolerance and frank diabetes occurred in association with hyperparathyroidism more often than would be expected by random coincidence [85]. It also had been shown that the elevated PTH concentrations in patients with primary hyperparathyroidism induced both mild peripheral insulin resistance and augmented insulin response to hyperglycemia. In the majority of reports, the data on insulin response are difficult to interpret because of the effects on insulin secretion of the hypercalcemia that accompany the elevated circulating PTH concentrations in patients with hyperparathyroidism. In one study, however, normal volunteers made hypercalcemic by PTH injection over 8 days demonstrated augmented insulin responses to glucose and to intravenous tolbutamide, while a control group rendered similarly hypercalcemic by calcium infusion failed to demonstrate an augmented insulin response to glucose [86]. To investigate the direct effects of PTH on pancreatic islets in vitro, Fadda et al. [87], before the description of PTHrP as an islet peptide,examined insulin secreation from isolated pancreatic islets in response to PTH-(1-34) and PTH- (l-84). These studies showed that PTH augmented both the first and second phases of secretion in response to 16.7 mM glucose.

The suggested link between parathyroid gland function and the pancreatic islet was met, quite appropriately, with skepticism and for two reasons. First, as noted above, it was very difficult to envision a physiological scenario in which PTH could be construed as participating in normal islet regulation. Second, studies such as that reported by Fadda et al. [87] generally required concentrations of PTH far in excess of those encountered in hyperparathyroidism to observe an effect. One was therefore forced to conclude either that these effects were nonphysiological and therefore meaningless or to postulate that there is another natural peptide of physiological import within the islet that might be mediating these effects in the islet. At the time these studies were performed, no such normal islet product was known. As is now obvious, islet derived PTHrP is a candidate worthy of consideration.

In 1992,Ishida et al,[88] reported that type 2 diabetics presented higher serum PTHrP levels than control subjects. However, in that study no stimulation tests were done to demonstrate whether PTHrP is released from the pancreas in response to insulin secretagogues like glucose or calcium. Extensive studies have demonstrated that an increase in the cytosolic calcium is essential for glucose-stimulated insulin release[89]. Indeed, one of the mature, secretory forms of PTHrP, called mid-region PTHrP,was demonstrated by Wu et. al. [90] to increase cytosolic calcium levels in a pancreatic b cell line. Increased cytosolic calcium levels have also been reported in insulinoma cells, supporting the notion that PTHrP is not only secreted by pancreatic cells, but might also play an autocrine or paracrine role within the islets themselves[91].In 2006,Shor et al [92] examined the effects of two stimulatory secretagogues -glucose and calcium-after an oral glucose load (75gr) to healthy controls. They reported that PTHrP and insulin rose in parallel although this response was not observed during the calcium load. Moreover , they found significant differences in basal serum PTHrP levels particularly in type 2 versus type 1 diabetics and healthy controls. Ishida et al[88], proposed that elevated PTHrP levels might play a compensatory role in calcium homeostasis in diabetic patients. They speculate that these patients often exhibit osteopenia and lower than normal PTH levels with a net result the preservation of normal serum calcium levels.

Performing PTHrP serum determinations in a fasting state in type 2 diabetics by our group [93] we have found that PTHrP was statistically significant correlated with glucose in type 2 diabetes **(r:0,992-p<0,0001)** and in normal subjects in the fasting state **(r:0,908-p<0,0001)**. Additionally, PTHrP serum levels exhibited a significant increase in type 2 diabetes compared to control subjects **(Diabetics-PTHrP(Median):380 pg/ml versus Normals-PTHrP(Median):180 pg/ml , p<0,001)**. Interestingly, PTHrP showed a positive correlation with insulin levels only among healthy individuals presumably due to defective glucose stimulated insulin secretion known to occur in type 2 diabetics.

In conclusion ,the recognition that PTHrP-a protein mostly indentified as a tumor product in cases of humoral malignant hypercalcemia, is found in almost every body tissue including the pancreas , where it is processed into multiple secreatory forms,co-packed with insulin , and secreted in a regulatory fashion in response to insulin secretagogeus , opens new directions in the autocrine/paracrine role of PTHrP in the islets of Langerhans and raises several questions for further experimentation in both type 1 and type 2 diabetes.

8. References

[1] Chang-Chen KJ.; Mullur R.; Bernal-Mizrachi E :Beta-cell failure as a complication of diabetes. Rev Endocr Metab Disord .,2008, 9, 329-343.

[2] Retnakaran R.;Qi Y.; Sermer M.; Connelly PW.; Hanley AJ.; Zinman B : Glucose intolerance in pregnancy anf future risk of pre-diabetes or diabetes. Diabetes Care., 2008, 31, 2026-2031.

[3] Nathan, D.M :Long-term complications of Diabetes Mellitus. N Engl J Med., 1993,328, 1676–1685.

[4] Legakis I.;Tsioras C.; Phenekos C : Decreased glucagon-like peptide 1 fasting levels in type 2 diabetes .Diabetes Care .,2003, 26, 252.

[5] Legakis I.;Mantouridis T.;Mountokalakis T : Positive correlation of galanin with glucose in type 2 diabetes . Diabetes Care., 2005, 28, 759-760.

[6] Mangin, M. A. C.; Webb. B. E.; Dreyer, J. T.; Posillico, K.; Ikeda, E. C.;Weir, A. F.; Stewart, N. H.; Bander, L. ;Milstone, D. E.; Barton, U. ;Francke, Broadus, A.E: Identification of a cDNA encoding a parathyroid hormone-like peptide from a human tumor associated with humoral hypercalcemia of malignancy. Proc. Natl. Acad. Sci. USA., 1988, 85, 597–601.

[7] Moseley, J. M.; M. Kubota, H.; Diefenbach-Jagger, R. E. H.;Wettenhall, B. E. Kemp.; L. J. Suva.; C. P. Rodda.; P. R. Ebeling.; P. J. Hudson.; J. D. Zajac and J. T. Martin : Parathyroid hormone-related protein purified from a human lung cancer cell line. Proc. Natl. Acad. Sci. USA,1987, 84, 5048–5052.

[8] Stewart, A. F. R.; Horst, L. J. ;Deftos, E. C. ;Cadman, R. Lang.; Broadus,A.E: Biochemical evaluation of patients with cancer-associated hypercalcemia. Evidence for humoral and non-humoral groups. N. Engl. J. Med., 1980, 303, 1377–1381.

[9] Strewler, G. J.; Stern, P.H.; Jacobs, J.W.; Eveloff,J.; Klein, R.F.;Leung, S.C.; Rosenblatt, M.;Nissenson, R.A: Parathyroid hormone-like protein from human renal carcinoma cells. Structural and functional homology with parathyroid hormone. J. Clin. Invest., 1987, 80, 1803–1807.

[10] Suva, L. J.;Winslow, G. A.; Wettenhall, R. E. ;Hammonds, R. G. ;Moseley, J. M.; Diefenbach-Jagger, H.; Rodda, C. P.; Kemp, B. E. ; Rodriguez, H.; Chen, E. Y. ;Hudson, P. J. ; Martin, J. T.;Wood, W. I :A parathyroid hormone-related protein

implicated in malignant hypercalcemia: cloning and expression. Science., 1987,237, 893-896.

[11] Karaplis, A. C.;Luz,A.; Glowacki, J.;Bronson,R.; Tybulewicz,V.; Kronenberg, H. M. ;R. C. Mulligan, R. C.: Lethal skeletal dysplasia from targeted disruption of the parathyroid hormone-related peptide gene. Genes Dev.,1994, 8, 277-289.

[12] Everhart-Caye, M.; Inzucchi, S.E.; Guinness-Henry, J.; Mitnick,M.A.; Stewart, A.F.: Parathyroid hormone (PTH)-related protein(1-36) is equipotent to PTH-(1-34) in humans. J. Clin. Endocrinol. Metab., 1996, 81, 199-208.

[13] Fraher, L. J.; Hodsman, A. B.;Jonas,K.; D. Saunders,D.; Rose,C.I.; Henderson, J.E.; Hendy, G.N.; Goltzman, D: A comparison of the in vivo biochemical responses to exogenous parathyroid hormone-(1-34) [PTH-(1-34)] and PTH-related peptide-(1-34) in man. J. Clin. Endocrinol. Metab., 1992, 75, 417-423.

[14] Horiuchi, N.;Caulfield, M.P.;Fisher, J.E.;Goldman, M.E.; McKee, R.L.; Reagan, J.E.; Levy, J.J;Nutt, R.F.; Rodan, S.B.; Schofield, T.L.; Clemens, T.L.; Rosenblatt, M : Similarity of synthetic peptide from human tumour to parathyroid hormone in vivo and in vitro. Science., 1987, 238, 1566-1568.

[15] Kemp, B. E.; Mosely, J.M.; Rodda, C.P.; Ebeling, P.R.; R. E. Wettenhall, H.; Stapleton, D.; Diefenbach-Jagger, H.; Ure, F.; Michelangali, V.P.; Simmons, H.A.; Raisz, L.G.; Martin, T.J: Parathyroid hormone-related protein of malignancy: active synthetic fragments. Science., 1987, 238, 1568-1570.

[16] Kovacs, C. S.; Lanske, B.; Hunzelman, J.L.; Guo, J.; Karaplis, A.C.; Kronenberg, H.M: Parathyroid hormonerelated peptide (PTHrP) regulates fetal placental calcium transport through a receptor distinct from the PTH/PTHrP receptor. Proc. Natl. Acad. Sci. USA., 1996, 93, 15233-15238.

[17] Potts, J. T. Jr.; Juppner, H. Parathyroid hormone and parathyroid hormone-related peptide in calcium homeostasis, bone metabolism, and bone development: the proteins, their genes, and receptors. In: Metabolic Bone Disease, edited by L. V. Avioli, L.V.; Krane, S.M. New York: Academic, 1997; pp. 51-94.

[18] Wu, T. L.; Vasavada, R.C.;Yang, K.; Massfelder, T.; Ganz, M.; Abbas, S.K.; Care, A.D.; Stewart, A.F: Structural and physiological characterization of the mid-region secretory species of parathyroid hormone-related protein. J. Biol. Chem., 1996, 271, 24371-24381.

[19] Goltzman, D.; Peytremann, A; Callahan, E.; Tregear, G.W.; Potts, Jr :Analysis of the requirements for parathyroid hormone action in renal membranes with the use of inhibiting analogues. J. Biol. Chem., 1975, 250, 3199-3203.

[20] Horiuchi, N.; Holick, M.F.; Potts, J.T.;Jr., Rosenblatt, M:A parathyroid hormone inhibitor in vivo: design and biologic evaluation of a hormone analog. Science., 1983, 220, 1053- 1055.

[21] Tregear, G. W.; Rietschoten, J.Van.; Greene, E.; Keutmann, H.T.; Niall, H.D.; Reit, B.; Parsons, J.A.; Potts, Jr : Bovine parathyroid hormone: minimum chain length of synthetic peptide required for biological activity. Endocrinology.,1973, 93, 1349-1353.

[22] Abou-Samra, A.-B.; Uneno, S.; Ju¨ppner, H.; Keutmann, H.; Potts, J.T.; Segre, G.V.;Nussbaum, S.R: Nonhomologous sequences of parathyroid hormone and the parathyroid hormone related peptide bind to a common receptor on ROS 17/2.8 cells. Endocrinology., 1989, 125, 2215-2217.

[23] Caulfield, M. P.; Rosenblatt. M.:Parathyroid hormone receptor interactions. Trends Endocrinol. Metab., 1990, 2, 164–168.

[24] Barden, J.; Cuthbertson, R.; Jia-Zhen, W.; Moseley, J.; Kemp,B.: Solution structure of parathyroid hormone related protein (residues 1–34) containing an Ala substituted for an Ile in position 15 (PTHrP[Ala15]-(1–34)). J. Biol. Chem., 1997, 273, 29572–29578.

[25] Marx, U.; Austermann, S.; Bayer, P.; Adermann, K.; Ejchart, A.; Sticht, H.; Walters, S.; Schmid, F.; Jaenicke, R.;Forssmann, W.; Rosch,P.: Structure of human parathyroid hormone 1–37 in solution. J. Biol. Chem., 1995, 270, 15194–15202.

[26] Pellegrini, M.; Royo, M.;Rosenblatt, M.; Chorev, M.; Mierke,D.: Addressing the tertiary structure of human parathyroid hormone-(1–34). J. Biol. Chem., 1998, 273, 10420–10427.

[27] Barden, J. A.; Kemp, B.E.: Stabilized NMR structure of the hypercalcemia of malignancy peptide PTHrP[Ala-26](1- 34)amide. Biochim. Biophys. Acta ., 1994, 1208, 256–262.

[28] Cohen, F. E.; Strewler, G.J.; Bradley, M.S.;Carlquist, M.; Nilsson, M.; Ericsson, M.; Ciardelli, T.L.;and R. A. Nissenson, R. A.: Analogues of parathyroid hormone modified at positions 3 and 6: effects on receptor binding and activation of adenylyl cyclase in kidney and bone. J. Biol. Chem., 1991, 266, 1997–2004.

[29] Gardella, T. J., M. D. Luck, A. K. Wilson, H. T. Keutmann, S. R. Nussbaum, J. T. Potts, Jr., and H. M. Kronenberg. Parathyroid hormone (PTH)/PTH-related peptide hybrid peptides reveal functional interactions between the 1–14 and 15–34 domains of the ligand. J. Biol. Chem.; 1995, 270: 6584–6588.

[30] Mannstadt M, Juppner H, Gardella J T: Receptors for PTH and PTHrP: their biological importance and functional properties. Am. J. Physiol.; 1999, 277, 665-675

[31] Ji, T. H.; Grossmann, M.; Ji,I.: G protein-coupled receptors. I. Diversity of receptor-ligand interactions. J. Biol. Chem., 1998, 273, 17299–17302.

[32] Segre, G. V.; Goldring,S.R.: Receptors for secretin, calcitonin, parathyroid hormone (PTH)/PTH-related peptide, vasoactive intestinal peptide, glucagon-like peptide 1, growth hormone-releasing hormone, and glucagon belong to a newly discovered G protein-linked receptor family. Trends Endocrinol. Metab.,1993, 4: 309–314.

[33] Ackerman AM.; Gannon M :Molecular regulation of pancreatic b-cell mass development ,maintenance and expansion . Journal of Molecular Endocrinology., 2007, 38, 193-206.

[34] Bhushan, A.; Itoh, N.; Kato, S.; Thiery, J.P.; Czernichow, P.; Bellusci, S.; Scharfmann, R.: Fgf10 is essential for maintaining the proliferative capacity of epithelial progenitor cells during early pancreatic organogenesis. Development ., 2001, 128 , 5109–5117.

[35] Spooner, B.S.; Walther, B.T.; Rutter,W.J.: The development of the dorsal and ventral mammalian pancreas *in vivo* and *in vitro*. Journal of Cell Biology., 1970, 47 , 235–246.

[36] Harrison, K.A.; Thaler, J.; Pfaff, S.L.; Gu, H.; Kehrl, J.H.: Pancreas dorsal lobe agenesis and abnormal islets of Langerhans in Hlxb9-deficient mice. Nature Genetics., 1999, 23, 71–75.

[37] Li, H.; Arber, S.; Jessell, T.M.; Edlund, H.: 1999 Selective agenesis of the dorsal pancreas in mice lacking homeobox gene *Hlxb9*. Nature Genetics., 1999, 23, 67–70.

[38] Ahlgren, U.; Pfaff, SL.; Jessell, T.M.; Edlund ,T.; Edlund, H.: Independent requirement for ISL1 in formation of pancreatic mesenchyme and islet cells. Nature., 1997, 385, 257-260.

[39] Guz,Y.; Montminy, M.; Stein, R.; Leonard, J.; Gamer, L.; Wright, C.; Teitelman, G.: Expression of murine STF-1, a putative insulin gene transcription factor, in beta cells of pancreas, duodenal epithelium and pancreatic exocrine and endocrine progenitors during ontogeny. Development., 1995, 121, 11-18.

[40] Melloul D.; Marshak S .; Cerasi E : Regulation of *pdx-1* gene expression. Diabetes., 2002, 51 , 320-325.

[41] Offield, M.F.; Jetton, T.L.; Labosky, P.A.; Ray, M.; Stein, R.W.; Magnuson, M.A.; Hogan, B.L.; Wright, C.V: PDX-1 is required for pancreatic outgrowth and differentiation of the rostral duodenum. Development., 1996, 122, 983-995.

[42] Stoffers, D.A.; Zinkin, N.T.; Stanojevic, V.; Clarke, W.L.; Habener,J.F: Pancreatic agenesis attributable to a single nucleotide deletion in the human *IPF1* gene coding sequence. Nature Genetics., 1997b, 15, 106-110.

[43] Krapp, A.; Knofler, M.; Ledermann, B.; Burki, K.; Berney, C.; Zoerkler, N.; Hagenbuchle, O.; Wellauer, P.K.: 1998 The bHLH protein PTF1-p48 is essential for the formation of the exocrine and the correct spatial organization of the endocrine pancreas. Genes and Developmen., 1998, 12 , 3752-3763.

[44] Kawaguchi, Y.; Cooper, B.; Gannon, M.; Ray, M.; MacDonald, R.J.; Wright, C.V.: The role of the transcriptional regulator Ptf1a in converting intestinal to pancreatic progenitors. Nature Genetics., 2002, 32, 128-134.

[45] Rhodes, C.J: 2005 Type 2 diabetes - a matter of beta-cell life and death? Science., 2005, 307, 380-384.

[46] [46] Scaglia, L.; Smith, F.; Bonner-Weir, S.: Apoptosis contributes to the involution of beta cell mass in the post partum rat pancreas. Endocrinology., 1995, 136 , 5461-5468.

[47] Vasavada, R.C.; Garcia-Ocaña, A.; Zawalich, W.S.; Sorenson, R.L.; Dann, P.; Syed, M.; Ogren, L.; Talamantes, F.; Stewart, A.F.: Targeted expression of placental lactogen in the beta cells of transgenic mice results in beta cell proliferation, islet mass augmentation, and hypoglycemia. Journal of Biological Chemistry., 2000, 275, 15399-15406.

[48] Cozar-Castellano, I.; Weinstock, M.; Haught, M.; Velazquez-Garcia, S.; Sipula, D.; Stewart, A.F.: Evaluation of beta-cell replication in mice transgenic for hepatocyte growth factor and placental lactogen: comprehensive characterization of the G1/S regulatory proteins reveals unique involvement of p21cip. Diabetes., 2006a, 55, 70-77.

[49] Garcia-Ocaña, A.; Takane, K.K.; Syed, M.A.; Philbrick, W.M.; Vasavada, R.C.; Stewart, A.F.: Hepatocyte growth factor overexpression in the islet of transgenic mice increases beta cell proliferation, enhances islet mass, and induces mild hypoglycemia. Journal of Biological Chemistry., 2000, 275 , 1226-1232.

[50] Garcia-Ocaña, A.; Vasavada, R.C.; Cebrian, A.; Reddy, V.; Takane, K.K.; Lopez-Talavera,J-C.; Stewart, A.F.: Transgenic overexpression of hepatocyte growth factor in the beta-cell markedly improves islet function and islet transplant outcomes in mice. Diabetes., 2001, 50 , 2752-2762.

[51] Sone, H.; Kagawa, Y.: Pancreatic beta cell senescence contributes to the pathogenesis of type 2 diabetes in high-fat diet-induced diabetic mice. Diabetologia., 2005, 48 , 58–67.

[52] Wang, Q.; Brubaker, P.L.: Glucagon-like peptide-1 treatment delays the onset of diabetes in 8 week-old *db/db* mice. Diabetologia., 2002, 45 , 1263–1273.

[53] Pick, A.; Clark, J.; Kubstrup, C,.; Levisetti, M.; Pugh, W.; Bonner-Weir, S.; Polonsky, K .:1998 Role of apoptosis in failure of beta-cell mass compensation for insulin resistance and beta-cell defects in the male Zucker diabetic fatty rat. Diabetes., 1998, 47, 358–364.

[54] Kubota, N.; Terauchi, Y.; Tobe, K.; Yano, W.; Suzuki, R.; Ueki, K.; Takamoto, I.; Satoh, H.; Maki, T.; Kubota, T: Insulin receptor substrate 2 plays a crucial role in beta cells and the hypothalamus. Journal of Clinical Investigation., 2004, 114 , 917–927.

[55] Hennige, A.M.; Burks, D.J.; Ozcan,U.; Kulkarni, R.N.; Ye, J.;Park, S.; Schubert, M.; Fisher, T.L.; Dow, M.A.; Leshan, R: Upregulation of insulin receptor substrate-2 in pancreatic beta cells prevents diabetes. Journal of Clinical Investigation., 2003, 112 , 1521–1532.

[56] Kitamura, T.; Nakae, J.; Kitamura, Y.; Kido, Y.;Biggs, W.H III.;Wright, C.V.E.; White,M.F.; Arden, K.C.; Accili, D: The forkhead transcription factor Foxo1 links insulin signaling to Pdx1 regulation of pancreatic beta cell growth. Journal of Clinical Investigation., 2002, 110, 1839–1847.

[57] Okamoto, H.; Hribal, M.L.; Lin, H.V.; Bennett, W.R.; Ward, A.; Accili, D: Role of the forkhead protein FoxO1 in beta cell compensation to insulin resistance. Journal of Clinical Investigation., 2006, 116 , 775–782.

[58] García-Ocaña A.; Vasavada CA .; Takane KK.; , Cebrian A .;Lopez-Talavera CJ ..; Stewart AF : Using ß-Cell Growth Factors to Enhance Human Pancreatic Islet Transplantation. Journ Endocr. Metab.,2001,86, 984-988.

[59] Broadus, A. E.; Stewart, A. F. in *The Parathyroids: Basic and Clinical Concepts* (Bilezikian, J. P., Levine, M. A., and Marcus, R., eds), Raven Press, New York, 1994; pp. 259-294.

[60] Orloff, J. J.; Reddy, D.; dePapp, A. E.; Yang, K. H.;Soifer, N. S.; Stewart, A. F. Endocrine Rev., 1994, 15, 40-60 .

[61] Jüppner, H.; Abou-Samra, A.-B.; Freeman, M.; Kong, X. F.; Schipani, E.; Richards, J.; Kolakowski, L. F.; Jr., Hock, J.; Potts, J. T.; Jr., Kronenberg, H.; Segre, G. V. Science., 1991, 254, 1024-1026.

[62] Porter, S.E.; Sorenson, R.L.; Dann, P.; García-Ocaña, A.; Stewart, A.F.; Vasavada,R.C.: 1998 Progressive pancreatic islet hyperplasia in the islet-targeted, PTH-related protein-overexpressing mouse. Endocrinology., 1998, 139, 3743–3751.

[63] Vasavada, R.C.; Cebrian, A.; García-Ocaña, A.: PTH-related protein (PTHrP): *in vivo* inhibition of streptozotocin-induced ß cell death in transgenic mice. Proceedings of the 82nd Annual Meeting of The Endocrine Society , Canada, 2000, p. 76.

[64] Philbrick, W.M.; Wysolmerski, J.J.; Galbraith, S.; Holt, E.; Orloff, J.J.; Yang, K.H.; Vasavada, R.C.;Weir, E.C.; Broadus, A.E.; Stewart, A.F.: 1996 Defining the physiologic roles of parathyroid hormone-related protein in normal physiology. Physiol Rev., 1996, 76, 127–173.

[65] Wysolmerski, J.J.; Stewart, A.F: The physiology of parathyroid hormone-related protein: an emerging role as a developmental factor. Ann Rev Physiol., 1998, 60, 431–460.

[66] Plawner, L.L.; Philbrick, W.M.; Burtis, W.J.; Broadus, A.E.; Stewart, A.F.: 1995 Secretion of parathyroid hormone-related protein: cell-specific secretion via the regulated *vs.* the constitutive secretory pathway. J Biol Chem., 1995, 270, 14078–14084.
[67] Deftos, L.J.; Burton, D.W.; Brandt, D.W: PTH-like protein is a secretory product of atrial myocytes. J Clin Invest., 1993, 92, 727–735.
[68] Ju¨ppner, H.; Abou-Samra, A-B.; Freeman, M.; Kong, X.F.; Schipani, E.; Richards, J.; Kolakowski, L.F. Jr.; Hock, J.; Potts, J.T. Jr.; Kronenberg, H.M.; Segre, G.V: A G protein-linked receptor for parathyroid hormone and parathyroid hormone-related peptide. Science., 1991, 254, 1024–1026.
[69] Abou-Samra, A-B.; Ju¨ppner, H.; Force, T.; Freeman, M.W.; Kong, X-F.; Schipani, E.; Urena, P.; Richards, J.; Bonventre, J.V.; Potts, J.T .Jr.; Kronenberg, H.M.; Segre, G.V: Expression cloning of a common receptor for parathyroid hormone and parathyroid hormone-related peptide from rat osteoblast-like cells: a single receptor stimulates intracellular accumulation of both cAMP and inositol triphosphates and increases intracellular free calcium. Proc Natl Acad Sci U S A., 1992, 89, 2732–2736.
[70] Stork, P.J.S.; Schmitt, J.M: Crosstalk between cAMP and MAP kinase signaling in the regulation of cell proliferation. Trends Cell Biol ., 2002, 12, 258–266.
[71] Burgering, B.M.T.; Bos, J.L: Regulation of Ras-mediated signalling: more than one way to skin a cat. Trends Biochem Sci., 1995, 20, 18–22.
[72] Vossler, M.R.; Yao, H.; York, R.D.; Pan, M-G.; Rim, C.S.; Stork, P.J.S: cAMP activates MAP kinase and Elk-1 through a B-Raf- and Rap1-dependent pathway. Cell ., 1997, 89, 73–82.
[73] Chen, T.; Cho, R.W.; Stork, P.J.S.; Weber, M.J: Elevation of cyclic adenosine 3′,5′-monophosphate potentiates activation of mitogen-activated protein kinase by growth factors in LNCaP prostate cancer cells. Cancer Res., 1991, 59, 213–218.
[74] Miller, C.P.; McGehee, R.E.; Habener, J.F: IDX-1: a new homeodomain transcription factor expressed in rat pancreatic islets and duodenum that transactivates the somatostatin gene. EMBO J., 1994, 13, 1145–1156.
[75] Leonard, J.; Peers, B.; Johnson, T.; Ferreri, K.; Lee, S.; Montminy, M.: Characterization of somatostatin transactivating factor-1, a novel homeobox factor that stimulates somatostatin expression in pancreatic islet cells. Mol Endocrinol., 1993, 7, 1275–1283.
[76] Jonsson, J.; Carlsson, L.; Edlund,T.; Edlund, H: Insulin promoter factor-1 is required for pancreas development in mice. Nature., 1994, 371, 606–609.
[77] Ahlgren, U.; Pfaff, S.; Jessell, T.M.; Edlund, T.; Edlund, H.: 1997 Independent requirement for ISL1 in formation of pancreatic mesenchyme and islet cells. Nature., 1997, 385, 257–260.
[78] Finegood, D.T.; Scaglia, L.; Bonner-Weir, S.: Perspectives in diabetes dynamics of ß-cell mass in the growing rat pancreas. Estimation with a simple mathematical model. Diabetes., 1995, 44, 249–256.
[79] Otonkoski, T.; Cirulli, V.; Beattie, G.M.; Mally, M.I.; Soto, G.; Rubin, J.S.; Hayek, A: A role for hepatocyte growth factor/scatter factor in fetal mesenchyme-induced pancreatic ß-cell growth. Endocrinology., 1996, 137, 3131–3139.
[80] Rafaeloff, R.; Pittenger, G.L.; Barlow, S.W.; Qin, X.F.; Yan ,B.; Rosenberg. L.; Duguid, W.P.; Vinik, A.I.: Cloning and expression of the pancreatic islet neogenesis-

associated protein (INGAP) gene and its expression in islet neogenesis in hamsters. J Clin Invest., 1997, 99, 2100–2109.
[81] Gaich, G.; Orloff, J.J.; Atillasoy, E.J.; Burtis, W.J.; Ganz, M.B.; Stewart, A.F: Amino-terminal parathyroid hormone-related protein: specific binding and cytosolic calcium responses in at insulinoma cells. Endocrinology., 1992, 132, 1402–1409.
[82] Drucker, DJ: Glucagon-like peptides: regulators of cell proliferation, differentiation, and apoptosis. Mol Endocrinol., 2003, 7 , 161 –171,
[83] Vasavada, R.C.; Cavaliere, C.; D'Ercole, A.J.; Dann, P.; Burtis, W.J.; Madlener, A.L.; Zawalich, K.; Zawalich, W.; Philbrick, W.; Stewart, A.F.: Overexpression of parathyroid hormone-related protein in the pancreatic islets of transgenic mice causes islet hyperplasia, hyperinsulinemia, and hypoglycemia. J Biol Chem ., 1996, 271 ,1200 –1208.
[84] Baggio, L.; Adatia, F.; Bock, T.; Brubaker, P.L.; Drucker, D.J.: Sustained expression of exendin-4 does not perturb glucose homeostasis, ß-cell mass, or food intake in metallothionein-preproexendin transgenic mice. J Biol Chem., 2000, 275 , 34471 – 34477.
[85] Ijunghall, S.; M. Palmer, G.; Akerstrom, Wide, L: Diabetes mellitus, glucose tolerance and insulin response to glucose in patients with primary hyperparathyroidism before and after parathyroidectomy. Eur. J. Clin. Invest., 1983, 13, 373-377.
[86] Kim, H.; R. K. Kalkhoff, N. V. ; Costrini, J. M.; Cerletty.; Jacobson,M.: Plasma insulin disturbances in primary hyperparathyroidism. J. Clin. Invest., 1971, 50, 2596-2605.
[87] Fadda, G. Z.; M. Ak&ial, L. G.;Lipson.; Massry, S.G.: Direct effect of parathyroid hormone on insulin secretion from pancreatic islets. Am. J. Physiol., 1990, 258 (Endocrinol Metab. 21), E975-E984.
[88] Ishida, H.; Suzuki, K.; Someya, Y.:Possible compensatory role of parathyroid hormone –related peptide on maintenance of calcium homeostasis in patients with non-insulin –dependant diabetes mellitus. Acta Endocrinologica., 1993,129, 519-524.
[89] De Marinis, L.; Merlini, G. ; Makhoul, O.; Barbarino, A.: Calcium antagonists and hormone release :IV.Role of calcium in glucose-stimulated early phase insulin in vivo. J Endocrinol Invest., 1982 ,5, 121-4.
[90] Wu, T.L.; Vasavada, R.C.; Yang, K.; Massfclder, T.; Ganz, M.; Abbas, S.K .: Structural and physiologic characterization of the mid-region secretory species of parathyroid hormone –related protein. J Biol Chem., 1996, 271, 24371-24381.
[91] Drucker, D.J .;Asa, S.L.; Henderson, J.; Glotzman, D.: The PTHrP gene is expressed in the normal and neoplastic human endocrine pancreas . Mol Endocrinol ., 1989, 1589-1595.
[92] Shor, R.; Halabe, A.; Aberbuh, E.;Matas, Z.;Fux, A.;Boaz, M.;Wainstein, J.: PTHrP and insulin levels following oral glucose and calcium administration. European Journal of Internal Medicine., 2006, 17, 408-411.
[93] Legakis, I.;Mantouridis, T.: Positive correlation of PTH-related peptide with glucose in type 2 diabetes. Exp Diabetes Res., 2009,31.

4

Impaired Vascular BK Channel Function in Type 2 Diabetes Mellitus

Tong Lu and Hon-Chi Lee
Division of Cardiovascular Diseases, Department of Internal Medicine, Mayo Clinic
USA

1. Introduction

Diabetes mellitus has become a global epidemic. According to the World Health Organization estimate, about 285 millions people worldwide, corresponding to 6.4% of the world's population, have diabetes in 2010. By 2030, this figure will be more than doubled (http://www.worlddiabetesday.org/media/press-materials/diabetes-data).

Diabetes mellitus is a major cause of morbidity and mortality and is associated with increased risks of cardiovascular diseases, stroke, nephropathy, neuropathy, retinopathy and other microvascular complications. Type 2 diabetes mellitus is characterized by obesity, glucose intolerance, insulin resistance, hyperinsulinemia, hyperglycemia, dyslipidemia and hypertension, and accounts for 90% of the total cases of diabetes mellitus. Although the clinical course of type 2 diabetes is usually less aggressive compared to its type 1 counterpart, the end results are equally devastating even with intensive glycemic control.

The causes of diabetic vascular dysfunction are multifactorial, and involve endothelial-dependent and -independent mechanisms. The role of endothelial-dependent vascular dysfunction in diabetes is well-known, and it is related to increased activity/bioavailability of vasoconstrictors such as reactive oxygen species (ROS), reactive nitrogen species (RNS), endothelin-1 (ET-1), angiotensin II (Ang II) and thromoxane A_2 (TXA_2), and reduced activity/bioavailability of endothelium-derived relaxing factors (EDRFs) such as nitric oxide (NO), carbon monoxide (CO), prostacyclin (PGI_2) and endothelium-derived hyperpolarizing factors (EDHFs) (Avogaro et al., 2006; De Vriese et al., 2000; Xu & Zou, 2009). The role of endothelial-independent vascular dysfunction in diabetes mellitus, however, has received less attention, and it is by no means less important, because vascular smooth muscle physiology is profoundly modulated by diabetes mellitus.

A major ionic mechanism that facilitates vascular smooth muscle relaxation is the activation of the large conductance Ca^{2+}-activated K^+ (BK) channels. Because of their large conductance and high density in vascular smooth muscle cells, BK channels are a key determinant of vascular tone, regulating tissue perfusion in response to changes in membrane potential and intracellular Ca^{2+} homeostasis (Ledoux et al., 2006). Substantial experimental and clinical evidence exists indicating that vascular BK channel function is impaired in type 2 diabetes (Feng et al., 2008; Liu et al., 2008). Multiple mechanisms are known to produce BK channel dysfunction in diabetes mellitus. In this article, we will describe the cellular and molecular mechanisms that underlie vascular BK channel dysfunction in type 2 diabetes. We will also provide a detailed treatise on the altered BK channel gating associated with type 2 diabetes.

2. Vascular BK channel structure and function

The BK channel α subunit is encoded by the Slo1 gene ($K_{Ca}1.1$, KCNMA1) and the functional channel has a homotetrameric assembly. The BK-α subunit shares homology with all voltage-gated K^+ channels containing a backbone of six transmembrane domains (S1 to S6) in which the S1-S4 constitute the voltage-sensing unit and the S5-P loop-S6 form the ion permeation domain which encompasses the conserved K^+ selectivity filter (TVGYG) (Cui et al., 2009; Ma et al., 2006). In addition, it has unique structural features. It has an additional transmembrane domain, S0, so the N-terminus is extracellular, and the C-terminus has 4 hydrophobic segments (S7 to S10) that contain two regulators of conductance for potassium (RCK1 and RCK2) (Fig. 1) (Jiang et al., 2002). Functionally, two high-affinity Ca^{2+} sensing regions with Ca^{2+} concentration at half-maximal effect (EC_{50}) in the 10^{-6} M range have been proposed. One is the Ca^{2+} bowl (889-QFLDQDDDD-897) in RCK2 (Bao et al., 2004; Schreiber et al., 1999; Xia et al., 2002) and the other (D362/D367) is located in RCK1 (Xia et al., 2002; Zeng et al., 2005). The RCK1s and RCK2s from the homotetrameric channel form an octameric gating ring which regulates K^+ efflux through allosteric control by the Ca^{2+}-bowl and the voltage sensor (Yuan et al., 2010). The extracellular N-terminus of BK-α subunit is important for functional coupling with BK-β subunit (Meera et al., 1997). In fact, the BK-α subunit S0, S1, S2, S3, and S6 are all implicated for functional and physical interaction with BK-β subunits (Lee & Cui, 2010; Morrow et al., 2006; Orio et al., 2006).

The BK-β_1 subunit is the predominant subtype in vascular smooth muscle cells. It contains two transmembrane (TM1 and TM2) domains connected by a relatively large extracellular loop which can reach the inner mouth of the channel central pore, and can modulate scorpion toxin and tetraethylammonium (TEA) binding and regulate channel permeability (Hanner et al., 1997; Meera et al., 2000; Shen et al., 1994). The TM1 is thought to interact with the S2 of an adjacent BK-α subunit and the TM2 with S0 of another adjacent BK-α subunit (Fig. 1) (Liu et al.,). BK-β_1 subunits are abundantly expressed in vascular smooth muscle cells. BK channel activity is profoundly regulated by BK-β_1 which significantly enhances the channel voltage- and Ca^{2+}-sensitivity (Cox & Aldrich, 2000; McManus et al., 1995; Meera et al., 1996; Xia et al., 1999), modulates channel kinetics (Nimigean & Magleby, 1999; Tanaka et al., 1997; Zeng et al., 2003) and stabilizes BK-α expression (Toro et al., 2006). The importance of BK-β_1 subunits in the regulation of vascular physiology is underscored by the β_1 subunit knockout mice, in which Ca^{2+} sparks are uncoupled to BK channels in the vascular smooth muscle cells, and these animals are hypertensive (Brenner et al., 2000; Pluger et al., 2000). In addition, there is a compensatory increase in vascular BK-β_1 expression in spontaneously hypertensive rats (Chang et al., 2006), while a gain-of-function mutation in BK-β_1 (E65K) is associated with low prevalence of diastolic hypertension in humans (Fernandez-Fernandez et al., 2004; Kelley-Hedgepeth et al., 2008; Nielsen et al., 2008) and with reduced risk of myocardial infarction and stroke, particularly in elderly women (Senti et al., 2005).

BK channels maintain smooth muscle cell Ca^{2+} homeostasis and regulate vascular tone through a negative feedback mechanism. Activation of the voltage-gated Ca^{2+} channels in vascular smooth muscle cells triggers Ca^{2+} release from the sarcoplasmic reticulum (Ca^{2+} sparks) which activates the BK channels in its vicinity and gives rise to the spontaneous transient outward currents (STOCs). STOCs hyperpolarize the cellular membrane potential, which in turn inactivates the voltage-gated Ca^{2+} channels, thereby relaxes the vascular smooth muscles (Brenner et al., 2000; Lohn et al., 2001; Pluger et al., 2000). In addition, the presence of splice variants of BK-α subunits (Xie & McCobb, 1998) contributes to the diversity of BK channel function in the body.

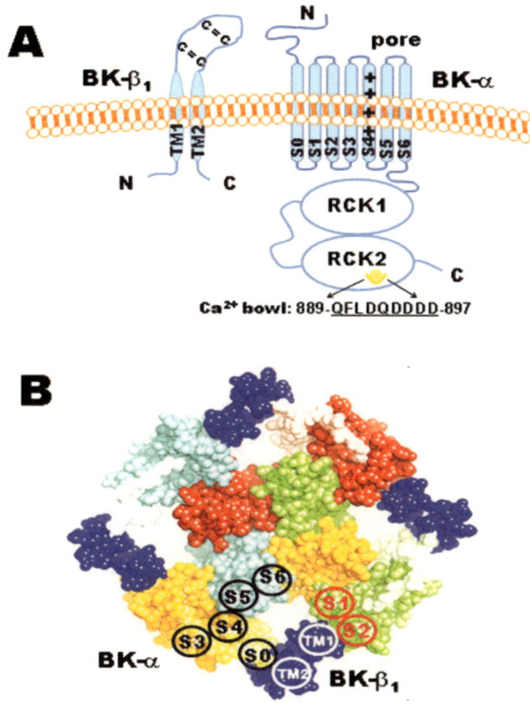

Fig. 1. Vascular BK channel structure. A: Membrane topology of BK-α and BK-β_1 subunits. Domain boundaries and the Ca^{2+} bowl are indicated. S0-S6 corresponds to the seven transmembrane domains of BK-α subunit; TM1 and TM2 represent the transmembrane domains of BK-β_1 subunit. B: Orientation of BK-α and BK-β_1 subunits in tetrameric BK channels, where the TM1 interacts with the S0 of adjacent BK-α and the TM2 interacts with the S2 of another adjacent BK-α. (Fig. 1B was adapted from Liu et al., 2010).

3. Regulation of vascular BK channel activity by signaling molecules

BK channels are targets of many signaling molecules and biological vasoactive mediators, which include protein kinases (Barman et al., 2004; Chae et al., 2005; Schopf et al., 1999; Tian et al., 2004), protein tyrosine kinases (Alioua et al., 2002; Lu et al., 2010), phospholipids (Vaithianathan et al., 2008), polyunsaturated fatty acid metabolites of the cytochrome P-450 epoxygenase (Campbell et al., 1996; Lauterbach et al., 2002; Lu et al., 2001; Wang et al. 2011; Zhang et al., 2001), the lipoxygenase (Obara et al., 2002; Zink et al., 2001) and the cyclooxygenase pathways (Burnette and White, 2006; Tanaka et al., 2004; Yamaki et al., 2001), reactive oxygen species (ROS) (Lu et al., 2006; Tang et al., 2004), reactive nitrogen species (RNS) (Liu et al., 2002; Lu et al., 2006), nitric oxide (NO) (Mandala et al., 2007; Wu et al., 2002), carbon monoxide (CO) (Dong et al., 2007; Wu et al., 2002), heme (Jaggar et al., 2005; Tang et al., 2003), angiotensin II (Ang II) (Minami et al., 1995; Zhang et al., 2010), endothelin -1 (ET-1) (Minami et al., 1995) and steroid hormones (Han et al., 2008; Lovell et al., 2004). It is worthwhile to point out that the regulation of BK channels by these signaling molecules is frequently complicated by the exhibition of signal cross-talk, with species and tissue specificity.

4. Impaired vascular BK channel function in the early stages of type 2 diabetes – Deficiency in the bioavailability of BK channel activating vasodilators

A commonly used animal model for the study of type 2 diabetes is the Zucker Diabetic Fatty (ZDF) rats, which are derived from selective inbreeding of Zucker Obese rats with the highest blood glucose levels (Shafrir, 1992). There animals exhibit many features found in patients with non-insulin dependent diabetes mellitus, including obesity, insulin resistance, hyperglycemia, hypertriglyceridemia, hypercholesterolemia (Corsetti et al., 2000; Shafrir, 1992), and microvascular pathology (Oltman et al., 2009; Oltman et al., 2008; Yang et al., 2000). ZDF rats have been used for studying insulin resistance (Kuhlmann et al., 2003; Srinivasan and Ramarao, 2007; Zhou et al., 1999), and vascular dysfunction (Oltman et al., 2009; Oltman et al., 2008; Zhou et al., 2005). We found that vascular BK channel function is impaired in ZDF rats and that the culprits change with progression of the disease.

In the early stages of diabetes development (2 to 4 weeks with blood glucose >300 mg/dl), BK channel-mediated vasodilatation in ZDF rats was impaired. Fig. 2A shows that arachidonic acid (AA) produced 50% less dilatation in the isolated coronary arteries from ZDF rats, compared to those from Lean control rats. The AA effects were significantly inhibited by preincubation with indomethacin (the cyclooxygenase inhibitor) in Lean rat vessels but not in ZDF rat vessels. Exposure of freshly isolated coronary smooth muscle cells to 1 μM AA produced a 4-fold increase in whole-cell K^+ currents in Lean rats, while these effects were significantly blunted in those from ZDF rats (Fig. 2B). The effects of AA on K^+ current activation were inhibited by preincubation with indomethacin, suggesting that the vasoactive molecules were cyclooxygenase products of AA (Lu et al., 2005).

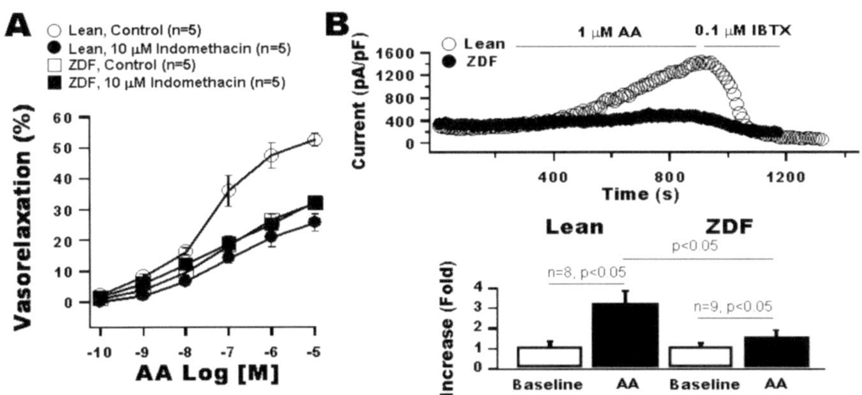

Fig. 2. Reduced arachidonic acid (AA)-mediated dilatation of coronary arteries and BK channel activation of coronary arterial smooth muscle cells from ZDF rats with 8 weeks of diabetes. A: Effects of AA on coronary arterial relaxation in Lean and ZDF rats with and without a 30-min incubation with indomethacin (10 μM). Compared to Lean rats, AA-mediated vasorelaxation was diminished in ZDF rats and the AA effects were abolished by preincubation with indomethacin. B: Time course of the effect of 1 μM AA on coronary smooth muscle K^+ currents in Lean control rats and ZDF rats. Group results on the increase in BK current density (iberiotoxin sensitive component) before and after exposure to AA are represented by the bar graphs. (adapted from Lu et al., 2005)

The reduced AA-induced vasodilatation and diminished BK channel activation resulted from deficient PGI_2 bioavailability in the ZDF vasculature (Lu et al., 2005). Protein expression of PGI_2 synthase (PGIS) was down-regulated by 65% in the coronary arteries of ZDF rats (Fig. 3A), leading to a 6.8-fold reduction in the conversion of AA to 6-keto $PGF_{1\alpha}$, the stable product of PGI_2 metabolism, in ZDF vessels (Fig. 3B). Exposure to the stable PGI_2 analog, iloprost (1 μM), produced similar BK channel activation in coronary smooth muscle cells from Lean control rats and ZDF rats, indicating that the ability of BK channels to respond to agonist activation was intact.

The biophysical properties of BK channel were intact during the early stages of diabetes in ZDF rats. Whole-cell BK current density and current-voltage relationships were not different between coronary smooth muscle cells from Lean control and ZDF rats (Fig. 4A and 4B). Determination of BK channel sensitivity to voltage- and Ca^{2+}-mediated activation of single channels in inside-out excised membrane patches also showed similar opening probability (Po)-voltage and Po-Ca^{2+} relationships between Lean and ZDF rats (Fig. 4C and 4D). There was no significant difference in the voltage at half maximal activation ($V_{0.5}$) or in the equivalent charge movement (z) value between Lean and ZDF rats. The Ca^{2+} EC_{50} and the Hill coefficient (which reflects the cooperativity of Ca^{2+} binding) for the Po-Ca^{2+} curves were likewise similar between the two groups, suggesting that in the early stage of type 2 diabetes, the voltage- and Ca^{2+}-dependent activation of BK channels were intact in ZDF rats.

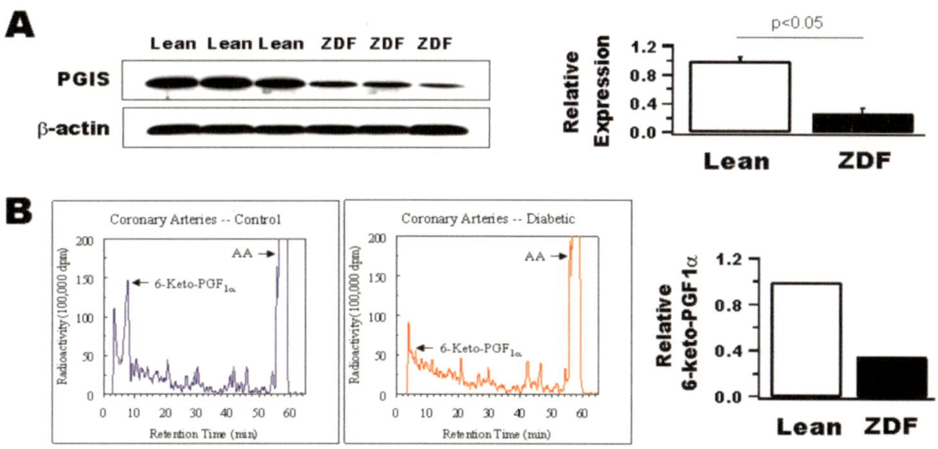

Fig. 3. Decreased PGI_2 synthase (PGIS) expression and PGI_2 production in coronary arteries from ZDF rats. A: Immunoblot with statistical analysis of PGIS expression in arteries of Lean and ZDF rats. B: Analysis of AA metabolism in coronary arteries from Lean rats and ZDF rats. Isolated vessels from 3 pairs of Lean and ZDF rats were incubated with 5 μM [^3H] AA (specific activity 1 μCi/nM) for 1 h at 37°C. Lipids were extracted and analyzed by HPLC. The major peak at 7.5 min has the same retention time as a 6-keto-$PGF_{1\alpha}$ standard, the stable product of PGI_2 that was significant decreased in ZDF rat vessels. (adapted from Lu et al., 2005).

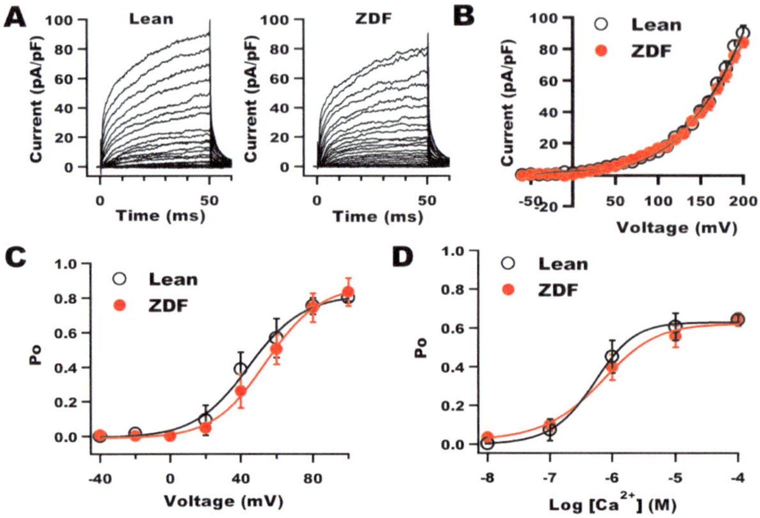

Fig. 4. Normal BK channel activity from the coronary smooth muscle cells of ZDF rats with 8-week development of hyperglycemia. A: Representative tracings of whole-cell BK currents (iberiotoxin-sensitive components) from freshly isolated coronary smooth muscle cells of Lean and ZDF rats. BK currents were elicited with 10 mV increments from -40 mV to +200 mV with a holding potential of -60 mV in the presence of 0.2 μM free Ca^{2+} in the pipette solution. B: The current-voltage (I-V) relationships of BK channels from Lean and ZDF rats. C: Ca^{2+} dose-dependent curves obtained from inside-out single BK channel currents recorded at +60 mV from coronary smooth muscle cells of Lean and ZDF rats. D: The open probability-voltage (Po-V) relationship obtained from inside-out single BK channel currents of Lean and ZDF rats in the presence of 1 μM free Ca^{2+} in the bath solution. There were no significant differences in current density, Ca^{2+}-sensitivtiy and voltage-sensitivity of BK channels between ZDF rats and age-matched Lean rats.

We also found that AA-induced dilatation was impaired in the small mesenteric arteries of ZDF rats at 4 weeks after the development of diabetes. The effects of AA were dependent on lipoxygenase activity and ZDF vessels showed an 81% downregulation in 12-lipoxygenases protein expression accompanied by a 54% reduction in AA conversion to its vasoactive product, 12-hydroxyeicosatetraenoic acid (Zhou et al., 2005). Moreover, AA-mediated vasodilatation in Lean rats was partially abolished by iberiotoxin, while exogenous application of 12-hydroxyeicosatetraenoic acid produced similar vasodilatation in Lean control and ZDF rat vessels, suggesting that the impaired AA-induced dilatation in mesentery arteries of ZDF rats is due to the deficiency of 12-lipoxygenase generated vasodilating metabolites (Zhou et al., 2005). Hence, during the early stages of type 2 diabetes, a common feature that impairs BK channel-mediated vasodilatation is the reduced bioavailability of BK channel activating vasodilators.

5. Impaired vascular BK channel function in the advanced stages of type 2 diabetes – Altered channel intrinsic biophysical properties

5.1 Reduced Ca^{2+}-dependent BK channel activation in ZDF rats with advanced diabetes

With further progression in type 2 diabetes, the biophysical properties of BK channel were altered, giving rise to BK channelopathy. Fig. 5A illustrates the normalized BK channel Po-V curves in the coronary smooth muscle cells from ZDF rats with 8 months of hyperglycemia and from age-matched Lean control rats. Inside-out BK currents were elicited from freshly isolated coronary smooth muscle cells in the absence of Ca^{2+} and in the presence of 1 μM free Ca^{2+} in the bath solution. Without Ca^{2+}, the Po-V relationships from Lean and ZDF rats were identical, indicating that the intrinsic voltage-dependent activation of BK channels remained unchanged. In the presence of 1 μM free Ca^{2+}, the Po-V relationships were leftward shifted in both Lean and ZDF rats, but there was a significant lag in the effects of Ca^{2+} on the shift in the Po-V relationship in ZDF rats, suggesting a decreased Ca^{2+}-dependent BK channel activation in these animals. Changes in the intrinsic free energy of Ca^{2+}-binding ($\Delta\Delta Ca^{2+}$) that contributes to BK channel activation can be estimated, based on the shift of Po-V relationship from 0 to 1 μM free Ca^{2+} in Lean and ZDF rats, using the equation: $\Delta\Delta Ca^{2+} = -\Delta(zeV_{0.5})$, where z is the number of equivalence charge movement, e is the elementary charge (Shi et al., 2002). There was a 62.3% reduction in the change in free energy for Ca^{2+}-binding to BK channels in ZDF rats. Any decrease in the free energy for Ca^{2+}-binding must be associated with reduced Ca^{2+}-sensitivity and/or Ca^{2+} cooperativity in BK channel function. These results indicated that Ca^{2+}-dependent activation was less favorable in ZDF rats at an advanced stage of type 2 diabetes.

Since the intrinsic voltage-sensitivity of BK channel was not significantly changed in ZDF rats 1 to 8 months after developing hyperglycemia, according to our experimental results (unpublished observations), the Ca^{2+} EC_{50} value can be used to evaluate BK channel Ca^{2+}-sensitivity. Fig. 5B shows the Ca^{2+} dose-dependent curves of coronary arterial BK channel activation from Lean and ZDF rats with 6 months of diabetes. In ZDF rats, there was reduced maximal channel Po, a rightward shifted Po-V relationship with a smaller value of the Hill coefficient, compared to those in Lean rats. Hence, impaired BK channel function in ZDF rats at advanced stages of type 2 diabetes was due to reduced free energy for Ca^{2+} binding to the channel with reduced Ca^{2+} cooperativity and reduced sensitivity to Ca^{2+} -mediated activation.

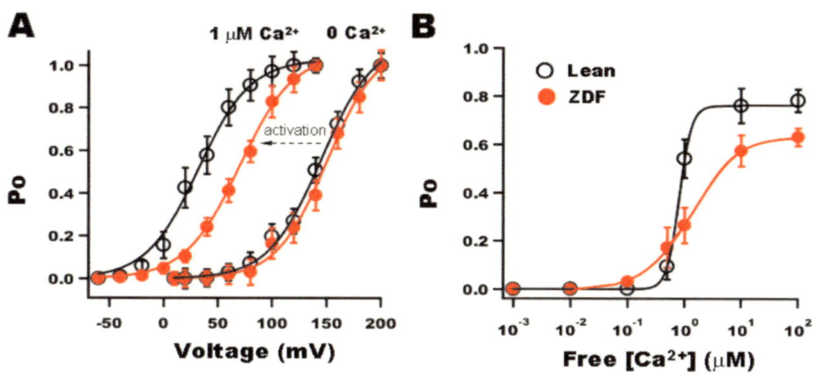

Fig. 5. Impaired Ca^{2+}-dependent BK channel activation in the coronary smooth muscle cells from ZDF rats 8 months after development of diabetes. A: The Po-V relationships of BK channels from ZDF rats and age-matched Lean rats in the absence of and in the presence of 1 μM free Ca^{2+} in the bath solution. Less Ca^{2+}-dependent leftward shift was observed in ZDF rats, compared with Lean rats. B: Ca^{2+} dose-dependent curve of BK channel activation from Lean and ZDF rats. Reduced maximal channel Po, increased Ca^{2+} EC_{50} and decreased slope steepness were found in ZDF rats, indicating that BK channel Ca^{2+}-sensitvity and Ca^{2+}-coopratività were impaired in ZDF rats. (adapted from Lu et al., 2008).

5.2 Altered vascular BK channel kinetics in ZDF rats with advanced diabetes

To better understand the altered Ca^{2+}-dependent BK channel activation in ZDF rats, we examined the Ca^{2+}-dependent gating properties in ZDF rats and age-matched Lean rats. We compared single channel gating between Lean and ZDF rats at various Ca^{2+} concentrations from 1 μM to 100 μM with a testing potential of +60 mV. Fig. 6 illustrates typical tracings of inside-out single-channel BK currents in Lean and ZDF rats with expanded details. In the presence of 1 μM Ca^{2+}, BK channel Po was much higher in Lean rats than in ZDF rats. An increase of Ca^{2+} to 10 and 100 μM markedly increased the channel Po in both Lean (Fig. 6A) and ZDF rats (Fig. 6B). However, increased cytoplasmic Ca^{2+} enhanced Po in Lean rats by significantly prolonging the mean channel open durations without altering the channel mean closed durations. In contrast, increased cytoplasmic Ca^{2+} augmented Po in ZDF rats by significantly abbreviating channel mean closed durations without a marked increase in channel mean open durations (Fig. 6C and 6D). These results indicated that there was an altered gating response to activation by Ca^{2+} in vascular BK channels in ZDF rats. Because normal intracellular Ca^{2+} concentration can reach >10 μM, especially in the vicinity of the microdomains where calcium sparks are elicited, these fundamental changes in BK channel properties are physiologically relevant.

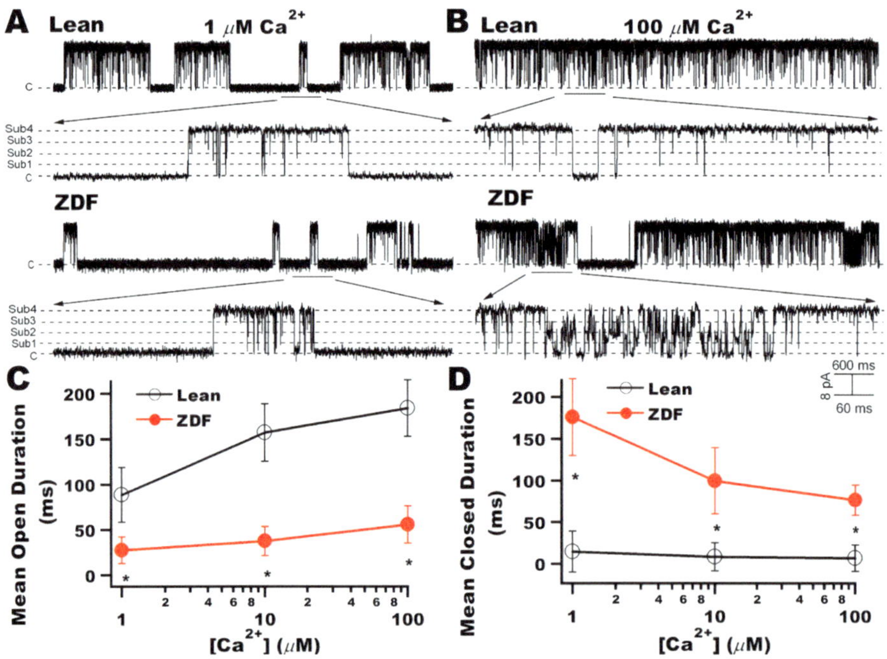

Fig. 6. Altered single BK channel openings in ZDF rats 6 months after development of diabetes. Representative inside-out single BK channel currents were recorded at +60 mV from freshly isolated coronary smooth muscle cells of ZDF rats and age-matched Lean rats in the presence of 1 μM Ca^{2+} (A) and 100 μM Ca^{2+} (B). Plots of relationships between Ca^{2+} concentrations and mean burst durations (C) and mean closed times (D) of BK channels in Lean and ZDF rats are shown. Compared with Lean rats, ZDF rats had shorter mean burst open durations and longer mean closed durations. Data are presented as mean ± SE. *$p < 0.05$ vs. Lean (n = 6). (adapted from Lu et al., 2008).

BK channel gating kinetics is known to contain multiple components of open and closed dwell-times. Based on single BK channel kinetic analysis from our group and other laboratories, the best fit of the open dwell-time distribution histograms showed three components: fast (τo_1), intermediate (τo_2) and slow (τo_3); the closed dwell-time distribution histograms showed four components: fast (τc_1), intermediate (τc_2), slow (τc_3) and very slow (τc_4) (Fig. 7) (Lu et al., 2001; Lu et al., 2008; McManus & Magleby, 1988; McManus & Magleby, 1991). Compared to Lean rats, BK channels from the coronary arterial smooth muscle cells of ZDF rats had shorter open dwell-times and longer closed dwell-times, in agreement with the lower channel opening probability observed in ZDF rats (Fig. 5). These changes in BK channel gating were consistent with reduced free energy for Ca^{2+}-dependent channel activation, favoring BK channel closure in ZDF rats.

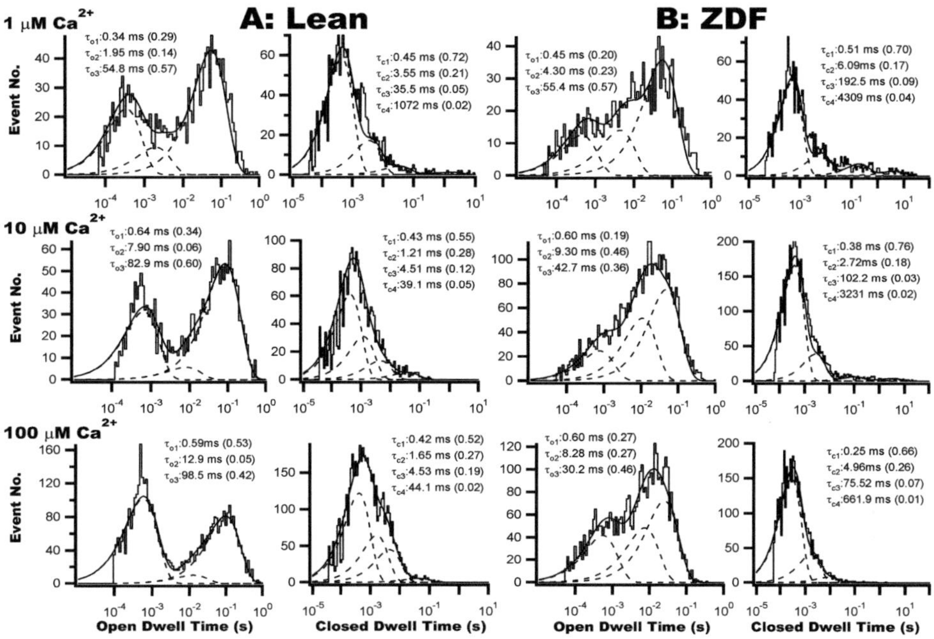

Fig. 7. Altered Ca^{2+}-dependent kinetics of BK channel from ZDF rats after 8 months of diabetes. Representative histograms of single BK channel open and closed dwell-time durations in the presence of 1 μM, 10 μM and 100 μM free Ca^{2+} in the bath solution. Dwell-time distributions were best fitted with three open dwell-time components (τo) and four closed dwell-time components (τc). The values of each time constants and its relative weight (in parentheses) are shown in each histogram. Dashed lines represent distribution of exponential components, determined by the logarithm likelihood ratio test.

An intriguing observation during single BK channel recordings in coronary smooth muscle cells from ZDF rats with 8 months of diabetes was the conspicuous increased encounter of subconductance openings (Fig. 8A). Amplitude histograms fitted with a Gaussian function clearly showed four levels of subconductance and channel state transition appeared to be slow with subconductance constituting ¾ of full channel opening seen 20% of the time (Fig. 8B and 8C), while BK channel subconductance openings was less frequently observed in Lean rats. Although the underlying mechanism of BK channel subconductance openings is not fully understood, this may be due to the conformational changes that each subunit of the tetrameric channel has to make from a closed state to an open state as the channel opens (Chapman & VanDongen, 2005). Normally, such transitions of conformational states are too transient to be discerned (Ferguson et al., 1993). However, conditions that cause slowing of the tetrameric conformational transitions would result in prolonged sojourn of intermediate state conformations and lead to discernible subconductance openings. The reduced Ca^{2+} cooperativity and Ca^{2+} sensitivity in BK-α subunits of ZDF rats with advanced diabetes could cause slowing of the conformational transitions of the heteromeric states. The cooperative conformational changes of the channel subunits can be estimated from the relationship between the number of subconductance states and their relative frequencies. As shown in Fig. 8D, the relative frequency was plotted against each subconductance state in Lean and ZDF rats, which were fitted by a single exponential function: $y=\omega\cdot\exp(\psi\cdot x)$, where ω is the fitting constant and ψ is the coefficient of subunit conformational change. The coefficient of BK channel subunit conformational change was estimated to be 3.3 in Lean rats and 1.4 in ZDF rats, in agreement with the reduction of the Hill coefficient of the Ca^{2+} dose-dependent curve from 4.1 in Lean rats to 1.1 in ZDF rats (Fig. 5B). Hence, these observations suggested that changes in Ca^{2+}-cooperativity and in subunit conformations in BK channels could be coupled, but such coupling was impaired in ZDF rats with more frequent subconductance openings.

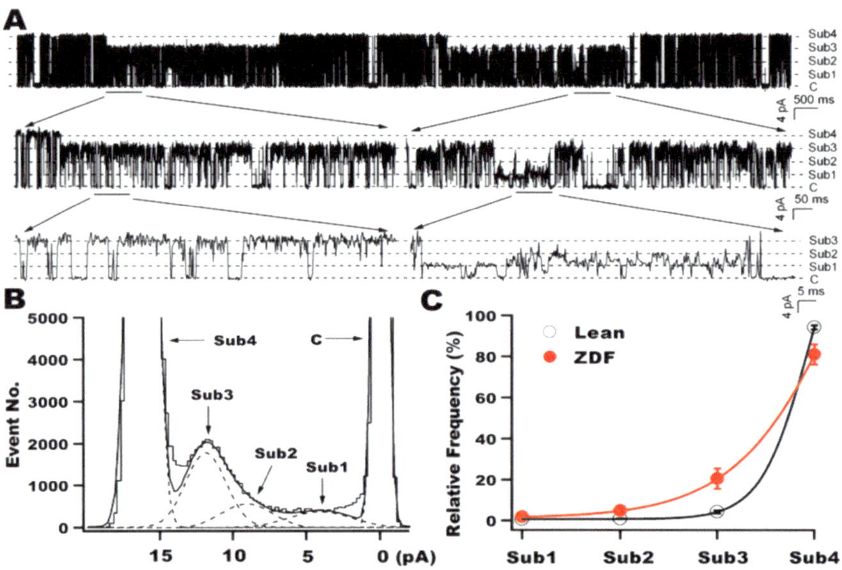

Fig. 8. Increased BK channel subconductance openings in ZDF rats with advanced diabetes. A: Representative single BK current recordings were obtained at +60 mV in the presence of 1 μM free Ca^{2+}, with selected segments that showed expanded details, demonstrating the presence of 4 sublevels of openings. B: Amplitude histogram was fitted using a Gaussian function and showed four peaks with unitary amplitudes of 4 pA (Sub1), 8 pA (Sub2), 12 pA (Sub3) and 16 pS (Sub4 or fully open). The relative frequencies of each subconductance state were calculated by the area under each component of the Gaussian function. C: Relative frequencies were plotted against subconductance states, and the relationships were fitted using a single exponential function. The coefficient of subconductance conformational changes was estimated to be 3.3 in Lean rats (n=3) and 1.4 in ZDF rats (n=3). (adapted from Lu et al., 2008).

5.3 Downregulation of vascular BK-β_1 subunit expression in ZDF rats with advanced diabetes

BK-β_1 subunits play an important role in the regulation of channel Ca^{2+}- and voltage-sensitivity. Fig. 9 shows the loss of BK-β_1-mediated channel activation in ZDF rats with 6 months of diabetes. Dehydrosoyasaponin-1 (DHS-1) is a cell-impermeable BK-β_1 subunit-specific activator, enhancing BK channel activity by acting on the cytoplasmic surface of the membrane. DHS-1 (0.1 μM) applied to the bath solution in inside-out excised membrane patches significantly increased the Po of BK channels in Lean rats, but not those in ZDF rats (Fig. 9A and 9B). A 2.1-fold reduction in BK-β_1 protein expression was observed in ZDF rats while BK-α expression was unchanged (Fig. 9C and 9D). The downregulation of vascular BK-β_1 expression appears to be a common feature in BK channelopathy for both type 1 and type 2 diabetes (Dong et al., 2008; Lu et al., 2008; McGahon et al., 2007; Zhang et al., 2010). Since the BK-β_1 subunit is known to modulate the Ca^{2+}- and voltage-dependent activation of BK channels and the subconductance activity of BK channel is also thought to be regulated by BK-β_1 subunits (Nimigean & Magleby, 1999), we can conclude that the vascular BK channelopathy in type 2 diabetes is produced by the downregulation of BK-β_1 expression.

In addition to changes in the BK-β_1-mediated channel regulation, the BK-α subunit may also undergo alterations in intrinsic properties as a result of prolonged diabetes. For example, hyperglycemia is known to enhance production of ROS, and H_2O_2 has been shown to directly inhibit BK channel function through redox modulation of the BK-α C911 residue

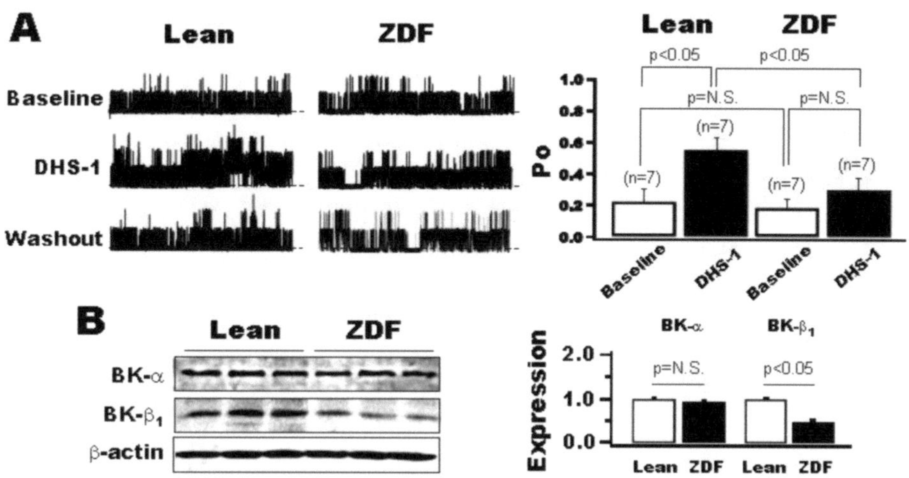

Fig. 9. Impaired the β_1-mediated channel activation and reduced BK-β_1 expression in the arteries of ZDF rats 8 weeks after the development of diabetes. A: Inside-out single BK currents recorded in the coronary smooth muscle cells from ZDF rats and age-matched Lean rats at +60 mV in the presence of 0.5 μM free Ca^{2+} at baseline, with application of 0.1 μM DHS-1, followed by drug wash out. Bar graphs show a significant DHS-1-induced increase in BK channel Po in Lean rats, but not in ZDF rats. B: Immunoblot analysis shows significant decrease in BK-β_1 expression but not that of BK-α expression in the aortas from ZDF rats, compared to those from Lean rats. (adapted from Lu et al., 2008)

(Lu et al., 2006; Tang et al., 2004). Also, the molecular mechanism that underlies the downregulation of BK-β_1 in type 2 diabetes is unknown. However, we have recently reported that in type 1 diabetes and in human coronary smooth muscle cells cultured with high glucose, BK-β_1 protein degradation was significantly accelerated through upregulated ubiquitin-proteasomal pathway (Zhang et al., 2010). Taken together, it is most likely that the above mechanisms could contribute to vascular BK channel dysfunction in type 2 diabetes, although direct confirmation will be necessary using appropriate tissues from human and animal models with type 2 diabetes mellitus.

6. Summary

Vascular BK channel function is impaired in type 2 diabetic animals. During the early stages of diabetic development, abnormal BK channel function is likely due to reduced activity and bioavailability of vasodilators (e.g., PGI_2, 12-hydroxyeicosatetraenoic acid) or increased activity and bioavailability of vasoconstrictors (e.g., Ang II, ROS). However, the BK channel biophysical properties remain intact. During advanced stages of type 2 diabetes, vascular BK channel gating properties, especially those pertaining to Ca^{2+}-dependent kinetics, are altered. These changes in BK channel gating are associated with reduced BK-β_1 subunit expression and increased BK-α subunit post-translational modification, contributing to BK channelopathy and vascular complications in type 2 diabetes. These results suggest that the potential therapeutic targets for restoring BK channel function are dependent on progression of the disease. Hence, a better understanding on the fundamental mechanisms of BK channel dysfunction in association with type 2 diabetes may help us provide better approaches for the treatment of diabetic vascular complications and improve the quality of life in these patients.

7. References

Alioua A, Mahajan A, Nishimaru K, Zarei MM, Stefani E and Toro L (2002) Coupling of c-Src to large conductance voltage- and Ca^{2+}-activated K^+ channels as a new mechanism of agonist-induced vasoconstriction. *Proceedings of the National Academy of Sciences of the United States of America* 99(22):14560-14565.

Avogaro A, Fadini GP, Gallo A, Pagnin E and de Kreutzenberg S (2006) Endothelial dysfunction in type 2 diabetes mellitus. *Nutriton, Metabolism and Cardiovascular Diseases* 16 Suppl 1:S39-45.

Bao L, Kaldany C, Holmstrand EC and Cox DH (2004) Mapping the BK_{Ca} channel's "Ca^{2+} bowl": side-chains essential for Ca^{2+} sensing. *The Journal of general physiology* 123(5):475-489.

Barman SA, Zhu S and White RE (2004) PKC activates BK_{Ca} channels in rat pulmonary arterial smooth muscle via cGMP-dependent protein kinase. *American Journal of Physiology Lung Cellular Molecular Physiology* 286(6):L1275-1281.

Brenner R, Perez GJ, Bonev AD, Eckman DM, Kosek JC, Wiler SW, Patterson AJ, Nelson MT and Aldrich RW (2000) Vasoregulation by the beta1 subunit of the calcium-activated potassium channel. *Nature* 407(6806):870-876.

Burnette JO and White RE (2006) PGI_2 opens potassium channels in retinal pericytes by cyclic AMP-stimulated, cross-activation of PKG. *Experimental eye research* 83(6):1359-1365.

Campbell WB, Gebremedhin D, Pratt PF and Harder DR (1996) Identification of epoxyeicosatrienoic acids as endothelium-derived hyperpolarizing factors. *Circulation research* 78(3):415-423.

Chae KS, Martin-Caraballo M, Anderson M and Dryer SE (2005) Akt activation is necessary for growth factor-induced trafficking of functional K_{Ca} channels in developing parasympathetic neurons. *Journal of neurophysiology* 93(3):1174-1182.

Chang T, Wu L and Wang R (2006) Altered expression of BK channel beta1 subunit in vascular tissues from spontaneously hypertensive rats. *American journal of hypertension* 19(7):678-685.

Chapman ML and VanDongen AM (2005) K channel subconductance levels result from heteromeric pore conformations. *The Journal of general physiology* 126(2):87-103.

Corsetti JP, Sparks JD, Peterson RG, Smith RL and Sparks CE (2000) Effect of dietary fat on the development of non-insulin dependent diabetes mellitus in obese Zucker diabetic fatty male and female rats. *Atherosclerosis* 148(2):231-241.

Cox DH and Aldrich RW (2000) Role of the beta1 subunit in large-conductance Ca^{2+}-activated K^+ channel gating energetics. Mechanisms of enhanced Ca^{2+} sensitivity. *The Journal of general physiology* 116(3):411-432.

Cui J, Yang H and Lee US (2009) Molecular mechanisms of BK channel activation. *Cellular and Molecular Life Science* 66(5):852-875.

De Vriese AS, Verbeuren TJ, Van de Voorde J, Lameire NH and Vanhoutte PM (2000) Endothelial dysfunction in diabetes. *British journal of pharmacology* 130(5):963-974.

Dong DL, Zhang Y, Lin DH, Chen J, Patschan S, Goligorsky MS, Nasjletti A, Yang BF and Wang WH (2007) Carbon monoxide stimulates the Ca^{2+}-activated big conductance K channels in cultured human endothelial cells. *Hypertension* 50(4):643-651.

Dong L, Zheng YM, Van Riper D, Rathore R, Liu QH, Singer HA and Wang YX (2008) Functional and molecular evidence for impairment of calcium-activated potassium channels in type-1 diabetic cerebral artery smooth muscle cells. *Journal of* Cerebral Blood Flow *&* Metabolism 28(2):377-386.

Feng J, Liu Y, Clements RT, Sodha NR, Khabbaz KR, Senthilnathan V, Nishimura KK, Alper SL and Sellke FW (2008) Calcium-activated potassium channels contribute to human coronary microvascular dysfunction after cardioplegic arrest. *Circulation* 118(14 Suppl):S46-51.

Ferguson WB, McManus OB and Magleby KL (1993) Opening and closing transitions for BK channels often occur in two steps via sojourns through a brief lifetime subconductance state. *Biophysical journal* 65(2):702-714.

Fernandez-Fernandez JM, Tomas M, Vazquez E, Orio P, Latorre R, Senti M, Marrugat J and Valverde MA (2004) Gain-of-function mutation in the KCNMB1 potassium channel subunit is associated with low prevalence of diastolic hypertension. *The Journal of clinical investigation* 113(7):1032-1039.

Han DH, Chae MR, Jung JH, So I, Park JK and Lee SW (2008) Effect of testosterone on potassium channel opening in human corporal smooth muscle cells. *The journal of sexual medicine* 5(4):822-832.

Hanner M, Schmalhofer WA, Munujos P, Knaus HG, Kaczorowski GJ and Garcia ML (1997) The beta subunit of the high-conductance calcium-activated potassium channel contributes to the high-affinity receptor for charybdotoxin. *Proceedings of the National Academy of Sciences of the United States of America* 94(7):2853-2858.

Jaggar JH, Li A, Parfenova H, Liu J, Umstot ES, Dopico AM and Leffler CW (2005) Heme is a carbon monoxide receptor for large-conductance Ca^{2+}-activated K^+ channels. *Circulation research* 97(8):805-812.

Jiang Y, Lee A, Chen J, Cadene M, Chait BT and MacKinnon R (2002) Crystal structure and mechanism of a calcium-gated potassium channel. *Nature* 417(6888):515-522.

Kelley-Hedgepeth A, Peter I, Kip K, Montefusco M, Kogan S, Cox D, Ordovas J, Levy D, Reis S, Mendelsohn M, Housman D and Huggins G (2008) The protective effect of KCNMB1 E65K against hypertension is restricted to blood pressure treatment with beta-blockade. *Journal of human hypertension* 22(7):512-515.

Kuhlmann J, Neumann-Haefelin C, Belz U, Kalisch J, Juretschke HP, Stein M, Kleinschmidt E, Kramer W and Herling AW (2003) Intramyocellular lipid and insulin resistance: a longitudinal in vivo 1H-spectroscopic study in Zucker diabetic fatty rats. *Diabetes* 52(1):138-144.

Lauterbach B, Barbosa-Sicard E, Wang MH, Honeck H, Kargel E, Theuer J, Schwartzman ML, Haller H, Luft FC, Gollasch M and Schunck WH (2002) Cytochrome P450-dependent eicosapentaenoic acid metabolites are novel BK channel activators. *Hypertension* 39(2 Pt 2):609-613.

Ledoux J, Werner ME, Brayden JE and Nelson MT (2006) Calcium-activated potassium channels and the regulation of vascular tone. *Physiology* 21(1):69-78.

Lee US and Cui J (2010) BK channel activation: structural and functional insights. *Trends in neurosciences* 33(9):415-423.

Liu G, Niu X, Wu RS, Chudasama N, Yao Y, Jin X, Weinberg R, Zakharov SI, Motoike H, Marx SO and Karlin A (2010) Location of modulatory beta subunits in BK potassium channels. *The Journal of general physiology* 135(5):449-459.

Liu Y, Sellke EW, Feng J, Clements RT, Sodha NR, Khabbaz KR, Senthilnathan V, Alper SL and Sellke FW (2008) Calcium-activated potassium channels contribute to human skeletal muscle microvascular endothelial dysfunction related to cardiopulmonary bypass. *Surgery* 144(2):239-244.

Liu Y, Terata K, Chai Q, Li H, Kleinman LH and Gutterman DD (2002) Peroxynitrite inhibits Ca^{2+}-activated K^+ channel activity in smooth muscle of human coronary arterioles. *Circulation research* 91(11):1070-1076.

Lohn M, Lauterbach B, Haller H, Pongs O, Luft FC and Gollasch M (2001) Beta-1-subunit of BK channels regulates arterial wall [Ca^{2+}] and diameter in mouse cerebral arteries. *Journal of Applied Physiology* 91(3):1350-1354.

Lovell PV, King JT and McCobb DP (2004) Acute modulation of adrenal chromaffin cell BK channel gating and cell excitability by glucocorticoids. *Journal of neurophysiology* 91(1):561-570.

Lu T, He T, Katusic ZS and Lee HC (2006) Molecular mechanisms mediating inhibition of human large conductance Ca^{2+}-activated K^+ channels by high glucose. *Circulation research* 99(6):607-616.

Lu T, Katakam PV, VanRollins M, Weintraub NL, Spector AA and Lee HC (2001) Dihydroxyeicosatrienoic acids are potent activators of Ca^{2+}-activated K^+ channels in isolated rat coronary arterial myocytes. *Journal of Physiology* 534(Pt 3):651-667.

Lu T, Wang XL, He T, Zhou W, Kaduce TL, Katusic ZS, Spector AA and Lee HC (2005) Impaired arachidonic acid-mediated activation of large-conductance Ca^{2+}-activated K^+ channels in coronary arterial smooth muscle cells in Zucker Diabetic Fatty rats. *Diabetes* 54(7):2155-2163.

Lu T, Ye D, He T, Wang XL, Wang HL and Lee HC (2008) Impaired Ca^{2+}-dependent activation of large-conductance Ca^{2+}-activated K^+ channels in the coronary artery smooth muscle cells of Zucker Diabetic Fatty rats. *Biophysical journal* 95(11):5165-5177.

Lu T, Zhang DM, Wang XL, He T, Wang RX, Chai Q, Katusic ZS and Lee HC (2010) Regulation of coronary arterial BK channels by caveolae-mediated angiotensin II signaling in diabetes mellitus. *Circulation research* 106(6):1164-1173.

Ma Z, Lou XJ and Horrigan FT (2006) Role of charged residues in the S1-S4 voltage sensor of BK channels. *The Journal of general physiology* 127(3):309-328.

Mandala M, Heppner TJ, Bonev AD and Nelson MT (2007) Effect of endogenous and exogenous nitric oxide on calcium sparks as targets for vasodilation in rat cerebral artery. *Nitric Oxide* 16(1):104-109.

McGahon MK, Dash DP, Arora A, Wall N, Dawicki J, Simpson DA, Scholfield CN, McGeown JG and Curtis TM (2007) Diabetes downregulates large-conductance Ca^{2+}-activated potassium beta-1 channel subunit in retinal arteriolar smooth muscle. *Circulation research* 100(5):703-711.

McManus OB, Helms LM, Pallanck L, Ganetzky B, Swanson R and Leonard RJ (1995) Functional role of the beta subunit of high conductance calcium-activated potassium channels. *Neuron* 14(3):645-650.

McManus OB and Magleby KL (1988) Kinetic states and modes of single large-conductance calcium-activated potassium channels in cultured rat skeletal muscle. *The Journal of physiology* 402:79-120.

McManus OB and Magleby KL (1991) Accounting for the Ca^{2+}-dependent kinetics of single large-conductance Ca^{2+}-activated K^+ channels in rat skeletal muscle. *The Journal of physiology* 443:739-777.

Meera P, Wallner M, Jiang Z and Toro L (1996) A calcium switch for the functional coupling between alpha (hSlo) and beta subunits (Kv,ca beta) of maxi K channels. *FEBS letters* 385(1-2):127-128.

Meera P, Wallner M, Song M and Toro L (1997) Large conductance voltage- and calcium-dependent K^+ channel, a distinct member of voltage-dependent ion channels with seven N-terminal transmembrane segments (S0-S6), an extracellular N terminus, and an intracellular (S9-S10) C terminus. *Proceedings of the National Academy of Sciences of the United States of America* 94(25):14066-14071.

Meera P, Wallner M and Toro L (2000) A neuronal beta subunit (KCNMB4) makes the large conductance, voltage- and Ca^{2+}-activated K^+ channel resistant to charybdotoxin and iberiotoxin. *Proceedings of the National Academy of Sciences of the United States of America* 97(10):5562-5567.

Minami K, Hirata Y, Tokumura A, Nakaya Y and Fukuzawa K (1995) Protein kinase C-independent inhibition of the Ca^{2+}-activated K^+ channel by angiotensin II and endothelin-1. *Biochemical pharmacology* 49(8):1051-1056.

Morrow JP, Zakharov SI, Liu G, Yang L, Sok AJ and Marx SO (2006) Defining the BK channel domains required for beta1-subunit modulation. *Proceedings of the National Academy of Sciences of the United States of America* 103(13):5096-5101.

Nielsen T, Burgdorf KS, Grarup N, Borch-Johnsen K, Hansen T, Jorgensen T, Pedersen O and Andersen G (2008) The KCNMB1 Glu65Lys polymorphism associates with reduced systolic and diastolic blood pressure in the Inter99 study of 5729 Danes. *Journal of hypertension* 26(11):2142-2146.

Nimigean CM and Magleby KL (1999) The beta subunit increases the Ca^{2+} sensitivity of large conductance Ca^{2+}-activated potassium channels by retaining the gating in the bursting states. *The Journal of general physiology* 113(3):425-440.

Obara K, Koide M and Nakayama K (2002) 20-Hydroxyeicosatetraenoic acid potentiates stretch-induced contraction of canine basilar artery via PKC alpha-mediated inhibition of K_{Ca} channel. *British journal of pharmacology* 137(8):1362-1370.

Oltman CL, Davidson EP, Coppey LJ, Kleinschmidt TL and Yorek MA (2009) Treatment of Zucker diabetic fatty rats with AVE7688 improves vascular and neural dysfunction. *Diabetes, obesity & metabolism* 11(3):223-233.

Oltman CL, Kleinschmidt TL, Davidson EP, Coppey LJ, Lund DD and Yorek MA (2008) Treatment of cardiovascular dysfunction associated with the metabolic syndrome and type 2 diabetes. *Vascular pharmacology* 48(1):47-53.

Orio P, Torres Y, Rojas P, Carvacho I, Garcia ML, Toro L, Valverde MA and Latorre R (2006) Structural determinants for functional coupling between the beta and alpha subunits in the Ca^{2+}-activated K^+ (BK) channel. *The Journal of general physiology* 127(2):191-204.

Pluger S, Faulhaber J, Furstenau M, Lohn M, Waldschutz R, Gollasch M, Haller H, Luft FC, Ehmke H and Pongs O (2000) Mice with disrupted BK channel beta1 subunit gene feature abnormal Ca^{2+} spark/STOC coupling and elevated blood pressure. *Circulation research* 87(11):E53-60.

Schopf S, Bringmann A and Reichenbach A (1999) Protein kinases A and C are opponents in modulating glial Ca^{2+} -activated K^+ channels. *Neuroreport* 10(6):1323-1327.

Schreiber M, Yuan A and Salkoff L (1999) Transplantable sites confer calcium sensitivity to BK channels. *Nature Neuroscience* 2(5):416-421.

Senti M, Fernandez-Fernandez JM, Tomas M, Vazquez E, Elosua R, Marrugat J and Valverde MA (2005) Protective effect of the KCNMB1 E65K genetic polymorphism against diastolic hypertension in aging women and its relevance to cardiovascular risk. *Circulation research* 97(12):1360-1365.

Shafrir E (1992) Animal models of non-insulin-dependent diabetes. *Diabetes/metabolism reviews* 8(3):179-208.

Shen KZ, Lagrutta A, Davies NW, Standen NB, Adelman JP and North RA (1994) Tetraethylammonium block of Slowpoke calcium-activated potassium channels expressed in Xenopus oocytes: evidence for tetrameric channel formation. *Pflugers Arch* 426(5):440-445.

Shi J, Krishnamoorthy G, Yang Y, Hu L, Chaturvedi N, Harilal D, Qin J and Cui J (2002) Mechanism of magnesium activation of calcium-activated potassium channels. *Nature* 418(6900):876-880.

Srinivasan K and Ramarao P (2007) Animal models in type 2 diabetes research: an overview. *The Indian journal of medical research* 125(3):451-472.

Tanaka Y, Meera P, Song M, Knaus HG and Toro L (1997) Molecular constituents of maxi KCa channels in human coronary smooth muscle: predominant alpha + beta subunit complexes. *The Journal of physiology* 502 (Pt 3):545-557.

Tanaka Y, Yamaki F, Koike K and Toro L (2004) New insights into the intracellular mechanisms by which PGI2 analogues elicit vascular relaxation: cyclic AMP-independent, Gs-protein mediated-activation of MaxiK channel. *Current medicinal chemistry* 2(3):257-265.

Tang XD, Garcia ML, Heinemann SH and Hoshi T (2004) Reactive oxygen species impair Slo1 BK channel function by altering cysteine-mediated calcium sensing. *Nature Structure Molecular Biology* 11(2):171-178.

Tang XD, Xu R, Reynolds MF, Garcia ML, Heinemann SH and Hoshi T (2003) Haem can bind to and inhibit mammalian calcium-dependent Slo1 BK channels. *Nature* 425(6957):531-535.

Tian L, Coghill LS, McClafferty H, MacDonald SH, Antoni FA, Ruth P, Knaus HG and Shipston MJ (2004) Distinct stoichiometry of BK_{Ca} channel tetramer phosphorylation specifies channel activation and inhibition by cAMP-dependent protein kinase. *Proceedings of the National Academy of Sciences of the United States of America* 101(32):11897-11902.

Toro B, Cox N, Wilson RJ, Garrido-Sanabria E, Stefani E, Toro L and Zarei MM (2006) KCNMB1 regulates surface expression of a voltage and Ca^{2+}-activated K^+ channel via endocytic trafficking signals. *Neuroscience* 142(3):661-669.

Vaithianathan T, Bukiya A, Liu J, Liu P, Asuncion-Chin M, Fan Z and Dopico A (2008) Direct regulation of BK channels by phosphatidylinositol 4,5-bisphosphate as a novel signaling pathway. *The Journal of general physiology* 132(1):13-28.

Wang RX, Chai Q, Lu T and Lee HC (2011) Activation of vascular BK channels by docosahexaenoic acid is dependent on cytochrome P450 epoxygenase activity. *Cardiovascular research* 90(2):344-52.

Wu L, Cao K, Lu Y and Wang R (2002) Different mechanisms underlying the stimulation of K_{Ca} channels by nitric oxide and carbon monoxide. *The Journal of clinical investigation* 110(5):691-700.

Xia XM, Ding JP and Lingle CJ (1999) Molecular basis for the inactivation of Ca^{2+}- and voltage-dependent BK channels in adrenal chromaffin cells and rat insulinoma tumor cells. *Journal Neuroscience* 19(13):5255-5264.

Xia XM, Zeng X and Lingle CJ (2002) Multiple regulatory sites in large-conductance calcium-activated potassium channels. *Nature* 418(6900):880-884.

Xie J and McCobb DP (1998) Control of alternative splicing of potassium channels by stress hormones. *Science (New York, NY* 280(5362):443-446.

Xu J and Zou MH (2009) Molecular insights and therapeutic targets for diabetic endothelial dysfunction. *Circulation* 120(13):1266-1286.

Yamaki F, Kaga M, Horinouchi T, Tanaka H, Koike K, Shigenobu K, Toro L and Tanaka Y (2001) MaxiK channel-mediated relaxation of guinea-pig aorta following stimulation of IP receptor with beraprost via cyclic AMP-dependent and -independent mechanisms. *Naunyn-Schmiedeberg's archives of pharmacology* 364(6):538-550.

Yang YS, Danis RP, Peterson RG, Dolan PL and Wu YQ (2000) Acarbose partially inhibits microvascular retinopathy in the Zucker Diabetic Fatty rat (ZDF/Gmi-fa). *Journal of Ocular Pharmacology and Therapeutics* 16(5):471-479.

Yuan P, Leonetti MD, Pico AR, Hsiung Y and MacKinnon R (2010) Structure of the human BK channel Ca^{2+}-activation apparatus at 3.0 A resolution. *Science (New York, NY* 329(5988):182-186.

Zeng XH, Xia XM and Lingle CJ (2003) Redox-sensitive extracellular gates formed by auxiliary beta subunits of calcium-activated potassium channels. *Nature structural biology* 10(6):448-454.

Zeng XH, Xia XM and Lingle CJ (2005) Divalent cation sensitivity of BK channel activation supports the existence of three distinct binding sites. *The Journal of general physiology* 125(3):273-286.

Zhang DM, He T, Katusic ZS, Lee HC and Lu T (2010) Muscle-specific F-box only proteins facilitate BK channel beta1 subunit downregulation in vascular smooth muscle cells of diabetes mellitus. *Circulation research* 107(12):1454-1459.

Zhang Y, Oltman CL, Lu T, Lee HC, Dellsperger KC and VanRollins M (2001) EET homologs potently dilate coronary microvessels and activate BK_{Ca} channels. *American journal of physiology* 280(6):H2430-2440.

Zhou W, Wang XL, Kaduce TL, Spector AA and Lee HC (2005) Impaired arachidonic acid-mediated dilation of small mesenteric arteries in Zucker diabetic fatty rats. *American journal of physiology* 288(5):H2210-2218.

Zhou YP, Cockburn BN, Pugh W and Polonsky KS (1999) Basal insulin hypersecretion in insulin-resistant Zucker diabetic and Zucker fatty rats: role of enhanced fuel metabolism. *Metabolism: clinical and experimental* 48(7):857-864.

Zink MH, Oltman CL, Lu T, Katakam PV, Kaduce TL, Lee H, Dellsperger KC, Spector AA, Myers PR and Weintraub NL (2001) 12-lipoxygenase in porcine coronary microcirculation: implications for coronary vasoregulation. *American Journal of Physiology - Heart & Circulatory Physiology* 280(2):H693-704.

Part 2

Endothelial Cells and Type 2 Diabetes

5

Endothelial Progenitor Cell Dysfunction in Diabetes Mellitus Type-2: Focus on Nitric Oxide System

Saher Hamed
Department of Cardiology, Rambam Health Care Campus, Haifa & Cardiovascular Research Laboratory, Rappaport Faculty of Medicine, Technion Haifa, Israel

1. Introduction

Diabetes mellitus type-2 (DM-2) is a global epidemic that is associated with a large economic burden, an increased risk of cardiovascular disease, poor outcomes as a result of vascular occlusion, and premature mortality. The clinical hallmark of DM-2 is hyperglycemia - with an etiology which involves genetic, environmental, and behavioral elements. Vascular endothelial function is impaired in DM-2. The underlying cause for the clinical severity of vascular occlusive disease in DM-2 patients has been partly attributed to impaired collateral vessel development due to altered function of mature endothelial cells (Abaci et al., 1999). Furthermore, increasing evidence suggest that new blood-vessel formation in adults may also involve bone marrow (BM)-derived endothelial progenitor cells (EPCs) (Asahara et al., 1997). The ability of DM-2 patients to develop coronary collaterals is diminished due to a diabetes-associated reduction in EPC count and an impairment of EPC mobilization (Lambiase et al., 2004). The deleterious effects of hyperglycemia on the vasculature are further exacerbated in DM-2 patients with elevated plasma lipid levels (Kanter et al., 2007). Several studies have shown that hyperglycemia or oxidized low-density lipoprotein (oxLDL) can reduce EPC count as well as impair EPC migration and proliferation by exerting harmful effects on the phosphatidylinositol-3 kinase (PI 3-K)/protein kinase B (PKB/Akt)/endothelial nitric oxide synthase (eNOS)/nitric oxide (NO) signaling cascade (Callaghan et al., 2005; Chen et al., 2007; Krankel et al., 2005; Ma et al., 2006).
This review presents and discusses the underlying metabolic alterations to the molecular mechanisms that are responsible for decreased EPC count and functionality in DM-2. The involvement of the NO system in this phenomenon is highlighted.

2. Endothelial Progenitor Cells (EPCs)

In 1997, BM-derived $CD34^+$/vascular endothelial growth factor receptor $(VEGFR)\text{-}2^+$ monocytes were first isolated from human blood by Asahara and co-workers and grown in culture under conditions that yielded colonies of cells which were characterized by the expression of surface markers of mature endothelial cells - CD31, E-selectin, von Willebrand factor (vWF), eNOS - and by the uptake of fluorescent-tagged acetylated LDL (Asahara et al., 1997). It was later discovered that these BM-derived cells are very important for the maintenance of endothelial integrity and function, as well as for postnatal new blood vessel formation (Rafii & Lyden, 2003). EPCs can be quantified by the number of circulating $CD34^+/VEGFR\text{-}2^+$ or $CD34^+/VEGFR\text{-}2^+/CD133^+$ cells, or by the number of colonies of adherent cells that can be obtained from circulating mononuclear cells (MNCs) that express mature endothelial cell markers (Peichev et al., 2000). The number of EPCs and their functionality level can serve as surrogate markers of endothelial function and cardiovascular diseases because these measures are indicative of the balance between endothelial integrity and repair.

2.1 Isolation and identification of EPCs

There are different sources for endothelial cells: hematopoietic stem cells, myeloid cells, circulating mature endothelial cells (which may also shed off the vessel wall), and other circulating progenitor cells. Therefore, there are no exact definitions for the origin and identification of EPCs isolated after culturing peripheral blood (PB)-MNCs in a medium that favors endothelial differentiation (Urbich & Dimmeler, 2004). A rare population of **highly proliferative endothelial colony-forming cells** from umbilical cord blood and from adult PB-MNCs that exhibit all the properties of progenitor cells **were also identified (**Ingram et al., 2004; Yoder et al., 2007). Furthermore, the outgrowth of endothelial cells from cultures of BM-derived PB-MNCs had an expansion rate that was more than a 1000-fold of that of circulating endothelial cells originating from vessel walls.

Two isolated types of EPCs derived from human PB have been described: early EPCs and late EPCs which have comparable angiogenic capabilities but different proliferation rates and survival behaviors (Hur et al., 2004). Early EPCs have a spindle-shaped phenotype but they do not give rise to endothelial outgrowth. These cells have also been referred to as monocyte-derived circulating angiogenic cells expressing CD14 (Gulati et al., 2003). Late EPCs have a cobblestone appearance and are similar to the circulating BM-derived cells that give rise to endothelial outgrowth (Gulati et al., 2003; Lin et al., 2004). Although they also have different gene expression profiles, which lead to different functions *in vitro*, they equally contribute to new blood vessel formation *in vivo*: early EPCs secrete angiogenic cytokines, and late EPCs supply a sufficient number of endothelial cells (Hur et al., 2004).

Three general approaches for identifying EPCs have been suggested by these studies: (1) isolating PB-MNCs from the blood, and then culturing them on fibronectin-coated tissue culture plates with various endothelial growth factors, (2) utilizing monoclonal antibodies and fluorescence-activated cell sorting (FACS) analysis to enumerate specific cell populations, and (3) using *in vitro* colon-forming cell assays. Some studies suggested that no specific or unique marker can be used to define EPCs in humans and experimental animals (Griese et al., 2003; Kocher et al., 2001; Timmermans et al., 2009).

2.2 EPCs and vascular risk factors

EPC count and function - mobilization, proliferation and attachment - inversely correlate with cardiovascular risk factors. This is demonstrated by the finding that the count and migratory ability of circulating EPCs of patients with coronary artery disease (CAD) are substantially lower than those of age-matched healthy individuals or individuals with high serum LDL cholesterol levels (Vasa et al., 2001). A powerful positive correlation between EPC colony number and endothelium-dependent vasodilatation was found in 45 men with varying cardiovascular risk, while a powerful negative correlation was found in these men between EPC colony number and the Framingham risk score (Hill et al., 2003). The EPC count in patients with poor coronary collateral circulation was reported to be lower than that of healthy individuals (Lambiase et al., 2004). In addition, an increased EPC count is associated with a reduced risk of death from a first major cardiovascular event, revascularization surgery, and hospitalization (Werner et al., 2005). The results of these studies indicate that EPCs are important for vascular health, thus advocating research into the underlying mechanisms that are responsible for impaired EPC count and function in various vascular diseases.

2.3 DM-2, vascular complications and EPCs

The pathophysiology of DM-2-associated vascular damage is complex, multi-factorial, and not fully understood. A two- to fourfold increased risk of cardiovascular events exists in adults with DM-2 compared with those without DM-2 (Fox et al., 2004) and DM-2 is directly implicated in various cardiovascular diseases that include stroke, ischemic heart disease, and peripheral vascular disease. The vascular complications in DM-2 patients can be caused by macro-angiopathy which mainly consists of accelerated atherosclerosis that affects the coronary, carotid, and peripheral arteries (Goldberg, 2003).

Cardiovascular disease in individuals with DM-2 is associated with endothelial dysfunction which is manifested by reduced bioavailability of endothelial cell-derived NO, resistance to the non-metabolic effects of insulin, hyperglycemia, hyperlipidemia, and oxidative stress (Anderson, 2003; Griendling et al., 2003), and with a decreased ability of the endothelium to regenerate and maintain its integrity (McVeigh et al., 1992). One of the important mechanisms for endothelial dysfunction and vascular diseases is reduced availability and downregulation of EPCs (Quyyumi, 2004). Decreased number and impaired function of EPCs can be involved early in endothelial dysfunction and atherogenesis, and later, in impaired collateralization after artery occlusive diseases, leading to clinical manifestations of vascular diseases (Landmesser et al., 2004).

Both type 1 diabetes mellitus and DM-2 are associated with reduced numbers and impaired function of EPCs; EPCs isolated from patients with DM-2 displayed impaired proliferation, adhesion, and attachment to activated human umbilical vein endothelial cells and the proliferation of EPCs the same diabetic patients was inversely correlated with their plasma glycated hemoglobin (HbA1c) levels, suggesting a relationship between the patients' glycemic control and EPC number and proliferation (Tepper et al., 2002). The EPC count in DM-2 patients with peripheral arterial disease (PAD) was shown to be substantially lower than that of healthy subjects, non-diabetic patients with vascular disease, and DM-2 patients without vascular disease (Fadini et al., 2005). The same study also showed that the reduced EPC number was associated with the severity of PAD in the DM-2 patients, and was inversely correlated with the patients' plasma glucose levels, and the number of cardiovascular risk factors. These findings led to the suggestion that EPC count could serve as a biomarker of peripheral atherosclerosis in DM-2 (Fadini et al., 2006). In another study, the same group demonstrated that the circulating $CD34^+$ cell count is inversely correlated with a cardiovascular risk profile and can be used to identify EPCs in diabetes (Fadini et al., 2006a). Although these studies demonstrated the existence of severe EPC impairment DM-2 patients with vascular diseases, they did not provide much information regarding the mechanisms that lead to the severe reduction in EPC numbers in diabetic patients. It was suggested, however, that the severe reduction in circulating EPC counts may be caused by a combination of hyperglycemia and adverse metabolites produced by diabetes which in turn could lead to accelerated endothelial dysfunction, atherogenecity, and subsequent severe vascular diseases. The contribution of clustered risk factors to EPC dysfunction is further discussed below.

2.4 EPCs and the PI 3-K/Akt pathway

The molecular mechanisms that underlie the homing and recruitment of BM-derived EPCs for the remodeling of vascular tissues remain unclear, but there is strong evidence that EPCs promote vascular repair and new blood vessel formation. EPC recruitment, mobilization and proliferation are regulated by the PI 3-K/Akt pathway (Morello et al., 2009). Exercise and drugs, such as hydroxymethylglutaryl-coenzyme A reductase inhibitors (statins), erythropoietin, estrogens, and vascular endothelial growth factor (VEGF), are known activators of the PI 3-K/Akt protein kinase pathway which increase circulating EPC count, proliferation and migration (Bahlmann et al., 2004; Dimmeler et al., 2001). Statin- and VEGF-induced EPC proliferation and differentiation were abolished *in vitro* and *in vivo* by pharmacological inhibition of PI 3-K as well as by the overexpression of a dominant negative Akt construct (Dimmeler et al., 2001). Furthermore, since compounds that stimulate the PI 3-K/Akt protein kinase pathway can also activate eNOS (Fulton et al., 1999), an association between eNOS and EPC count and activity appears to be essential because the expression of eNOS is necessary for the mobilization of stem and progenitor cells (Aicher et al., 2003), and disturbances in the PI 3-K/Akt/eNOS/NO signaling pathway or one of its members may result in EPC dysfunction.

2.5 The NO system and EPCs

EPCs participate in formation of new blood vessels. They are mobilized from BM stem cell niches to the peripheral circulation by NO and eNOS (Aicher et al., 2003; Ozuyaman et al., 2005). Nitric oxide is a biologically active unstable radical that is synthesized in vascular endothelial cells by eNOS, and its bioavailability depends on the balance between its production and inactivation (Wattanapitayakul et al., 2000). Asymmetric dimethylarginine (ADMA) – an endogenous NOS inhibitor - may lead to endothelial dysfunction and inhibition of angiogenesis *in vivo* (Boger & Bode-Boger 2000), and it has been suggested as a surrogate marker for cardiovascular events or deaths, as high circulating ADMA levels were correlated with decreased EPC mobilization, differentiation, and proliferation in patients with CAD (Thum et al., 2005).

One of the determinants of vascular damage in DM-2 is decreased NO bioavailability. DM-2 patients have a lower overall systemic fraction of L-arginine that is converted to NO compared with that found in healthy individuals (Avogaro et al., 2003). An additional factor that leads to diminished NO bioavailability in blood vessels of DM-2 patients is the reduction in the essential eNOS cofactor - (6R)-5,6,7,8-tetrahydro-L-biopterin (BH4) - which leads to the uncoupling of eNOS in blood vessels (Bauersachs & Schäfer , 2005). The migration of EPCs taken from DM-2 patients was normalized after treatment with an NO donor drug (Segal et al., 2006). Moreover, an NO-dependent mechanism was responsible for restoring EPC homing in diabetic wounds in mice which were treated with stromal derived factor-1 alpha (SDF1α), (Gallagher et al., 2007). Inactivation of NAD(P)H oxidase restored NO bioavailability and the *in vivo* re-endothelialization capacity of EPCs from diabetic patients (Sorrentino et al., 2007). Our group recently reported that the proliferation of glucose-stressed EPCs can be restored by preserving the bioavailability of NO with superoxide dismutase (SOD), emphasizing the importance of NO and oxidative stress to EPC count and proliferation (no self citation is allowed..).

NO bioavailability in sites of active vascularization seems to be critical for EPC biology and function. Vasorelaxant prostanoids such as prostacyclin (PGI_2) or its derivatives exert protective effects on endothelial cells by mechanisms that partly involve cyclic adenosine monophosphate (cAMP)-mediated NO formation (Niwano et al., 2003). Indeed, it was demonstrated that PGI_2 analogues such as Beraprost or Iloprost increase EPC number and migration in human and in ischemic tissues of experimental animal models (di Stefano et al., 2008; Miyahara et al., 2006). It was suggested that by mediating its beneficial effects on angiogenesis and repairing vascular walls, PGI_2 has a direct effect on EPC functions in an autocrine or paracrine manner through an NO dependent mechanism (Kawabe et al., 2010). In this regard, NO-dependent vasoprotective agents such as prostacyclin or statins could have a significant therapeutic role in cardiovascular diseases under pathological conditions, such as diabetes where the count and migratory activity of EPCs are impaired.

3. Suggested mechanisms for EPC impairment in DM-2

3.1 Effect of hyperglycemia

Hyperglycemia induces a reduction of the number of EPCs, their survival ability and impairs their proliferative and migratory capacity. Several mechanisms are involved in this process: some mechanisms cause a reduction in NO bioavailability (Krankel et al., 2005) and an deterioration by activating p38 mitogen-activated protein kinase (Kuki et al., 2006). Oxidative stress induced by hyperglycemia has also been suggested as a potential mechanism for reduced EPC count and impairment (Callaghen et al., 2005) and is discussed below. Contrary to the concept of oxidative stress-induced EPC damage through the NO system, *in vitro* down-regulation of eNOS expression and phosphorylation by high glucose concentrations resulted in reduced numbers and activity of early and late EPCs through mechanisms that were not associated with oxidative stress (Chen et al., 2007). Despite differences in gene expression and *in vitro* function between early and late EPCs (Hur et al., 2004), it was demonstrated that eNOS is an important target for high glucose adverse effects on EPC number and activity. While, eNOS deactivation in diabetic EPCs resulted in excessive superoxide anion production and in reduced NO bioavailability (Thum et al., 2007), implying an intimate relationship between oxidative stress and EPC damage, it is still unclear if high glucose-associated eNOS damage causes oxidative stress or if it is the high glucose-associated oxidative stress that causes eNOS deactivation. The different protocols used for EPC isolation and culture in the presence of high glucose might therefore play a significant role in determining the outcomes of EPC function *in vitro*.

Enhanced oxidative stress in DM-2 patients was shown to damage the protein signaling pathways that lead to NO production (Cohen & Tong 2010).

We recently showed that an inverse relationship exists between the reduced NO bioavailability in EPCs from DM-2 patients and the patients' plasma glucose and HbA1c levels. This reduction in NO bioavailability could be attributed to enhanced oxidative stress in DM-2 patients, which is known to damage the protein signaling pathways that lead to NO production (Cohen & Tong, 2010).

3.2 Effect of reactive oxygen species-induced oxidative stress

EPC dysfunction in diabetic patients can be also caused by excessive generation of reactive oxygen species (ROS) also leads to (Galasso et al., 2006). We showed that prolonged exposure of EPCs to high glucose concentrations *in vitro* increased superoxide anion production and reduced NO bioavailability. Several processes that are related to glucose stress in EPCs take place: glucose auto-oxidation, increased protein kinase C (PKC), and NAD(P)H oxidase activity lead to generation of superoxide anions. In addition, eNOS uncoupling due to BH4 deficiency or/and to increased PKC activity also lead to excessive superoxide anion production and to reduced NO bioavailability. All these processes impair EPC number and function (Thum et al., 2007). This was demonstrated by the inhibition of NAD(P)H oxidase activity in EPCs from DM-2 patients that restored their NO bioavailability and function (Sorrentino et al., 2007).
Reduced extracellular SOD activity has been shown to be closely associated with increased vascular oxidative stress, and has been implicated in the endothelial dysfunction of patients with hypertension (Giansante & Fiotti, 2006), congestive heart failure, and CAD (Landmesser et al., 2000). Ceradini *et al.* demonstrated that prevention of hyperglycemia-induced ROS generation significantly improved EPC-induced revascularization in ischemic tissues in genetically-engineered diabetic mice that overexpressed SOD, or after treating diabetic mice with SOD (Ceradini et al., 2008). Neutralization of the $p66^{ShcA}$ gene, which regulates the apoptotic response to oxidative stress, prevented high glucose-induced EPC impairment *in vitro* (di Stefano et al., 2008). Human EPCs have high intracellular expression levels of manganese SOD, which plays a crucial role in protecting these cells against oxidative stress (Dernbach et al., 2004; He et al., 2004). However, it should be argued that if the increased SOD activity of EPCs from DM-2 patients is sufficient to neutralize the high levels of superoxide anion that are observed in these patients. Ohshima *et al.* demonstrated that antioxidant therapy with SOD in diabetic mice reduced oxidative stress, and increased EPC count and potential to differentiate into endothelial cells (Ohshima et al., 2009). We reported that treating glucose-stressed EPCs with SOD restored their proliferative ability through an NO-dependent mechanism and we suggested that the extent of the interaction between NO and superoxide anion is important to the development of EPC dysfunction since the resultant product, peroxynitrite, can reduce the EPC count and impair their proliferation. This could provide a possible mechanism for the development of cardiovascular disease in patients with DM-2. Tao and colleagues demonstrated that augmentation of SOD expression in human EPCs by shear stress can accelerate the neutralization of superoxide anions (Tao et al., 2007). Therefore, it is possible that the addition of SOD, which catalyzes the dismutation of superoxide into oxygen and hydrogen peroxide, prevented the formation of peroxynitrite, thereby increasing NO bioavailability in EPCs (Figure 1). Our data and that of others revealed a significant mechanism that could account for the reduction of NO bioavailability in EPCs, in addition to the already known mechanism of downregulation of eNOS expression and activation by high glucose concentrations (Callaghan et al., 2005).

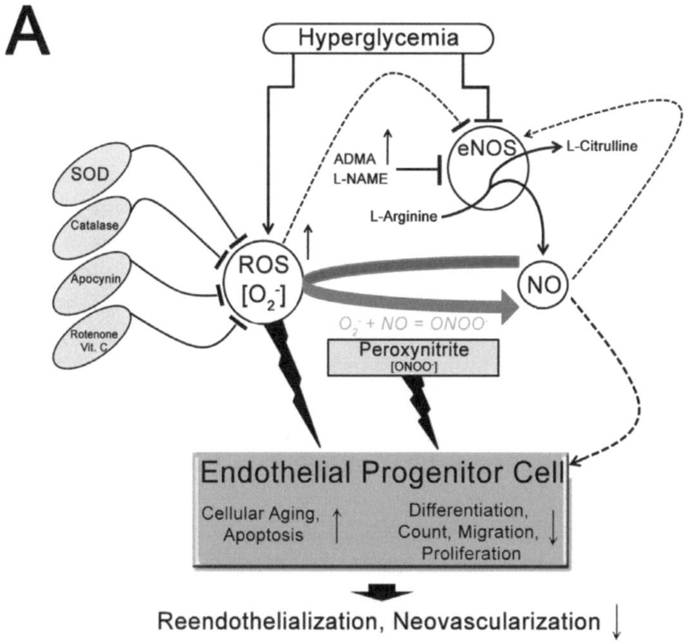

Fig. 1. Schematic representation of the role of ROS-mediated mechanisms in hyperglycemia-induced EPC dysfunction. ROS are generated in hyperglycemia. The interaction between ROS and NO produces peroxynitrite which together with free ROS impairs the count and function of EPCs. ADMA, asymmetric dimethyl-arginine; eNOS, endothelial NO synthase; LDL, low density lipoproteins; oxLDL, oxidized LDL; NO, nitric oxide; ROS, reactive oxygen species; SOD, superoxide dismutase. injury; interaction; ----- partial effect.

3.3 Effect of clustered risk factors

Hyperglycemia alone seems to be insufficient to cause severe vascular complications such as stimulating macrophage proliferation in atherosclerotic lesions (Lamharzi et al., 2004) in DM-2 patients. Rather, a combination of hyperglycemia and adverse diabetes metabolites, such as hyperlipidemia and advanced glycation end products, could most likely explain the severe reduction in circulating EPC counts in DM-2 patients, that lead to accelerated endothelial dysfunction, atherogenecity, and subsequent severe vascular diseases (Fadini et al., 2005; 2006; 2006a). Vascular disease in DM-2, therefore, appears to be related to hyperglycemia with a cluster of risk factors that include hypertension, smoking, hypercholesterolemia, dyslipidemia, and obesity (Caballero, 2003).

High serum levels and abnormalities of lipids that include triglycerides and LDL are associated with an increased risk of CAD in DM-2 patients (Shimada et al., 2004). Hyperlipidemia in apoE-deficient mice caused a low circulating EPC count, which correlated with enhanced atherosclerosis (Xu et al., 2003), while lipid aphaeresis treatment of patients with refractory hyperlipidemia stimulated EPC proliferation and increased eNOS activity (Patschan et al., 2009).

Several *in vitro* studies on EPCs from DM-2 patients revealed that oxLDL reduced EPC survival, count, and function, as well as their eNOS activity and NO bioavailability

(Imanishi et al., 2004; Ma et al., 2006). Elevated oxLDL levels exacerbate hyperglycemia-impaired EPC migration; we recently showed that DM-2 patients with CAD have high plasma oxLDL levels, which were inversely correlated with EPC migration and NO production. We also found that EPC migration and NO production were profoundly impaired in DM-2 patients with CAD compared with EPC migration and NO production in healthy individuals, DM-2 patients without CAD, and CAD patients without DM-2. These findings led us to propose that the combination of hyperglycemia and elevated plasma oxLDL levels account for the low EPC count and impaired EPC migration in these patients by involving the Akt/eNOS signaling pathway (Figure 2). The results from our study may only be relevant for some uncontrolled DM-2 patients with CAD because concomitant elevated circulating glucose and oxLDL levels are not usually found in well-controlled DM-2 patients with or without CAD, but can be seen in some uncontrolled DM-2 patients after consuming meals that are rich in carbohydrates and unsaturated fat. Concomitant elevated circulating glucose and oxLDL levels are also observed in some stress conditions, such as in inflammation or infection, and during hospitalization.

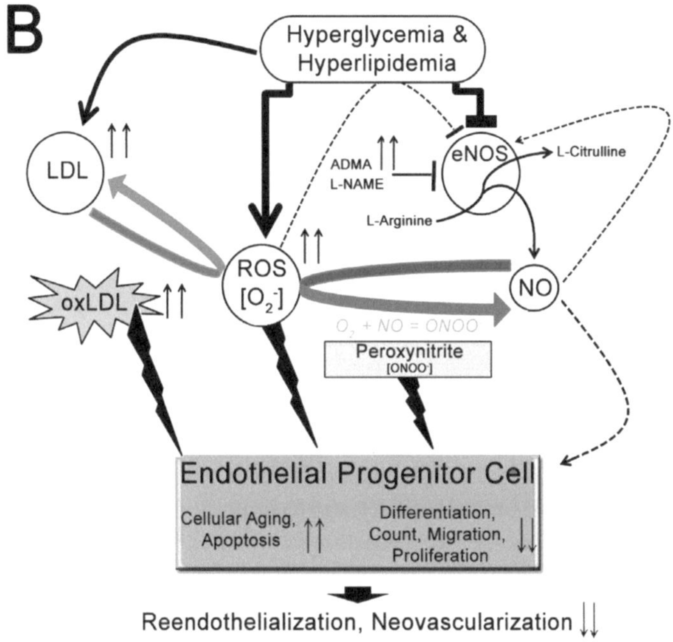

Fig. 2. Schematic representation of combined hyperlipidemia and hyperglycemia-induced EPC dysfunction. Hyperlipidemia or hyperglycemia impairs the count and function of EPCs, while together they aggravate this impairment. More ROS are generated in the presence of both hyperlipidemia and hyperglycemia. The interaction between high ROS levels and NO produces high peroxynitrite levels, and the interaction between high ROS and high levels of LDL produces high levels of oxLDL, which together with free ROS induce severe impairment of the count and function of EPCs. ADMA, asymmetric dimethyl-arginine; eNOS, endothelial NO synthase; LDL, low density lipoproteins; oxLDL, oxidized LDL; NO, nitric oxide; ROS, reactive oxygen species; SOD, superoxide dismutase. , injury; interaction; ----- partial effect.

4. Conclusions

Hyperglycemia-induced oxidative stress plays an important role in EPC dysfunction in DM-2. The combination of elevated plasma/serum oxLDL levels and hyperglycemia that may be seen in some uncontrolled DM-2 patients further aggravates the impaired EPC migration and NO production observed in hyperglycemia alone. The mechanisms that are responsible for the reduced number and impaired function of EPCs in DM-2 are partially linked to the PI 3-K/Akt/eNOS/NO signaling pathway. Therefore, we suggest that either this pathway or the interaction between hyperglycemia and hyperlipidemia in DM-2 patients, who have vascular diseases, are potential therapeutic targets for abolishing the impaired function of EPCs. The use of antioxidants and/or other medications, such as prostacyclin or statins, can enhance EPC number and function and restore their capacity for forming new blood vessels, at least through NO-dependent mechanisms.

5. Acknowledgments

This research was supported by grants from the Israel Ministry of Science Culture & Sport, and the Planning and Finance Committee for Higher Education.

6. References

Abaci, A., Oguzhan, A., Kahraman, S., Eryol, N.K., Unal, S., Arinç, H., *et al.* (1999). Effect of diabetes mellitus on formation of coronary collateral vessels. *Circulation,* 99:2239-2242.

Aicher, A., Heeschen, C., Mildner-Rihm, C., Urbich, C., Ihling, C., Technau-Ihling, K. *et al.* (2003). Essential role of endothelial nitric oxide synthase for mobilization of stem and progenitor cells. *Nat Med,* 9:1370-1376.

Anderson, T.J. (2003). Nitric oxide, atherosclerosis and the clinical relevance of endothelial dysfunction. *Heart Fail Rev,* 8:71-86.

Asahara, T., Murohara, T., Sullivan, A., Silver, M., van der Zee, R., Li, T. *et al.* (1997). Isolation of putative progenitor endothelial cells for angiogenesis. *Science,* 275:964-967.

Avogaro, A., Toffolo, G., Kiwanuka, E., de Kreutzenberg, S.V., Tessari, P. & Cobelli, C. (2003). L-arginine-nitric oxide kinetics in normal and type 2 diabetic subjects: a stable-labelled 15N arginine approach. *Diabetes,* 52:795-802.

Bahlmann, F.H., De Groot, K., Spandau, J.M., Landry, A.L., Hertel, B., Duckert, T. *et al.* (2004). Erythropoietin regulates endothelial progenitor cells. *Blood,* 103:921-926.

Bauersachs, J. & Schäfer, A. (2005). Tetrahydrobiopterin and eNOS dimer/monomer ratio--a clue to eNOS uncoupling in diabetes? *Cardiovasc Res,* 65:768-769.

Boger, R.H. & Bode-Boger, S.M. (2000). Asymmetric dimethylarginine, derangements of the endothelial nitric oxide synthase pathway, and cardiovascular diseases. *Semin Thromb Hemost,* 26:539-545.

Caballero, A.E., (2003). Endothelial dysfunction in obesity and insulin resistance: a road to diabetes and heart disease. *Obes Res,* 11:1278-1289.

Callaghan, M.J., Ceradini, D.J. & Gurtner, G.C. (2005). Hyperglycemia-induced reactive oxygen species and impaired endothelial progenitor cell function. *Antioxid Redox Signal*, 7:1476-1482.

Ceradini, D.J., Yao, D., Grogan, R.H., Callaghan, M.J., Edelstein, D., Brownlee, M. *et al.* (2008). Decreasing intracellular superoxide corrects defective ischemia-induced new vessel formation in diabetic mice. *J Biol Chem,* 283:10930-10938.

Chen, Y.H., Lin, S.J., Lin, F.Y., Wu, T.C., Tsao, C.R., Huang, P.H. *et al.* (2007). High glucose impairs early and late endothelial progenitor cells by modifying nitric oxide-related but not oxidative stress-mediated mechanisms. *Diabetes*, 56:1559-1568.

Cohen, R.A. & Tong, X. (2010). Vascular oxidative stress: the common link in hypertensive and diabetic vascular disease. *J Cardiovasc Pharmacol*, 55:308-316.

Dernbach, E., Urbich, C., Brandes, R.P., Hofmann, W.K., Zeiher, A.M. & Dimmeler, S. (2004) Antioxidative stress-associated genes in circulating progenitor cells: evidence for enhanced resistance against oxidative stress. *Blood*, 104:3591–3597.

Dimmeler, S., Aicher, A., Vasa, M., Mildner-Rihm, C., Adler, K., Tiemann, M., *et al.* (2001). HMG-CoA reductase inhibitors (statins) increase endothelial progenitor cells via the PI 3-kinase/Akt pathway. *J Clin Invest*, 108:391-397.

Di Stefano, R., Barsotti, M.C., Melillo, E., Iorio, M., Santoni, T., Armani, C. *et al.* (2008). The prostacyclin analogue iloprost increases circulating endothelial progenitor cells in patients with critical limb ischemia. *Thromb Haemost*, 100:871-877.

Di Stefano, V., Cencioni, C., Zaccagnini, G., Magenta, A., Capogrossi, M.C. & Martelli, F. (2009) p66ShcA modulates oxidative stress and survival of endothelial progenitor cells in response to high glucose. *Cardiovasc Res*, 82:421-429.

Fadini, G.P., Miorin, M., Facco, M., Bonamico, S., Baesso, I., Grego, F., *et al.* (2005). Circulating endothelial progenitor cells are reduced in peripheral vascular complications of type 2 diabetes mellitus. *J Am Coll Cardiol*, 45:1449-1457.

Fadini, G.P., Sartore, S., Albiero, M., Baesso, I., Murphy, E., Menegolo, M., *et al.* (2006). Number and function of endothelial progenitor cells as a marker of severity for diabetic vasculopathy. *Arterioscler Thromb Vasc Biol*, 26:2140-2146.

Fadini, G.P., de Kreutzenberg, S.V., Coracina, A., Baesso, I., Agostini, C., Tiengo, A. *et al.* (2006a). Circulating CD34+ cells, metabolic syndrome, and cardiovascular risk. *Eur Heart J*, 27:2247-2255.

Fox, C.S., Coady, S., Sorlie, P.D., Levy, D., Meigs, J.B., D'Agostino, R.B. Sr., *et al.* (2004). Trends in cardiovascular complications of diabetes. *JAMA*, 292:2495-2499.

Fulton, D., Gratton, J.P., McCabe, T.J., Fontana, J., Fujio, Y., Walsh, K. *et al.* (1999). Regulation of endothelium-derived nitric oxide production by the protein kinase Akt. *Nature*, 399:597-601.

Galasso, G., Schiekofer, S., Sato, K., Shibata, R., Handy, D.E., Ouchi, N. *et al.* (2006). Impaired angiogenesis in glutathione peroxidase-1-deficient mice is associated with endothelial progenitor cell dysfunction. *Circ Res*, 98:254-261.

Gallagher, K.A., Liu, Z.J., Xiao, M., Chen, H., Goldstein, L.J., Buerk, D.G. *et al.* (2007). Diabetic impairments in NO-mediated endothelial progenitor cell mobilization and homing are reversed by hyperoxia and SDF-1 alpha. *J Clin Invest*, 117:1249-1259.

Giansante, C. & Fiotti, N. (2006). Insights into human hypertension: the role of endothelial dysfunction. *J Hum Hypertens*, 20:725-726.

Goldberg, R.B. (2003). Cardiovascular disease in patients who have diabetes. *Cardiol Clin*, 21:399-413.

Griendling, K.K. & FitzGerald, G.A. (2003). Oxidative stress and cardiovascular injury: Part I: basic mechanisms and in vivo monitoring of ROS. *Circulation*, 108:1912-1916.

Griese, D.P., Ehsan, A., Melo, L.G., Kong, D., Zhang, L., Mann, M.J. *et al.* (2003). Isolation and transplantation of autologous circulating endothelial cells into denuded vessels and prosthetic grafts: implications for cell-based vascular therapy. *Circulation*, 108:2710-2715.

Gulati, R., Jevremovic, D., Peterson, T.E., Chatterjee, S., Shah, V., Vile, R.G. *et al.* (2003). Diverse origin and function of cells with endothelial phenotype obtained from adult human blood. *Circ Res*, 93:1023-1025.

He, T., Peterson, T.E., Holmuhamedov, E.L., Terzic, A., Caplice, N.M., Oberley, L.W. *et al.* (2004). Human endothelial progenitor cells tolerate oxidative stress due to intrinsically high expression of manganese superoxide dismutase. *Arterioscler Thromb Vasc Biol*, 24:2021-2027.

Hill, J.M., Zalos, G., Halcox, J.P., Schenke, W.H., Waclawiw, M.A., Quyyumi, A.A. *et al.* (2003). Circulating endothelial progenitor cells, vascular function, and cardiovascular risk. *N Engl J Med*, 348:593-600.

Hur, .J, Yoon, C.H., Kim, H.S., Choi, J.H., Kang, H.J., Hwang, K.K. *et al.* (2004). Characterization of two types of endothelial progenitor cells and their different contributions to neovasculogenesis. *Arterioscler Thromb Vasc Biol*, 24:288-293.

Ingram, D.A., Mead, L.E., Tanaka, H., Meade, V., Fenoglio, A., Mortell, K. *et al.* (2004). Identification of a novel hierarchy of endothelial progenitor cells using human peripheral and umbilical cord blood. *Blood*, 104:2752-2760.

Imanishi, T., Hano, T., Sawamura, T. & Nishio, I. (2004). Oxidized low-density lipoprotein induces endothelial progenitor cell senescence, leading to cellular dysfunction. *Clin Exp Pharmacol Physiol* 31:407-413.

Kanter, J.E., Johansson, F., LeBoeuf, R.C. & Bornfeldt, K.E. (2007). Do glucose and lipids exert independent effects on atherosclerotic lesion initiation or progression to advanced plaques? *Circ Res*, 100:769-781.

Kawabe, J., Yuhki, K., Okada, M., Kanno, T., Yamauchi, A., Tashiro, N. *et al.* (2010). Prostaglandin I2 promotes recruitment of endothelial progenitor cells and limits vascular remodeling. *Arterioscler Thromb Vasc Biol*, 30:464-470.

Kocher, A.A., Schuster, M.D., Szabolcs, M.J., Takuma, S., Burkhoff, D., Wang, J. *et al.* (2001). Neovascularization of ischemic myocardium by human bone-marrow-derived angioblasts prevents cardiomyocyte apoptosis, reduces remodeling and improves cardiac function. *Nat Med*, 7:430-436.

Krankel, N., Adams, V., Linke, A., Gielen, S., Erbs, S., Lenk, K. *et al.* (2005). Hyperglycemia reduces survival and impairs function of circulating blood-derived progenitor cells. *Arterioscler Thromb Vasc Biol*, 25:698-703.

Kuki, S., Imanishi, T., Kobayashi, K., Matsuo, Y., Obana, M. & Akasaka, T. (2006). Hyperglycemia accelerated endothelial progenitor cell senescence via the activation of p38 mitogen-activated protein kinase. *Circ J*, 70:1076-1081.

Lambiase, P.D., Edwards, R.J., Anthopoulos, P., Rahman, S., Meng, Y.G., Bucknall, C.A. *et al.* (2004). Circulating humoral factors and endothelial progenitor cells in patients with differing coronary collateral support. *Circulation,* 109:2986-2992.

Lamharzi, N., Renard, C.B., Kramer, F., Pennathur, S., Heinecke, J.W., Chait, A. *et al.* (2004). Hyperlipidemia in concert with hyperglycemia stimulates the proliferation of macrophages in atherosclerotic lesions: potential role of glucose-oxidized LDL. *Diabetes*, 53:3217-3225.

Landmesser, U., Merten, R., Spiekermann, S., Büttner, K., Drexler, H. & Hornig, B. (2000). Vascular extracellular superoxide dismutase activity in patients with coronary artery disease: relation to endothelium-dependent vasodilation. *Circulation,* 101:2264-2270.

Landmesser, U., Engberding, N., Bahlmann, F.H., Schaefer, A., Wiencke, A., Heineke, A., *et al.* (2004). Statin-induced improvement of endothelial progenitor cell mobilization, myocardial neovascularization, left ventricular function, and survival after experimental myocardial infarction requires endothelial nitric oxide synthase. *Circulation,* 110:1933-1939.

Lin, Y., Weisdorf, D.J., Solovey, A. & Hebbel, R.P. (2000). Origins of circulating endothelial cells and endothelial outgrowth from blood. *J Clin Invest,* 105:71-77.

Ma, F.X., Zhou, B., Chen, Z., Ren, Q., Lu, S.H., Sawamura, T. *et al.* (2006). Oxidized low density lipoprotein impairs endothelial progenitor cells by regulation of endothelial nitric oxide synthase. *J Lipid Res*, 47:1227-1237.

McVeigh, G.E., Brennan, G.M., Johnston, G.D., McDermott, B.J., McGrath, L.T., Henry, W.R. *et al.* (1992). Impaired endothelium-dependent and independent vasodilation in patients with type 2 (non-insulin-dependent) diabetes mellitus. *Diabetologia*, 35:771-776.

Miyahara, Y., Ohnishi, S., Obata, H., Ishino, K., Sano, S., Mori, H. *et al.* (2006) Beraprost sodium enhances neovascularization in ischemic myocardium by mobilizing bone marrow cells in rats. *Biochem Biophys Res Commun*, 349:1242-1249.

Morello, F., Perino, A. & Hirsch, E. (2009). Phosphoinositide 3-kinase signalling in the vascular system. *Cardiovasc Res*, 82:261-271.

Niwano, K., Arai, M., Tomaru, K., Uchiyama, T., Ohyama, Y. & Kurabayashi, M. (2003). Transcriptional stimulation of the eNOS gene by the stable prostacyclin analogue beraprost is mediated through cAMP-responsive element in vascular endothelial cells: close link between PGI2 signal and NO pathways. *Circ Res*, 93:523-530.

Ohshima, M., Li, T.S., Kubo, M., Qin, S.L. & Hamano, K. (2009). Antioxidant therapy attenuates diabetes-related impairment of bone marrow stem cells. *Circ J,* 73:162-166.

Ozuyaman, B., Ebner, P., Niesler, U., Ziemann, J., Kleinbongard, P., Jax, T. *et al.* (2005). Nitric oxide differentially regulates proliferation and mobilization of endothelial progenitor cells but not of hematopoietic stem cells. *Thromb Haemost,* 94:770-772.

Patschan, D., Patschan, S., Henze, E., Wessels, J.T., Koziolek, M. & Müller, G.A. (2009). LDL lipid apheresis rapidly increases peripheral endothelial progenitor cell competence. *J Clin Apher*, 24:180-185.

Peichev, M., Naiyer, A.J., Pereira, D., Zhu, Z., Lane, W.J., Williams, M. *et al.* (2000). Expression of VEGFR-2 and AC133 by circulating human CD34(+) cells identifies a population of functional endothelial precursors. *Blood,* 95:952-958.

Quyyumi, A.A. (2004). Circulating endothelial progenitor cells as novel biological determinants of vascular function and risk. *Can J Cardiol,* 20:44B-48B.

Rafii, S. & Lyden, D. (2003). Therapeutic stem and progenitor cell transplantation for organ vascularization and regeneration. *Nat Med,* 9:702-712.

Segal, M.S., Shah, R., Afzal, A., Perrault, C.M., Chang, K., Schuler, A. *et al.* (2006). Nitric oxide cytoskeletal-induced alterations reverse the endothelial progenitor cell migratory defect associated with diabetes. *Diabetes,* 55:102-109.

Shimada, K., Mokuno, H., Matsunaga, E., Miyazaki, T., Sumiyoshi, K., Miyauchi, K. *et al.* (2004). Circulating oxidized low-density lipoprotein is an independent predictor for cardiac event in patients with coronary artery disease. *Atherosclerosis,* 174:343-347.

Sorrentino, S.A., Bahlmann, F.H., Besler, C., Müller, M., Schulz, S., Kirchhoff, N. *et al.* (2007). Oxidant Stress Impairs In Vivo Reendothelialization Capacity of Endothelial Progenitor Cells From Patients With Type 2 Diabetes Mellitus. *Circulation,* 116:163-173.

Tao, J., Yang, Z., Wang, J.M., Wang, L.C., Luo, C.F., Tang, A.L. *et al.* (2007). Shear stress increases Cu/Zn SOD activity and mRNA expression in human endothelial progenitor cells. *J Hum Hypertens,* 21:353-358.

Tepper, O.M., Galiano, R.D., Capla, J.M., Kalka, C., Gagne, P.J., Jacobowitz, G.R. *et al.* (2002). Human endothelial progenitor cells from type II diabetics exhibit impaired proliferation, adhesion, and incorporation into vascular structures. *Circulation,* 106:2781-2786.

Thum, T., Tsikas, D., Stein, S., Schultheiss, M., Eigenthaler, M., Anker, S.D. *et al.* (2005). Suppression of endothelial progenitor cells in human coronary artery disease by the endogenous nitric oxide synthase inhibitor asymmetric dimethylarginine. *J Am Coll Cardiol,* 46:1693-1701.

Thum, T., Fraccarollo, D., Schultheiss, M., Froese, S., Galuppo, P., Widder, J.D. *et al.* (2007). Endothelial nitric oxide synthase uncoupling impairs endothelial progenitor cell mobilization and function in diabetes. *Diabetes,* 56:666-674.

Timmermans, F., Plum, J., Yoder, M.C., Ingram, D.A., Vandekerckhove, B. & Case, J. (2009). Endothelial progenitor cells: identity defined? *J Cell Mol Med,* 13:87-102.

Urbich, C. & Dimmeler, S. (2004) Endothelial progenitor cells: characterization and role in vascular biology. *Circ Res,* 95:343-353.

Vasa, M., Fichtlscherer, S., Aicher, A. Adler, K., Urbich, C., Martin, H. *et al.* (2001). Number and migratory activity of circulating endothelial progenitor cells inversely correlate with risk factors for coronary artery disease. *Circ Res,* 89:E1-7.

Wattanapitayakul, S.K., Weinstein, D.M., Holycross, B.J. & Bauer J.A. (2000). Endothelial dysfunction and peroxynitrite formation are early events in angiotensin-induced cardiovascular disorders. *FASEB J,* 14:271-278.

Werner, N., Kosiol, S., Schiegl, T., Ahlers, P., Walenta, K., Link, A. *et al.* (2005). Circulating endothelial progenitor cells and cardiovascular outcomes. *N Engl J Med,* 353:999-1007.

Xu, Q., Zhang, Z., Davison, F. & Hu, Y. (2003) Circulating progenitor cells regenerate endothelium of vein graft atherosclerosis, which is diminished in ApoE-deficient mice. *Circ Res,* 93:e76-86.

Yoder, M.C., Mead, L.E., Prater, D., Krier, T.R., Mroueh, K.N., Li, F. *et al.* (2007). Redefining endothelial progenitor cells via clonal analysis and hematopoietic stem/progenitor cell principals. *Blood,* 109:1801-1809.

6

Glycaemic Control and Protection of the Vasculature from Glucose Toxicity

Hong Ding and Chris R. Triggle
Weill Cornell Medical College in Qatar
Qatar

1. Introduction

Diabetes, notably type 2 diabetes, is a major and prevalent health problem with a minimal current estimate of 250 million sufferers worldwide, a prediction of 366 million by 2030 and, based on the evidence of numerous reports, we can also anticipate an excessive morbidity and mortality rate in this population primarily as a result of cardiovascular disease (Kannel & McGee, 1979; Wild et al., 2004). As reflected by the data from the 1991 United Kingdom Prospective Diabetes Study, UKPDS, with 5102 subjects with type 2 diabetes, and the 1993 Diabetes Control and Complications Trial, DCCT, with 1441 type 1 diabetics, the established dogma for the best form of management for patients with diabetes is tight glycaemic control (DCCT 1993; UKPDS 1991, 1998). Such conclusions have been re-emphasised as reflected by a report by Standl and colleagues (2009) indicating that the incidence of cardiovascular events associated with diabetes is reduced by 10-15% per 1% reduction in absolute glycated haemoglobin, HBA_{1c}, levels. In addition, the Emerging Risk Factors Collaboration (ERFC) study, a collaborative meta-analysis of 102 prospective studies, made the observation that the pre-existence of diabetes enhanced the risk of vascular disease more than two fold (ERFC, 2010). Furthermore, the ERFC study of 820,900 participants also concluded that a 50-year-old with diabetes died approximately 6 years earlier than a person without diabetes and that diabetes was moderately associated (but not necessarily causality) with death from certain cancers such as liver, pancreas, bladder, breast, colorectal, lung and ovary as well as other causes including infectious diseases, degenerative disorders and others (ERFC, Seshasai et al 2011). Nonetheless, a 'glucocentric' approach to the treatment of diabetes was delivered a setback with the results, released in 2007, from the Action to Control Cardiovascular Risk in Diabetes, ACCORD study of 10,251 patients. The intensified glucose lowering arm of the ACCORD study with 5,128 patients targeted glycated haemoglobin, HBA_{1c}, of <6% was discontinued when it became apparent that such an intensive regimen resulted in a significantly higher all-cause risk of death of 22% and a 35% increase in cardiovascular mortality (Gerstein et al., ACCORD, 2008). In contrast, data from the Action in Diabetes and Vascular Disease, ADVANCE, that was released shortly after that from the ACCORD study provided no evidence of an increased mortality amongst the 11,140 high-risk patients who were randomly assigned to either standard or intensive glucose control (HbA_{1c} of 6.5 or less) in the study, but also reported a 10% reduction in combined micro- and macrovascular events (ADVANCE 2008). Similarly for the Investigators in the Veterans Affairs Diabetes Trial,

VADT, wherein 1791 military veterans were subjected to either an intensive or a standard therapy for glycaemic control no significant increase in mortality was noted, but there was no significant reduction in microvascular events excepting a reduction in the progression of albuminuria (Duckworth et al., 2009).

Although, initially, it appeared that no one particular subgroup in the ACCORD study had a particularly higher mortality, independent concerns have been raised concerning an elevated cardiovascular risk with some of the drugs used in these studies, for instance as reported in the Rosiglitazone Evaluated for Cardiac Outcomes and Regulation of glycaemia in Diabetes, RECORD, study (Goldfine 2008; Komajda 2010). New information also indicates that additional post-hoc subgroup analysis from the ACCORD trial may be helpful in the identification of sub-groups (Calles-Escandon, 2010). In addition, the meta analysis performed by the Collaborators on Trials of Lowering Glucose, CONTROL, on the data from the ACCORD, ADVANCE, UKPDS and the VDAT trials concluded that a more intensive glucose-lowering regimen did reduce, albeit modestly, major cardiovascular events in patients with type 2 diabetes, but increased major hypoglycaemic episodes (Turnbull et al., 2009). Issues over the make up of the patient groups versus the onset of diabetes have also been raised, as have questions over the benefits of intensive glycaemic control versus cholesterol and/or blood pressure lowering (ACCORD 2010a,b; Emanuele, 2010; Nilsson 2010; Yudkin & Richter, 2010). A 2009 meta analysis of 5 trials that addressed intensive control of glucose and cardiovascular outcomes indicated that intensive compared with standard glycaemic control did significantly reduce coronary events without an increased risk of death; however, population variability may be evident regarding the optimum mechanism, speed, and extent of reduction (Ray et al., 2009). Putting all of these data sets together and considering the conclusions from a number of meta-analysis and subgroup analysis that have been completed and reviewed one can conclude that the management of glycaemia remains central to the treatment of patients with diabetes and important for reducing cardiovascular disease risk, but individualised treatment is to be preferred (Mazzone, 2010). This conclusion is supported by the 2011 recommendations made by the American Association of Clinical Endocrinologists (AACE) (Handlesman et al., 2011). Nonetheless questions remain as to how to optimise the treatment protocols for the better protection of patients with diabetes from cardiovascular disease as well as stroke.

To summarize, although further analysis and potentially new studies are required what does remain clear is that the morbidity and mortality associated with diabetes predominantly reflect cardiovascular pathophysiological sequelae that result in a 2- to 4-fold increase in the incidence of coronary artery disease, a 10-fold increase in peripheral vascular diseases and a 3- to 4-fold increase mortality rate that, primarily, reflect a doubling of the risk of vascular disease (Grundy et al 2002; ERFC 2010).

2. Diabetes, cardiovascular disease and endothelial dysfunction

Changes in the function of the endothelium are argued to be early indicators of the onset of vascular disease including that associated with diabetes and, as an example, are apparent prior to the detection of atherosclerotic plaque development (McLenachan et al., 1990; Werns et al., 1989). Endothelial dysfunction is frequently defined as a reduced endothelium-dependent vasodilatation (EDV) response to either an endothelium-dependent vasodilator, such as acetylcholine or bradykinin, or to flow-mediated vasodilatation. This functional definition of endothelial dysfunction is one that can be readily demonstrated using the methodology first described by Furchgott and Zawadzki in their 1980 in vitro study of endothelium-dependent relaxation to acetylcholine in rabbit aortae and has been extended to include wire and pressure myography studies in small arteries from animals as well as man. In humans, both non-invasive and invasive techniques have been applied to measure both vasodilator and flow-mediated vasodilatation and the data generated have advanced our understanding of the pathophysiology of coronary artery disease in humans (Anderson et al., 1995; Bohm et al., 2005). It is not just the vasodilatation response that is decreased or lost, but, in addition, an increased expression of adhesion molecules including the soluble adhesion molecules, sE-Selectin and sICAM-1, pro-inflammatory molecules, altered regulation of smooth muscle cell proliferation and the development of a procoagulatory state. Increased levels of the soluble adhesion molecules, sE-Selectin and sICAM-1, and also the endothelium-specific marker, soluble thrombomodulin have been determined by biomarkers for the risk and severity of diabetes-associated coronary artery disease and cardiovascular disease in general (Constans 2006; Thorand 2006). Thus, a revised and broader definition of 'endothelial dysfunction' is required and has been suggested by Triggle & Ding (2010):

"Endothelial dysfunction reflects a reduced (EDV) response to either an endothelium-dependent vasodilator, such as acetylcholine (or bradykinin), or to flow-mediated vasodilatation that is accompanied by elevated expression of adhesion molecules, enhanced vascular smooth muscle proliferation and the development of a hypercoagulatory state."

Endothelial dysfunction has been demonstrated in a number of studies to be both an early indicator of vascular disease and a predictor of a future cardiovascular event (see Esper et al., 2006). Furthermore, endothelial dysfunction in diabetes has been linked to hyperglycaemia- and hyperlipidaemia (hypertriglceridemia)-induced oxidative stress as demonstrated in both human and animal studies (Ceriello et al., 2002; Monnier et al., 2006; Triggle et al., 2005). Furthermore, high glucose induces both premature senescence and reduces total numbers of endothelial progenitor cells (EPCs) and thus impairs both repair and angiogenic processes (Balestrieri et al., 2008). Endothelial cells normally have a relatively long turnover rate that has been stated to be approximately three years, however, damage to the endothelium results in replacement by regenerated cells that may not have the same properties as normal endothelial cells (Brandes et al., 2005; Vanhoutte, 2010).

2.1 Hyperglycaemia and endothelial dysfunction

Elevated glucose levels acutely as well chronically affect vascular function. Acute effects include a rapid loss of flow-mediated EDV in humans with a pronounced delayed recovery in type 2 diabetes that most likely reflects a glucose-induced uncoupling of endothelial nitric oxide synthase (eNOS) secondarily to the oxidation of the key eNOS co-factor tetrahydrobiopterin (BH_4) (Ihlemann, 2003; Kawano et al, 1999; reviewed by Ding & Triggle, 2010). A key observation is the ratio BH_4 to BH_2 (oxidised product of BH_4) that is critical for eNOS function as BH_4 and BH_2 bind with equal affinity to eNOS and hyperglycaemia promotes BH_4 oxidation (Crabtree et al., 2008). Studies with the db/db leptin receptor mutant diabetic mouse also substantiate the important role of the BH_4/BH_2 ratio in endothelial function (Pannirselvam et al., 2002; 2003; 2006). Simply supplementing with BH_4 in the presence of hyperglycaemia may not improve eNOS function, or at best only acutely, as persistent hyperglycaemia will, via enhanced superoxide production, oxidise BH_4 to BH_2. Interestingly ascorbic acid, but not vitamin E, helps stabilize BH_4 and increases eNOS

activity of aortic endothelial cells from ApoE-deficient mice (d'Uscio et al., 2003) and also porcine endothelial cells (Huang et al., 2000).
Under hyperglycaemic conditions the glycolytic and oxidative phosphorylation pathways are overloaded and the result is the shunting of glucose and the intermediates of glucose metabolism, namely fructose 1,6 biphosphate and glyceraldehyde 3 phosphate, into pro-oxidative stress pathways such as hexosamine metabolism, sorbitol metabolism, protein kinase C activation, α-ketoaldehyde formation and methyglyoxol/advanced glycated end product (AGE) formation (Robertson, 2005). In addition, glucose in the physiological range of 4 to 10mM, following metabolism and protein kinase C activation, rapidly depresses voltage-gated potassium channel, Kv, currents in rat mesenteric myocytes and inhibits Kv channel modulation by endothelin-1 (Rainbow et al., 2006). Kv channels are key regulators of vascular tone (Knot and Nelson, 1995; Cole et al., 2005) and thus glucose-induced reduction of Kv channel activity would have profound effects on blood flow, glucose disposal and ultimately could contribute to the development of insulin resistance and hyperglycaemia-linked vascular disease (Straub and Nelson, 2006). Calcium homeostasis is also affected and exposure of primary endothelial cells for 24-72 hours to high glucose also alters Store-Operated Ca^{2+} Entry (SOCE) and has been associated with changes in expression of the Transient Receptor Potential Channel 1 (TRPC1) (Bishara and Ding, 2010). Comparable changes have been reported in the expression levels of TRPC1 and also another Store-Operated Ca^{2+} Channel protein, STIM1, in the coronary artery of of the Ossabaw pig model of diabetes (Edwards et al., 2010). An increase in expression levels of TRPC1 has also been associated with vascular disease and injury thus suggesting that alterations in SOCE may be closely associated with the development of vascular disease and thus, potentially, another target for therapeutic intervention (Kumar et al., 2006; van Breemen et. al., 2006).

2.2 Postprandial hyperglycaemia is an important risk factor

The importance of postprandial regulation of blood glucose as a determinant of the impact of hyperglycaemia on vascular function is receiving increasing attention (Ceriello 2005; Woerle et al., 2007; Aryangat & Gerich 2010) and another confounding influence seems to be that the impact of oscillating levels of glucose on endothelial function may be more damaging than sustained high glucose (Ceriello 2008a). Indeed, a high postprandial glucose 'spike' starting from a lower basal fasting glucose may be more damaging than that produced by the equivalent 'spike' level, but starting from a higher basal glucose simply because it is the extent of the change in glucose that determines the degree of endothelial dysfunction (Ceriello, 2008b). Data from the RIAD study (Risk Factors in Impaired Glucose Tolerance for Atherosclerosis and Diabetes) also indicated that the postprandial glucose 'spike' is a better predictor of carotid artery intima-media thickness (a measure of atherosclerosis) than fasting glucose or HbA1c (Hanefield et al., 2000; Temelkova-Kurtschiev et al., 2000). Thus, collectively these data indicate that reducing the extent of post-prandial excursions in blood glucose should reduce cardiovascular events.

2.3 Consequences of chronic hyperglycaemia

Chronic exposure to high glucose results in the non-enzymatic formation of AGEs, alters proteasome function, as well as produces epigenetic changes in histone methylation and demethylation that, secondary to glucose-induced elevated oxidative stress, result in persistent gene activation that likely forms the basis for the development of 'hyperglycaemic memory' (Brasacchio et al., 2009; Cognali, 2008; Queisser et al., 2010; Vlassara & Palace, 2002). Hyperglycaemic memory is a serious consequence of a lack of adequate glycaemic control as, despite restoration of normoglycaemia, vascular disease continues to progress (reviewed by Triggle & Ding, 2010). Figure 1 summarizes the potential contributions of AGEs and epigenetic changes to the development of hyperglycaemic memory, pancreatic beta cell dysfunction and vascular disease:

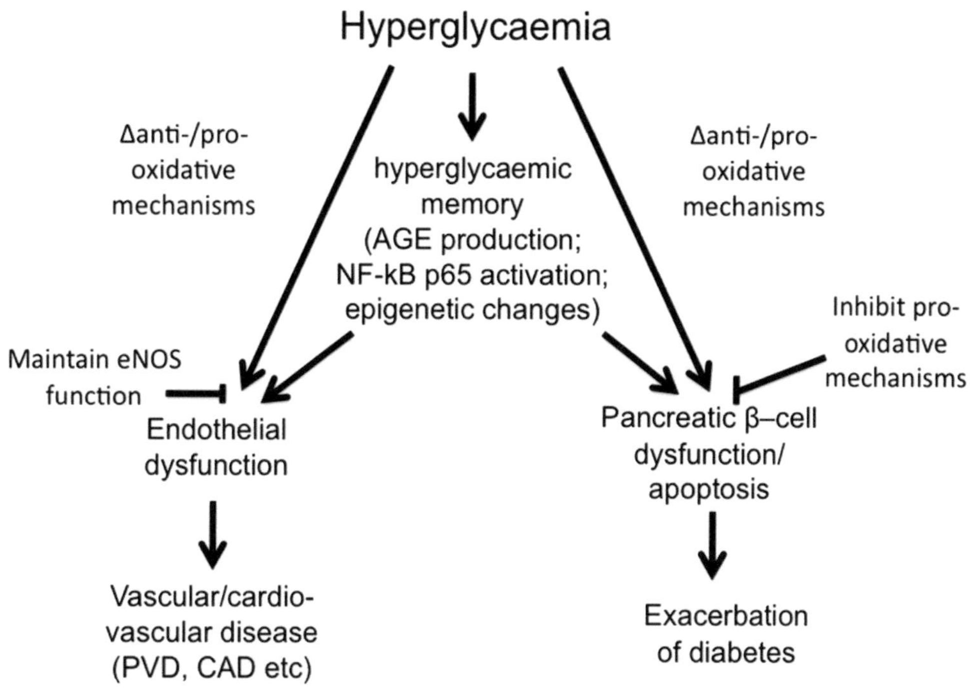

Fig. 1. Hyperglycaemia induces both endothelial and pancreatic β-cell dysfunction. The long-term sequelae of hyperglycaemia results in cardiovascular disease include peripheral vascular disease (PVD) and coronary artery disease (CAD).

If AGEs are important contributors to hyperglycaemic memory then arguably tight and aggressive glycaemic control should be translated into better protection against future cardiovascular events (Chalmers & Cooper, 2008). In addition, early treatment designed to reduce cellular reactive species, glycation and the build up of AGEs should minimize long-term diabetic complications (Ceriello, 2009). Glucose toxicity is also linked to pancreatic β-cell apoptosis that may involve several pathways including links to oxidative stress, endoplasmic (ER) stress, changes in the expression of the antiapoptotic protein Bcl-2 and epigenetic changes in the promoter for nuclear factor kappa B (NF-KB) subunit p65 (Eizirik et al., 2008; El-Osta et al., 2008; McKenzie et al., 2010; Robertson 2004).

2.4 Antioxidant therapy and diabetic vascular disease

Although many animal studies clearly indicate that oxidative stress results in endothelial dysfunction (see reviews by Ding & Triggle 2010; Triggle & Ding 2010) antioxidant therapy in humans has been demonstrated to be ineffective in reducing mortality [MRC/BHF, 2002]. In the MRC/BHF randomised study 20,536 individuals with various prior cardiovascular disease morbidities were recruited into 69 hospitals and were treated with either a statin, antioxidant vitamin therapy (600 mg E, 250 mg C and 20 mg beta-carotene daily or a placebo). Nonetheless, protection of endothelial function as is evident by a reduction in oxidative stress as well as enhanced levels of the dimeric 'coupled' eNOS can be demonstrated by provision of the precursor of BH_4, sepiapterin, at least in endothelial cells in culture (Ding et al., 2007; Aljofan & Ding, 2010). The role of antioxidant dietary adjuncts and therapy in prevention and treatment remains a highly important clinical question and Dusting and Triggle (2005) argued that there is a need for re-thinking of the choice of antioxidants as well as better-designed studies. Thus, further studies of the benefits of antioxidants and, in the cellular setting, appropriately targeted antioxidants to the cellular source(s) of excessive free radical production are clearly justified. It is thus of value to reflect on the apparent benefits of the natural phenolic resveratrol on lifespan in a number of organisms, including yeast, worms, flies as well as mice on a high fat diet (see Baur et al. 2005). The cellular basis for the protective effect of compounds such as the polyphenol antioxidant, resveratrol, in diabetes may be linked to activation of AMP-activated protein kinase (AMPK) - the so-called metabolic master switch that has multiple targets facilitating, for instance, glucose uptake in muscle, fatty acid oxidation and inhibition of glucose production by the liver (Um et al., 2010).

Antioxidant enzyme levels are low in pancreatic β cells and chronic oxidative stress is thought to be a major contribution to β cell dysfunction in diabetes (Robertson, 2004; Tiedge et al., 1997). These data suggest that antioxidant therapy should benefit β cell function; however, the efficacy of the common antioxidants available either from dietary or supplement sources may simply not be high enough to have significant benefit (Robertson, 2004). Furthermore, with the exception of the PPAR-gamma agonists and incretin-mimetics that do have protective and/or trophic effects, direct beneficial effects of most anti-diabetic agents on β cells have not been clearly documented (Bonora 2008).

2.5 Endoplasmic Reticulum (ER) stress and diabetes

The ER plays a critical role in protein folding and sorting and stress will impair these functions resulting in the *'Unfolded Protein Response'*, or UPR, that, initially, despite an increase load on the protein folding machinery, helps to maintain homeostasis. Prolonged ER stress, which may include oxidative stress secondary to the contribution of molecular oxygen to disulphide bond formation, results in cell death via apoptosis and there is increasing evidence that ER stress plays an important role in the aetiology of many diseases including diabetes and atherosclerosis (Eizirik et al., 2008; Hosoi and Ozawa, 2010; Tabas 2010; Tu and Weissman 2004). It is also now recognised that UPR is regulated by a signal transduction pathway with three major components: 1/ inositol requiring 1 (IRE1); 2/ Protein kinase RNA-like ER kinase (PERK); 3/ Activating Transcription factor 6 (ATF6) that can all contribute to ER stress. As our knowledge on ER stress expands so do avenues for interventions that may slow the progression of a disease (Patil & Walker 2001; Eizirik et al., 2008).

Notably in response to obesity, post-prandial hyperglycaemia and the development of insulin resistance the insulin producing pancreatic β-cell is exposed to considerable stress as newly formed pro-insulin is directed to the ER for appropriate folding. ER stress in the pancreatic β-cell results in progressive pancreatic β-cell dysfunction and death (Fonesca et al., 2009). The loss of pancreatic β-cell function is a key contributor to the later stages of type 2 diabetes and results in the requirement for insulin therapy. A key mediator of ER stress-induced apoptosis is the transcription factor CHOP (also known as GADD153), which under normal conditions has a low expression level, but levels increase with increasing ER stress (Eizirik et al., 1993; Oyadomari & Mori, 2004). Similarly the endothelial cell, just like the pancreatic β-cell, when exposed to hyperglycaemia responds with an increase in ER stress that seems to be secondary to mitochondria metabolism and superoxide generation (Sheikh-Ali et al., 2010a). Of additional interest and relevant to the protective role of resveratrol is that ER stress in endothelial cell is enhanced with the deletion of AMPKα2 and that certain antioxidants can reduce ER stress (Dong et al., 2010; Sheikh-Ali et al., 2010b).

3. What can we learn from other mammalian species?

The "thrifty" gene hypothesis ('Diabetes Mellitus: A "Thrifty" Genotype Rendered Detrimental by "Progress"?'), as originally proposed by Neel, argues that we are descended from hunter-gatherers who survived and evolved despite having to cope with an unpredictable availability of food and therefore survival was based on "selectivity" to store energy as fat (Neel, 1962). Europeans have maintained a comparatively lower prevalence of diabetes than most other populations and, perhaps, this can be related to the fact that Europeans have arguably been exposed to relatively stable food supply and "modern" technology for a comparatively longer period than other ethnic groups. However, support for this latter speculation is reduced by evidence that Australians and North Americans of European descent have significantly higher rates of diabetes than their European counterparts (Diamond 2003; Dunstan et al., 2002; Harris et al., 1998). Various explanations can be provided to explain such differences and whether we accept a "thrifty (like) gene", or a "drifty gene" hypothesis, or even the role(s) of environmental influences such as bacteria and viruses, continues to be debated (Diamond 2003: Prentice et al., 2008; Speakman, 2008; Zinn, 2010). Of relevance to the thrifty gene debate are data from studies of domesticated pigs and cattle that have been bred for countless centuries to store energy for future human consumption and yet do not, or only rarely, develop diabetes (Gerstein & Waltman 2006). These observations provide a basis for a tentative conclusion that it is possible to provide 'protection' against diet- and hyperglycaemia-induced vascular disease in mammals despite exposure to ample food supply and limited exercise and thus warrant further studies of the comparative physiology/genetics of these species (Venn-Watson et al., 2011). Nonetheless, as reflected in the Ossabaw pig colony on Ossabaw Island, (Georgia, USA) in as little as 500 years domestic pigs exposed to a feast and famine environment do become prone to the development of metabolic syndrome and diabetes when these feral pigs are provided the same diet as their domesticated cousins (Gerstein and Waltman, 2006; Whitfield 2003). Studies with Ossabaw pigs are providing insights into the pathophysiology of vascular disease associated with metabolic syndrome and diabetes (Edwards et al., 2010). The one-humped camel, *Camelus dromedaries*, is a desert animal that can withstand both a harsh climate and limited supplies of food and water, but, similar to the Ossabaw pig, when exposed to a high calorie diet develops signs of diabetes (Ali et al., 2006). On the other hand milk from *Camelus dromedaries* has been known through ethnomedical practice and recent clinical trials to lessen the insulin requirements of diabetics (Mohamad et al., 2009). Whether the anti-diabetic factor in camel milk, which might be insulin or an insulin-like factor, also provides some protection to the camel when exposed to a high carbohydrate diet is unknown.

It is of interest to note that certain mammalian species, specifically the bottlenose dolphin, *Tursiops truncates*, can maintain high post-prandial glucose levels and a diabetic-like state that is probably essential for the dolphin to maintain adequate brain levels of glucose and yet not, apparently, truly develop diabetes (Venn-Watson & Ridgway, 2007). About 55 million years ago dolphins, pigs and ungulates shared a common ancestor that was a herbivore and the possible link between elevated blood glucose levels in dolphins may relate to the need to maintain adequate glucose levels for an enlarged brain size and function (Thewissen & Mador, 1999; Venn-Watson et al., 2007; 2011). Miller and Colagiuri (1994) have advanced the hypothesis that for Homo sapiens the low carbohydrate and high protein carnivorous diet that existed for about 2 million years up until the end of the last ice age disadvantaged the insulin-sensitive phenotype in favour of insulin resistance. Europeans have, on the other hand, been exposed to a long period of agricultural development and thus the selection process for insulin resistance was relaxed with the result that present-day Europeans are more resistant to type 2 diabetes than most other ethnic groups (Miller & Colagiuri, 1994).

The more generally held view is the present obesity/diabetes pandemic has resulted from a combination of greater food availability, reduced physical activity and genetic susceptibility. We should, however, be cautious about accepting this view without considering other influences (Zinn 2010). A hypothesis advanced by Klimentidis et al (2011) is based on the "Canary in the coal mine" analogy and notes that similar trends in body weight increase have been observed in some domesticated and non-domesticated mammals including feral rats trapped in urban Baltimore that showed a 5.7% increase in body weight per decade. The data presented by Klimentidis et al (2011) is suggestive of environmental influences such as endocrine-disrupters and infectious diseases that may have epigenetic effects on mammalian genomes. Nonetheless the close link between diet, a sedentary lifestyle, obesity and cardiovascular disease in humans is difficult to deny. Alternatively, or in addition, the "thrifty phenotype" hypothesis argues that poor foetal and infant nutrition that negatively affect growth result in permanent changes in glucose homeostasis that result in the development of the metabolic syndrome and type 2 diabetes (Hales and Barker, 2001). Calorie restriction on the other hand has been shown to increase longevity in rats and, more recently, studies in non-mammalian species that include yeast and invertebrate species, have linked longevity to the SIRT1, the mammalian homolog of Sir2 (silent information regulator 2 and originally termed MARI, Mating-Type Regulator-1). In *Saccharomyces*, *Caenorhabditis elegans* and *Drosophila* Sir2 mediates the effects of calorie restriction on life extension and therefore has been associated with the regulation of longevity (Dali-Youcef, et al., 2007). Collectively these data have led to the hypothesis that, in mammals, SIRT1, by virtue of the key role it plays in post-transcriptional regulation, is the central co-ordinator of metabolic regulation and insulin sensitivity and obesity (Holness et al., 2010). SIRT1 as a target for the treatment of metabolic diseases is discussed in more detail later in this chapter.

Regardless of the genetic basis for susceptibility to obesity and diabetes evidence for atherosclerotic changes linked to a high fat diet is clearly shown in human remains from several ancient societies including the mummies of Egyptian pharaohs, priests and other privileged members of the Egyptian society back to at least 1500 AD (David et al., 2010). These findings seem to parallel those in a society, such as the USA today, where the impact of diet is clearly evident on the prevalence of obesity that from 1976--1980 to 2007--2008, increased from 15% to 34% among adults and from 5% to 17% among children and adolescents (Freedman et al., 2008). Perhaps *Homo sapiens,* unlike *Sus scrofa domesticus,* have not evolved, or adapted, sufficiently such that its cardiovascular system cannot withstand the abuse of a diabetogenic/atherogenic diet? The debate continues as to whether diabetes in *Homo sapiens* reflects a 'thrifty' genotype or simply a genetic drift - the 'drifty' gene hypothesis with, perphaps, the latter being supported by the Ossabaw pig example (Prentice et al., 2008; Speakman 2008)?

4. How to proceed?

The results from the ACCORD study questioned the benefits of an overly intensive glycaemic control regimen and yet data from animal studies as well the UKPDS & DCCT data indicate that hyperglycaemia is detrimental to vascular function and increases morbidity and mortality. Thus, the question arises: "Can we, in addition to pursuing a more modest reduction in blood glucose levels and HBA_{1c}, determine new approaches to protect the cardiovascular system against glucose toxicity?" In other words: "Are there new therapeutic approaches that can provide improved cardiovascular protection?" Most therapeutic interventions targeting cardiovascular disease modulate endothelial function indirectly via targeting the risk factors linked to endothelial dysfunction. Thus, for hypertension, angiotensin converting enzyme inhibitors (ACEIs) and angiotensin receptor blockers (ARBs) are widely used and for dislipidemia the lipid-lowering statins. Many of these drugs have been reported to have pleiotropic effects that improve endothelial function and their actions have been reviewed (Dobarro et al., 2009). A number of the drugs that are used as anti-hypoglycaemic agents for the treatment of type 2 diabetes also have been reported to have direct and/or indirect effects to improve endothelial function.

4.1 Metformin

Metformin, a first-line and most widely prescribed drug for the treatment of type 2 diabetes, has has been demonstrated to not only correct hyperglycaemia but also to improve endothelial function in human subjects (Mather et al., 2001). Metformin also seems more effective in obese patients with the recent observation suggesting that metformin, a substrate for organic cation transporters, OCTs, and notably OCT1, reduces adipogenesis as a result of an increased action in adipocytes from obese patients that could be linked to an elevated expression of OCTs (Rotella et al., 2006; Moreno-Navarrete, 2011). The therapeutic efficacy of metformin thus makes it an ideal drug to study in terms of its cellular mode(s) of action and, in particular, although effective a high level of non-fatal gastrointestinal side effects can reduce patient compliance. Metformin, at least in part, mediates its' cellular action(s) via the activation of AMPK with the reported involvement of mitochondrial-derived reactive nitrogen species and the requirement of eNOS expression (Mather et al., 2001; Zhou et al., 2001; Zou et al., 2004). The ability of metformin to reduce hepatic glucose output has been credited to an action via the LKB1 (a serine/threonine kinase)-AMPK/SIRT1 pathways and inhibition of key glucogenic genes in the liver (Zhou et al., 2001; Shaw et al., 2005). The role of SIRT1 and GCN5 (a histone acetyltransferase), two regulators of gluconeogenic gene expression via the modulation of cAMP-response element binding protein (CREB), in the action of metformin are of particular interest because AMPK is known to activate SIRT1 which, via deacetylase of key targets, including LKB1, may mediate the beneficial effects of metformin (Canto et al., 2009;

Caton et al., 2011; Lan et al., 2008). As discussed later in this chapter SIRT1 is a key target of interest for the treatment of metabolic disorders.

AMPK-independent actions on hepatic gluconeogenesis and endothelial function have also been reported suggesting that the beneficial actions of metformin in type 2 diabetes result from effects on several targets including a protective action on complex I and the mitochondrial permeability transition pore (PTP) (Detaille et al., 2005; Foretz et al., 2011; Zhou et al 2001). Thus, conceivably, metformin has multiple actions on cell metabolism via AMPK, SIRT1 and GCN5.

4.2 The incretins

Recent advances in new medications for the treatment of type 2 diabetes include the introduction of modulators of the incretin pathway such as the glucagon-like peptide-1 (GLP-1), exenatide, and the dipeptidyl peptidase-4 (DPP-4) inhibitor, sitagliptin, has increased the armamentarium for the treatment of type 2 diabetes with favourable clinical results (Chia and Egan, 2008; Hansen et al., 2009). Exenatide, however, is inconvenient to use as the drug requires sub-cutaneous administration and is also associated with a high frequency of nausea (>50%) and vomiting (17%), however, use is associated with improved β-cell function and weight loss (Chia & Egan, 2008). Sitagliptin is orally effective, weight neutral, well tolerated, but has been associated with a relatively high incidence of nasopharyngitis (6.4%) and headache (5.1%) (Amori et al., 2007). Incretin mimetics have not been shown to have direct vascular protective actions although the ability of GLP-1 to inhibit cytokine, lipid and glucose induced apoptosis of β-cells would infer that incretin mimetics should at least indirectly infer protection via improved β-cell function (Hvidberg et al., 1994).

4.3 Fibroblast Growth Factor 21 (FGF21)

The human genome encodes 22 members of the Fibroblast Growth Factor superfamily and Fibroblast Growth Factor 21 (FGF21) lacks mitogenic activity and is a high profile prospect and/or target as a novel therapeutic agent for the treatment of metabolic diseases by virtue of its ability to lower plasma glucose, triglycerides as well as improve insulin sensitivity (Kharitonenkov et al., 2005; Kharitonenkov and Shanafelt 2009; Kharitonenkov and Larsen 2011). FGF21 has been reported to enhance insulin-independent uptake via GLUT1 into adipocytes and skeletal muscle and dramatically reduce blood glucose levels in the ob/ob, leptin-resistant, diabetic mouse (Kharitonenkov et al., 2005; Mashili et al., 2011). Although the liver was assumed to be the source of FGF21, brown adipose tissue, skeletal muscle and, possibly, other tissues can also express FGF21 thus inferring hepatokine, adipokine and myokine functions (Hondares et al., 2011; Mashili et al., 2011). βKlotho, a type 1 transmembrane glycoprotein and a coreceptor for FGF21, is expressed in the mouse aorta suggesting that FGF21 may contribute to the regulation of blood vessel function (Fon Tracer et al., 2010). FGF21 expression is regulated by both PPAR alpha and gamma activation and preclinical assessment of FGF21 indicates a lack of any major side effects (Kharitonenkov and Shanafelt); Hondares et al., 2011). FGF21 has important endocrine-functions in the regulation of glucose and lipid homeostasis that include an increase in the expression of GLUT1 (Mashili et al., 2011; Berglund et al., 2009). Elevated plasma levels of FGF21 are seen in humans with type 2 diabetes and mouse models where "FGF21 resistance" is associated with a reduced response to the blood glucose and triglyceride lowering and insulin sensitizing actions of FGF21 (Kharitonenkov et al., 2005; Berglund et al., 2009). To date there is a lack of any functional data on the effects of FGF21 on vascular function, but, via the ability of FGF21 to enhance insulin sensitivity and improve glucose disposal, FGF21 will indirectly protect the vasculature against glucose toxicity. Evidence indicating that FGF21 regulates metabolic homeostasis and enhances mitochondrial oxidative function in adipocytes via activation of AMPK and SIRT1 suggests that the effects of FGF21 should also be pursued in vascular tissue (Chau et al., 2010).

4.4 Sirtuins

The sirtuins are a seven-member family (SIRT1-7) of NAD^+-dependent protein deacetylases and ADP-ribosyltransferases associated with the regulation of a wide range of biological processes ranging from apoptosis, adipocyte and muscle differentiation, and energy expenditure to gluconeogenesis and, SIRT1 in particular, has been implicated as the central epigenetic controller of metabolism (Michan and Sinclair, 2007; Holness et al., 2010). SIRT1 gain of function in mice has been shown to increase insulin sensitivity in mice fed a high fat diet or backcrossed onto leptin resistant db/db diabetic mice (Banks et al., 2008). Overexpression of SIRT1 in the liver of diabetic and obese leptin deficient ob/ob mice reduces insulin resistance and reduces expression of X-box binding protein-1 (XBP-1), a key transcription factor that regulates ER stress (Li et al., 2011). Furthermore, treatment of EPCs with high glucose downregulated EPC numbers, reduced SIRT1 expression levels and increased expression levels of the acetylated Forkhead transcription factor, FoxO1 (Balestrieri et al., 2008).

SIRT1 has an ubiquitous distribution and exerts its effects on metabolism via deacetylation-mediated activation of the peroxisome proliferator-activated receptor-gamma (PPARγ) transcription co-activator, PGC-1α (Michan and Sinclair, 2007). PGC-1α increases fatty acid utilisation in muscle, whereas in the liver gluconeogenesis is regulated by SIRT1-mediated deacetylation and the subsequent nuclear retention of FoxO1. FoxO1 regulates the expression of gluconeogenic enzymes and the actions of FoxO1 are suppressed by insulin (Jackson et al., 2000). The transcriptional activity of FoxO1 is inhibited by SIRT1-mediated deacetylation (Yang et al., 2005). FoxO1 transcriptional activity is also regulated by XBP-1s, which, in addition to being involved in the upregulation of genes that reduce ER stress, promotes proteasome-mediated degradation of FoxO1 (Zhou et al., 2011).

SIRT1, PGC-1α, and FoxO1 are all targets for intensive investigation as potential additions to the armamentarium of drugs for the treatment of obesity, diabetes and cardiovascular disease (Alcain & Villalba, 2009; Borradaile & Pickering, 2009; Brandes, 2008; Lavu et al., 2008; Liang & Ward, 2006; Milne et al., 2007; Nagashima et al., 2010; Zhou et al., 2011). For instance, small molecule inhibitors of FoxO1 have been reported to have a hypoglycaemic effect in diabetic db/db mice (Nagashima et al., 2011; Tanaka et al., 2010). The oral hypoglycaemic agent, metformin, a first line choice for the treatment of type 2 diabetes, also has SIRT1, as previously discussed, as one of its potential targets (Caton et al., 2011; Lan et al., 2008). Interestingly, the polyphenol antioxidant resveratrol has also been associated with positive effects on longevity, activation of SIRT1, and beneficial effects on mice fed a high calorie diet (Bauer et al., 2006).

The overexpression of SIRT1 is cardioprotective and endothelium-specific overexpression of SIRT1 decreases atherosclerotic lesions in apoE null mice (Alcendor et al., 2007; Zhang et al., 2008). Of particular interest in the Zhang et al study (2008) was the observation that calorie restriction increased whereas a high-fat diet decreased the expression of SIRT1; however, SIRT1 overexpression overcame high-fat induced endothelial dysfunction and enhanced the expression of eNOS. Furthermore, in a cell culture protocol, the overexpression of SIRT1 was protective against apoptosis (Zhang et al., 2008). The constitutively active serine/threonine protein kinase, LKB1, has been reported to be a binding partner and intracellular target for SIRT1 in porcine aortic endothelial cells and SIRT1-mediated deacetylation of LKB1 may be a key pathway for promoting proliferation and retarding endothelial senescence via limiting LKB1/AMPK activation as a result of proteasome-mediated degradation of LKB1 (Zu et al., 2010).

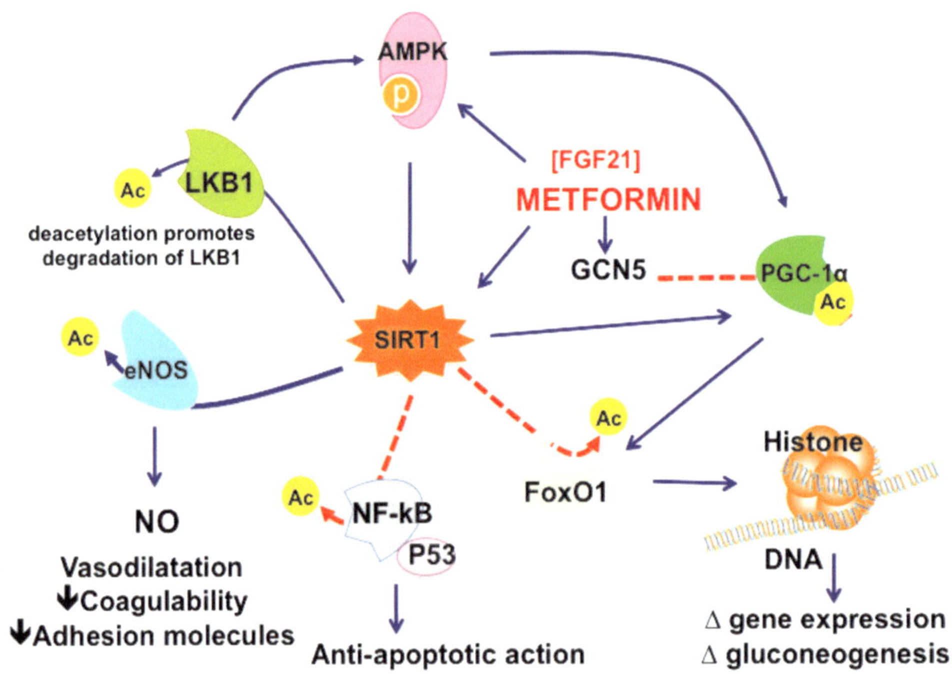

Fig. 2. Summarises the key cellular pathways that are involved with the effects of metformin and FGF21 on endothelial function and gluconeogenesis. SIRT1 can activate, as depicted by a solid blue arrow, a target via deacetylation (Ac), or inactivate via deacetylation (Ac) as depicted by a dotted red arrow. Thus, SIRT1 can via deacetylation, enhance eNOS activity, reduce apoptosis via inactivation of NF-kB and p53, reduce endothelial cell senescence via the acetyl transferase GCN5 deacetylation and subsequent degradation of LKB1 thus limiting phosphorylation-mediated AMPK activation, and also, in the liver, decrease, gluconeogenesis via deactylation of FoxO1. Metformin and FGF21 may have direct effects on both SIRT1 and AMPK and SIRT1 and metformin, via GCN5, can activate PGC-1α thus promoting fatty acid utilization.

Metformin, as already mentioned, is currently the most widely used oral hypoglycaemic agent and possesses insulin-sensitizing actions and also has proven endothelial protective actions in humans subjects with diet-treated type 2 diabetes (Mather et al., 2001). Mather et al (2001) measured blood flow responses to intraarterial administration of endothelium-dependent (acetylcholine) versus endothelium-independent (sodium nitroprusside) and nitrate-independent (verapamil) vasodilators using forearm plethysmography. Subjects who received metformin demonstrated statistically significant improved responses to acetylcholine versus placebo, but not nitroprusside-stimulated or verapamil-stimulated blood flow. Several studies indicate that one of the targets for metformin is SIRT1, possibly in part also involving AMPK, with subsequent multiple target actions that include an inhibition of hepatic gluconeogenesis (Caton et al., 2010; Detaille et al., 2005; Foretz et al., 2011; Zhou et al., 2001). SIRT1 activation has also been shown to increase the generation of NO via the deacetylation of eNOS at lysines 496 and 506 (Mattagajasingh et al., 2007) thus providing a cellular basis for the improvement of acetylcholine-mediated forearm blood flow in human subjects with diabetes that was reported by Mather et al (2001). Thus, metformin provides us a valuable prototype drug to serve as a template for the development of new and possibly more specific drugs with fewer side effects that target the key cellular pathway(s).

5. Conclusion

Good glycaemic control remains an important target in the treatment of diabetes, however, new approaches to the treatment of diabetes, metabolic diseases and glucose toxicity that offer improved benefits over existing treatments are required. Studies of the beneficial effects of FGF21 on metabolism and, in particular, glucose utilization as well as elucidation of the metabolic and cell survival pathways regulated by SIRT1 and its cellular targets, such as FoxO1, appear to be worthy avenues for further study.

6. References

ACCORD. (2008). The Action to Control Cardiovascular Risk in Diabetes Study Group Effects of intensive glucose lowering in type-2 diabetes. New Engl J Med 358:2560-2572.

ACCORD Study Group. (2010a). Effects of Combination Lipid Therapy in Type 2 Diabetes Mellitus. NEJM 2010 e-pub March 14th. 10.1056/NEJMoa1001282).

ACCORD Study Group. (2010b). Effects of Intensive Blood-Pressure Control in Type 2 Diabetes Mellitus. NEJM 2010 e-pub March 14th. 10.1056/NEJMoa1001286).

ADVANCE (2008). The Advance Collaborative Group Intensive blood glucose control and vascular outcomes in patients with type 2 diabetes. New Engl J. Med 358:2560-2572.

Alcendor RR, Gao S, Zhai P, Zablocki D, Holle E, Yu X, Tian B, Wagner T, Vatner SF, Sadoshima J. (2007). Sirt1 regulates aging and resistance to oxidative stress in the heart. Circ Res. 100(10): 1512-1521.

Ali MA, Nyberg F, Chandranath SI, Ponery AS, Adem A, Adeghate E. (2006). Effect of high-calorie diet on the prevalence of diabetes mellitus in the one-humped camel (Camelus dromedarius). Ann N Y Acad Sci. 1084:402-410.

Alcaín FJ, Villalba JM. (2009a). Sirtuin inhibitors. Expert Opin Ther Pat. 19(3):283-394.

Alcaín FJ, Villalba JM. (2009b) Sirtuin activators. Expert Opin Ther Pat. 19(4):403-414.

Aljofan M, Ding H. (2010). High glucose increases expression of cyclooxygenase-2, increases oxidative stress and decreases the generation of nitric oxide in mouse microvessel endothelial cells. J Cell Physiol. 222:669-675.

Amori RE, Lau J, Pittas AG. (2007). Efficacy and safety of incretin therapy in type 2 diabetes: systematic review and meta-analysis. JAMA. 298(2):194-206.

Anderson TJ, Uehata A, Gerhard MD, Meredith IT, Knab S, Delagrange D, Lieberman EH, Peter Ganz P, Creager MA, Yeung AC, Selwyn AP (1995) Close relation of endothelial function in the human coronary and peripheral circulations. J Am Coll Cardiol. 26:1235-1241.

Aryangat AV, Gerich JE. (2010). Type 2 diabetes: postprandial hyperglycaemia and increased cardiovascular risk. Vasc Health & Risk Management 6:145-155.

Balestrieri ML, Rienzo M, Felice F, Rossiello R, Grimaldi V, Milone L, Casamassimi A, Servillo L, Farzati B, Giovane A, Napoli C. (2008). High glucose downregulates endothelial progenitor cell number via SIRT1. Biochim Biophys Acta. 1784(6):936-945.

Banks AS, Kon N, Knight C, Matsumoto M, Gutiérrez-Juárez R, Rossetti L, Gu W, Accili D. (2008). SirT1 gain of function increases energy efficiency and prevents diabetes in mice. Cell Metab.;8(4):333-341.

Baur JA, Pearson KJ, Price NL, Jamieson HA, Lerin C, Kalra A, Prabhu VV, Allard JS, Lopez-Lluch G, Lewis K, Pistell PJ, Poosala S, Becker KG, Boss O, Gwinn D, Wang M, Ramaswamy S, Fishbein KW, Spencer RG, Lakatta EG, Le Couteur D, Shaw RJ, Navas P, Puigserver P, Ingram DK, de Cabo R, Sinclair DA. (2006). Resveratrol improves health and survival of mice on a high-calorie diet. Nature. 444:337-342.

Berglund ED, Li CY, Bina HA, Lynes SE, Michael MD, Shanafelt AB, Kharitonenkov A, Wasserman DH. (2009). Fibroblast growth factor 21 controls glycemia via regulation of hepatic glucose flux and insulin sensitivity. Endocrinology. 150:4084-4093.

Bishara NB, Ding H. (2010). Glucose enhances expression of TRPC1 and calcium entry in endothelial cells. Am J Physiol Heart Circ Physiol. 298:H171-H178.

Böhm F, Ahlborg G, Pernow J. (2002). Endothelin-1 inhibits endothelium-dependent vasodilatation in the human forearm: reversal by ETA receptor blockade in patients with atherosclerosis. Clin Sci (Lond) 102:321-327.

Bonora E. (2008). Protection of pancreatic beta-cells: is it feasible? Nutr Metab Cardiovasc Dis. 18:74-83.

Booth GL, Kapral MK, Fung K, Tu JV. (2006). Relation between age and cardiovascular disease in men and women with diabetes compared with non-diabetic people: a population-based retrospective cohort study. Lancet. 368(9529):29-36.

Borradaile NM, Pickering JG. (2009). NAD(+), sirtuins, and cardiovascular disease. Curr Pharm Des. 15(1):110-117.

Brandes RP, Fleming I, Busse R. (2005). Endothelial aging. Cardiovasc Res. 66(2):286-294.

Brandes RP. (2008). Activating SIRT1: a new strategy to prevent atherosclerosis? Cardiovasc Res. 80(2):163-164.

Brasacchio D, Okabe J, Tikellis C, Balcerczyk A, George P, Baker EK, Calkin AC, Brownlee M, Cooper ME, El-Osta A. (2009). Hyperglycemia induces a dynamic cooperativity of histone methylase and demethylase enzymes associated with gene-activating epigenetic marks that coexist on the lysine tail. Diabetes; 58:1229-1236.

Calles-Escandón J, Lovato LC, Simons-Morton DG, Kendall DM, Pop-Busui R, Cohen RM, Bonds DE, Fonseca V, Ismail-Beigi F, Banerji MA, Failor A, Hamilton B. (2010).

Effect of intensive compared with standard glycemia treatment strategies on mortality by baseline subgroup characteristics: The ACCORD trial. Diabetes Care. 33(4):721-727.

Cantó C, Gerhart-Hines Z, Feige JN, Lagouge M, Noriega L, Milne JC, Elliott PJ, Puigserver P, Auwerx J. (2009). AMPK regulates energy expenditure by modulating NAD+ metabolism and SIRT1 activity. Nature. 458(7241):1056-1060.

Caton PW, Nayuni NK, Kieswich J, Khan NQ, Yaqoob MM, Corder R. (2010). Metformin suppresses hepatic gluconeogenesis through induction of SIRT1 and GCN5. J Endocrinol. 205(1):97-106.

Ceriello A, Taboga C, Tonutti L, Quagliaro L, Piconi L, Bais B, Da Ros R, Motz E. (2002). Evidence for an independent and cumulative effect of postprandial hypertriglyceridemia and hyperglycemia on endothelial dysfunction and oxidative stress generation: effects of short- and long-term simvastatin treatment. Circulation. 106(10):1211-1218.

Ceriello A. (2005). Postprandial hyperglycemia and diabetes complications: is it time to treat? Diabetes. 54(1):1-7.

Ceriello A, Esposito K, Piconi L, Ihnat MA, Thorpe JE, Testa R, Boemi M, Giugliano D.(2008). Oscillating glucose is more deleterious to endothelial function and oxidative stress than mean glucose in normal and type 2 diabetic patients. Diabetes. 57(5):1349-1354.

Ceriello A, Esposito K, Piconi L, Ihnat M, Thorpe J, Testa R, Bonfigli AR, Giugliano D. (2008).Glucose "peak" and glucose "spike": Impact on endothelial function and oxidative stress. Diabetes Res Clin Pract. 82(2):262-267.

Ceriello A, Ihnat MA, Thorpe JE. (2009). Clinical review 2: The "metabolic memory": is more than just tight glucose control necessary to prevent diabetic complications? J Clin Endocrinol Metab. 94(2):410-415.

Chalmers J, Cooper ME. (2008). UKPDS and the legacy effect. N Engl J Med. 359:1618-1620.

Chau MD, Gao J, Yang Q, Wu Z, Gromada J. (2010). Fibroblast growth factor 21 regulates energy metabolism by activating the AMPK-SIRT1-PGC-1alpha pathway. Proc Natl Acad Sci U S A. 107(28):12553-12558.

Chia CW, Egan JM. (2008). Incretin-based therapies in type 2 diabetes mellitus. J Clin Endocrinol Metab. 93(10):3703-3716.

Cole WC, Chen TT, Clement-Chomienne O. (2005). Myogenic regulation of arterial diameter: role of potassium channels with a focus on delayed rectifier potassium current. Can J Physiol Pharmacol. 83:755-765.

Constans J, Conri C. (2006). Circulating markers of endothelial function in cardiovascular disease. Clin Chim Acta 368:33-47.

Corgnali M, Piconi L, Ihnat M, Ceriello A. (2008). Evaluation of gliclazide ability to attenuate the hyperglycaemic 'memory' induced by high glucose in isolated human endothelial cells. Diabetes Metab Res Rev. 24:301-309.

Crabtree MJ, Smith CL, Lam G, Goligorsky MS, Gross SS. (2008). Ratio of 5,6,7,8-tetrahydrobiopterin to 7,8-dihydrobiopterin in endothelial cells determines glucose-elicited changes in NO vs. superoxide production by eNOS. Am J Physiol Heart Circ Physiol. 294(4):H1530-H1540.

Dali-Youcef N, Lagouge M, Froelich S, Koehl C, Schoonjans K, Auwerx J. (2007). Sirtuins: the 'magnificent seven', function, metabolism and longevity. Ann Med. 39(5):335-345.

David AR, Kershaw A, Heagerty A. (2010). Atherosclerosis and diet in ancient Egypt. Lancet. 375(9716):718-719.

d'Uscio LV, Milstien S, Richardson D, Smith L, Katusic ZS. (2003). Long-term vitamin C treatment increases vascular tetrahydrobiopterin levels and nitric oxide synthase activity. Circ Res. 92(1):88-95.

DCCT: (1993). The Diabetes Control and Complications Trial Research Group: The effect of intensive treatment of diabetes on the development and progression of long-term complications in insulin-dependent diabetes mellitus. N Engl J Med 329:977-986.

Detaille D, Guigas B, Chauvin C, Batandier C, Fontaine E, Wiernsperger N, Leverve X. (2005). Metformin prevents high-glucose-induced endothelial cell death through a mitochondrial permeability transition-dependent process. Diabetes. 54(7):2179-2187.

Diamond J. (2003). The double puzzle of diabetes. Nature. 423(6940):599-602.

Ding H, Aljofan M, Triggle CR. (2007). Oxidative stress and increased eNOS and NADPH oxidase expression in mouse microvessel endothelial cells. J Cell Physiol. 212:682-689.

Ding H, Triggle CR. (2010). Endothelial dysfunction in diabetes: Multiple targets for treatment. Pflügers Archiv Eur J Physiol. 459(6):977-994.

Dobarro D, Gómez-Rubín MC, Sanchez-Recalde A, Moreno R, Galeote G, Jimenez-Valero S, Calvo L, López de Sá E, López-Sendón JL. (2009). Current pharmacological approach to restore endothelial dysfunction. Cardiovasc Hematol Agents Med Chem. 7(3):212-222.

Dong Y, Zhang M, Liang B, Xie Z, Zhao Z, Asfa S, Choi HC, Zou MH. (2010). Reduction of AMP-activated protein kinase {alpha}2 increases endoplasmic reticulum stress and atherosclerosis in vivo. Circulation. 121(6):792-803.

Duckworth W, Abraira C, Moritz T, Reda D, Emanuele N, Reaven PD, Zieve FJ, Marks J, Davis SN, Hayward R, Warren SR, Goldman S, McCarren M, Vitek ME, Henderson WG, Huang GD; VADT Investigators. (2009). Glucose control and vascular complications in veterans with type 2 diabetes. N Engl J Med. 360:129-139.

Dunstan DW, Zimmet PZ, Welborn TA, Cameron AJ, Shaw J, de Courten M, Jolley D, McCarty DJ; Australian Diabetes, Obesity and Lifestyle Study (AusDiab). (2002. The Australian Diabetes, Obesity and Lifestyle Study (AusDiab)--methods and response rates. Diabetes Res Clin Pract. 57(2):119-129.

Dusting GJ, Triggle C. (2005). Are we over oxidized? Oxidative stress, cardiovascular disease, and the future of intervention studies with antioxidants. Vasc Health Risk Manag. 1(2):93-97.

Dyson MC, Alloosh M, Vuchetich JP, Mokelke EA, Sturek M. (2006). Components of metabolic syndrome and coronary artery disease in female Ossabaw swine fed excess atherogenic diet. Comp Med. 56(1):35-45.

Edwards, JM, Neeb ZP, Alloosh MA, Long X, Bratz IN, Peller CR, Byrd JP, Kumar S, Obukhov AG, Sturek M. (2010). Exercise training decreases store-operated Ca2+entry associated with metabolic syndrome and coronary atherosclerosis. Cardiovasc Res. 85(3):631-640.

Eizirik DL, Björklund A, Cagliero E. (1993). Genotoxic agents increase expression of growth arrest and DNA damage--inducible genes gadd 153 and gadd 45 in rat pancreatic islets.Diabetes. 42(5):738-745.

Eizirik DL, Cardozo AK, Cnop M. (2008). The role for endoplasmic reticulum stress in diabetes mellitus. Endocr Rev. 29:42-61

El-Osta A, Brasacchio D, Yao D, Pocai A, Jones PL, Roeder RG, Cooper ME, Brownlee M. (2008) Transient high glucose causes persistent epigenetic changes and altered gene expression during subsequent normoglycemia. J Exp Med 205:2409-2417.

Emanuele NV. (2010). Duration of diabetes, glucose control and cardiovascular risk. Diabetologia. 53:214-215.

Emerging Risk Factors Collaboration [ERFC], Sarwar N, Gao P, Seshasai SR, Gobin R, Kaptoge S, Di Angelantonio E, Ingelsson E, Lawlor DA, Selvin E, Stampfer M, Stehouwer CD, Lewington S, Pennells L, Thompson A, Sattar N, White IR, Ray KK, Danesh J. (2010). Diabetes mellitus, fasting blood glucose concentration, and risk of vascular disease: a collaborative meta-analysis of 102 prospective studies. Lancet. 375(9733):2215-2222.

Emerging Risk Factors Collaboration [ERFC], Seshasai SR, Kaptoge S, Thompson A, Di Angelantonio E, Gao P, Sarwar N, Whincup PH, Mukamal KJ, Gillum RF, Holme I, Njølstad I, Fletcher A, Nilsson P, Lewington S, Collins R, Gudnason V, Thompson SG, Sattar N, Selvin E, Hu FB, Danesh J. (2011). Diabetes mellitus, fasting glucose, and risk of cause-specific death. N Engl J Med. 364(9):829-41. Erratum in: N Engl J Med. 2011 Mar 31;364(13):1281.

Esper RJ, Nordaby RA, Vilariño JO, Paragano A, Cacharrón JL, Machado RA. (2006). Endothelial dysfunction: a comprehensive appraisal. (2006). Cardiovasc Diabetol. 23;5:4.

Fonseca SG, Burcin M, Gromada J, Urano F. (2009). Endoplasmic reticulum stress in beta-cells and development of diabetes. Curr Opin Pharmacol. 9(6):763-770.

Foretz M, Hébrard S, Leclerc J, Zarrinpashneh E, Soty M, Mithieux G, Sakamoto K, Andreelli F, Viollet B. (2010). Metformin inhibits hepatic gluconeogenesis in mice independently of the LKB1/AMPK pathway via a decrease in hepatic energy state. J Clin Invest. 120(7):2355-2369.

Fon Tacer K, Bookout AL, Ding X, Kurosu H, John GB, Wang L, Goetz R, Mohammadi M, Kuro-o M, Mangelsdorf DJ, Kliewer SA. (2010). Research resource: Comprehensive expression atlas of the fibroblast growth factor system in adult mouse. Mol Endocrinol. 2010; 24:2050-2064.

Freedman DS; Centers for Disease Control and Prevention (CDC). (2011). Obesity - United States, 1988-2008. MMWR Surveill Summ. 60 Suppl:73-77.

Furchgott RF, Zawadzki JV. (1980). The obligatory role of endothelial cells in the relaxation of arterial smooth muscle by acetylcholine. Nature 288:373-376.

Jackson JG, Kreisberg JI, Koterba AP, Yee D, Brattain MG. (2000). Phosphorylation and nuclear exclusion of the forkhead transcription factor FKHR after epidermal growth factor treatment in human breast cancer cells. Oncogene. 19(40):4574-4581.

Liang H, Ward WF. Liang H, Ward WF. (2006). PGC-1alpha: a key regulator of energy metabolism Adv Physiol Educ.30(4):145-151.

Gerstein HC, Waltman L. (2006). Why don't pigs get diabetes? Explanations for variations in diabetes susceptibility in human populations living in a diabetogenic environment. CMAJ. 174:25-26.

Goldfine AB. (2008). Assessing the cardiovascular safety of diabetes therapies. N Engl J Med. 359:1092-1095.

Grundy SM, Howard B, Smith S Jr, Eckel R, Redberg R, Bonow RO. (2002). Prevention Conference VI: Diabetes and Cardiovascular Disease: Executive Summary: Conference Proceeding for Healthcare Professionals From a Special Writing Group of the American Heart Association. Circulation 105:2231-2239.

Hales CN, Barker DJ. (2001). The thrifty phenotype hypothesis. Br Med Bull. 60:5-20.

Handelsman Y, Mechanick JI, Blonde L, Grunberger G, Bloomgarden ZT, Bray GA, Dagogo-Jack S, Davidson JA, Einhorn D, Ganda O, Garber AJ, Hirsch IB, Horton ES, Ismail-Beigi F, Jellinger PS, Jones KL, Jovanovič L, Lebovitz H, Levy P, Moghissi ES, Orzeck EA, Vinik AI, Wyne KL. (2011). AACE Task Force for Developing Diabetes Comprehensive Care Plan. American Association of Clinical Endocrinologists Medical Guidelines for Clinical Practice for developing a diabetes mellitus comprehensive care plan. Endocr Pract. 17 Suppl 2:1-53.

Hanefeld M, Koehler C, Henkel E, Fuecker K, Schaper F, Temelkova-Kurktschiev T. (2000). Post-challenge hyperglycaemia relates more strongly than fasting hyperglycaemia with carotid intima-media thickness: the RIAD Study. Risk Factors in Impaired Glucose Tolerance for Atherosclerosis and Diabetes. Diabet Med. 17(12):835-840.

Hansen KB, Vilsbøll T, Knop FK. (2010). Incretin mimetics: a novel therapeutic option for patients with type 2 diabetes - a review. Diabetes Metab Syndr Obes. 3:155-163.

Harris MI, Flegal KM, Cowie CC, Eberhardt MS, Goldstein DE, Little RR, Wiedmeyer HM, Byrd-Holt DD. (1998). Prevalence of diabetes, impaired fasting glucose, and impaired glucose tolerance in U.S. adults. The Third National Health and Nutrition Examination Survey, 1988-1994. Diabetes Care. 21(4):518-524.

Holness MJ, Caton PW, Sugden MC. (2010). Acute and long-term nutrient-led modifications of gene expression: potential role of SIRT1 as a central co-ordinator of short and longer-term programming of tissue function. Nutrition. 26(5):491-501.

Hondares E, Iglesias R, Giralt A, Gonzalez FJ, Giralt M, Mampel T, Villarroya F. Thermogenic activation induces FGF21 expression and release in brown adipose tissue. *J Biol Chem*. 2011; Feb 13. [Epub ahead of print]

Hosoi T, Ozawa K. (2010). Endoplasmic reticulum stress in disease: mechanisms and therapeutic opportunities. Clin Sci 118:18-29.

Huang A, Vita JA, Venema RC, Keaney JF Jr. (2000). Ascorbic acid enhances endothelial nitric-oxide synthase activity by increasing intracellular tetrahydrobiopterin. J Biol Chem. 275(23):17399-17406.

Hummasti S, Hotamisligil GS. (2010). Endoplasmic reticulum stress and inflammation in obesity and diabetes. Circ Res. 107(5):579-591.

Hvidberg A, Nielsen M T, Hilsted J, Orskov C, Holst JJ. (1994). "Effect of glucagon-like peptide-1 (proglucagon 78-107amide) on hepatic glucose production in healthy man", Metabolism 43(1): pp. 104–108.

Ihlemann N, Rask-Madsen C, Perner A, Dominguez H, Hermann T, Køber L, Torp-dersen C. (2003). Tetrahydrobiopterin restores endothelial dysfunction induced by an oral glucose challenge in healthy subjects. Am J Physiol Heart Circ Physiol. 285:H875-H882.

Jabbour S, Ziring B. (2011). Advantages of extended-release metformin in patients with type 2 diabetes mellitus. Postgrad Med. 123(1):15-23.

Kannel WB, McGee DL. (1979). Diabetes and glucose tolerance as risk factors for cardiovascular disease: the Framingham Study. Diabetes Care 2:120-126.

Kawano H, Motoyama T, Hirashima O, Hirai N, Miyao Y, Sakamoto T, Kugiyama K, Ogawa H, Yasue H. (1999). Hyperglycemia rapidly suppresses flow-mediated endothelium-dependent vasodilation of brachial artery. J Am Coll Cardiol 34:146-154.

Kharitonenkov A, Shiyanova TL, Koester A, Ford AM, Micanovic R, Galbreath EJ, Sandusky GE, Hammond LJ, Moyers JS, Owens RA, Gromada J, Brozinick JT, Hawkins ED, Wroblewski VJ, Li DS, Mehrbod F, Jaskunas SR, Shanafelt AB. (2005). FGF-21 as a novel metabolic regulator. J Clin Invest. 115:1627-1635.

Kharitonenkov A, Shanafelt AB. (2009). FGF21: a novel prospect for the treatment of metabolic diseases. Curr Opin Investig Drugs. 10:359-364.

Kharitonenkov A, Larsen P. (2011). FGF21 reloaded: challenges of a rapidly growing field. Trends Endocrinol Metab. 22:81-86.

Kharitonenkov A, Shanafelt AB. (2009). FGF21: a novel prospect for the treatment of metabolic diseases. Curr Opin Investig Drugs. 10:359-364.

Kharitonenkov A, Larsen P. (2011). FGF21 reloaded: challenges of a rapidly growing field. Trends Endocrinol Metab. 22:81-86.

Klimentidis YC, Beasley TM, Lin HY, Murati G, Glass GE, Guyton M, Newton W, Jorgensen M, Heymsfield SB, Kemnitz J, Fairbanks L, Allison DB. (2011). Canaries in the coal mine: a cross species analysis of the plurity of obesity epidemics. Proc Biol Sci.;278(1712):1626-1632.

Knot, HJ & Nelson, MT. (1995). Regulation of membrane potential and diameter by voltage-dependent K+ channels in rabbit myogenic cerebral arteries. Am J Physiol. 269(1 Pt 2):H348-H355.

Komajda M, McMurray JJ, Beck-Nielsen H, Gomis R, Hanefeld M, Pocock SJ, Curtis PS, Jones NP, Home PD. (2010). Heart failure events with rosiglitazone in type 2 diabetes: data from the RECORD clinical trial. Eur Heart J. 31(7):824-831.

Kume S, Uzu T, Kashiwagi A, Koya D. (2010). SIRT1, a calorie restriction mimetic, in a new therapeutic approach for type 2 diabetes mellitus and diabetic vascular complications. Endocr Metab Immune Disord Drug Targets. 10(1):16-24.

Kumar B, Dreja K, Shah SS, Cheong A, Xu SZ, Sukumar P, Naylor J, Forte A, Cipollaro M, McHugh D, Kingston PA, Heagerty AM, Munsch CM, Bergdahl A, Hultgårdh-Nilsson A, Gomez MF, Porter KE, Hellstrand P, Beech DJ. (2006). Upregulated TRPC1 channel in vascular injury in vivo and its role in human neointimal hyperplasia. Circ Res. 98(4):557-563.

Lan F, Cacicedo JM, Ruderman N, Ido Y. (2008). SIRT1 modulation of the acetylation status, cytosolic localization, and activity of LKB1. Possible role in AMP-activated protein kinase activation. J Biol Chem. 283(41):27628-27635.

Lavu S, Boss O, Elliott PJ, Lambert PD. (2008). Sirtuins--novel therapeutic targets to treat age-associated diseases. Nat Rev Drug Discov. 7(10):841-853. Review. Erratum in: Nat Rev Drug Discov. 2009 8(6):516.

Li Y, Xu S, Giles A, Nakamura K, Lee JW, Hou X, Donmez G, Li J, Luo Z, Walsh K, Guarente L, Zang M. (2011). Hepatic overexpression of SIRT1 in mice attenuates endoplasmic reticulum stress and insulin resistance in the liver. FASEB J. 2011 Feb 24. [Epub ahead of print]

C. M. McCay, CM, Crowell, MF, Maynard LA (1935). The Effect of Retarded Growth Upon the Length of Life Span and Upon the Ultimate Body Size. *J. Nutr.* 10(1):63-79.

McKenzie, MD, Jamieson, E, Jansen, ES, Scott, CL, Huang, DCS, Bouillet, P, Allison, J, Kay, TWH, Strasser, A, Thomas, HE. (2010). Glucose Induces Pancreatic Islet Cell Apoptosis That Requires the BH3-Only Proteins Bim and Puma and Multi-BH Domain Protein Bax Diabetes 59: 644-652.

Mashili FL, Austin RL, Deshmukh AS, Fritz T, Caidahl K, Bergdahl K, Zierath JR, Chibalin AV, Moller DE, Kharitonenkov A, Krook A. (2011). Direct effects of FGF21 on glucose uptake in human skeletal muscle: implications for type 2 diabetes and obesity. Diabetes Metab Res Rev. 27:286-297.

Masoro EJ. (2005). Overview of caloric restriction and ageing. Mech Ageing Dev. 126(9):913-22.

Mather KJ, Verma S, Anderson TJ. (2001). Improved endothelial function with metformin in type 2 diabetes mellitus. J Am Coll Cardiol. 37(5):1344-1350.

Mattagajasingh I, Kim CS, Naqvi A, Yamamori T, Hoffman TA, Jung SB, DeRicco J, Kasuno K, Irani K. (2007). SIRT1 promotes endothelium-dependent vascular relaxation by activating endothelial nitric oxide synthase. Proc Natl Acad Sci U S A. 104(37):14855-14860.

Mazzone T. (2010). Intensive glucose lowering and cardiovascular disease prevention in diabetes: reconciling the recent clinical trial data. Circulation. 122:2201-2211.

McLenachan JM, Vita J, Fish DR, Treasure CB, Cox DA, Ganz P, Selwyn AP. (1990). Early evidence of endothelial vasodilator dysfunction at coronary branch points. Circulation. 82:1169-1173.

Michan S, Sinclair D. (2007). Sirtuins in mammals: insights into their biological function. Biochem J. 404(1):1-13.

Miller JC, Colagiuri S. (1994). The carnivore connection: dietary carbohydrate in the evolution of NIDDM. Diabetologia. 37(12):1280-1286.

Milne JC, Lambert PD, Schenk S, Carney DP, Smith JJ, Gagne DJ, Jin L, Boss O, Perni RB, Vu CB, Bemis JE, Xie R, Disch JS, Ng PY, Nunes JJ, Lynch AV, Yang H, Galonek H, Israelian K, Choy W, Iffland A, Lavu S, Medvedik O, Sinclair DA, Olefsky JM, Jirousek MR, Elliott PJ, Westphal CH. (2007). Small molecule activators of SIRT1 as therapeutics for the treatment of type 2 diabetes. Nature. 450(7170):712-716.

Mohamad RH, Zekry ZK, Al-Mehdar HA, Salama O, El-Shaieb SE, El-Basmy AA, Al-said MG, Sharawy SM. (2009). Camel milk as an adjuvant therapy for the treatment of type 1 diabetes: verification of a traditional ethnomedical practice. J Med Food. 12(2):461-465.

Monnier L, Mas E, Ginet C, Michel F, Villon L, Cristol JP, Colette C. (2006). Activation of oxidative stress by acute glucose fluctuations compared with sustained chronic hyperglycemia in patients with type 2 diabetes. JAMA. 295(14):1681-1687.

Moreno-Navarrete JM, Ortega FJ, Rodríguez-Hermosa JI, Sabater M, Pardo G, Ricart W, Fernández-Real JM. (2011). OCT1 Expression in adipocytes could contribute to increased metformin action in obese subjects. Diabetes. 60(1):168-176.

MRC/BHF Heart Protection Study (2002). Antioxidant vitamin supplementation in 20,536 high-risk individuals: a randomised placebo-controlled trial *The Lancet* 360:23-33.

Nagashima T, Shigematsu N, Maruki R, Urano Y, Tanaka H, Shimaya A, Shimokawa T, Shibasaki M. (2010). Discovery of novel forkhead box O1 inhibitors for treating type 2 diabetes: improvement of fasting glycemia in diabetic db/db mice. Mol Pharmacol. 78(5):961-970.

Neel JV (1962). "Diabetes mellitus: a "thrifty" genotype rendered detrimental by "progress"?" Am. J. Hum. Genet. 14:353–62.

Nilsson PM. (2010). ACCORD and Risk-Factor Control in Type 2 Diabetes. N Engl J Med. 362(17):1628-1630.

Oyadomari S, Mori M. (2004). Roles of CHOP/GADD153 in endoplasmic reticulum stress. Cell Death Differ. 11(4):381-389.

Pannirselvam M, Verma S, Anderson TJ, Triggle CR. (2002). Cellular basis of endothelial dysfunction in small mesenteric arteries from spontaneously diabetic (db/db -/-) mice: role of decreased tetrahydrobiopterin bioavailability. Br J Pharmacol 136:255-263.

Pannirselvam M, Simon V, Verma S, Anderson T, Triggle CR. (2003). Chronic oral supplementation with sepiapterin prevents endothelial dysfunction and oxidative stress in small mesenteric arteries from diabetic (db/db) mice. Br J Pharmacol 140:701-706.

Pannirselvam M, Ding H, Anderson TJ, Triggle CR. (2006). Pharmacological characteristics of endothelium-derived hyperpolarizing factor-mediated relaxation of small mesenteric arteries from db/db mice. Eur J Pharmacol 551:98-107.

Patil C, Walter P. (2001). Intracellular signaling from the endoplasmic reticulum to the nucleus: the unfolded protein response in yeast and mammals. Curr Opin Cell Biol. 13(3):349-355.

Potente M, Dimmeler S. (2008). Emerging roles of SIRT1 in vascular endothelial homeostasis. Cell Cycle. 7(14):2117-2122.

Prentice AM, Hennig BJ, Fulford AJ. (2008). Evolutionary origins of the obesity epidemic: natural selection of thrifty genes or genetic drift following predation release? Int J Obes (Lond). 32(11):1607-1610.

Queisser, MA, Yao, D, Geisler, S, Hammes, H-P, Lochnit, G, Schleicher, ED, Brownlee, M, Preissner, KT. (2010). Hyperglycemia Impairs Proteasome Function by Methylglyoxal. Diabetes 59: 670-678.

Rainbow RD, Hardy ME, Standen NB, Davies NW (2006) Glucose reduces endothelin inhibition of voltage-gated potassium channels in rat arterial smooth muscle cells. J Physiol. 575:833-844.

Ray KK, Seshasai SR, Wijesuriya S, Sivakumaran R, Nethercott S, Preiss D, Erqou S, Sattar N. (2009). Effect of intensive control of glucose on cardiovascular outcomes and death in patients with diabetes mellitus: a meta-analysis of randomised controlled trials. Lancet. 373(9677):1765-1772.

Robertson RP. (2004). Chronic oxidative stress as a central mechanism for glucose toxicity in pancreatic islet beta cells in diabetes. J Biol Chem. 279:42351-42354.

Rotella CM, Monami M, Mannucci E. (2006). Metformin beyond diabetes: new life for an old drug. Curr Diabetes Rev. 2(3):307-315.

Shaw RJ, Lamia KA, Vasquez D, Koo SH, Bardeesy N, Depinho RA, Montminy M, Cantley LC. N. (2005). The kinase LKB1 mediates glucose homeostasis in liver and therapeutic effects of metformin. Science. 310(5754):1642-1646.

Sheikh-Ali M, Sultan S, Alamir AR, Haas MJ, Mooradian AD. (2010a). Hyperglycemia-induced endoplasmic reticulum stress in endothelial cells. Nutrition. 26(11-12):1146-1150

Sheikh-Ali M, Sultan S, Alamir AR, Haas MJ, Mooradian AD. (2010b). Effects of antioxidants on glucose-induced oxidative stress and endoplasmic reticulum stress in endothelial cells. Diabetes Res Clin Pract. 87(2):161-6.

Speakman JR. (2008). Thrifty genes for obesity, an attractive but flawed idea, and an alternative perspective: the 'drifty gene' hypothesis. Int J Obes (Lond). 32(11):1611-1617.

Standl E, Müller M, Schnell O. (2009). The impact of glucose-lowering therapy on cardiovascular outcomes. Best Pract Res Clin Endocrinol Metab. 23(3):401-411.

Straub SV, Nelson MT. (2006). A spoonful of sugar helps the KV channel activity go down. J Physiol. 575(3):691.

Tabas I. (2010). The role of endoplasmic reticulum stress in the progression of atherosclerosis. Circ Res. 107(7):839-850.

Tanaka H, Nagashima T, Shimaya A, Urano Y, Shimokawa T, Shibasaki M. (2010). Effects of the novel Foxo1 inhibitor AS1708727 on plasma glucose and triglyceride levels in diabetic db/db mice. Eur J Pharmacol. 645(1-3):185-191.

Temelkova-Kurktschiev TS, Koehler C, Henkel E, Leonhardt W, Fuecker K, Hanefeld M. (2000). Postchallenge plasma glucose and glycemic spikes are more strongly associated with atherosclerosis than fasting glucose or HbA1c level. Diabetes Care. 23(12):1830-1834.

Thewissen JG, Madar SI. (1999). Ankle morphology of the earliest Cetaceans and its implications for the phylogenetic relations among ungulates. Syst Biol. (1):21-30.

Thorand B, Baumert J, Döring A, Schneider A, Chambless L, Löwel H, Kolb H, Koenig W. (2006). Association of cardiovascular risk factors with markers of endothelial dysfunction in middle-aged men and women. Results from the MONICA/KORA Augsburg Study. Thromb Haemost 95:134-141.

Tiedge M, Lortz S, Drinkgern J, Lenzen S. (1997). Relation between antioxidant enzyme gene expression and antioxidative defense status of insulin-producing cells. Diabetes. 46:1733-1742.

Triggle CR, Ding H. (2010). A review of endothelial dysfunction in diabetes: A focus on the contribution of a dysfunctional eNOS. J. American Society for Hypertension 2010. 4(3):102-115.

Triggle CR, Howarth A, Cheng ZJ, Ding H. (2005). Twenty-five years since the discovery of endothelium-derived relaxing factor (EDRF): does a dysfunctional endothelium contribute to the development of type 2 diabetes? Can J Physiol Pharmacol. 83(8-9):681-700.

Tu BP, Weissman JS. (2004). Oxidative protein folding in eukaryotes: mechanisms and consequences. J Cell Biol. 164(3):341-346.

Turnbull FM, Abraira C, Anderson RJ, Byington RP, Chalmers JP, Duckworth WC, Evans GW, Gerstein HC, Holman RR, Moritz TE, Neal BC, Ninomiya T, Patel AA, Paul SK, Travert F, Woodward M. (2009). Intensive glucose control and macrovascular outcomes in type 2 diabetes. Diabetologia 52:2288-2298.

UKPDS: UK Prospective Diabetes Study (UKPDS) Group: UK Prospective Diabetes Study (UKPDS). VIII. (1991). Study design, progress and performance. Diabetologia 34:877-890.

UKPDS 28: a randomized trial of efficacy of early addition of metformin in sulfonylurea-treated type 2 diabetes. (1998). U.K. Prospective Diabetes Study Group. Diabetes Care. 21:87-92.

Um J-H, Park S-J, Kang H, Yang S, Foretz M, McBurney MW, Kim MK, Viollet B, Chung JH. (2010). AMP-Activated Protein Kinase–Deficient Mice Are Resistant to the Metabolic Effects of Resveratrol Diabetes 59:554-563.

van Breemen C, Poburko D, Okon EB. (2006). TRP proteins: a new dimension in the treatment of occlusive vascular disease. Circ Res. 98(4):446-447.

Vanhoutte PM. (2010). Regeneration of the endothelium in vascular injury. Cardiovasc Drugs Ther. 24(4):299-303.

Venn-Watson SK, Ridgway SH. (2007). Big brains and blood glucose: common ground for diabetes mellitus in humans and healthy dolphins. Comp Med. 57:390-395.

Venn-Watson S, Carlin K, Ridgway S. (2011). Dolphins as animal models for type 2 diabetes: sustained, post-prandial hyperglycemia and hyperinsulinemia. Gen Comp Endocrinol. 170(1):193-199.

Vlassara H, Palace MR. (2002). Diabetes and advanced glycation endproducts. J Intern Med. 251(2):87-101.

Wang Y, Liang Y, Vanhoutte PM. (2011). SIRT1 and AMPK in regulating mammalian senescence: A critical review and a working model. FEBS Lett. 585(7):986-994.

Werns SW, Walton JA, Hsia HH, Nabel EG, Sanz ML, Pitt B. (1989). Evidence of endothelial dysfunction in angiographically normal coronary arteries of patients with coronary artery disease. Circulation 79:287-291.

Whitfield J. (2003). Fat pigs ape obese humans Nature Science News on line doi:10.1038/news030804-5

Wild S, Roglic G, Green A, Sicree R, King H. (2004). Global prevalence of diabetes: estimates for the year 2000 and projections for 2030. Diabetes Care. 27(5):1047-1053.

Woerle HJ, Neumann C, Zschau S, Tenner S, Irsigler A, Schirra J, Gerich JE, Göke B. (2007). Impact of fasting and postprandial glycemia on overall glycemic control in type 2 diabetes Importance of postprandial glycemia to achieve target HbA1c levels. Diabetes Res Clin Pract. 77(2):280-285.

Yang Y, Hou H, Haller EM, Nicosia SV, Bai W. (2005). Suppression of FOXO1 activity by FHL2 through SIRT1-mediated deacetylation. EMBO J. 24(5):1021-1032.

Yudkin JS, Richter B. (2010). Using individual patient data in meta-analyses of glucose-lowering studies. Diabetologia. 53:216-217.

Zhang QJ, Wang Z, Chen HZ, Zhou S, Zheng W, Liu G, Wei YS, Cai H, Liu DP, Liang CC. (2008). Endothelium-specific overexpression of class III deacetylase SIRT1 decreases atherosclerosis in apolipoprotein E-deficient mice. Cardiovasc Res. 80(2):191-199.

Zhou G, Myers R, Li Y, Chen Y, Shen X, Fenyk-Melody J, Wu M, Ventre J, Doebber T, Fujii N, Musi N, Hirshman MF, Goodyear LJ, Moller DE. (2001). Role of AMP-activated protein kinase in mechanism of metformin action. J Clin Invest. 108(8):1167-1174.

Zhou Y, Lee J, Reno CM, Sun C, Park SW, Chung J, Lee J, Fisher SJ, White MF, Biddinger SB, Ozcan U. (2011). Regulation of glucose homeostasis through a XBP-1-FoxO1 interaction. Nat Med. 17(3):356-365.

Zinn AR. (2010). Unconventional wisdom about the obesity epidemic. Am J Med Sci. 340(6):481-491.

Zou MH, Kirkpatrick SS, Davis BJ, Nelson JS, Wiles WG 4th, Schlattner U, Neumann D, Brownlee M, Freeman MB, Goldman MH. (2004). Activation of the AMP-activated protein kinase by the anti-diabetic drug metformin in vivo. Role of mitochondrial reactive nitrogen species. J Biol Chem. 279(42):43940-43951.

Zu Y, Liu L, Lee MY, Xu C, Liang Y, Man RY, Vanhoutte PM, Wang Y. (2010). SIRT1 promotes proliferation and prevents senescence through targeting LKB1 in primary porcine aortic endothelial cells. Circ Res. 106(8):1384-1393.

7

Endothelial Dysfunction and Therapeutic Intervention in Type 2 Diabetes

Fernando Grover Páez
Centro Universitario de Ciencias de la Salud, Universidad de Guadalajara
México

1. Introduction

Diabetes mellitus (DM) is a major risk factor for micro and macrovascular complications (Kannel & McGee, 1979; King & Sheetz, 2002), and is associated with endothelial dysfunction, premature atherosclerosis (Johnstone et al., 1993; Nathan et al., 2003; Williams et al., 2005), and a reduced capability of neovascularization in ischemic conditions (Abaci et al., 1999). Hyperglycemia increases the production of superoxide (O2-) and reduces the bioavailability of nitric oxide (NO) resulting in the development of endothelial dysfunction in diabetic patients (Creager et al., 2003; Loomans et al., 2005). Exposure to oxidative stress induces a pro-inflammatory response and increases endothelial cell apoptosis, which leads to a disturbance in the endothelial monolayer. The denuded vessel wall is highly pro-atherogenic, so fast regeneration of the endothelium is essential to prevent formation of atherosclerotic plaques (Dimmeler et al., 2002; Dimmeler & Zeiher, 2004).
Patients with type 2 diabetes suffer disturbances in the intermediate metabolism of carbohydrates, proteins and lipids, caused by poor insulin secretion what leads to chronically sustained hyperglycemia. As a result, insulin-resistance develops in target organs and at peripheral sites, the main cause of the pathogenesis related to type 2 diabetes (Cerrato, 2004). Hyperinsulinemia promotes atherogenesis through cell proliferation at the vascular wall which produces endothelial damage (Mátthael & Stumvall, 2001). These endothelial alterations induce the early appearance of atherosclerosis, altering vascular homeostasis mainly due to the interaction of nitric oxide (NO) and free oxygen radicals. As a consequence of this interaction the endothelial anti-inflammatory and vasodilator properties are perturbed which leads to endothelial cell death, proliferation and inadequate restructuring of the vascular walls (Galle et al., 2003). While endothelial damage and the underlying inflammatory processes are often detected later, endothelial damage occurs before the atherosclerotic plate can be identified (Bots et al., 1997). There are many biomarkers for inflammation and early endothelial dysfunction that can be used to identify endothelial damage in order to prevent cardiovascular disease (CD), including: high sensitivity C reactive protein (hs-CRP), homocysteine, microalbuminuria, glycosylated hemoglobin (A1c), Von Willebrand factor and plasminogen-activator inhibitor type 1 (Reinhart et al., 2002). Elevated hs-CRP appears to be a strong predictor for future cardiovascular events (Tornel et al., 2003). On the other hand, much interest has been generated in determining serum homocysteine levels due to the relationship with CD (de Luis et al., 2004). Indeed, elevated serum homocysteine levels have been associated with a

greater risk of developing thrombosis, as well as an increase in the production of hydrogen peroxide and in the oxidation of low-density lipoprotein cholesterol (LDL-C), leading to endothelial damage (Retterstol et al., 2003). At the same time, while microalbuminuria is an important risk factor for nephropathy in type 1 diabetes patients, in type 2 diabetes patients it serves as a predictor of CD (Festa et al., 2000).

Over the last two decades it has become evident that the endothelium is not an inert, single-cell lining covering the internal surface of blood vessels, but in fact plays a crucial role in regulating vascular tone and structure. Importantly, a healthy endothelium inhibits platelet and leukocyte adhesion to the vascular surface and maintains a balance of profibrinolytic and prothrombotic activity (Libby, 2002). Endothelial dysfunction has received increasing attention as a potential contributor to the pathogenesis of vascular disease in diabetes mellitus. Under physiological conditions, there is a balanced release of endothelial-derived relaxing and contracting factors, but this delicate balance is altered in diabetes and atherosclerosis, thereby contributing to further progression of vascular and end-organ damage (Tan et al., 2002).

Hyperglycemia is the major causal factor in the development of endothelial dysfunction in diabetes mellitus. Although the mechanisms underlying this phenomenon are likely to be multifactorial. Insulin resistance has been described in several diseases that increase cardiovascular risk and mortality, such as diabetes, obesity, hypertension, metabolic syndrome, and heart failure. Increasing evidence suggests that the progression of insulin resistance to type 2 diabetes parallels the progression of endothelial dysfunction to atherosclerosis. Insulin resistance is closely linked with visceral adiposity, and early data suggested that free fatty acids were responsible for this association (Boden & Shulman, 2002). More recently, other plasma biomarkers produced by adipose tissue, including TNF and resistin, have been shown to have elevated levels during obesity and to mediate insulin resistance. Conversely, the expression and secretion of adiponectin, an adipocyte-specific protein that enhances insulin-mediated glucose uptake, is inversely correlated with fat mass (Lyon et al., 2003). Several studies have demonstrated that nitric oxide (NO)-mediated vasodilation is abnormal in patients with type 2 diabetes (Williams et al., 1996). Brachial artery responses were found to be abnormal to both endogenous and exogenous NO donors, suggesting that there was increased inactivation of NO, possibly caused by enhanced metabolism of NO or abnormal vascular smooth muscle cell (VSMC) responses to NO because of alterations in signal transduction in the guanylate cyclase pathway. Obese patients without frank type 2 diabetes have been shown also to have abnormal endothelial function (Perticone et al., 2001; Steinberg et al., 1996).

Diminished capacity of NOS to generate NO has been demonstrated experimentally when ECs are exposed either in vitro or in vivo to a diabetic environment (Cosentino & Luscher, 1998; Huszka et al., 1997; Huvers et al., 1999; Lambert et al., 1996). The EC is then a target of the diabetic milieu and endothelial dysfunction is thought to play an important role in the vasculopathy of this disease state. A large body of evidence in humans indicates that endothelial dysfunction is closely associated to microangiopathy and atherosclerosis in both types 1 and 2 diabetes mellitus (Cosentino & Luscher, 1998). This association is particularly true in those patients with type 1 diabetes who have either early (microalbuminuria) or late (macroalbuminuria) nephropathy. In these patients, a great variety of markers indicate endothelial dysfunction: poor EC-dependent vasodilation, increased blood levels of von Willebrand factor (vWF), thrombomodulin, selectin, PAI-1, type IV collagen, and t-PA (Cosentino & Luscher, 1998; Furchgott & Zawadzki, 1980; Schneider et al., 2002). Once established, EC dysfunction can, in turn, induce alterations in vessels that worsen vasculopathy and progress disease. Hyperglycemia may lead to intracellular changes in the redox state resulting in depletion of the cellular NADPH pool. Overexpression of growth factors has also been implicated in diabetes with proliferation of both endothelial cells and vascular smooth muscle, possibly promoting neovascularization. The diabetic state is typified by an increased tendency for oxidative stress and high levels of oxidized lipoproteins, especially the so-called small, dense low-density lipoprotein. The high levels of fatty acids and hyperglycemia have also both been shown to induce an increased level of oxidation of phospholipids as well as proteins. In humans it is associated with a prothrombotic tendency as well as increased platelet aggregation, with tumor necrosis factor implicated as a link between insulin resistance, diabetes, and endothelial dysfunction; a hypothesis has been advanced that insulin and/or insulin precursors may be atherogenic. The general consensus is that the occurrence of endothelial cell dysfunction in type 1 diabetes signifies a very high risk of micro- and macroangiopathy, and although the diabetic state predisposes to endothelial cell dysfunction in this disease, it is not sufficient to cause it. It is more likely that other agents (genes, environment) have a role in determining which patients will develop aggressive angiopathy and hence endothelial cell dysfunction. Irrespective of whether endothelial cell dysfunction is a cause or a consequence of vascular injury in type 1 diabetes, it is hoped that therapeutic efforts aimed at restoring endothelial cell function to normal will affect the natural history of vasculopathy in type 1 diabetes (Cosentino & Luscher, 1998). Impaired endothelium-dependent vasodilatation has been demonstrated in various vascular beds of different animal models of diabetes and in humans with type 1 and 2 diabetes. Several mechanisms of endothelial dysfunction have been reported, including impaired signal transduction or substrate availibility, impaired release of endothelium-derived relaxing factors (EDRF), increased destruction of EDRF, enhanced release of endothelium-derived constricting factors and decreased sensitivity of the vascular smooth muscle to EDRF. The principal mediators of hyperglycemia-induced endothelial dysfunction may be activation of protein kinase C, increased activity of the polyol pathway, nonenzymatic glycation and oxidative stress. Both insulin and glucose play a role in ET-1 release. Insulin activates ET-1 production by endothelial cells, and hyperglycemia leads to the formation of advanced glycation end products (AGEs) that promote ET-1 production by endothelial cells through the activation of transcription factor NF-kB. Diabetic patients, both those with type I diabetes and those with insulin resistance, present increased ET-1 plasma concentrations. AGEs are known to trigger vascular inflammation and endothelial dysfunction. The hyperglycemia associated with diabetes can lead to modification of macromolecules, for example, by forming AGEs. By binding surface receptors such as RAGE (receptor for AGE), these AGE-modified proteins can augment the production of proinflammatory cytokines and other inflammatory pathways in vascular endothelial cells. Beyond the hyperglycemia, the diabetic state promotes oxidative stress mediated by reactive oxygen species and carbonyl groups (Cosentino & Luscher, 1998; Huszka et al., 1997; Huvers et al., 1999; Lambert et al., 1996 Furchgott & Zawadzki, 1980; Schneider et al., 2002; Quehenberger et al., 2000; O'Brien et al., 1997).

In patients with a high risk of developing CD, such as diabetic patients, it is important to improve endothelial function since vascular damage may continue even when good glycemic control has been achieved (Volpe et al., 2007). Accordingly, some therapeutic strategies have been directed towards the stimulation of distinct processes that may reestablish the function of the endothelium, including the use of 3-hydroxy-3-methylglutaryl coenzyme A reductase inhibitors (Endemann & Schiffrin, 2004), the angiotensin converting enzyme (ACE) inhibitors (Schachinger et al., 2000), selective blockade of the AT1 receptor of angiotensin-II (ARBs) (Behrendt & Ganz, 2002) and folic acid supplementation (Libby et al., 2002), antioxidants (Beckman et al., 2003), antidiabetics (Lund et al., 2008), insulin (Vehkavaara et al., 2000) and others (Grover-Páez et al., 2007). All these strategies are aimed at decreasing the progress of atherosclerotic disease

Herein, we review the literature about endothelial dysfunction in diabetes mellitus with regards to its pathogenesis at molecular and clinical level, and possible available mode of therapy.

2. Normal endothelial cell (EC) function

The EC is no longer considered a simple barrier. In fact it is a complex organ, with paracrin and autocrin function, which provides a "first line" physiological defense against atherosclerosis. The EC lines the internal lumen of all the vasculature and serves as an interface between circulating blood and vascular smooth muscle cells (VSMC). In addition to serving as a physical barrier between the blood and tissues, the EC facilitates a complex array of functions in intimate interaction with the VSMC, as well as cells within the blood compartment (De Meyer & Herman, 1997).

The last two decades of research have established unambiguously that the EC has a critical role in overall homeostasis whose functions are integrated by a complicated system of chemical mediators. This system exerts effects on both the surrounding VSMC and the cells in the blood that lead to one or more of the following alterations: (1) vasodilatation or vasoconstriction to regulate organ blood, (2) maintenance of fluidity of blood and avoidance of bleeding, (3) proinflammatory or anti-inflammatory changes, and (4) growth and/or changes in the phenotypic characteristics of VSMC (Wautier et al., 1996). During the last decade, a multitude of experimental arguments have led to the concept that NO is not only involved in the control of vasomotor tone but also in vascular homeostasis and neuronal and immunological functions. Endogenous NO is produced through the conversion of the amino acid, l-arginine to l-citrulline by the enzyme, NO-synthase (NOS) from which several isoforms have recently been isolated, purified, and cloned. NOS-type I (isolated from brain) and type III (isolated from ECs) are termed "constitutive-NOS" and produce picomolar levels of NO from which only a small fraction elicits physiological responses. NO produced by NOS type III in the endothelium diffuses to the vascular smooth muscle (VSM) where it activates the enzyme guanylate cyclase. The concomitant increase in cyclic GMP then induces relaxation of the VSM. The EC produces mediators that induce vasoconstriction, including endothelin (Haefliger, 1992) [46], prostaglandins (Viberti, 1989) and angiotensin II (ANG-II) (Studdy, 1983) and regulates vascular tone by maintaining a balance between vasodilation (NO production) and vasoconstriction (eg, A-II generation). ANG-II is produced in local tissues by the EC (Mombouli, 1997) [49] and exerts regulatory effects upon several VSMC functional activities including contraction (ie, vasoconstriction), growth, proliferation, and differentiation. NOS also are regulated by local concentrations of bradykinin (Busse et al.,1993). This peptide acts with b2 receptors on the EC cell surface membrane, increasing the generation of NO via NOS activation. Interestingly, the local concentrations of bradykinin are regulated by the activity of angiotensin converting enzyme (ACE). ACE breaks down bradykinin into inactive peptides (Luscher et al., 1993). Furthermore the EC has a prominent role in maintaining blood fluidity and restoration of vessel wall integrity to avoid bleeding and plays a key role in the balance between the coagulation and fibrinolytic systems. In addition to its key role in growth and differentiation of the VSMC through the release of either promoters of growth and/or inhibitors of growth and differentiation and, as such, has an impact on vascular remodeling (Cowan & Langille, 1996). However, strong evidence suggests that promotion of VSM growth is mediated by local production of platelet growth factor (PGF) and ANG-II (Williams, 1998). The EC is also involved in the production of specific molecules that have a regulatory role in inflammation such as leukocyte adhesion molecule (LAM), intracellular adhesion molecule (ICAM) and vascular cell adhesion molecule (VCAM). These molecules are denominated "adhesion molecules" and function to attract and "anchor" those cells involved in the inflammatory reaction. Very recently it has been demonstrated that the atherosclerotic process is associated with an increased blood level of inflammation (acute phase proteins) markers (Biegelsen & Loscalzo, 1999).

2.1 Endothelial dysfunction

Since the actions of the EC are multiple and involve several systems, alterations in EC function may affect one or more of these systems, either simultaneously or at distinct time periods. Thus, no single definition of EC dysfunction covers the whole array of possible disruption in normal function. In consequence, endothelial dysfunction has been defined pragmatically. It basically involves either an increase (or a decrease) in any of the EC-related chemical messenger and/or by alteration in any of the functional changes. Some examples of EC dysfunction include an increased permeation of macromolecules (Aird, 2005; Forstermann & Munzel, 2006; Ross, 1993; Vita & Keaney, 2002), increased or decreased production of vasoactive factors producing abnormal vasoconstriction/vasodilation, and increased prothrombotic and/or procoagulant activity. However, the most commonly accepted EC dysfunction alteration pertains to abnormalities in the regulation of the lumen of vessels. In this context, EC dysfunction has been defined by blunting of the vasodilatory response to acetylcholine or hyperemia, both of which are known to produce NO-dependent vasodilation. In some specific circumstances, endothelial dysfunction has been defined by a paradoxical vasoconstrictive response to acetylcholine or similar pharmacological agents (i.e., metacholine). At the heart of the definition of EC dysfunction is the measurement of EC function.

Endothelial dysfunction is defined by an impaired vascular reactivity, but it also refers to a proinflammatory and prothrombotic state. A critical balance between endothelium-derived relaxing and contracting factors maintains vascular homeostasis. When this balance is disrupted, it predisposes the vasculature to vasoconstriction, leukocyte adherence, platelet activation, mitogenesis, pro-oxidation, thrombosis, impaired coagulation, vascular inflammation, and atherosclerosis. Endothelial dysfunction has been described in many cardiovascular and metabolic disorders such as hypertension, coronary heart disease, dyslipidemia, and type I and II diabetes. Endothelial dysfunction appears to precede the clinical manifestations of many of these cardiovascular disorders, hypertension for example, and also atherosclerosis, where abnormal vasoconstriction can be observed at the future site of plaque development (Aird, 2005; Endemann & Schiffrin, 2004; Forstermann & Munzel, 2006; Schachinger et al., 2000; Volpe et al., 2007). Thus, endothelial dysfunction is one of the earliest hallmarks of vascular abnormality.

Endothelial dysfunction is thought to precede the development of atherosclerosis. Indeed, in the presence of cardiovascular risk factors endothelial dysfunction can be detected before there is any angiographic evidence of disease or increased intima-media ratio on ultrasound examination. Many of the cardiovascular risk factors, including hyperlipidemia, hypertension, diabetes and smoking, are associated with overproduction of reactive oxygen species or increased oxidative stress, both of which reduce vascular nitric oxide bioavailability and promote cellular damage (Volpe et al., 2007). Hence, increased oxidative stress is considered to be a major mechanism involved in the pathogenesis of endothelial cell dysfunction and may serve as a common pathogenic mechanism of the effect of risk factors on the endothelium (Aird, 2005; Schachinger et al., 2000).

2.2 Endothelial dysfunction and atherosclerosis

Atherosclerosis is regarded as a dynamic and progressive disease arising from the combination of endothelial dysfunction and inflammation. Physiological laminar shear stress is of particular importance in protecting EC against abnormal activation. Endothelial activation can be observed under specific hemodynamic conditions such as prolonged low or oscillatory shear stress. These conditions are responsible for plaque formation and plaque vulnerability in mouse carotid artery. Both low and oscillatory shear stress increase ET-1 expression while decreasing endothelial NO synthase (eNOS) expression. The increase in ET-1 expression may lead to vascular inflammation, which is central to all stages of atherosclerosis. ET-1 induces expression of adhesion molecules on isolated endothelial cells, promotes vascular inflammation and excessive oxidative stress, and mediated nuclear factor-kB (NFkB) activation in monocytes. In a variety of animal models of atherosclerosis, signs of inflammation occur hand-in-hand with incipient lipid accumulation in the artery wall. For example, blood leukocytes, mediators of host defenses and inflammation, localize in the earliest lesions of atherosclerosis, not only in experimental animals but in humans as well. The basic science of inflammation biology applied to atherosclerosis has afforded considerable new insight into the mechanisms underlying this recruitment of leukocytes. The normal endothelium does not in general support binding of white blood cells. However, early after initiation of an atherogenic diet, patches of arterial endothelial cells begin to express on their surface selective adhesion molecules that bind to various classes of leukocytes. In particular, vascular cell adhesion molecule-1 (VCAM-1) binds precisely the types of leukocytes found in early human and experimental atheroma, the monocyte and T lymphocyte. Not only does VCAM-1 expression increase on endothelial cells overlying nascent atheroma, but mice genetically engineered to express defective VCAM-1 show interrupted lesion development (Aird, 2005; Behrendt & Ganz, 2002; Forstermann & Munzel, 2006; Ishizuka et al., 1999; Li et al., 1993). Interestingly, the foci of increased adhesion molecule expression overlap with sites in the arterial tree particularly prone to develop atheroma. Considerable evidence suggests that impaired endogenous atheroprotective mechanisms occur at branch points in arteries, where the endothelial cells experience disturbed flow. For example, absence of normal laminar shear stress may reduce local production of endothelium-derived NO. This endogenous vasodilator molecule also has anti-inflammatory properties and can limit expression of VCAM-1. In addition to inhibiting natural protective mechanisms, disturbed flow can augment the production of certain leukocyte adhesion molecules (eg, intercellular adhesion molecule-1 [ICAM-1]). Augmented wall stresses may also promote the production by arterial smooth muscle cells (SMCs) of proteoglycans that can bind and retain lipoprotein particles, facilitating their oxidative modification and thus promoting an inflammatory response at sites of lesion formation. Once adherent to the endothelium, the leukocytes penetrate into the intima.

Recent research has identified candidate chemoattractant molecules responsible for this transmigration. For example, monocyte chemoattractant protein-1 (MCP-1) appears responsible for the direct migration of monocytes into the intima at sites of lesion formation. A family of T-cell chemoattractants may likewise call lymphocytes into the intima. Once resident in the arterial wall, the blood-derived inflammatory cells participate in and perpetuate a local inflammatory response. The macrophages express scavenger receptors for modified lipoproteins, permitting them to ingest lipid and become foam cells. In addition to MCP-1, macrophage colony-stimulating factor (M-CSF) contributes to the differentiation of the blood monocyte into the macrophage foam cell. T cells likewise encounter signals that cause them to elaborate inflammatory cytokines such as γ-interferon and lymphotoxin (tumor necrosis factor [TNF]-β) that in turn can stimulate macrophages as well as vascular endothelial cells and SMCs. As this inflammatory process continues, the activated leukocytes and intrinsic arterial cells can release fibrogenic mediators, including a variety of peptide growth factors that can promote replication of SMCs and contribute to elaboration by these cells of a dense extracellular matrix characteristic of the more advanced atherosclerosis lesion. Inflammatory processes not only promote initiation and evolution of atheroma, but also contribute decisively to precipitating acute thrombotic complications of atheroma. Most coronary arterial thrombi that cause fatal acute myocardial infarction arise because of a physical disruption of the atherosclerotic plaque (Cybulsky et al., 2001; Forstermann & Munzel, 2006; Ishizuka et al., 1999; Lee et al., 2001; Libby et al., 2002; Quehenberger et al., 2000; Schneider et al., 2002).

3. Endothelial dysfunction and diabetes

The role of endothelial dysfunction in type 2 diabetes is more complicated than that for type 1. The effects of ageing, hyperlipidemia, hypertension and other factors add to the complexity of the problem. In contrast to patients with type 1 diabetes, endothelial dysfunction can also occur in patients with type 2 diabetes even when the patients have normal urinary albumin excretion. In fact, markers of endothelial dysfunction are often elevated years before any evidence of microangiopathy becomes evident (Gazis et al., 1999).
The insulin resistance syndrome encompasses a subnormal response to insulin-mediated glucose disposal and frequently elevated blood pressure, hyperlipidemia and dysfi binolysis, even without any clinically demonstrable alteration in plasma glucose concentrations (Steinberg et al., 1994). There is a growing body of evidence to suggest the coexistence of insulin resistance and endothelial dysfunction. Insulin-induced vasodilation, which is partially mediated by NO release, is impaired in obese individuals who do not have type 2 diabetes but whom display insulin resistance (Cleland et al., 2000).
Moreover, the obese state, a model of human insulin resistance, is associated with high levels of endothelin in plasma. Also blood concentrations of PAI-1 are high in patients with otherwise uncomplicated obesity (Calles-Escandón et al., 1996). Endothelial activation and acute-phase reaction correlate with insulin resistance and obesity in type 2 diabetic patients (Leinonen et al., 2003).
Abnormalities in vascular reactivity and biochemical markers of endothelial cell activation are present early in individuals at risk of developing type 2 diabetes. The vasodilatory responses to acetylcholine were reduced in healthy normoglycemic subjects who have first degree diabetic relatives. The plasma levels of endothelin-1 were significantly higher in subjects with impaired glucose tolerance and patients with type 2 diabetes without vascular

complications compared with healthy normoglycemic subjects with no history of type 2 diabetes in a first-degree relative (Caballero ET AL., 1999). In addition there is a significant association between endothelial dysfunction and insulin resistance in young first degree relatives of DM subjects independent of the classic cardiovascular risk factors (Balletshofer ET AL., 2000).

In a case-cohort study, using the Monitoring of Trends and Determinants in Cardiovascular Disease (MONICA)/ Cooperative Research, men and women with elevated levels of sE-selectin had a significantly increased risk of type 2 diabetes after multivariable adjustment. Hazard ratios (95% CIs) comparing tertile extremes of sE-selectin were 2.63 (1.79–3.88) and 1.71 (1.07–2.75) for men and women, respectively. Elevated levels of sICAM-1 were also associated with an increased risk of type 2 diabetes; however, the association was not independent of other diabetes risk factors including E-selectin, while vWF was not associated with risk of type 2 diabetes (Thorand et al., 2006). A prospective, nested case-control study within the Nurses' Health Study, has found elevated E-selectin and ICAM-1 levels can predict incident diabetes in logistic regression models conditioned on matching criteria and adjusted for body mass index (BMI), family history of diabetes, smoking, diet score, alcohol intake, activity index and postmenopausal hormone use. Adjustment for waist circumference instead of BMI or further adjustment for baseline levels of C-reactive protein, fasting insulin, and HbA1c or exclusion of cases diagnosed during the first 4 years of follow-up did not alter these associations (Meigs et al., 2004).

In the other hand, in diabetes, glycation, tissue oxidation and endothelial function are all abnormal and predisposing to microvascular complications but interrelationships are complex with glycation appearing most direct (Wen et al., 2002). The patients with microalbuminuria, unlike those without it, are characterized by longer course of diabetes, more pronounced lipid exchange disorder, more variable arterial pressure, higher pressure load index, elevated activity of lipid peroxidation (LP) processes and prominent disorder of NO-producing endothelial function. All improve with treatment (Ametov et al., 2005). The Endothelium-dependent vasodilation was impaired in the microalbuminuric patients compared with the normoalbuminuria patients and the healthy controls. Plasma PAI-1 and vWF levels increased in the microalbuminuric patients compared with the levels in the normoalbuminuric patients and in the healthy controls (Yu et al., 2005).

In addition, in type 2 diabetes mellitus as in type 1, increased calpain (calcium-dependent protease) activity in response to hyperglycemia may play a role in diabetic cardiovascular disease. Immunoprecipitation studies revealed that glucose induces loss of NO via a calpain-dependent decrease in the association of hsp90 with endothelial NOS. In addition, inhibition of calpain activity decreased endothelial cell surface expression of the pro-inflammatory adhesion molecules ICAM-1 and VCAM-1 during hyperglycemia (Stalker et al., 2003). Furthermore inhibition of PKC activity reduces leukocyte-endothelium interactions by suppressing surface expression of endothelial cell adhesion molecules in response to increased oxidative stress (Booth et al., 2002).

In diabetes associated with diabetic microangiopathy, compared with non diabetics, asymmetric dimethylarginine [ADMA]; an endogenous inhibitor of NOS, serum TNF-alpha and soluble TNF receptor I (sTNFR-I) has been assessed in a study which concludes that the serum sTNFR-I and VEGF levels were signifi cantly increased, but no difference in the serum TNF-alpha, sTNFR-II, and ADMA levels between uncomplicated diabetic patients and in non diabetics (Makino et al., 2005). Increased levels of vWF antigen, t-PA antigen and PAI-1 activity were seen in impaired glucose tolerance (IGT) and diabetics compared with

the normal glucose tolerance (NGT). Tissue factor pathway inhibitor TFPI activity and thrombomodulin levels were increased in all elderly subjects, with positive association between HbA (1c), TFPI activity and vWF antigen. Fasting blood glucose levels correlated with vWF antigen, t-PA antigen and PAI-1 activity, whereas urine albumin excretion correlated with TFPI activity, vWF antigen and PAI-1 activity. Serum insulin levels correlated strongly not only with vWF antigen and t-PA antigen but also with PAI-1 activity. This correlation did not change after further adjustment for serum glucose and HbA(1c), which may suggest that in the elderly subjects, impaired fibrinolysis is probably associated with insulin resistance (Leurs et al., 2002). The above reflect a prothrombotic state associated with an insulin resistance state, an increased vWF release, raised sP-Sel and TNFalpha levels and, may be, low NO bioavailability, which could lead to a higher risk of development of thrombotic events in hypertensive diabetic patients (Ouvina et al., 2001).
Besides this, NADPH oxidase gene expression is increased in circulating lymphomonocytes from patients with DM, and this increased gene expression is dependent upon metabolic control. Hyperglycemia can mediate its adverse effects through the activation of protein kinase C. Recent study has shown an increase in membrane-associated PKC beta 2 activity in monocytes from patients with DM. This activity was reduced by 40% in the euglycemic condition (Avogaro et al., 2001). Further more patients with Type 2 diabetes with good residual C-peptide secretion are better protected from endothelial dysfunction that those with poor C-peptide secretion (Manzella et al., 2003).

3.1 Hyperglycemia as the major causal factor in the development of endothelial dysfunction

Clinical trials have identified hyperglycemia as the key determinant in the development of chronic diabetic complications. The formation of advanced glycation end products (AGEs) is an important biochemical abnormality accompanying diabetes mellitus and, likely inflammation in general. Although the mechanisms underlying this phenomenon are likely to be multi-factorial, recent in-vivo and in- vitro studies have indicated a crucial role of the diacylglycerol (DAG)-protein kinase C (PKC) pathway in mediating this phenomenon. PKC may have multiple adverse effects on vascular function, including the activation of superoxide-producing enzymes such as the nicotinamide adenine dinicleotide phosphate (NADPH) oxidase as well as increased expression of a dysfunctional, superoxide-producing, uncoupled endothelial nitric oxide synthase (NOS III). PKC-mediated superoxide production may inactivate NO derived from endothelial NOS III, and may inhibit the activity and/or expression of the NO downstream target, the soluble guanylyl cyclase. The effects of AGEs on vessel wall homeostasis may account for the rapidly progressive atherosclerosis associated with diabetes. Driven by hyperglycemia and oxidant stress, AGEs form to a greatly accelerated degree in diabetes. Within the vessel wall, collagen-linked AGEs may "trap" plasma proteins, quench NO activity and interact with specific receptors to modulate a large number of cellular properties. On plasma low density lipoproteins (LDL), AGEs initiate oxidative reactions that promote the formation of oxidized LDL. The interaction of AGEs with endothelial, as well as with other cells accumulating within the atherosclerotic plaque, such as mononuclear phagocytes and smooth muscle cells, provides a mechanism to augment vascular dysfunction. Specifically, the interaction of AGEs with vessel wall component increases vascular permeability, the expression of procoagulant activity and the generation of reactive oxygen species, resulting in increased endothelial expression of endothelial leukocyte adhesion molecules (Farhangkhoee et al., 2006), while acute hyperglycemia and hyperinsulinemia induced vasodilatation is not accompanied by changes in microvascular permeability or endothelial markers. The effects of acute glycemia on plasma nitric oxide (NO; nitrite plus nitrate) levels, Cu-Zn Superoxide dismutase (Cu-Zn SOD) activity and thiobarbituric acid-reactive substances (TBARS) levels were studied in age-matched female subjects before and two hours after glucose loading. Plasma NO levels were significantly higher in subjects with diabetic glucose tolerance (DGT) than in subjects with normal glucose tolerance ($p < 0.001$) and impaired glucose tolerance (IGT) ($p < 0.05$) at baseline. TBARS levels were significantly elevated in subjects with DGT and IGT ($p < 0.001$ and $p < 0.001$). Cu-Zn SOD activities were significantly increased in subjects with NGT, and were significantly decreased in subjects with IGT and DGT ($p < 0.001$ and $p < 0.001$) after glucose loading; suggest that NO availability was decreased when the blood glucose levels were only moderately elevated above normal levels. This might be related with the enhanced oxidative stress (Konukoglu et al., 2003). Other studies examined the effect of acute hyperglycemia on endothelium-dependent vasodilation in patients with DM or impaired glucose metabolism in- vivo by plethysmography. The vasodilatory response to acetylcholine at infusion rates of 7.5, 15, and 30 microg/min was studied in the fasting state and at two levels of hyperglycemia, which were achieved by the infusion of glucose, insulin and somatostatin. The vasodilatory response to acetylcholine was measured by calculating the forearm blood fl ow ratio (FBFR), defined as the measured forearm blood flow at a specific acetylcholine infusion rate divided by the baseline forearm blood flow without acetylcholine infusion. The induction of hyperglycemia resulted in a significant reduction in FBFR for all rates of acetylcholine infusion and suggests the importance of hyperglycemia in the development of endothelial dysfunction observed in patients with DM or impaired glucose metabolism (Bhargava et al., 2003).

4. Endothelial dysfunction and therapeutic intervention

Several pharmacological interventions have been used to improve endothelial function in patients with type 2 diabetes mellitus in this part of the chapter we will mention the most important issues.

4.1 Antidiabetics

4.1.1 Metformin

Metformin is an oral anti-hyperglycaemic agent which enhances insulin sensitivity and lowers hepatic glucose output (Hundal & Inzucchi, 2003). In obese patients with T2DM, metformin is currently the drug of first choice due to its bilateral effect on glycaemic regulation and cardiovascular protection (Inzucchi 2002; (Union Kingdom Prospective Diabetes Study, [UKPDS], 1998 (UKPDS,1998). However, obese and non-obese patients with T2DM experience a similar cardiovascular risk (Adlerberth et al., 1998; Manson et al., 1991) and the use of metformin even in the non-obese patients with T2DM might be beneficial as well.

In predominantly obese patients with T2DM, metformin has previously been shown to decrease levels of vWf, sVCAM-1, ADMA, methylglyoxal (i.e. a major precursor in the formation of AGE) and albuminuria (Abbasi et al., 2004; Asagami et al., 2002; Amador-Licona et al., 2000; Beisswenger et al.,1999; De Jager et al., 2005; Nagi & Yudkin., 1993) and either decrease or having no significant effect (Abbasi et al., 2004; Asagami et al., 2002; Chu

et al., 2002; De Jager et al., 2005; Natali et al., 2004; Testa et al., 1996) on circulating levels of CRP, TNF-a, PAI-1-ag, t-PA-ag, sICAM-1 and sE-selectin.
Recent in vitro studies have suggested that metformin activates the intracellular 'fuel-sensor', i.e. the AMP activated kinase (AMPK). The activated AMPK, in turn, inhibits the TNF-a-induced activation of the nuclear transcription factor, NF-kB, and hereby the NF-kBinduced gene expression of sICAM-1, sVCAM and sE-selectin (Hattori et al., 2006; Isoda et al., 2006). In the other hand, in a recent study comparing metformin versus repaglinide, a decrease was observed in several CVD biomarkers, may be explained by actions of metformin via the pathway of AMPK, TNF-a and NF-kB. The changes from first-period baseline in the levels of TNF-α were not significantly different from zero during either of the two treatments.
Therefore, besides AMPK other, yet unknown, mechanisms (promoting, inhibitory and/or feedback) might contribute to the effect of metformin as well as repaglinide on CVD biomarkers. This is also underscored by the attenuating effect of metabolic variables on the treatment effects on several CVD biomarkers in that study

4.1.2 Thiazolidinediones

Thiazolidinediones enhances insulin-mediated glucose uptake into insulin target tissues, through activation of peroxisome proliferator-activated receptor (PPAR) (Mudaliar & Henry, 2001). They have direct effects on adipose tissue by suppression TNF and, possibly, leptin expression; suppress lipolysis and thus decrease plasma free fatty acid concentrations and increase plasma adiponectin levels (Hauner, 2002) and exert direct effects on insulin-mediated glucose transport in skeletal muscle and the heart (Bishop-Bailey, 2000).
Thiazolidinedione administration reverses insulin resistance and many components of the metabolic syndrome. Treatment is generally associated with increased HDL cholesterol levels; decreased blood pressure, plasma triglyceride levels, small dense LDL cholesterol particles, PAI-1 levels and albumin excretion rates; in addition to decreased glucose levels and reduced hemoglobin A1C levels (Freed et al., 2002). PPAR ligands also improve endothelial function (Dandona & Aljada, 2004). Several studies have demonstrated improvements in brachial artery reactivity in patients with diabetes. (Caballero et al., 2003).
Rosiglitazone, improves coronary artery endothelial function in patients with insulin resistances who have no traditional risk factors for atherosclerosis as well as no impaired glucose tolerance or diabetes (Quiñones et al., 2002). With an increase in insulin sensitivity and a drop in fasting insulin and free fatty acid levels, thiazolidinediones in combination with hormone therapy (HT) in postmenopausal women is, however, have shown in study to attenuates endothelial function (Honisett et al., 2004).
The mechanisms by which thiazolidinediones improve endothelial-dependent blood fl ow are unknown, but likely involve several effects. First, as described above; it has an important anti-inflammatory effects that involve decreasing circulating adipokines levels (eg, TNF, PAI-1, leptin), which are reflected by reduced high-sensitivity C-reactive protein levels; increasing adiponectin levels; decreasing vascular expression of adhesion molecules (Wakino et al., 2002). Second, insulin is a vasodilator stimulating expression of eNOS through the phosphatidylinositol 3-kinase (PI3K) pathway (Zeng et al., 2000). This effect of insulin is blunted in patients with insulin resistance (Kuboki et al., 2000). PPAR- is expressed in endothelial cells, and its ligands have been reported to enhance NO production, possibly by stimulating the PI3K pathway and hence expression of eNOS (Kim et al., 2002). Third, PPAR- ligands improve several components of the metabolic syndrome

that could adversely affect endothelial function, including low HDL cholesterol levels, high triglyceride and free fatty acid levels, hypertension and carbohydrate intolerance. PPAR-ligands also decrease oxidative stress and thus are able to improve the vascular balance between NO and vasoconstrictors (Bagi et al., 2004).

Rosiglitazone administration for 12 weeks was shown to improve insulin sensitivity and decrease asymmetric dimethylarginine levels. An endogenous inhibitor of NOS, is associated with reduced NO–mediated vasodilation and enhanced adherence of mononuclear cells to the endothelium (Stuhlinger et al., 2002). In recently performed a double-blind crossover trial of 12 patients with recently diagnosed type 2 diabetes concludes that insulin resistance is a major contributor toward endothelial dysfunction in type 2 diabetes; both endothelial dysfunction and insulin resistance are amenable to treatment by rosiglitazone (Pistrosch et al., 2005).

Recently studies have shown that Rosiglitazone ameliorated glomerular hyperfiltration in early type 2 diabetes, improved NO bioavailability and lessened renal end-organ damage in type 2 diabetes with microalbuminuria (Pistrosch et al., 2004) and Pioglitazone improves endothelial dysfunction independently from the observed benefits on insulin sensitivity and beta-cell function in patients with newly diagnosed type 2 diabetes and CAD and may exerts additional effects on endothelial function beyond metabolic control (Forst et al., 2005). Furthermore the GATE study may provide the rationale and impetus for the aggressive treatment of insulin-resistant patients with glitazone therapy (Hubacek et al., 2004).

Recently a study was published that used the addition of pioglitazone and ramipril to intensive insulin therapy in Type 2 diabetic patients that which showed that pioglitazone improves vascular dysfunction by different mechanisms.

In this study, they demonstrated that the addition of either the insulin sensitizer pioglitazone or the ACE-blocking agent ramipril further improves vascular dysfunction and markers of inflammation independent of glycemic control. their data indicate that pioglitazone primarily enhances endothelial-mediated, whereas ramipril augments endothelial-independent, vasodilation. These different vascular effects, combined with the observation that pioglitazone increases the vasodilator adiponectin concentration, while ramipril reduces the vasoconstrictor endothelin-1 levels, suggest that different and complementary mechanisms underlie the observed improvements in vascular reactivity. In agreement with previous studies, pioglitazone therapy also was accompanied by a reduction in plasma fatty acids and triglyceride concentrations, both of which may play a role in the correction of vascular dysfunction (Natali et al., 2004; Pfutzner et al., 2005; Wajcberg et al., 2007) [120-122]. Previous studies (Natali et al., 2004; Pfutzner et al., 2005) also have shown that pioglitazone can improve endothelial dysfunction independent of changes in blood glucose levels. Thus, it is likely that the beneficial effects of TZDs on vascular function are mediated by 1) direct effects on the vascular endothelium, 2) improved glycemic control, and 3) enhanced insulin-mediated glucose metabolism. Pioglitazone did not improve endothelial- independent vasodilation beyond that observed with intensive insulin therapy alone.

4.1.3 Meglitinides

Recently the repaglinide administration, showed that it improves brachial reactivity and declines oxidative stress indexes. in vitro through good control of postprandial glucose levels, in agreement with previous data (Ceriello, 2004; Gomes et al., 2004; Gross et al., 2003).

In addition, the relationship between changes in 2-h plasmaglucose levels and brachial reactivity is independent of the main metabolic parameters but is dependent on the TBARS and TEAC levels. The latter data, according to a previous study showing that endothelial dysfunction is present in the postprandial state in type 2 diabetic patients (Ceriello et al., 2004), they support the hypothesis that 2-h plasma glucose levels are the main factor determining oxidative stress and endothelial dysfunction and that a tight control of postprandial glucose excursion—as those found after repaglinide—is a key point for preventing endothelial dysfunction and macroangiopathy (Manzella et al., 2005).
Furthermore, because the modulation of vascular tone is mediated by NO and endothelium-derived hyperpolarizing factor (EDHF), and because the role of EDHF in modulating vascular smooth muscle contraction is mediated by KCa channels on vascular smooth muscle (Georgescu et al., 2001; Inokuchi et al., 2003), While Nateglinide an oral antidiabetic insulinotropic agent neither improved nor impaired myocardial blood flow in Type 2 diabetic patients (Bengel et al., 2005).

4.1.4 α-glucosidase inhibitors

4.1.4.1 Acarbose

Acarbose inhibits enzymes (glycoside hydrolases) needed to digest carbohydrates, to be specific, alpha-glucosidase enzymes in the brush border of the small intestines and pancreatic alpha-amylase. Pancreatic alpha-amylase hydrolyzes complex starches to oligosaccharides in the lumen of the small intestine, whereas the membrane-bound intestinal alpha-glucosidases hydrolyze oligosaccharides, trisaccharides, and disaccharides to glucose and other monosaccharides in the small intestine. Inhibition of these enzyme systems reduces the rate of digestion of complex carbohydrates.
There is a randomized Crossover Study with Acarbose, that shows the effects of a single administration of acarbose on postprandial glucose excursion and endothelial dysfunction in type 2 diabetic patients. In this study the authors hypothesize that acarbose might reduce macrovascular complication by avoiding endothelial injury in postprandial hyperglycemic status (Shimabukuro et al., 2006)].
A potential mechanism by which postprandial hyperglycemia impairs endothelial function is the generation of reactive oxygen species (ROS) (Sheetz & King, 2002). (Yano et al., 2004) reported that a short-time exposure (3 h) to 25 mmol/liter glucose increased intracellular ROS generation in cultured bovine aortic endothelial cells. Previously has been reported that nateglinide, a phenylalanine-derived insulin secretagogue, could also improve postchallenge endothelial function in type 2 diabetic patients (Shimabukuro et al., 2004).
Collectively, postprandial endothelial function could be improved by an intervention to reduce postprandial glucose peak at least in part. (Vallejo et al., 2005) reported that acetylcholine-induced endothelium-dependent relaxations were impaired in aortic and mesenteric vessels isolated from streptozotocin-induced diabetic rats, and such endothelial dysfunction was improved either with suppression of blood glucose levels by acarbose or with ROS suppression by superoxide dismutase. Taken together, it was still possible that suppression of postchallenge hyperglycemia by acarbose decreased generation of ROS and the ROS-mediated impairment of endothelial function, although we could not detect changes of urinary 8-epi-prostaglandin-F2, one reliable marker of whole-body oxygen stress, during the test meal loading. Previous studies showed that insulin can induce either vasodilation by

increasing NOx levels or vasoconstriction by stimulating endothelin-1 levels (Piatti et al., 2003) and the net balance between vasodilator and vasoconstrictor effects of insulin is altered in diabetic patients in favor of a relative vasoconstriction (Cardillo et al., 2002). In the study of (Shimabukuro et al., 2006), there were no significant differences in plasma NOx and endothelin-1 levels before and after meal ingestion in control and diabetic subjects. Because plasma levels of endothelin-1 may not truly reflect the activity of endothelin-1 and endothelin receptor subtype A (ETA)-dependent mechanism could be involved in vascular derangements of diabetic condition, additional future studies need to be done.

4.1.4.2 Miglitol

Miglitol has been launched as an α-GI, which possesses particular pharmacokinetics. Miglitol is absorbed rapidly and almost completely from the small intestine after oral administration (Ahr et al., 1997). Thus, it can strongly suppress the elevation of blood sugar levels shortly after a meal while causing relatively fewer side-effects in the digestive system such as abdominal bloating and diarrhea. The administration of miglitol has been demonstrated to suppress the progression of atherosclerosis associated with controlling fluctuations of blood sugar in apolipoprotein E knockout mice (Mita et al., 2007).

Recently (Makoto et al., 2010), reported the post-prandial effects of a single administration of miglitol and voglibose on endothelial function and changing levels of glucose, insulin, lipids, glucagon-like peptide (GLP)-1, and gastric inhibitory polypeptide (GIP) that were compared after a standard meal loading in 11 diabetic patients with CAD, using a placebo controlled cross-over design. They showed the changing levels of glucose, insulin and triglycerides at 60 min were significantly lower in the miglitol group than in the voglibose and placebo groups (all $P<0.01$). GLP-1 levels that were significantly higher at 120 min ($P<0.05$) and GIP levels were significantly lower at 30 min and 60 min ($P<0.05$) in the miglitol group compared to other treatments. The reactive hyperemia duration at 120 min was significantly maintained in the miglitol group compared to the other groups.

The precise mechanisms are still unidentified, but negative correlations between endothelial function and the indices of changing of post-prandial glucose levels were demonstrated. A previous study also reported the association between post-prandial endothelial function and post-prandial glucose levels (Shimabukuro et al., 2006). In addition, swings in glucose levels affect monocyte adhesion to the endothelium in animal models (Mita et al., 2007) and oscillating glucose levels cause much deleterious impairment on endothelial function rather than constant high glucose (Ceriello et al., 2008). Therefore, post-prandial endothelial function could, in part, be improved by amelioration of post-prandial glucose levels by administration of miglitol.

5. Insulin therapy

The UK Prospective Diabetes Study (UKPDS) showed that intensive blood glucose control with insulin or sulfonylureas, both of which significantly increase circulating free insulin concentrations, retards the development of microvascular complications. The incidence of myocardial infarction decreased by 16%, which was almost statistically significant ($P = .052$). Neither insulin nor sulfonylureas had adverse effects on cardiovascular outcome (Union Kingdom Prospective Diabetes Study, [UKPDS], 1998 (UKPDS, 1998).

Considering this, an "in vivo" study was reported (Vehkavaara et al., 2000), in which the endothelial function was measured in 18 type 2 diabetic patients previously treated with metformin (1000 mg BID, n514; 500 mg BID, n54) before and 6 months after combination therapy with bedtime human isophane insulin and metformin (effect of insulin therapy). A control group of 27 normal subjects was studied to determine whether endothelial function was abnormal in the type 2 diabetic patients.

In this study a total of 75 in vivo endothelial function tests (intrabrachial artery infusions of endothelium-dependent [acetylcholine] and -independent [sodium nitroprusside] vasoactive agents) were performed in 18 type 2 diabetic patients and 27 matched normal subjects. These tests were performed before and 6 months after combination therapy with insulin and metformin and before and 6 months after metformin therapy only. Before insulin therapy, blood flow responses to acetylcholine were significantly blunted in type 2 diabetic patients compared with normal subjects. During insulin therapy, the acetylcholine response increased by 44% ($P<0.05$). Insulin therapy also significantly increased the blood flow responses to both low and high doses of sodium nitroprusside. They conclude that insulin therapy improves endothelium-dependent and -independent vasodilatation. These data support the idea that insulin therapy has beneficial rather than harmful effects on vascular function.

In the Diabetes Mellitus Insulin Glucose Infusion in Acute Myocardial Infarction (DIGAMI) study, patients with an acute myocardial infarction, who received insulin acutely and chronically, had a 28% reduction in mortality rate compared with those of patients who continued their existing therapies Coronary endothelial dysfunction, defined as impaired vasodilatory response to intracoronary infusion of acetylcholine (ACh), is an independent predictor of vascular events even after adjustment for traditional cardiovascular risk factors (Schachinger et al., 2000; Suwaidi et al., 2000). Recently, these findings were extended to measurements performed across the forearm vascular bed (Heitzer et al., 2001; Perticone et al., 2001).

Regarding insulin, acute studies have shown that a physiological increase in the circulating insulin concentration potentiates ACh-induced but not sodium nitroprusside (SNP)-induced vasodilatation (Rask-Madsen et al., 2001; Taddei et al., 1995). In studies addressing effects of long-term insulin therapy on endothelial function, we have previously shown that endothelium-dependent and endothelium independent blood flow in forearm resistance vessels improves during 6 months of combination therapy with bedtime neutral protamine Hagedorn (NPH) insulin and metformin, while continuation of long-term metformin therapy had no effect on vascular function (Vehkavaara et al., 2000). In another study of patients with type 2 diabetes, 2 months of insulin therapy tended ($P<0.09$) to increase the blood flow response to ACh and restored the ability of insulin to acutely potentiate ACh-induced vasodilatation (Rask-Madsen et al., 2001).

Insulin glargine is a long-acting insulin analogue. Compared with regular human insulin in vitro, insulin glargine was, in one study, reported to have a 6.5-fold higher affinity for insulinlike growth factor 1 (IGF-1) receptors in transfected baby hamster kidney cells (Kurtzhals et al., 2000). In contrast to these results, a recent study found equivalent binding of insulin glargine and regular human insulin to insulin and IGF-1 receptors in skeletal muscle cells (Ciaraldi et al., 2001). IGF-1 is a potent stimulator of blood flow (Pendergrass et al., 1998). It is therefore not self-evident that effects of glargine on vascular function are similar to those of human insulin.

(Vehkavaara & Yki-Järvinen, 2004), determined the effects of 3.5 years of addition of insulin glargine to previous metformin therapy on in vivo endothelial function in patients with type

2 diabetes. The data were compared with data from a group of normal subjects. A total of 49 in vivo endothelial function tests, intrabrachial artery infusions of endothelium dependent (acetylcholine [ACh]) and endothelium-independent (sodium nitroprusside [SNP]) vasoactive agents, were performed in 11 patients with type 2 diabetes and 16 matched normal subjects. The tests in the type 2 diabetic patients were performed before and after 6 months and 3.5 years of combination therapy with insulin glargine and metformin. The study conclude that insulin glargine therapy improves endothelium-dependent and endothelium-independent vasodilatation. These data support the idea that long-term insulin therapy has beneficial rather than harmful effects on vascular function in type 2 diabetes.

6. Inhibition of renin angiotensin pathway

Angiotensin II has several pro-oxidative effects on the vasculature, decreasing NO bioavailability and resulting in vascular injury. ACE inhibitors are known to improve endothelial dysfunction, but the ability of angiotensin receptor blockers to improve endothelial dysfunction is less clear (Mancini et al., 1996). Both drug classes consistently prevent coronary artery (particularly in the case of ACE inhibitors), stroke, and diabetic microvascular complications of nephropathy and retinopathy (McFarlane et al., 2003).

Inhibition of the renin-angiotensin system is associated with reduced incidence of new-onset diabetes. In the Heart Outcomes Prevention Evaluation (HOPE) study) (Yusuf et al., 2001), the incidence of diabetes was 32% lower in the ramipril-treated group than in the placebo group. In the Losartan Intervention for Endpoint reduction in hypertension (LIFE) study (Dahlof et al., 2002), losartan was associated with 25% less new-onset diabetes compared with atenolol. The mechanisms responsible for the reduced incidence of diabetes observed during these trials are unknown, although possible mechanisms include increased plasma bradykinin levels, which improves insulin-mediated glucose uptake (Duka et al., 2001), improved endothelial function, increased vascular NO activity and reduced vascular inflammation.

Moreover, In view of the pathogenetic role of the imbalance between angiotensin II and NO in target-organ damage, it is a logical approach to target the renin-angiotensin system (RAS). Considering this, it has been observed that ACE inhibitors prevent the formation of angiotensin II from angiotensin I, whereas the angiotensin II receptor blockers (ARBs) specifically prevent the binding of angiotensin II to type 1 receptors (Burnier, 2001).

ACE inhibitors lead to accumulation of bradykinin, known to improve endothelial function, whereas ARBs elicit stimulation of the angiotensin II AT2 receptors and modulate peroxisome proliferator–activated receptor-receptors.

The clinical relevance of these additional effects of ACE inhibitors and ARBs is controversial. So far, the effects of ACE inhibitors and ARBs have been examined mainly in the peripheral circulation. Although small sample sizes have been used, significant improvement of endothelial function has been observed for both compounds used in the current trial.

Ramipril significantly improved renal endothelial function in normotensive, normoalbuminuric men with type 1 diabetes (Komerset al., 2000), and telmisartan increased endothelial function in treatment-naive hypertensive patients (Svolis et al., 2002). Recently, (Schmieder, 2007), reported the results head-to head comparisons examining the effects of RAS blockade on renal endothelial function in patients with type 2 diabetes and hypertension, who are known to have a very high risk of cardiovascular and renal morbidity (Delles et al., 2002; Schmieder, 2005). He studied in a multicenter, prospective, double-blind, forced-titration, randomized study, 96 patients with type 2 diabetes, hypertension, glomerular filtration rate 80 ml/min, and normo-or microalbuminuria were treated once daily with 40/80 mg telmisartan or 5/10 mg ramipril for 9 weeks. He concluded that in patients with type 2 diabetes, telmisartan and ramipril both increased NO activity of the renal endothelium significantly, which in turn may support the preservation of cardiovascular and renal function.

7. Statin and endothelial dysfunction

Several clinical trials have demonstrated that statin treatment not only reduces serum cholesterol levels in hypercholesterolemic patients, but also substantially decreases the risk of cardiovascular disease (Shepherd et al., 1995). In current clinical use, statins can reduce LDL cholesterol levels by an average of 20%-35%, with a corresponding 30%-35% reduction in major cardiovascular outcomes. Decreases in serum cholesterol levels could account for the observed risk reduction, since LDL cholesterol has a strong, well documented association with cardiovascular risk, and since plasma LDL apheresis has been shown to improve both endothelium-dependent vasodilation and cardiovascular risk in hypercholesterolemic patients (Tamai et al., 1997). Several studies, however, have shown that improvements in endothelial function can occur before reductions in serum cholesterol levels. These acute effects are in agreement with other studies that have reported improvements in endothelial function after statin administration that do not correlate with reductions in serum LDL cholesterol levels, and it has been observed that statins can decrease high-sensitivity C-reactive protein levels by 30%-40%, independent of their cholesterol lowering capacities (Ansell et al., 2003).

7.1 Rosuvastatin

In this context, the Justification for the Use of Statins in Prevention: an Intervention Trial Evaluating Rosuvastatin (JUPITER) Study (Ridker et al., 2008), that randomly assigned 17,802 apparently healthy men and women with low-density lipoprotein (LDL) cholesterol levels of less than 130 mg per deciliter (3.4 mmol per liter) and high-sensitivity C-reactive protein levels of 2.0 mg per liter or higher to rosuvastatin, 20 mg daily, or placebo and followed them for the occurrence of the combined primary end point of myocardial infarction, stroke, arterial revascularization, hospitalization for unstable angina, or death from cardiovascular causes. The trial was stopped after a median follow-up of 1.9 years (maximum, 5.0). Rosuvastatin reduced LDL cholesterol levels by 50% and high-sensitivity C-reactive protein levels by 37%.

The rates of the primary end point were 0.77 and 1.36 per 100 person-years of follow-up in the rosuvastatin and placebo groups, respectively (hazard ratio for rosuvastatin, 0.56 95% confidence interval [CI], 0.46 to 0.69; $P<0.00001$), with corresponding rates of 0.17 and 0.37 for myocardial infarction (hazard ratio, 0.46; 95% CI, 0.30 to 0.70; $P = 0.0002$), 0.18 and 0.34 for stroke (hazard ratio, 0.52; 95% CI, 0.34 to 0.79; $P = 0.002$), 0.41 and 0.77 for revascularization or unstable angina (hazard ratio, 0.53; 95% CI, 0.40 to 0.70; $P<0.00001$), 0.45 and 0.85 for the combined end point of myocardial infarction, stroke, or death from cardiovascular causes (hazard ratio, 0.53; 95% CI, 0.40 to 0.69; $P<0.00001$), and 1.00 and 1.25 for death from any cause (hazard ratio, 0.80; 95% CI, 0.67 to 0.97; $P = 0.02$). The conclusion of this trial is that in apparently healthy persons without hyperlipidemia but with elevated high-sensitivity C-reactive protein levels, rosuvastatin significantly reduced the incidence of major cardiovascular events.

7.2 Atorvastatin

Undoubtedly the most important study to demonstrate the pleiotropic effect of atorvastatin has been The Reversal of Atherosclerosis with Aggressive Lipid Lowering (REVERSAL) study (Nicholls et al., 2006), this clinical trial was carried out to determine the influence of increasing body mass index (BMI) on plasma lipids, C-reactive protein, plaque burden as determined by intravascular ultrasound, and the serial change in these parameters with a moderate or intensive lipid-lowering strategy. In this clinical trial patients were randomized to receive an intensive lipid-lowering strategy with 80 mg/day of atorvastatin and a pravastatin placebo or a moderate lipid-lowering strategy with 40 mg/day of pravastatin and an atorvastatin placebo. Treatments were administered for an 18-month period. Patients with a higher BMI were younger, more likely to be women, and had a greater prevalence of hypertension, diabetes, and the metabolic syndrome. Although a higher BMI was associated with a lower high-density lipoprotein level and higher triglyceride and C-reactive protein levels, there was no apparent influence of BMI on plaque burden. However, with the intensive lipid-lowering strategy, a greater BMI was associated with a lower proportionate decrease in low-density lipoprotein (49.1 ± 21.4% vs 43.0 ±22.4%, $p < 0.008$) and a greater proportionate decrease in C-reactive protein (39.7% vs 33.3%, $p <0.04$). Further, although moderate and intensive lipid-lowering strategies halted plaque progression in subjects with a lower BMI (median progression rates +1.5% and +1.2%, respectively), a significant effect on plaque progression rates was seen only with adoption of an intensive lipid lowering strategy in the most obese subjects (median progression rate -1.88% vs + 6.5% with the moderate lipid-lowering strategy, $p <0.01$). In conclusion, plaque progression in obese patients is attenuated using an intensive, but not moderate, lipid-lowering strategy. These results highlight the need for aggressive risk factor modification and a decrease in vascular inflammation in obese patients.

These findings provide further evidence in support of the concept that statins possess significant nonlipid-lowering properties in vivo (Takemoto & Liao, 2001). It is likely that statins inhibit the inflammatory cascade by multiple mechanisms. Statins decrease low-density lipoprotein (Schectman et al., 2004) and oxidative stress (Stoll et al., 2004), which are key promoters of inflammatory events. In addition, it is becoming increasingly recognized that statins may exert direct anti-inflammatory effects at the level of the arterial wall. Inhibition of isoprenylation by statins results in a decrease in the activation and nuclear translocation of the transcription factor, nuclear factor κB (Inoue et al., 2002). Nuclear factor κB plays a central role in directing inflammatory events. Similarly, statins inhibit the modification of proteins by myeloperoxidase-catalyzed reactive nitrogen species (Shishehbor et al., 2003). These species have been demonstrated to promote multiple inflammatory pathways. In support of this observation, atorvastatin therapy has been shown to decrease systemic levels of nitrotyrosine, a major product of myeloperoxidase-catalyzed pathways (Shishehbor et al., 2003). The ability of statins to modulate each of these inflammatory pathways in obese patients in vivo remains to be clarified.

8. The phosphodiesterase-5 inhibitors

PDE-5 inhibitors cause an accumulation of NO-driven cGMP and subsequent vasodilatation in the corpus cavernosum and in pulmonary vasculature, therefore pharmacological PDE-5 inhibition has become a widely used treatment for erectile dysfunction (Shabsigh, 2004) and pulmonary arterial hypertension (Galiè et al., 2005). Effects of the different PDE-5 inhibitors on vasomotor function have also been described (Schäfer et al., 2008; Teixeira et al., 2006). In recent years it has been demonstrated, that not only the vascular wall, but also myocardial tissue contains PDE-5 (Giordano et al., 2001; Senzaki et al., 2001), 183] and there has been considerable interest in the role of the NO-cGMP-protein kinase G (PKG) pathway in cardioprotection (Kukreja et al., 2004). Recent studies reported considerable myocardial protection (Salloum et al., 2006) and improvement of endothelial dysfunction (Gori et al., 2005) after ischaemia/reperfusion with pharmacological PDE-5 inhibition, which were mediated by cGMP-induced opening of ATP-sensitive K+ channels.

8.1 Sildenafil citrate

Sildenafil citrate, a potent PDE-5 inhibitor has been reported to improve the impaired endothelial function in smokers (Vlachopoulos et al., 2004), in patients with coronary artery disease (Halcox et al., 2002) and most recently in the setting of experimental diabetes (Schäfer et al., 2008). In addition, intracellular cGMP accumulation has been shown to reduce oxidative tissue injury in conditions associated with increased free radical release and oxidative stress (Abdollah et al., 2003) and even in diabetes mellitus (Milani et al., 2005).

Moreover, sildenafil citrate has been shown to display beneficial cardiovascular effects in patients with congestive heart failure and pulmonary hypertension, suggesting that it may have other systemic benefits involving the endothelium (Galie\` et al., 2005). Administration of sildenafil citrate in both humans and animals offers protection against ischemic phenomena and it reduces the possibility of myocardial infarction after inducing ischemia (Bremer et al., 2005). There is little data regarding the long term use of PDE-5 and the effects of this on different organs. However, there is evidence that sildenafil citrate may be useful as an additional pharmacological strategy to deal with endothelial dysfunction in individuals with a high risk of developing CAD, as is the case of diabetic patients.

We reported recently the results of a double-blind, randomized, controlled trial in 40 male patients, age 35–50, with type 2 diabetes. Subjects received sildenafil citrate 50 mg daily (n = 20) or placebo (n = 20) for 30 days. Levels of hs-CRP, microalbuminuria, homocysteine, A1c and erectile function were measured at baseline and to the end of the study. We found that men who received sildenafil citrate displayed a significant decrease in the microalbuminuria concentrations ($p < 0.01$) versus baseline, ($p = 0.02$) versus placebo and A1c ($p < 0.01$) versus baseline, ($p = 0.01$) versus placebo (Grover-Páez et al., 2007).

Vardenafil and Tadalafil have also shown beneficial effects on endothelial function in different clinical trials (Schäfer et al., 2008).

9. Other therapies

Other therapies such as the use of antioxidants like vitamin E (Economides et al., 2005; Paolisso et al., 2003), coenzyme Q (Hamilton et al., 2009), folic acid (Oostrom et al., 2009) and allopurinol (Butle et al., 2000, have also demonstrated in several clinical trials some benefits on endothelial function, however more evidence is required to recommend these treatment strategies as prevention of endothelial damage in patients with type 2 diabetes mellitus.

10. Conclusion

Since endothelial dysfunction is the fundamental substrate for atherosclerosis and cardiovascular disease in patients with type 2 diabetes mellitus, it is imperative to study integrally to the diabetic patient taking into account both, the clinical manifestations, and the inflammation markers like the hsCRP, homocysteine, microalbuminuria, as the most important.

It is therefore of interest to the clinician to know which are the current treatment strategies that have demonstrated a real benefit to decrease the endothelial damage or delay it, like the use of ACEIs, ARBs, statins, folic acid, 5-PDF inhibitors, antioxidants, among others and include them as part of the comprehensive treatment of diabetic patients in addition to giving up the harmful habits known such as physical inactivity and smoking.

11. References

Abaci A, Oguzhan A, Kahraman S, Eryol NK, Unal S, Arinc H, Ergin A: Effect of diabetes mellitus on formation of coronary collateral vessels. *Circulation 1999; 99(17):2239-224290..*

Abbasi F, Chu JW, McLaughlin T, Lamendola C, Leary ET & Reaven GM. Effect of metformin treatment on multiple cardiovascular disease risk factors in patients with type 2 diabetes mellitus. *Metabolism 2004;53: 159–164.*

Abdollahi M, Fooladian F, Emami B, Zafari K, Bahreini-Moghadam A. Protection by sildenafil and theophylline of lead acetate induced oxidative stress in rat submandibular gland and saliva. *Hum Exp Toxicol 2003; 22: 587–592.*

Adlerberth AM, Rosengren A & Wilhelmsen L. Diabetes and long term risk of mortality from coronary and other causes in middle aged Swedish men. A general population study. *Diabetes Care 1998; 21:539–545.*

Ahr HJ, Boberg M, Brendel E, Krause HP, Steinke W. Pharmacokinetics of miglitol. Absorption, distribution, metabolism, and excretion following administration to rats, dogs, and man. *Arzneimittel-forschung 1997; 47: 734 – 745.*

Aird WC. Spatial and temporal dynamics of the endothelium. *J Thromb Haemost 2005; 3:1392-1406.*

Amador-Licona N, Guizar-Mendoza J, Vargas E, Sanchez-Camargo G & Zamora-Mata L. The short-term effect of a switch from glibenclamide to metformin on blood pressure and microalbuminuria in patients with type 2 diabetes mellitus. *Arch Med Res 2000; 31:571–575.*

Ametov AS, Demidova TIu, Kosykh SA.. [NO synthesis in the vascular endothelium of patients with type II diabetes]. *Klin Med (Mosk)2005; 83(8):62–8*

Ansell BJ, Watson KE, Weiss RE, et al. hsCRP and HDL Effects of Statins Trial (CHEST): rapid effect of statin therapy on C-reactive protein and high-density lipoprotein levels. A clinical investigation. Heart Dis 2003; 5:2–7.

Asagami T, Abbasi F, Stuelinger M, Lamendola C, McLaughlin T, Cooke JP, Reaven GM & Tsao PS. Metformin treatment lowers asymmetric dimethylarginine concentrations in patients with type 2 diabetes. *Metabolism 2002; 51:843–846.*

Avogaro A, Miola M, Favaro A, et al.. Gemfibrozil improves insulin sensitivity and flow-mediated vasodilatation in type 2 diabetic patients. *Eur J Clin Invest 2001; 31:603–9.*

Balletshofer BM, Rittig K, Enderle MD, et al. Endothelial dysfunction is detectable in young normotensive first-degree relatives of subjects with type 2 diabetes in association with insulin resistance. *Circulation 2000; 101:1780–4.*

Bagi Z, Koller A, Kaley G.. Peroxisome proliferator-activated receptor activation increases NO bioavailability in coronary arterioles in type 2 diabetes by reducing oxidative stress. *Am J Physiol Heart Circ Physiol 2004; 286:H742–8.*

Beckman J A., A B. Goldfine, M B Gordon, L A. Garrett, J F. Keaney, Jr. and M A. Creager. Oral antioxidant therapy improves endothelial function in Type 1 but not Type 2 diabetes mellitus. *Am J Physiol Heart Circ Physiol 2003; 285:2392–2398*

Behrendt D, Ganz P. Endothelial function: from vascular biology to clinical applications. *Am J Cardiol 2002; 90: 40L-48L.*

Beisswenger PJ, Howell SK, Touchette AD, Lal S & Szwergold BS. Metformin reduces systemic methylglyoxal levels in type 2 diabetes. *Diabetes 1999; 48:198–202.*

Bengel FM, Abletshauser C, Neverve J, et al. Effects of nateglinide on myocardial microvascular reactivity in Type 2 diabetes mellitus - a randomized study using positron emission tomography. *Diabet Med 2005; 22:158–63.*

Bhargava K, Hansa G, Bansal M, et al. Endothelium-dependent brachial artery flow mediated vasodilatation in patients with diabetes mellitus with and without coronary artery disease. *J Assoc Physicians India 2003; 51:355–8.*

Biegelsen ES, Loscalzo J. Endothelial function and atherosclerosis. *Coron Artery Dis 1999; 10:241–56.*

Bishop-Bailey D.. Peroxisome proliferator-activated receptors in the cardiovascular system. *Br J Pharmacol 2000; 129:823–34.*

Boden G, Shulman GIFree fatty acids in obesity and type 2 diabetes: defining their role in the development of insulin resistance and beta cell dysfunction. *Eur J Clin Invest 2002; 32(Suppl 3):14–23.*

Booth G, Stalker TJ, Lefer AM, et al. Mechanisms of amelioration of glucose-induced endothelial dysfunction following inhibition of protein kinase C in vivo. *Diabetes 2002; 51:1556–64.*

Bots M L A, W. Hoes, P J Koudstaal, A Hofman, D E Grobbee. Common Carotid Intima-Media Thickness and Risk of Stroke and Myocardial Infarction.The Rotterdam Study. *Circulation. 1997;96:1432-1437*

Bremer Y, F Salloum, O Ockaili, E Chou, W Moskowitz, R Kukreja. Sildenafil citrate induces cardioprotective effects after ischemia/reperfusion injury in infant rabbits. *Pediatr Res 2005; 57:22–28.*

Burnier M: Angiotensin II type 1 receptor blockers. *Circulation 2001; 103:904–912.*

Busse R, Fleming I, Hecker M.. Signal transduction in endothelium dependent vasodilatation. *Eur Heart J 1993; 14 (Suppl I):2–9.*

Butler R, A D Morris, JJF. Belch, A Hill, A D Struthers. Allopurinol Normalizes Endothelial Dysfunction in Type 2 Diabetics With Mild Hypertension. Hypertension 2000; 35:746-751.

Caballero AE, Arora S, Saouaf R, et al. Microvascular and macrovascular reactivity is reduced in subjects at risk for type 2 diabetes. *Diabetes 1999; 48:1856–62.*

Caballero AE, Saouaf R, Lim SC, et al.. The effects of troglitazone, an insulin-sensitizing agent, on the endothelial function in early and late type 2 diabetes: a placebo-controlled randomized clinical trial. Metabolism 2003; 52:173–80.

Calles-Escandon J, Ballor D, Harvey-Berino J, et al. Amelioration of the inhibition of fi brinolysis in elderly, obese subjects by moderate energy intake restriction. Am *J Clin Nutr 1996; 64:7–11.*

Cardillo C, Campia U, Bryant MB, Panza JA. Increased activity of endogenous endothelin in patients with type II diabetes mellitus. *Circulation 2002; 106:1783–1787.*

Ceriello A, Cavarape a, Martinelli l, DaRos R, Marra G, Quagliaro L, Piconi l, Assoli R, Motz E: The post-prandial state in type 2 diabets and endothelial dysfunction: effects of insulin aspart. *Diabet Med 2004; 21:171–175.*

Ceriello A: Impaired glucose tolerance and cardiovascular disease: the possible role of post-prandial hyperglycemia. *Am Heart J 2004; 14 803–807.*

Ceriello A, Esposito K, Piconi L, Ihnat MA, Thorpe JE, Testa R, et al. Oscillating glucose is more deleterious to endothelial function and oxidative stress than mean glucose in normal and type 2 diabetic patients. *Diabetes 2008; 57: 1349 – 1354.*

Cerrato J, Hipoglucemia en la diabetes, fisiopatología, clínica y tratamiento. *Medicine 2004; 17:1029–1033.*

Chu NV, Kong AP, Kim DD, Armstrong D, Baxi S, Deutsch R, Caulfield M, Mudaliar SR, Reitz R, Henry RR & Reaven PD. Differential effects of metformin and troglitazone on cardiovascular risk factors in patients with type 2 diabetes. *Diabetes Care 2002; 25: 542–549.*

Ciaraldi TP, Carter L, Seipke G, Mudaliar S, Henry RR. Effects of the long-acting insulin analog insulin glargine on cultured human skeletal muscle cells: comparisons to insulin and IGF-1. *J Clin Endocrinol Metab 2001; 86:5838–5847.*

Cleland SJ, Petrie JR, Small M, et al. Insulin action is associated with endothelial function in hypertension and type 2 diabetes. *Hypertension 2000; 35 (1 Pt 2):507–11.*

Cosentino F, Luscher TF. Endothelial dysfunction in diabetes mellitus. *J Cardiovasc Pharmacol 1998; 32 (Suppl 3): S54-S61.*

Cowan DB, Langille BL.. Cellular and molecular biology of vascular remodeling. *Curr Opin Lipidol 1996; 7:94–100.*

Creager MA, Luscher TF, Cosentino F, Beckman JA: Diabetes and vascular disease: pathophysiology, clinical consequences, and medical therapy: Part I. *Circulation 2003; 108(12):1527-15323.*

Cybulsky MI, Iiyama K, Li H, et al. A major role for VCAM-1, but not ICAM-1, in early atherosclerosis. *J. Clin. Invest 2001; 107:1255-1262.*

Dahlof B, Devereux RB, Kjeldsen SE, et al. Cardiovascular morbidity and mortality in the Losartan Intervention For Endpoint reduction in hypertension study (LIFE): a randomised trial against atenolol. *Lancet 2002; 359:995–1003.*

Dandona P, Aljada A.. Endothelial dysfunction in patients with type 2 diabetes and the effects of thiazolidinedione antidiabetic agents. *J Diabetes Complications 2004; 18:91–102.*

De Jager J, Kooy A, Lehert P, Bets D, Wulffele MG, Teerlink T, Scheffer PG, Schalkwijk CG, Donker AJ & Stehouwer CD. Effects of short-term treatment with metformin on markers of endothelial function and inflammatory activity in type 2 diabetes mellitus: a randomized, placebo-controlled trial. *J Int Med 2005; 257: 100–109.*

De Luis DA, N Fernández, R. Aller. Homocisteína metabolismo y determinantes higiénico dietéticos. *Endocrinol Nutr 2004; 51:458–463.*
De Meyer GR, Herman AG. Vascular endothelial dysfunction. *Prog Cardiovasc Dis 1997; 39:325–42.*
Delles C, Jacobi J, Schlaich MP, John S, Schmieder RE: Assessment of endothelial function of the renal vasculature in human subjects. *Am J Hypertens 2002; 15:3–9.*
Dimmeler S, Haendeler J, Zeiher AM: Regulation of endothelial cell apoptosis in atherothrombosis. Current Opinion in Lipidology 2002; 13(5):531-536.
Dimmeler S, Zeiher AM: Vascular repair by circulating endothelial progenitor cells: the missing link in atherosclerosis?. *Journal of Molecular Medicine 2004; 82(10):671-677*
Duka I, Shenouda S, Johns C, et al. Role of the B(2) receptor of bradykinin in insulin sensitivity. *Hypertension 2001; 38:1355–60.*
Economides PA, L Khaodhiar, A Caselli, et al. The Effect of Vitamin E on Endothelial Function of Micro- and Macrocirculation and Left Ventricular Function in Type 1 and Type 2 Diabetic Patients. *Diabetes 2005; 54:204–211.*
Endemann DH, Schiffrin EL. Endothelial dysfunction. *J Am Soc Nephrol 2004; 15: 1983- 1992.*
Farhangkhoee H, Khan ZA, Kaur H, et al. Vascular endothelial dysfunction in diabetic cardiomyopathy: Pathogenesis and potential treatment targets. *Pharmacol Ther 2006; 111:384–99.*
Festa A, R D'Agostino, G Howard, L Mykkanen. Inflammation and microalbuminuria in nondiabetic and type 2 diabetic subjects: the insulin resistance atherosclerosis study. *Kidney Int 2000; 58:1703–1710.*
Forst T, Lubben G, Hohberg C, et al.. Infl uence of glucose control and improvement of insulin resistance on microvascular blood flow and endothelial function in patients with diabetes mellitus type 2. Microcirculation 2005; 12:543–50.
Forstermann U, Munzel T. Endothelial nitric oxide synthase in vascular disease: from marvel to menace. *Circulation 2006; 113:1708-1714.*
Freed MI, Ratner R, Marcovina SM, et al. Effects of rosiglitazone alone and in combination with atorvastatin on the metabolic abnormalities in type 2 diabetes mellitus. Am J Cardiol 2002; 90:947–52.
Furchgott RF, Zawadzki JV. The obligatory role of endothelial cells in the relaxation of arterial smooth muscle by acetylcholine. *Nature 1980; 288: 373-376.*
Galie` N, HA Ghofrani, A Torbicki, RJ Barst, LJ Rubin. Sildenafil use in pulmonary arterial hypertension (SUPER) study group. *N Engl J Med 2005; 353:2148–2157.*
Galiè N, Ghofrani HA, Torbicki A, Barst RJ, Rubin LJ, Badesch D et al. Sildenafil citrate therapy for pulmonary arterial hypertension. *N Engl J Med 2005; 353: 2148–2157.*
Galle J, T Quaschning, S. Seibold, C. Wanner, Endothelial dysfunction and inflammation: what is the link? *Kidney Int 2003; 84:545–549.*
Gazis A, White DJ, Page SR, et al. Effect of oral vitamin E (α-tocopherol) supplementation on vascular endothelial function in type 2 diabetes mellitus. *Diabet Med 1999; 16:304–11.*
Georgescu A, Popov D, Simionescu M. Mechanisms of decreased bradykinin-induced vasodilatation in experimental hyperlipemia-hyperglycemia: contribution of nitric oxide and Ca 2-actived Kchannel. *Fundam Clin Pharmacol 2001; 15:335–342.*
Giordano D, De Stefano ME, Citro G, Modica A, Giorgi M Expression of cGMP-binding cGMP-specific phosphodiesterase (PDE5) in mouse tissues and cell lines using an

antibody against the enzyme amino-terminal domain. *Biochim Biophys Acta 2001; 1539: 16–27.*

Gomes MB, Affonso FS, Cailleaux S, Almeida AL, Pinto LF, Tibirica E: Glucose levels observed in daily clinical practice induce endothelial dysfunction in the rabbit macro- and microcirculation. *Fundam Clin Pharmacol 2004; 18:339 -346.*

Gori T, Sicuro S, Dragoni S, Donati G, Forconi S, Parker JD. Sildenafil prevents endothelial dysfunction induced by ischemia and reperfusion via opening of adenosine triphosphate-sensitive potassium channels: a human in vivo study. *Circulation 2005; 111: 742–746.*

Grover-Páez F, G Villegas-Rivera, R Guillén-Ortíz. Sildenafil citrate diminishes microalbuminuria and the percentage of A1c in male patients with type 2 diabetes. *Diab Res Clinl Prac 2007; 78:136–140*

Gross ER, LaDisa JF, Weihrauch D, Olson LE, Kress TT, Hettrick DA, Pagel PS, Warltier DC, Kersten1 JR: Reactive oxygen species modulate coronary wall shear stress and endothelial function during hyperglycemia. *Am J Physiol Heart Circ Physiol 2003; 284:H1552–H1559.*

Haefliger IO, Flammer J, Luscher TF. Nitric oxide and endothelin-1are important regulators of human ophthalmic artery. *Invest Ophthalmol Vis Sci. 1992; 33:2340–3.*

Halcox JP, Nour KR, Zalos G, Mincemoyer RA,Waclawiw M, Rivera CE et al. The effect of sildenafil on human vascular function, platelet activation, and myocardial ischemia. *J Am Coll Cardiol 2002; 40: 1232–1240.*

Hamilton SJ, GT Chew, GF Watts. Coenzyme Q10 Improves Endothelial Dysfunction in Statin-Treated Type 2 Diabetic Patients. *Diabetes Care 2009; 32:810–812.*

Heitzer T, Schlinzig T, Krohn K, Meinertz T, Munzel T. Endothelial dysfunction, oxidative stress, and risk of cardiovascular events in patients with coronary artery disease. *Circulation 2001; 104:2673–2678*

Hattori Y, Suzuki K, Hattori S & Kasai K. Metformin inhibits cytokine-induced nuclear factor kappaB activation via AMP activated protein kinase activation in vascular endothelial cells. *Hypertension 2006; 47: 1183–1188.*

Hauner H.. The mode of action of thiazolidinediones. *Diabetes Metab Res Rev 2002; 18(Suppl 2):S10–15.*

Honisett SY, Stojanovska L, Sudhir K, et al.. Hormone therapy impairs endothelial function in postmenopausal women with type 2 diabetes mellitus treated with rosiglitazone. *J Clin Endocrinol Metab 2004; 89:4615–9.*

Hubacek J, Verma S, Shewchuk L, et al.. Rationale and design of the Glitazones and the Endothelium (GATE) study: evaluation of rosiglitazone on endothelial function in patients with diabetes. *Can J Cardiol 2004; 20:1449–53.*

Hundal RS & Inzucchi SE. Metformin: new understandings, new uses. *Drugs 2003; 63:1879–1894.*

Huvers FC, De Leeuw PW, Houben AJ, et al. Endothelium-dependent vasodilatation, plasma markers of endothelial function, and adrenergic vasoconstrictor responses in type 1 diabetes under near-normoglycemic conditions. *Diabetes 1999; 48:1300-1307.*

Huszka M, Kaplar M, Rejto L, et al. The association of reduced endothelium derived relaxing factor-NO production with endothelial damage and increased in vivo platelet activation in patients with diabetes mellitus. *Thromb Res 1997; 86: 173-180.*

Inokuchi K, Hirooka Y, Shimokawa H, Sakay K, Kishi T, Ito K, Kimura Y, Tekeshita A: Role of endothelium-derived hyperpolarizing factor in human forearm circulation. *Hypertension 2003; 42:919 –924.*

Inoue I, Itoh F, Aoyagi S, Tazawa S, Kusama H, Akahane M, Mastunaga T, Hayashi K, et al. Fibrate and statin synergistically increase the transcriptional activities of PPARalpha/RXRalpha and decrease the transactivation of NFkappaB. *Biochem Biophys Res Commun 2002; 290:131–139*

Inzucchi SE. Oral antihyperglycemic therapy for type 2 diabetes -scientific review. *J Am Med Assoc 2002; 287:360–372.*

Ishizuka T, Takamizawa-Matsumoto M, Suzuki K, et al. Endothelin-1 enhances vascular cell adhesion molecule-1 expression in tumor necrosis factor alpha-stimulated vascular endothelial cells. *Eur J Pharmacol 1999; 369:237-245*

Isoda K, Young JL, Zirlik A, MacFarlane LA, Tsuboi N, Gerdes N,Schönbeck U & Libby P. Metformin inhibits proinflammatory responses and nuclear factor-kB in human vascular wall cells. Arteriosclerosis, Thrombosis, and Vascular Biology 2006; 26: 611–617.

Johnstone MT, Creager SJ, Scales KM, Cusco JA, Lee BK, Creager MA: Impaired endothelium-dependent vasodilation in patients with insulin-dependent diabetes mellitus. *Circulation 1993; 88(6):2510-2516.*

Kannel WB, McGee DL: Diabetes and cardiovascular disease. The Framingham study. *JAMA 1979; 241(19):2035-2038.*

Kim Y-B, Ciaraldi TP, Kong A, et al.. Troglitazone but not metformin restores insulin-stimulated phosphoinositide 3-kinase activity and increases p110_ protein levels in skeletal muscle of type 2 diabetic subjects. Diabetes 2002; 51:443–8.

Komers R, Komersova K, Kazdova L, Ruzickova J, Pelikanova T: Effect of ACE inhibition and angiotensin AT1 receptor blockade on renal and blood pressure response to L-arginine in humans. *J Hypertens 2000; 18:51–5984.*

Konukoglu D, Dogan E, Turhan MS, et al. Impaired glucose tolerance: its relevance to early endothelial dysfunction. *Horm Metab Res 2003; 35:607–10.*

Kuboki K, Jiang ZY, Takahara N, et al.. Regulation of endothelial constitutive nitric oxide synthase gene expression in endothelial cells and in vivo: a specifi c vascular action of insulin. Circulation 2000; 101:676–81.

Kukreja RC, Ockaili R, Salloum F, Yin C, Hawkins J, Das A et al. Cardioprotection with phosphodiesterase-5 inhibition–a novel preconditioning strategy. *J Mol Cell Cardiol 2004; 36: 165–173.*

Kurtzhals P, Schaffer L, Sorensen A, Kristensen C, Jonassen I, Schmid C, Trub T. Correlations of receptor binding and metabolic and mitogenic potencies of insulin analogs designed for clinical use. *Diabetes 2000; 49:999–1005.*

Lambert J, Aarsen M, Donker AJ, Stehouwer CD. Endothelium-dependent and independent vasodilation of large arteries in normoalbuminuric insulin-dependent diabetes mellitus. *Arterioscler Thromb Vasc Biol 1996; 16:705-711.*

Lee RT, Yamamoto C, Feng Y, et al. Mechanical strain induces specific changes in the synthesis and organization of proteoglycans by vascular smooth muscle cells. *J. Biol. Chem 2001; 276:13847- 13851.*

Leinonen E, Hurt-Camejo E, Wiklund O, et al. Insulin resistance and adiposity correlate with acute-phase reaction and soluble cell adhesion molecules in type 2 diabetes. *Atherosclerosis 2003; 166:387–94.*

Leurs PB, Stolk RP, Hamulyak K, et al.. Tissue factor pathway inhibitor and other endothelium-dependent hemostatic factors in elderly individuals with normal or impaired glucose tolerance and type 2 diabetes. *Diabetes Care 2002; 25:1340–5.*

Li H, Cybulsky MI, Gimbrone MA Jr, et al. An atherogenic diet rapidly induces VCAM-1, a cytokine regulatable mononuclear leukocyte adhesion molecule, in rabbit endothelium. *Arterioscler Thromb 1993; 13:197-204.*

Libby P, Ridker PM, Maseri A. Inflammation in atherosclerosis. *Circulation 2002; 105: 1135-1143.*

Libby P. Inflammation in atherosclerosis. *Nature 2002*; 420:868–74.

Loomans CJ, De Koning EJ, Staal FJ, Rabelink TJ, Zonneveld AJ: Endothelial progenitor cell dysfunction in type 1 diabetes: another consequence of oxidative stress? *Antioxidants & redox signaling 2005; 7(11–12):1468-1475.*

Lund S S., L Tarnow, C D. Stehouwer, C G. Schalkwijk, T Teerlink, J Gram. Impact of metformin versus repaglinide on non-glycaemic cardiovascular risk markers related to inflammation and endothelial dysfunction in non-obese patients with type 2 diabetes. *Eur J Endo 2008; 158:631–641*

Luscher TF, Tanner FC, Tschudi MR, et al. Endothelial dysfunction in coronary artery disease. *Annu Rev Med 1993; 44:395–418.*

Lyon CJ, Law RE, Hsueh WA. Mini review: adiposity, inflammation, and atherogenesis. *Endocrinology 2003; 144:2195–200.*

Mancini GB, Henry GC, Macaya C, et al. Angiotensin-converting enzyme inhibition with quinapril improves endothelial vasomotor dysfunction in patients with coronary artery disease. The TREND (Trial on Reversing ENdothelial Dysfunction) Study. *Circulation 1996; 94:258–65.*

Makino N, Maeda T, Sugano M, et al. High serum TNF-alpha level in Type 2 diabetic patients with microangiopathy is associated with eNOS down-regulation and apoptosis in endothelial cells. *J Diabetes Complications 2005; 19:347–55.*

Makoto Hiki, Kazunori Shimada, Takashi Kiyanagi, Kosuke Fukao, Kuniaki Hirose, Hiromichi Ohsaka. Single Administration of α-Glucosidase Inhibitors on Endothelial Function and Incretin Secretion in Diabetic Patients With Coronary Artery Disease. *Circ J 2010; 74: 1471 - 1478.*

Manson JE, Colditz GA, Stampfer MJ, Willett WC, Krolewski A, Rosner B, Arky RA, Speizer FE & Hennekens CH. A prospective study of maturity-onset diabetes mellitus and risk of coronary heart disease and stroke in women. *Arch Int Med 1991; 151: 1141–1148.*

Manzella D, Ragno E, Abbatecola AM, et al.. Residual C-peptide secretion and endothelial function in patients with Type II diabetes. *Clin Sci 2003; 105:113–18.*

Manzella D, Grella R, Abbatecola AM, et al. Repaglinide administration improves brachial reactivity in type 2 diabetic patients. Diabetes Care 2005; 28:366–71.

Mátthael,S M Stumvall, Pathophysiology and pharmacological treatment of insulin resistance. *Endocr Rev 2001; 6: 585–618.4.*

McFarlane SI, Kumar A, Sowers JR.. Mechanisms by which angiotensin-converting enzyme inhibitors prevent diabetes and cardiovasculardisease. *Am J Cardiol 2003; 91:30H–37H*

Meigs JB, Hu FB, Rifai N, et al. Biomarkers of endothelial dysfunction and risk of type 2 diabetes mellitus. *JAMA 2004; 291:1978–86.*

Milani E, Nikfar S, Khorasani R, Zamani MJ, Abdollahi M. Reduction of diabetes-induced oxidative stress by phosphodiesterase inhibitors in rats. Comp Biochem *Physiol C Toxicol Pharmacol 2005; 140: 251–255.*

Mita T, Otsuka A, Azuma K, Uchida T, Ogihara T, Fujitani Y, et al. Swings in blood glucose levels accelerate atherogenesis in apolipoprotein E-deficient mice. *Biochem Biophys Res Commun 2007; 358:679 - 685.*

Mombouli JV.. ACE inhibition, endothelial function and coronary artery lesions. Role of kinins and nitric oxide. *Drugs 1997; 54 (Suppl 5):12–22.*

Mudaliar S, Henry RR. New oral therapies for type 2 diabetesmellitus: the glitazones or insulin sensitizers. *Annu Rev Med 2001; 52:239–57.*

Nagi DK & Yudkin JS. Effects of metformin on insulin resistance, risk factors for cardiovascular disease, and plasminogen activator inhibitor in NIDDM subjects. A study of two ethnic groups. *Diabetes Care 1993; 16:621–629.*

Natali A, Baldeweg S, Toschi E, Capaldo B, Barbaro D, Gastaldelli A, Yudkin JS & Ferrannini E. Vascular effects ofimproving metabolic control with metformin or rosiglitazone in type 2 diabetes. *Diabetes Care 2004; 27: 1349–1357.*

Nathan DM, Lachin J, Cleary P, Orchard T, Brillon DJ, Backlund JY, O'Leary DH, Genuth S: Intensive diabetes therapy and carotid intima-media thickness in type 1 diabetes mellitus. *N Engl J Med 2003; 348(23):2294-2303.*

Nicholls SJ, E Murat , I Sipahi, et al. Effects of Obesity on Lipid-Lowering, Anti-Inflammatory, and Antiatherosclerotic Benefits of Atorvastatin or Pravastatin in Patients With Coronary Artery Disease (from the REVERSAL Study). *Am J Cardiol 2006; 97:1553–1557.*

O'Brien SF, Watts GF, Playaford DA, et al. Low-density lipoprotein size, high-density lipoprotein concentration, and endotelial dysfunction in non-insulin-dependent diabetes. *Diab Med 1997; 14:974-978.*

Oostrom O van, D PV de Kleijn, J O Fledderus, M Pescatori, A Stubbs, A Tuinenburg, et al. Folic acid supplementation normalizes the endothelial progenitor cell transcriptome of patients with type 1 diabetes: a case-control pilot study. Cardiovascular *Diabetology 2009; 47: 1-11.*

Ouvina SM, La Greca RD, Zanaro NL, et al.. Endothelial dysfunction, nitric oxide and platelet activation in hypertensive and diabetic type II patients. *Thromb Res 2001; 102:107–14.*

Paolisso G, MR Tagliamonte, M Barbieri, et al. Chronic Vitamin E Administration Improves Brachial Reactivity and Increases Intracellular Magnesium Concentration in Type II Diabetic Patients. *J Clin Endocrinol Metab 2000; 85: 109–115.*

Pendergrass M, Fazioni E, Collins D, Defronzo RA. IGF-I increases forearm blood flow without increasing forearm glucose uptake. *Am J Physiol 1998; 275:E345–E350.*

Perticone F, Ceravolo R, Candigliota M, et al. Obesity and body fat distribution induce endothelial dysfunction by oxidative stress: protective effect of vitamin C. *Diabetes 2001; 50:159–65.*

Perticone F, Ceravolo R, Pujia A, Ventura G, Iacopino S, Scozzafava A, Ferraro A, Chello M, Mastroroberto P, Verdecchia P, Schillaci G. Prognostic significance of endothelial dysfunction in hypertensive patients. *Circulation 2001; 104:191–196.*

Piatti P, Fragasso G, Monti LD, Setola E, Lucotti P, Fermo I. Acute intravenous l-arginine infusion decreases endothelin-1 levels and improves endothelial function in patients with angina pectoris and normal coronary arteriograms: correlation with asymmetric dimethylarginine levels. *Circulation 2003; 107:429–436.*

Pfutzner A, Marx N, Lubben G, Langenfeld M, Walcher D, Konrad T, Forst T: Improvement of cardiovascular risk markers by pioglitazone is independent from glycemic control: results from the Pioneer Study. *J AmColl Cardiol 2005; 45:1925–1931.*

Pistrosch F, Passauer J, Fischer S, et al. In type 2 diabetes, Rosiglitazone therapy for insulin resistance ameliorates endothelial dysfunction independent of glucose control. *Diabetes Care 2004; 27:484–90.*

Pistrosch F, Herbrig K, Kindel B, et al.. Rosiglitazone improves glomerular hyperfiltration, renal endothelial dysfunction, and microalbuminuria of incipient diabetic nephropathy in patients. *Diabetes 2005; 54:2206–11.*

Quehenberger P, Bierhaus A, Fasching P, et al. Endothelin 1 transcription is controlled by nuclear factor-kappaB in AGE-stimulated cultured endothelial cells. *Diabetes 2000; 49: 1561-1570.*

Quiñones MJ, Hernandez-Pampaloni M, Chon Y, et al.. Improvement of coronary artery endothelial dysfunction in insulin resistant patients after treatment with insulin-sensitizing thiazolidinediones. *Diabetes 2002; 51:A172.*

Rask-Madsen C, Ihlemann N, Krarup T, Christiansen E, Kober L, Nervil KC, Torp-Pedersen C. Insulin therapy improves insulin-stimulated endothelial function in patients with type 2 diabetes and ischemic heart disease. *Diabetes 2001; 50:2611–2618.*

Reinhart K, O Baker, F Brunkhorst, Markers of endothelial damage in organ dysfunction and sepsis, *Crit Care Med 2002; 30:5302–5312.*

Retterstol L, B Paus, A Bakken. Plasma total homocysteine levels and prognosis in patients with previous premature myocardial infarction: a 10-year follow-up study. *J Int Med 2003; 253:284–292.*

Ridker PM, E Danielson, FAH Fonseca, et al. Rosuvastatin to Prevent Vascular Events in Men and Women with Elevated C-Reactive Protein. N Engl J Med 2008; 359:2195-207151.

Ross R. The pathogenesis of atherosclerosis: a perspective for the 1990s. Nature 1993; 362: 801-809.

Salloum FN, Ockaili RA, Wittkamp M, Marwaha VR, Kukreja RC. Vardenafil: a novel type 5 phosphodiesterase inhibitor reduces myocardial infarct size following ischemia/reperfusion injury via opening of mitochondrial K(ATP) channels in rabbits. *J Mol Cell Cardiol 2006; 40: 405–411*

Satu Vehkavaara, Sari Ma¨kimattila, Anna Schlenzka, Juha Vakkilainen, Jukka Westerbacka, Hannele Yki-Ja¨rvinen. Insulin Therapy Improves Endothelial Function in Type 2 Diabetes. *Arterioscler Thromb Vasc Biol 2000; 20:545-550*

Satu Vehkavaara, Hannele Yki-Järvinen. 3.5 Years of Insulin Therapy With Insulin Glargine Improves In Vivo Endothelial Function in Type 2 Diabetes. *Arterioscler Thromb Vasc Biol 2004; 24:325-330.*

Senzaki H, Smith CJ, Juang GJ, Isoda T, Mayer SP, Ohler A et al. Cardiac phosphodiesterase 5 (cGMP-specific) modulates beta adrenergic signaling in vivo and is down-regulated in heart failure. *FASEB J 2001; 15: 1718–1726.*

Schachinger V, Britten MB, Zeiher AM. Prognostic impact of coronary vasodilator dysfunction on adverse long-term outcome of coronary heart disease. *Circulation 2000; 101:1899–1906.*

Schäfer A, Fraccarollo D, Pförtsch S, Flierl U, Vogt C, Pfrang J et al. Improvement of vascular function by acute and chronic treatment with the PDE-5 inhibitor sildenafil in experimental diabetes mellitus. *Br J Pharmacol 2008; 153: 886–893.*

Shabsigh R. Therapy of ED: PDE-5 Inhibitors. *Endocrine 2004; 23: 135–141.*

Schachinger V, Britten MB, Zeiher AM. Prognostic impact of coronary vasodilator dysfunction on adverse long-term outcome of coronary heart disease. *Circulation 2000; 101: 1899-1906*

Shepherd J, Cobbe SM, Ford I, et al. Prevention of coronary heart disease with pravastatin in men with hypercholesterolemia. West of Scotland Coronary Prevention Study Group. *N Engl J Med 1995; 333:1301–7.*

Schectman G, Hiatt J. Dose-response characteristics of cholesterol lowering drug therapies: implications for treatment. *Ann Intern Med 1996; 125:990 –1000.*

Sheetz MJ, King GL. Molecular understanding of hyperglycemia's adverse effects for diabetic complications. *JAMA 2002; 288:2579–2588.*

Shimabukuro M, Higa N, Takasu N, Tagawa T, Ueda S. A single dose of nateglinide improves postprandial endothelial dysfunction in type 2 diabetic patients. *Diabet Med 2004; 21:983–986.*

Shimabukuro Michio, Namio Higa, Ichiro Chinen, Ken Yamakawa, and Nobuyuki Takasu. Effects of a Single Administration of Acarbose on Postprandial Glucose Excursion and Endothelial Dysfunction in Type 2 Diabetic Patients: A Randomized Crossover Study. (J Clin Endocrinol Metab 2006; 91: 837–842.

Schmieder RE: Optimizing therapeutic strategies to achieve renal and cardiovascular risk reduction in diabetic patients with angiotensin receptor blockers. *J Hypertens 2005; 23:905–911,*

Schmieder RE. Impact of Telmisartan Versus Ramipril on Renal Endothelial Function in Patients With Hypertension and Type 2 Diabetes. *Diabetes Care 2007; 30:1351–1356.*

Schneider JG, Tilly N, Hierl T, et al. Elevated plasma endothelin-1 levels in diabetes mellitus. *Am J Hypertens 2002; 15:967-972.*

Shishehbor MH, Brennan ML, Aviles RJ, Fu X, Penn MS, Sprecher DL, Hazen SL. Statins promote potent systemic antioxidant effects through specific inflammatory pathways. *Circulation 2003; 108:426–431.*

Shishehbor MH, Aviles RJ, Brennan ML, Fu X, Goormastic M, Pearce GL, Gokce N, Keaney JF Jr, Penn MS, Sprecher DL, et al. Association of nitrotyrosine levels with cardiovascular disease and modulation by statin therapy. JAMA 2003; 289:1675–1680.

Stalker TJ, Skvarka CB, Scalia R. A novel role for calpains in the endothelial dysfunction of hyperglycemia. *FASEB J 2003; 17:1511–13.*

Stoll LL, McCormick ML, Denning GM, Weintraub NL. Antioxidant effects of statins. *Drugs Today (Barc) 2004; 40:975–990.*

Suwaidi JA, Hamasaki S, Higano ST, Nishimura RA, Holmes DRJ, Lerman A. Long-term follow-up of patients with mild coronary artery disease and endothelial dysfunction. *Circulation. 2000; 101:948–954.*

Svolis KA, Lemboussi DSP, Svolis AA, Stellas L, Bakopoulos C, Patronis A, Giannoulaki E: Telmisartan, an angiotensin II type 1 receptor blocker, improves endothelial function in patients with chronic heart failure (Abstract). *J Am Coll Cardiol 2002; 39 (Suppl. B):266B.*

Taddei S, Virdis A, Mattei P, Natali A, Ferrannini E, Salvetti A. Effect of insulin on acetylcholine-induced vasodilatation in normotensive subjects and patients with essential hypertension. *Circulation 1995; 92:2911–2918.*

Sheetz MJ, King GL: Molecular understanding of hyperglycemia's adverse effects for diabetic complications. *JAMA 2002; 288(20):2579-2588.*

Steinberg HO, Brechtel G, Johnson A, et al. Insulin-mediated skeletal muscle vasodilation is nitric oxide dependent. A novel action of insulin to increase nitric oxide release. *J Clin Invest 1994; 94:1172–9.*

Steinberg HO, Chaker H, Leaming R, et al. Obesity/insulin resistance is associated with endothelial dysfunction: implications for the syndrome of insulin resistance. *J Clin Invest 1996; 97:2601–10.*

Studdy PR, Lapworth R, Bird R. Angiotensin-converting enzyme and its clinical significance–a review. *J Clin Pathol 1983; 36:938–47.*

Stuhlinger MC, Abbasi F, Chu JW, et al.. Relationship between insulin resistance and an endogenous nitric oxide synthase inhibitor. JAMA 2002; 287:1420–6.

Tan KC, Chow WS, Ai VH, et al. Effects of angiotensin II receptor antagonist on endothelial vasomotor function and urinary albumin excretion in type 2 diabetic patients with microalbuminuria. *Diabetes Metab Res Rev 2002; 18:71–6.*

Testa R, Bonfigli AR, Piantanelli L, Manfrini S, Testa I & Gregorio F. Relationship between plasminogen activator inhibitor type-1 plasma levels and the lipoprotein(a) concentrations in noninsulin-dependent diabetes mellitus. *Diab Res Clin Prac 1996; 33: 111–118.*

Thorand B, Baumert J, Chambless L, et al. MONICA/KORA Study Group. Elevated markers of endothelial dysfunction predict type 2 diabetes mellitus in middle-aged men and women from the general population. *Arterioscler Thromb Vasc Bio 2006; 26:398–405.*

Tornel,PL J Abellán, A Cano, P Martínez, La proteína C reactiva como marcador del riesgo cardiovascular, *Hipertensión 2003; 20:74–81.*

Takemoto M, Liao JK. Pleiotropic effects of 3-hydroxy-3-methylglutaryl coenzyme A reductase inhibitors. *Arterioscler Thromb Vasc Biol 2001; 21:1712–1719.*

Tamai O, Matsuoka H, Itabe H, et al. Single LDL apheresis improves endothelium-dependent vasodilatation in hypercholesterolemic humans. *Circulation 1997; 95:76–82.*

Teixeira CE, Priviero FB, Webb RC Differential effects of the phosphodiesterase type 5 inhibitors sildenafil, vardenafil, and tadalafil in rat aorta. *J Pharmacol Exp Ther 2006; 316: 654–661.*

UK Prospective Diabetes Study (UKPDS) Group. Effect of intensive blood–glucose control with metformin on complications in overweight patients with type 2 diabetes (UKPDS 34). *Lancet 1998; 352:854–865.*

UK Prospective Diabetes Study Group. Intensive blood-glucose control with sulphonylureas or insulin compared with conventional treatment and risk of complications in patients with type 2 diabetes (UKPDS 33). *Lancet 1998; 352:837- 853.*

Vehkavaara S, Si Ma¨kimattila, A Schlenzka, Ja Vakkilainen, J Westerbacka, H Yki-Ja¨rvinen. Insulin Therapy Improves Endothelial Function in Type 2 Diabetes. *Arterioscler Thromb Vasc Biol 2000;20:545-550.*

Viberti GC, Benigni A, Bognetti E, et al.. Glomerular hyperfiltration and urinary prostaglandins in type 1 diabetes mellitus. *Diabet Med 1989; 6:219–23.*

Vita JA, Keaney JF. Endothelial function: a barometer for cardiovascular risk? *Circulation 2002; 106: 640-642.*

Volpe Massimo, Castello Lorenzo, Cosentino Francesco. Effects of Olmesartan on Endothelial Function. *High Blood Pressure Cardiov Prevention 2007; 14 (4): 221-227.*

Vallejo S, Angulo J, Peiro C, Cercas E, Sanchez-Ferrer A, Nevado J. Treatment with acarbose may improve endothelial dysfunction in streptozotocin-induced diabetic rats. *J Cardiovasc Pharmacol 2000; 36:255–262.*

Vlachopoulos C, Tsekoura D, Alexopoulos N, Panagiotakos D, Aznaouridis K, Stefanadis C). Type 5 phosphodiesterase inhibition by sildenafil abrogates acute smoking-induced endothelial dysfunction. *Am J Hypertens 2004; 17: 1040–1044.*

Vehkavaara S, Mäkimattila S, Schlenzka A, Vakkilainen J, Westerbacka J, Yki-Järvinen H. Insulin therapy improves endothelial function in type 2 diabetes. *Arterioscler Thromb Vasc Biol 2000; 20:545–550.*

Wautier JL, Zoukourian C, Chappey O, et al. Receptor mediated endothelial cell dysfunction in diabetic vasculopathy. Soluble receptor for advanced glycation end products blocks hyperpermeability in diabetic rats. *J Clin Invest, 1996; 97:238–*

Wakino S, Law RE, Hsueh WA.. Vascular protective effects by activation of nuclear receptor PPAR. *J Diab Com 2002; 16:46–9.*

Williams SB, Cusco JA, Roddy MA, Johnstone MT, Creager MA: Impaired nitric oxide-mediated vasodilation in patients with non-insulin-dependent diabetes mellitus. *Journal of the American College of Cardiology 1996; 27(3):567-574.*

Wajcberg E, Sriwijilkamol A, Musi N, De-Fronzo R, Cersosimo E: Relationship Between vascular reactivity and lipids in Mexican American with T2DM treated with pioglitazone. *J Clin Endocrinol Metab 2007; 92:1256–1262.*

Wen Y, Skidmore JC, Porter-Turner MM, et al. Relationship of glycation, antioxidant status and oxidative stress to vascular endothelial damage in diabetes. *Diabetes Obes Metab 2002; 4:305–8.*

Williams B. A potential role for angiotensin II-induced vascular endothelial growth factor expression in the pathogenesis of diabetic nephropathy? Miner Electrolyte *Metab 1998; 24:400–5.*

Yano M, Hasegawa G, Ishii M, Yamasaki M, Fukui M, Nakamura N, Yoshikawa T. Short-term exposure of high glucose concentration induces generation of reactive oxygen species in endothelial cells: implication for the oxidative stress associated with postprandial hyperglycemia. Redox Rep 2004: 9:111-116.

Yu Y, Suo L, Yu H, et al.. Insulin resistance and endothelial dysfunction in type 2 diabetes patients with or without microalbuminuria. *Diabetes Res Clin Pract 2004; 65:95–104.*

Yusuf S, Gerstein H, Hoogwerf B, et al.. Ramipril and the development of diabetes. *JAMA 2001; 286:1882–5.*

Zeng G, Nystrom FH, Ravichandran LV, et al.. Roles for insulin receptor, PI3-kinase, and Akt in insulin-signaling pathways related to production of nitric oxide in human vascular endothelial cells. *Circulation 2000; 101:1539–45.*

Part 3

Genetics of Type 2 Diabetes

8

Using Gene Expression Signatures to Dissect Insulin Resistance Subtypes

Brad Hayward, Nicky Konstantopoulos and Ken R. Walder
Metabolic Research Unit, School of Medicine, Deakin University
Australia

1. Introduction

It is now apparent that many diseases such as diabetes are more complex and heterogeneous than had been thought just a decade ago. Combinations of varying causative factors, as well as interactions between environmental and genetic factors all play a role in the onset of the disease. This complexity has hindered the development of new effective treatment options for patients, and makes understanding the onset of the disease difficult. This chapter will focus on a new technology to study diabetes using a novel unbiased approach, and to develop individualised therapeutics for patients with diabetes.

1.1 Type 2 diabetes

Diabetes mellitus is characterised by dysregulation of a number of metabolic processes as a result of abnormal insulin secretion and/or signalling (Saltiel and Pessin, 2002). Insulin, secreted by the pancreas, is a potent anabolic hormone involved in the regulation of glucose homeostasis as well as lipid and protein metabolism (Saltiel and Pessin, 2002). There are two main types of diabetes mellitus. Type 1 diabetes (T1D), is caused by a defect in insulin secretion by the pancreas, and can be treated by administration of exogenous insulin. T1D is often caused by an autoimmune disorder, where the insulin-secreting β-cells of the pancreas are destroyed, however, additional environmental causes such as viruses may also be involved (Tisch and McDevitt, 1996). In contrast, type 2 diabetes (T2D) is characterised by resistance to the action of insulin in key metabolic tissues such as skeletal muscle, liver and adipose tissue, coupled with reduced insulin secretion caused by impaired β-cell function in the pancreas (McKinlay and Marceau, 2000; NIDDK, 2009).

T2D accounts for over 90% of all reported cases of diabetes (Taylor, 1999). The disease is characterised by peripheral insulin resistance, hyperglycaemia and defective insulin secretion. Defective insulin signalling in peripheral tissues including muscle, adipose tissue and the liver, adversely affects whole body glucose homeostasis. Impaired insulin signalling, coupled with the eventual exhaustion of β-cell insulin production, leads to T2D (Fig. 1). Unlike type 1 diabetes, where insulin therapy can provide effective relief, T2D requires treatment of insulin resistance, in addition to insulin secretion defects.

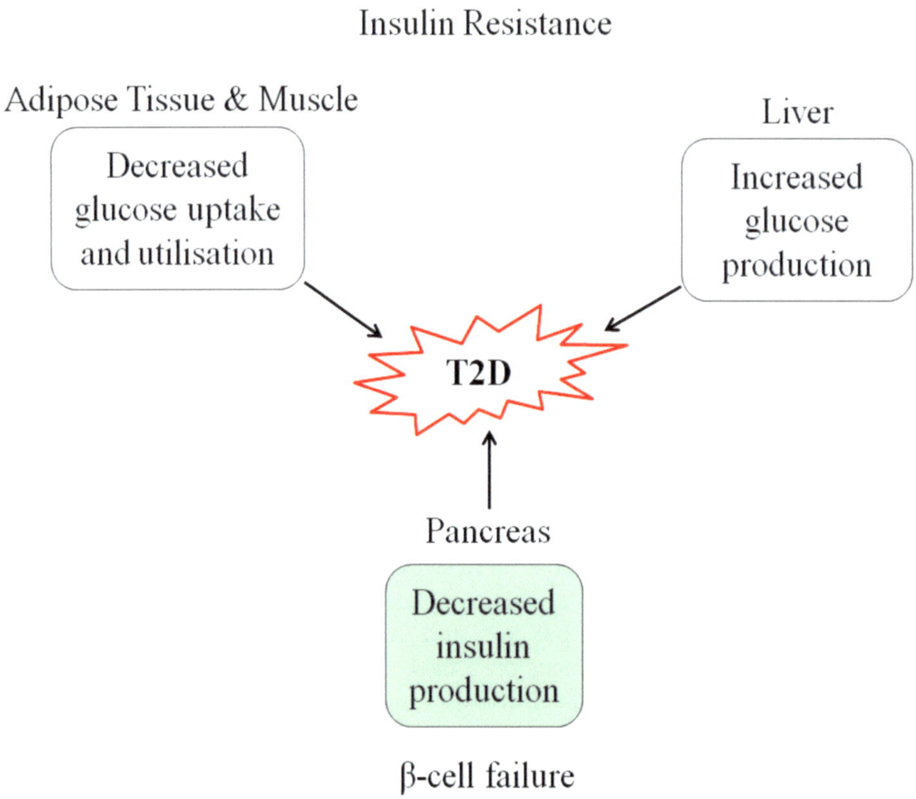

Fig. 1. A simplified overview of the pathogenesis of type 2 diabetes, encompassing insulin resistance in muscle, adipose tissue and liver, as well as impaired insulin secretion by the β-cells of the pancreas. Adapted from (Baudry et al., 2002).

1.2 Prevalence and cost of diabetes

There are currently 25.8 million people in the United States living with diabetes, and this accounts for 8.3% of the population (CDC, 2011). This alarming figure is growing rapidly, with 1.9 million people being newly diagnosed in 2010 alone (CDC, 2011). Diabetes represents a significant health burden to the US, both in terms of the number of patients currently living with diabetes, and the huge number of patients estimated to develop diabetes in the coming years. It has been estimated that there are currently 79 million adults in the US who are pre-diabetic (as determined by fasting blood glucose or HbA1c levels). The costs associated with managing the diabetes epidemic were recently estimated at $174 billion annually, and this figure is set to increase in the coming years. The projected increase in the prevalence of diabetes, coupled with the already significant economic costs associated with the disease, make the development of alternative effective treatments an urgent priority.

2. Diagnosis and treatment of type 2 diabetes

2.1 Diagnosis of type 2 diabetes

Diagnosis of T2D, and its precursor insulin resistance, is made difficult by the lack of symptoms early in the development of the disease, and many cases go undiagnosed. The

Australian Diabetes, Obesity and Lifestyle study found that half of all subjects studied who were suffering from T2D had not been previously diagnosed (Dunstan et al., 2002). Predictors of risk for the development of T2D and cardiovascular disease include body mass index (BMI), ethnic origin, blood pressure and cholesterol levels (Gavin et al., 2003). Current clinical guidelines for the diagnosis of diabetes however are based upon blood glucose measures. The World Health Organisation (WHO) standard criteria for diagnosis of T2D involve fasting plasma glucose (FPG) and the response to an oral glucose tolerance test (OGTT). FPG is a measure of plasma glucose after 8 hours of fasting, while the OGTT measures plasma glucose 2 hours following an intake of 75 g glucose. The current guidelines are outlined in Table 1.

	FPG	OGTT
NGT	< 6.1 mmol/L	< 7.8 mmol/L
IGT	< 7.0 mmol/L	7.8 - 11.1 mmol/L
IFG	6.1 - 6.9 mmol/L	< 7.8 mmol/L
Diabetes	≥ 7.0 mmol/L	≥ 11.1 mmol/L

Abbreviations used: NGT - normal glucose tolerance, IGT - impaired glucose tolerance, IFG - impaired fasting glucose (WHO/IDF, 2006).

Table 1. WHO guidelines for the diagnosis of diabetes and other hyperglycaemic states.

IGT and IFG are both strong indicators of risk for the development of T2D, with individuals suffering from both conditions placed at even higher risk (Gavin et al., 2003). IGT is characterised by peripheral insulin resistance, while defects in insulin secretion coupled with increased hepatic glucose output characterise IFG (Davies et al., 2000). While the associated health risks, prevalence and distribution vary for IGT and IFG (Unwin et al., 2002), the risk of developing T2D is similar for both, and increases further when both IGT and IFG are present (Gavin et al., 2003).

2.2 Current anti-diabetic treatments

The development of both insulin resistance and impaired glucose tolerance, conditions which precede the onset of T2D, are closely linked with obesity (Sharma, 2006). Excess visceral fat, and the hormones and inflammatory factors it releases, coupled with excess free fatty acid release have been implicated in the development of T2D (Mlinar et al., 2007). For obese patients exhibiting these symptoms, changes to healthier eating patterns and increases in exercise can result in improvements to glucose tolerance. However this approach often fails within the first year of treatment, and therefore the use of various medications is usually required (Nathan et al., 2006). Lifestyle changes immediately following the diagnosis of T2D can often be successful in the early treatment of the disease. Unfortunately, a lack of diagnosis, coupled with difficulties in maintaining lifestyle changes, means that this is not a treatment option which will be effective in the long term for all patients (Nathan et al., 2006).

Metformin is an oral antidiabetic agent, based upon the molecule biguanide. Its mechanism of action involves a reduction in hepatic gluconeogenesis, leading to a reduction in blood glucose levels (Knowler et al., 2002). This can also have the associated benefit of reducing blood insulin levels. Metformin has a number of side effects including gastrointestinal symptoms and has been linked with rare cases of lactic acidosis which can be fatal, although evidence for this has been contradicted in some studies (Salpeter et al., 2006). Metformin is one of only two oral anti-diabetic agents on the WHO list of essential medicines. The second oral anti-diabetic to be listed by WHO is the drug family known as the sulfonylureas, the most commonly used drug of which is glibenclamide. The sulfonylureas mechanism of action involves enhancing insulin secretion (Groop, 1992). For this reason, the sulfonylureas show their best efficacy in the early stages of the disease when β-cell function is still viable. Side effects associated with the sulfonylureas include hypoglycaemia due to their long half life in plasma, and weight gain.

The glinides are a family of drugs with a mechanism of action similar to the sulfonylureas, in that they bind to the same receptor - although at a different binding site - to induce insulin secretion from the β-cells of the pancreas. The glinides have an advantage over the sulfonylureas in that they have a shorter half life in blood plasma. As such, some glinides pose a lower risk of hypoglycaemia then some of the sulfonylureas (Kristensen et al., 2000).

Thiazolidinediones (TZDs or glitazones) are an insulin sensitizing family of compounds. TZDs are ligands for the nuclear transcription factor peroxisome proliferator-activated receptor γ (PPARγ). It is through transcriptional regulation of PPARγ that this family of compounds increase the sensitivity of muscle, liver and adipose tissue to the effects of insulin (Yki-Jarvinen, 2004). However, this family of drugs has been linked to some serious long term side effects. Troglitazone, first approved for use in T2D patients in 1997, was withdrawn from the market in 2000 after it was linked to a number of cases of liver dysfunction and failure (Watkins, 2005). The widely used alternative rosiglitazone has in recent years been linked to increased cardiovascular disease (Nissen and Wolski, 2010). The drug has been withdrawn from sale in the UK and New Zealand. While still available in the US, rosiglitazone is currently branded with additional safety warnings and restrictions on its use, and sales in recent years have fallen significantly (GlaxoSmithKline, 2010).

Exogenous insulin is a very important therapeutic agent for the treatment of diabetes, capable of increasing blood insulin levels when β-cell function has been impaired, and can be given in increasing amounts to overcome insulin resistance. However, insulin is also associated with increases in weight gain, as well as risk of hypoglycaemia if monitoring of blood glucose levels is not rigorously performed.

Glucagon-like peptide 1 agonists (GLP-1 agonists) are mimics of a protein secreted by the L-cells of the small intestine. They act on GLP-1 receptors in pancreatic β-cells, inducing insulin release. GLP-1 agonists have also been shown to stimulate β-cell proliferation (Drucker, 2003, 2005) and suppress glucagon release and gastric motility, while inducing weight loss. Side effects of GLP-1 agonists include a decrease in gastric motility, responsible for the nausea commonly experienced by patients (Kendall et al., 2005).

Amylin is a β-cell hormone co-secreted with insulin. Amylin lowers blood glucose levels by inhibiting glucagon secretion following a meal, and induces satiety by acting upon the area postrema (AP) neurons within the brain stem (Potes and Lutz, 2010). While amylin forms aggregates which make it unsuitable as a therapeutic agent, amylin agonists such as pramlintide can effectively simulate the effects of the physiological amylin. Like GLP-1 agonists, amylin agonists can also induce nausea in patients (Schmitz et al., 2004).

2.3 Problems and adverse effects of current drug therapies

As highlighted above, the currently used range of antidiabetic medicines have a number of adverse side effects, including hypoglycaemia, fluid retention and weight gain, and gastrointestinal symptoms. As T2D generally progresses over time to a worsening in glycaemic control, the need to utilise multiple therapies together is unfortunately the reality for many patients with T2D (Nathan et al., 2006). Difficulties in managing T2D are exacerbated by the fact that the various drugs available have a wide range of effects in individual patients, in terms of the magnitude of both efficacy and side effects. In addition to these factors, many of the current drugs used to treat T2D lose their efficacy over time (Cohen and Horton, 2007). Therefore, the focus of new treatments has to be on how to personally tailor pharmacotherapy to suit each patient's characteristics.

We believe that the reason why current therapies are not effective in all patients is that they do not address the heterogeneous nature of T2D. A number of different subtypes of insulin resistance have been described, in a number of different tissues and due to varying insults. If effective treatments for T2D are to be developed, there is a need to gain a better understanding of the different subtypes of insulin resistance. Then, the development of new treatment regimes which specifically target the various subtypes of insulin resistance will be possible - enabling the development of a personalised medicine approach to T2D.

3. Insulin resistance subtypes

3.1 Insulin resistance subtypes

Insulin resistance is a major risk factor for the development of T2D (Lillioja et al., 1993). Combating insulin resistance is therefore a key to developing effective treatments for T2D. The etiology of T2D is multifactorial, with both genetic and environmental factors involved (Bergman and Ader, 2000). Likewise, the onset of insulin resistance is multifactorial and can occur in different tissues and arise from multiple causes as depicted in Fig. 2. There are numerous known insults to insulin signalling and action. Insults to insulin action can be both endogenous, such as inflammatory cytokines released in response to a fatty meal, and exogenous, such as the fatty acids themselves, which can lead to the development of insulin resistance. These subtypes can be mimicked in cell culture based models, as shown in Table 2.

Subtype	Causative agents
Inflammation	Cytokines: eg. Some interleukins, TNFα
ER Stress	Tunicamycin, Thapsigargin
Glucocorticoid	Dexamethasone
Hyperinsulinemia	Chronic elevated insulin levels
Oxidative stress	ROS: eg. Superoxide anions
Hyperlipidemia	Long chain, saturated FFAs: eg. Palmitate (16:0) (Chavez and Summers, 2003)

Table 2. Proposed subtypes of insulin resistance and the insults which can lead to their genesis in cell models.

While there are a number of factors which may lead to the development of insulin resistance in various tissues, they do not necessarily develop in complete isolation, and signalling crosstalk between the various models mentioned above occurs. For example, hyperlipidemia induced insulin resistance has also been linked to increased generation of the inflammatory cytokine TNF-α through activation of proinflammatory transcription factor NF-κβ (Itani et al., 2002; Jove et al., 2006).

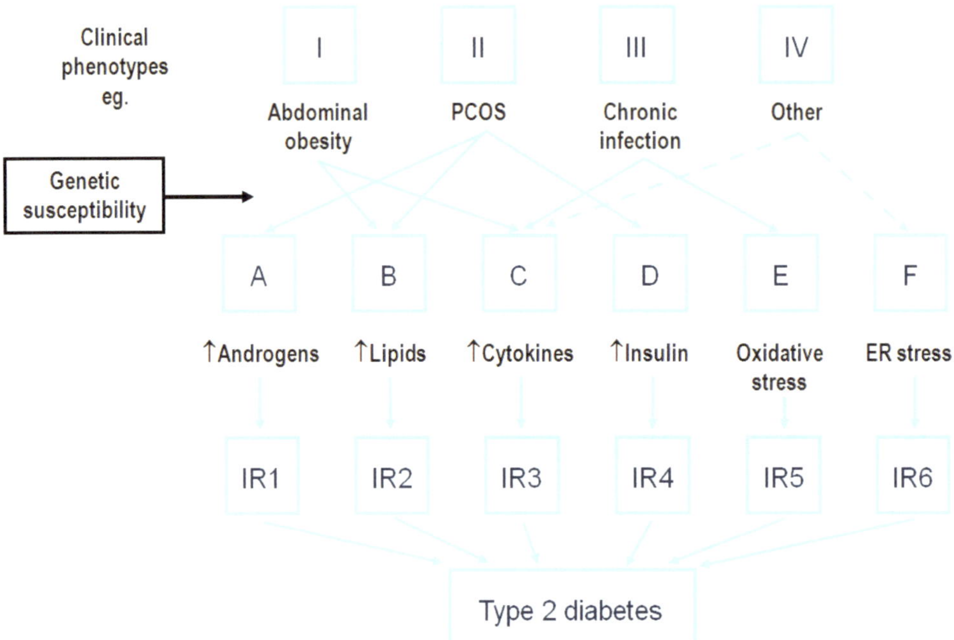

Fig. 2. The multifactorial nature of T2D. Multiple clinical phenotypes such as abdominal obesity, polycystic ovary (PCOS) and Cushing's syndromes, lipodystrophies, chronic levels of hyperinsulinemia, acromegaly (elevated growth hormone) and chronic infection are all associated with insulin resistance. The links between the causes of insulin resistance associated with these phenotypes is not obvious since multiple pathways have been implicated in the development of insulin resistance, such as hyperlipidemia, elevated levels of pro-inflammatory cytokines and/or induction of oxidative or endoplasmic reticulum (ER) stress pathways which may be activated individually or concurrently. Superimposed on this network of interactions is the genetic variability of each individual that confers a differential susceptibility to each insult, adding another layer of complexity. However, all of these insults can cause insulin resistance, albeit via different mechanisms.

We propose that there may be multiple factors contributing to insulin resistance in an individual. We aim to identify a "signature" or "profile" for each of the causative agents of insulin resistance. Profiling of patients could then allow the determination of which subtypes of insulin resistance each individual has. One such subtype of insulin resistance is that caused by increased saturated fatty acid levels in some obese individuals. We hypothesise that we can use the profiles to identify a main contributing subtype to a patient's insulin resistance. Then we will aim to specifically target that subtype (or subtypes) in an individual for longer term and personalised management of their metabolic dysregulation. This will be discussed in further detail below.

3.2 Obesity

The most commonly associated disorder linked with the onset of insulin resistance is obesity (Cummings and Schwartz, 2003; Granberry and Fonseca, 1999). Obesity is widespread in the western world, with the recent US National Health and Nutrition Examination Survey

(NHANES) finding that 67% of Americans aged 20 and above are overweight or obese, with 34% being obese (NCHS, 2008). The WHO estimates that in 2005 there were 1.6 billion adults worldwide who were overweight, at least 400 million of who were obese. These numbers are projected to increase to 2.3 billion overweight and at least 700 million obese adults by 2015 (WHO, 2006). The increasing epidemic of obesity will further increase the prevalence of insulin resistance and T2D within society, making the development of effective treatments a critical challenge for the 21st century.

As one of the primary risk factors for the development of T2D, obesity warrants extensive study as a target for the development of additional and alternative therapies. The defining characteristic of obesity is increased adiposity. Increased availability of free fatty acids (FFA) in patients with obesity plays a critical role in the development of insulin resistance (DeFronzo, 2004). There are numerous factors in obesity which can lead to increases in circulating free fatty acids, including exceeding the storage capacity of adipose tissue by excess caloric intake (Langeveld and Aerts, 2009), and adipose tissue stimulation by the paracrine tumour necrosis factor alpha (TNFα) which induces triglyceride metabolism and free fatty acid release (Ruan and Lodish, 2003). Insulin resistance in adipose tissue can also lead to excess fatty acid release, due to suppression of the antilipolytic effects of insulin (Ruan and Lodish, 2003). The direct effects of increased circulating free fatty acids on macrophages to stimulate release of pro-inflammatory cytokines such as TNFα and IL-6 has also been recently described (for a review see (Bilan et al., 2009)). The onset of insulin resistance caused by free fatty acids is therefore highly complex, and although direct action upon target tissues have been described, there are secondary actions upon other tissue types which further complicate the pathology of the disease. Given the increasing prevalence of obesity around the world, dissecting the mechanisms by which free fatty acids contribute to insulin resistance may identify new avenues for effective treatment regimes

4. Previous approaches at characterising insulin resistance

4.1 Classical single target-based approaches

Classical approaches for dissecting insulin resistance involve targeting signalling defects in both *in vitro* and *in vivo* models of insulin resistance. These approaches - including western blotting for proteins and PCR for genetic data have enhanced our knowledge of insulin resistance and the mechanisms by which insulin signalling is impaired. However such approaches rely upon previous knowledge to build a network of signalling connections, and implicating signalling defects in the observed *in vitro* or *in vivo* model being observed. As is becoming increasingly clear, signalling networks within cells are far more complicated than previously thought. Single insults (such as fatty acids) not only impact upon insulin signalling directly, but also on numerous signalling cascades such as inflammatory pathways, which may be either distally related to insulin signalling or not related at all. This will result in activation of many kinases, and modification of transcription of a number of genes, in the process of the cell reaching an equilibrium state.

We now know that the single target or pathway approaches provide too narrow a window to appreciate the changes induced in complex disease states. While the contribution of the single target / pathway approaches cannot be denied, in terms of expanding our knowledge base, a wider approach is now required for the development of the next line of therapies.

4.2 Endpoint-based approaches

Endpoint-based approaches have been significant in developing our understanding of the development of diabetes. Utilising insulin signalling endpoints such as hepatic glucose output or muscle glucose transport can provide a more global overview of the cellular state compared with the phosphorylation of a single kinase amongst a signalling network. The discovery of new therapies targeted against endpoints allow us to bypass the upstream complexity that hinders the target-based approaches.

4.3 'Omics' approaches

The development of powerful platform technologies such as microarrays has led to a vast increase in the utilisation of the 'omics' type studies. Current mass spectroscopy techniques allow for the study of nearly the entire lipid or protein fraction of a sample, allowing characterisation of disease states in an unprecedented way. The requirement to investigate and treat many diseases with multifactorial natures has necessitated the need for more powerful technologies to give researchers a "global" view of disease states. The search for effective early diagnostic tools, insight into the development of disease states, and the development of new therapies are increasingly relying on one or more of these new platform approaches.

In the context of obesity, lipidomic approaches are proving to be very useful in identifying characteristic changes in tissue-specific lipid profiles of patients with T2D (Meikle and Christopher, 2011), which has been made possible by advances in mass spectroscopy techniques. Advances have also been applied to the proteomic field. Techniques such as Stable Isotope Labeling by Amino acids in Cell culture (SILAC) are proving to be powerful in furthering our knowledge of insulin signalling cascades in both normal and insulin resistant states, by allowing the investigation of a large number of proteins at once across multiple samples (Hanke and Mann, 2009).

4.4 Genomics-based approaches

Developed in the mid 90's for the analysis of the expression of multiple genes in parallel (Schena et al., 1995), microarray technology can now be used to assess the expression of tens of thousands of genes in a sample simultaneously. This provides a powerful tool to assess whole cell transcriptional events for any given cell or tissue in any biological state. Microarray technology has a range of applications including identifying disease-causing genes, identifying targets for new therapies and prediction of drug responsiveness (Jayapal and Melendez, 2006).

Two major applications for microarray technology involve examining gene sets for pathway analysis, and examining differentially expressed genes between two or more experimental conditions (Kauffmann and Huber, 2010). Gene set enrichment analysis (GSEA) involves taking a gene list , ranked according to the difference in expression between the phenotypes or treatments being investigated. The goal of GSEA is to determine whether members of specific gene sets (grouped on functional similarity), are ranked together towards the top or bottom of the list. GSEA therefore indicates whether a correlation exists between differential expression of that set of genes, and the specific phenotype being investigated (Oron et al., 2008; Subramanian et al., 2005). This pathway analysis approach to dissecting disease is complimented well by proteomic approaches which can similarly be used for pathway analysis.

The second of the two applications involves performing microarray analysis on gene sets from multiple experimental conditions, and can be used to identify differentially expressed genes in differing disease states. This 'shotgun' style approach to genome analysis can yield previously unknown information about the regulation of disease states at the transcriptional level, which can have important implications for understanding the pathophysiology of disease. The set of differentially expressed genes can also be used for a diagnostic approach to the disease. Applying Bayesian Linear statistical modelling to gene sets allows for selection of a relatively small gene set which can characterise the particular biological state of the cell or tissue being investigated (Smyth, 2004). This process statistically evaluates which set of genes have the greatest differential expression between the conditions tested, and identifies a 'fingerprint' indicative of the biological state of the cell or tissue involved, known as a gene expression signature (GES). Previously, GESs have been applied to the field of cancer research, for applications such as classifying tumour types and predicting tumour response to chemotherapy. By classifying tumours into distinct types, and with knowledge of how each type will respond to particular therapies, clinicians are therefore able to treat patients more effectively by personalising treatment regimes (Lee et al., 2007). Personalised medicine approaches such as this are becoming increasingly important tools in fighting diseases and the use of GES are likewise increasing in disease research.

5. Gene expression signatures

5.1 Gene expression signatures as a diagnostic tool

First described in 2000, GESs were developed in the field of cancer research. The differences in patient response to therapies led researchers to believe that groups of cancers that were not able to be histologically characterised were actually a heterogeneous group of tumours. Seeking a non-biased method for classification, gene expression data was investigated to search for patterns which could differentiate classes of B-cell lymphomas with differing patient survival rates (Alizadeh et al., 2000). The main outcome of the study was the finding of two subgroups, classified on the basis of differential gene expression of hundreds of genes, with differing survival outcomes for patients. This early study was instrumental in highlighting the use of gene expression data as a disease classification tool. The power of the GES approach is that entire genome datasets are narrowed down to the smallest number of genes capable of robustly characterising differences between biological samples. Using complex statistical analysis of large datasets, the prediction power of these small subsets of genes has been shown to be equivalent to the whole dataset. Once developed, the GES tool allows for rapid, reliable characterisation of various cellular states, which has a number of important applications.

Accurate classification of disease states plays a vital role in diagnosis and treatment. GESs have been successfully used in a number of different cancer types including breast (Nuyten et al., 2008; van de Vijver et al., 2002), gastric (Cui et al., 2011), lung, colon and ovarian cancer (Mettu et al., 2010) to aid in prediction of survival, and to guide clinicians in choice of treatments for their patients. Recently, GESs have even been applied to predicting the likelihood of side effects in patients treated by acute radiotherapy (Mayer et al., 2011).

Using GES technology for prediction and/or classification however represents only part of its potential. The use of GESs for the discovery and development of new therapies is perhaps the most promising application of this technology. The use of GESs to develop new therapies is especially powerful when a specific endpoint is known, but intermediate signalling steps or the molecular targets have not been identified. Provided a model for the disease of interest has been developed, high throughput screening of small molecule libraries can be performed by assessing the effects of those agents on the mRNA levels of the genes identified as the GES. The GES approach has been used in a number of cancer models to identify new therapies, which have increased efficacy over current treatments. For acute myelogenous leukemias, the identification of inducers of terminal differentiation has opened up new therapeutic avenues previously unavailable (Stegmaier et al., 2004). For the treatment of Ewing sarcomas, the targeting of the EWS/FLI oncoprotein had previously been unsuccessful with screening approaches, until the GES approach was used successfully to identify cytosine arabinoside as a modulator of the EWS/FLI oncoprotein (Stegmaier et al., 2007).

What makes GESs unique is that the GES genes are not limited to genes known to be involved in the particular physiological process being investigated. A GES is the minimal set of genes that best defines the difference between two biological samples - be that a disease state or the physiological response to a particular drug or chemical. While it is possible that a GES gene plays a role in the specific model being investigated, it is also possible it does not, and thus any conclusions based upon the identity of genes in the GES must be confirmed with subsequent studies.

6. Overview of GES development

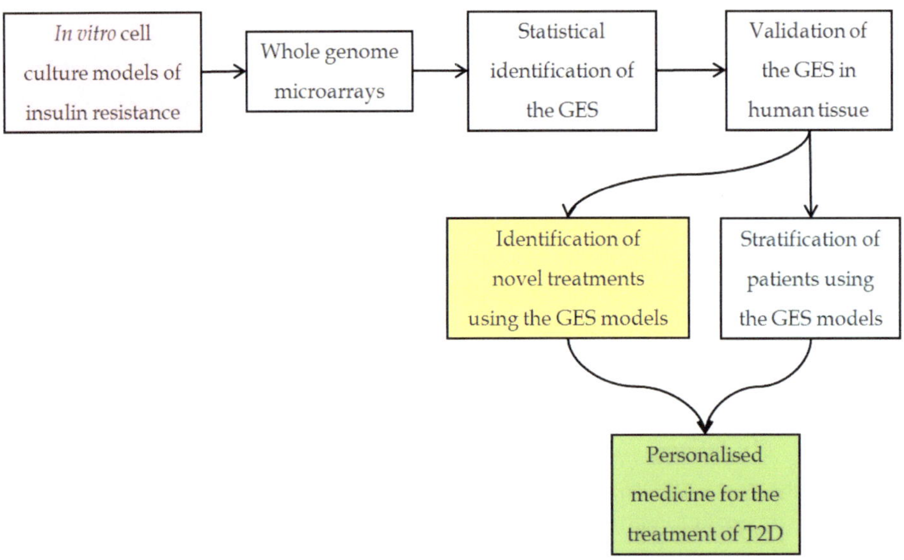

Fig. 3. Development procedure for a GES for insulin resistance, based upon (Stegmaier et al., 2004). mRNA is extracted from *in vitro* cell culture models of insulin resistance, and analysed using whole genome microarrays. The GES genes are identified, and validated in human tissues. The validated GES can then be used to identify novel treatments, as well as stratify patients. This allows for the personalised treatment of T2D.

6.1 Application to dissecting insulin resistance subtypes

We propose that GESs can be applied to dissect and study insulin resistance subtypes. The GES methodology described here can be undertaken in either animal tissues or cell culture models. Due to the high reproducibility required when extracting the data from relevant platform technology (for example, microarray), we have found that working in cell culture systems is the most robust and consistent approach. Once the GES is developed from a cell culture model, the biological relevance of an *in vitro*-derived GES requires validation in human tissue. Validation of the GES in human cohorts tests for a correlation between the homeostasis model assessment (HOMA) measures of insulin resistance, based upon plasma glucose and insulin levels (Matthews et al., 1985), and similarity to the GES profile for each subject. If it can be shown that those patients whose expression profiles were most similar to the GES showed a greater degree of insulin resistance as indicated by the HOMA score, the GES is considered to be valid in human tissue. The modelling of insulin resistance subtypes in the GES models involves the use of a specific insult to induce insulin resistance which are known to cause insulin resistance in individuals. Such insults include saturated fatty acids (PA) or mediators of chronic inflammation (TNFα).

The development of a GES in cell culture requires modelling three distinct cellular states relating to insulin sensitivity. The first state is that of a 'healthy', insulin sensitive cell. The second state is that of a 'diseased', insulin resistant cell. This is achieved by treatment of the target cells with the insulin resistance insult such as TNFα or PA. The third state represents a 'recovered from disease' state, which is achieved by treating insulin resistant cells with a cocktail of antidiabetic agents to restore insulin action. The definition of these three states is deliberate and critical to the integrity of the GES. Insulin resistance in this model system is measured using a key endpoint of insulin action, such as glucose uptake in muscle or adipose tissue, or glucose production in the liver, and will be discussed in further detail below (see section 6.2).

To apply the GES approach to insulin resistance, firstly we assessed the significant changes in gene expression levels between the 'healthy' insulin-responsive cells, and the 'insulin resistant' cells to identify the genes which change in response to the insulin resistance-inducing insult. In order to determine which genes are being affected due to insulin resistance and not non-specific changes induced by the insult *per se*, the changes induced by the 'recovered from disease' state was then assessed. Only those genes whose expression levels were significantly changed in the 'diseased' state, and then changed again in the reverse direction in the 'recovered from disease' state are used for the development of the GES. It is this group of genes whose expression are linked to the insulin resistant state of the cell or tissue.

6.2 Characterising insulin resistance *in vitro*

In order to effectively model insulin resistance *in vitro*, an endpoint measure of insulin action is required. Cell-based models offer a number of assays which can be used to determine insulin signalling in both sensitive and insulin resistant states. *In vitro* models of insulin resistance can be developed in each of the main insulin sensitive tissues; muscle, adipose and liver. One key measure of insulin action in muscle and adipose cells is glucose uptake. In liver cells, regulation of gluconeogenesis by insulin is one of the key endpoints of insulin action. These assays work by measuring the relevant endpoint (glucose uptake or gluconeogenesis) in the presence and absence of an insulin resistance insult to characterise insulin resistance. As the *in vitro* cell culture model must be manipulated from healthy to diseased and then restored, a robust and large dynamic range is needed in the bioassay used to measure the insulin resistance endpoint parameter.

Reversal of insulin resistance involves assessing a wide range of known insulin sensitisers in the model of choice. A combination therapy which is able to fully reverse insulin resistance is selected, based upon its ability to not only reverse insulin resistance, but also avoid negatively impacting upon cellular viability. Combination therapy is required, as this will ensure that the GES is characteristic of an insulin resistant state which has been reversed by a multi-target approach. There is a greater chance that in drug development the GES will identify novel therapies, rather than the individual therapies used in its creation - as may happen with a single treatment GES. Potential reversers of insulin resistance include known antidiabetic drugs such as the biguanide metformin, TZDs, chemical chaperones such as tauroursodeoxycholic acid (TUDCA) (Iglesias et al., 2002), antioxidants such as N-acetylcysteine (NAC) (Houstis et al., 2006), and NSAIDs such as aspirin (Sinha et al., 2004; Yuan et al., 2001).

6.2.1 Personalised treatment for patients

The GES holds promise for personalised treatments for patients by allowing the stratification of patients based on subgroups of insulin resistance. Once patients are sub grouped, treatments can be personalised to their individual diagnosis, leading to improved health outcomes. The subgrouping of patients according to the GES involves measuring the expression levels of the GES genes in the patient. Regardless of which tissue or cell type the GES is derived from, a non-invasive, easy to obtain sample is needed to facilitate screening of as many individuals as possible. A blood sample is ideal for these requirements. Lymphocyte gene expression profiles have been shown to correlate well with gene expression profiles of insulin responsive tissues including liver and adipose tissue (Iida et al., 2006). We propose that by measuring the expression levels of the GES genes in a patients white blood cells we can subtype patients according to one or more GES. The GES which best correlates with the gene expression pattern of a patient's white blood cells will therefore indicate a specific avenue of treatment for that patient (see Fig. 4).

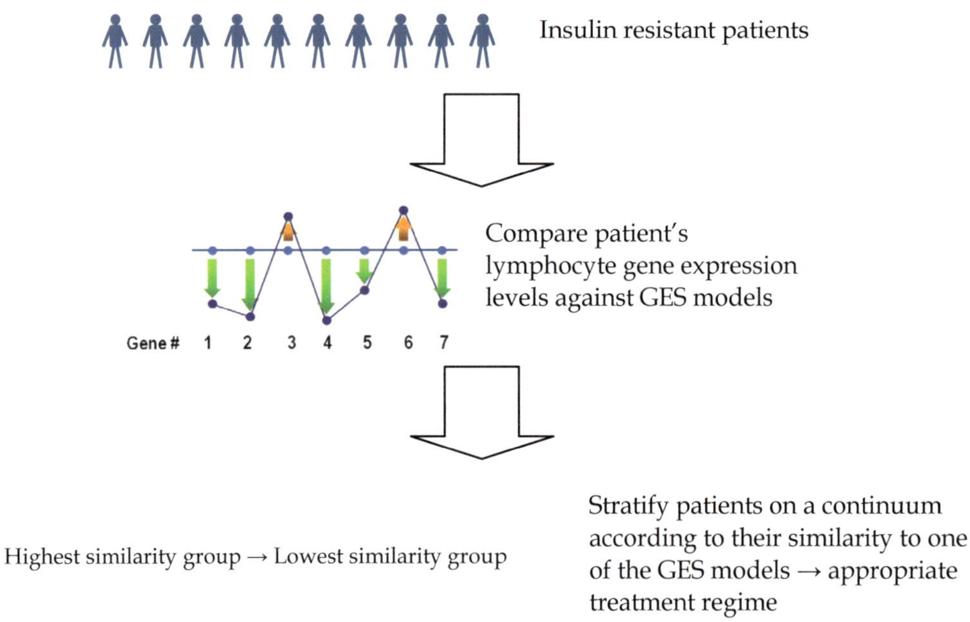

Fig. 4. Stratification of patients according to their similarities to the GES models of insulin resistance.

6.2.2 Development of "targeted" therapies

The GES can be used to aid in the development of new therapies for T2D, by allowing for high throughput screening for new drugs with insulin sensitising and antidiabetic properties. Screening involves treating cells with chemical libraries, which can include previously known and marketed drugs. After screening the GES genes in the treated cells, the key analysis is comparing the GES genes in the treated cells with the GES profile of the specific model being used. Those chemicals which mimic the GES profile of successful reversal of insulin resistance are identified as the most promising candidate drugs. These drugs can then be validated both *in vitro* and *in vivo* to assess their efficacy. We propose that new therapies identified via this approach may show increased efficacy in treating patients subtyped by the same gene expression signature. The subtyping of patients according to gene expression signatures, as well as the potential for targeted therapies against each subtype, represents a personalised medicine approach for the treatment of insulin resistance and T2D.

6.3 Proof of principle: Inflammation-induced cellular "insulin resistance"

As proof of principle, we recently developed a GES for TNFα-induced insulin resistance (Konstantopoulos et al., 2011). Using 3T3-L1 adipocytes as the cell-based model, we identified 3325 genes whose expression was altered by the induction of insulin resistance by TNFα. Of those genes, only 1022 showed altered expression by the reversal of insulin resistance with the insulin sensitisers aspirin and troglitazone. From those 1022 genes, a set of 5 genes were selected whose combined expression profile gave the highest predictive power to differentiate the insulin resistant state, and the re-sensitised state.

As described above, GESs can be used for screening of patients with T2D. We evaluated this by assessing whether the *in vitro*-derived GES for TNFα could characterise insulin resistant subtypes in a human cohort. We used lymphocytes from the San Antonio Family Heart Study (Mitchell et al., 1996), and measured the expression of 47,289 transcripts in 1,240 individuals from 42 extended families (Goring et al., 2007). The TNFα GES of 5 genes was detected in the human profile dataset, and GES score assigned - comprising the sum of the absolute values of the standardised expression units of each of the 5 genes. This was tested for association with HOMA measures of insulin resistance for each subject. Those patients whose expression profiles were most similar to the TNFα GES showed a higher degree of insulin resistance as indicated by the HOMA score ($P<0.001$) (Konstantopoulos et al., 2011). This correlation is consistent with the use of GES technology to characterise an insulin resistant subtype in this population.

In vitro screening of compound libraries has also been used in this model, assessing the ability of a given compound to affect the genes identified in the GES (Fig. 5). Screening for those compounds whose effects on the target genes mirrored the expression profile observed in the gene expression signature was successful in identifying known and novel insulin sensitising agents such as non-steroidal anti-inflammatory agents, β-adrenergic antagonists, beta-lactams and sodium channel blockers (Konstantopoulos et al., 2011).

Investigation of the GES genes, and their role in insulin resistance has also yielded positive outcomes. We conducted a series of studies to assess what role (if any) the GES genes might play in the development of insulin resistance. Our investigation of the GES gene STEAP4 was mirrored by the results of data published at that time which showed that STEAP4 protects against inflammation and metabolic dysfunction (Wellen et al., 2007). This highlighted the utility of the GES in gene discovery related to the particular biological state being investigated, and is further proof of the power of this technique in investigating disease states.

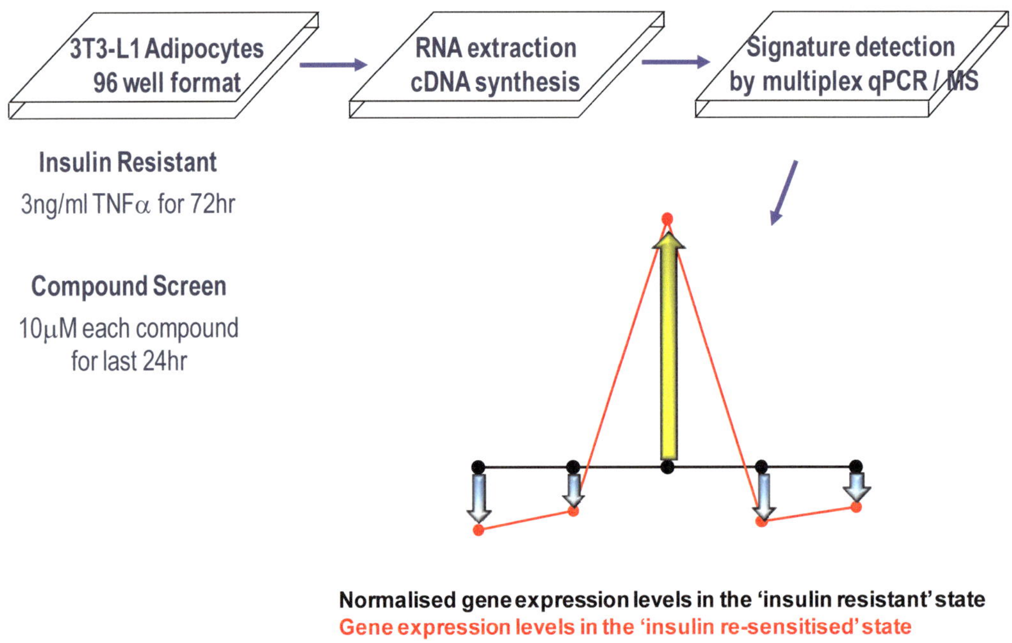

Fig. 5. GES screen of a chemical library. Screening involves assessing the effects of compounds on the GES profile in insulin resistant cells.

6.4 Identification of palmitate-derived GES from liver cells

Following the development of the TNFα GES, a GES for palmitic acid (PA) induced insulin resistance is currently being developed. The cell model has been established in FAO liver cells, with insulin resistance achieved after incubating the cells with 75μM PA for 48h. This insulin resistant phenotype has been reversed by treating PA treated cells with 0.25mM metformin and 2mM sodium salicylate (NAS) in the final 24 hours of PA incubation (Fig. 6). This model has been developed using the same statistical modelling as the TNFα GES. The identity of the GES genes for this model is currently being determined.

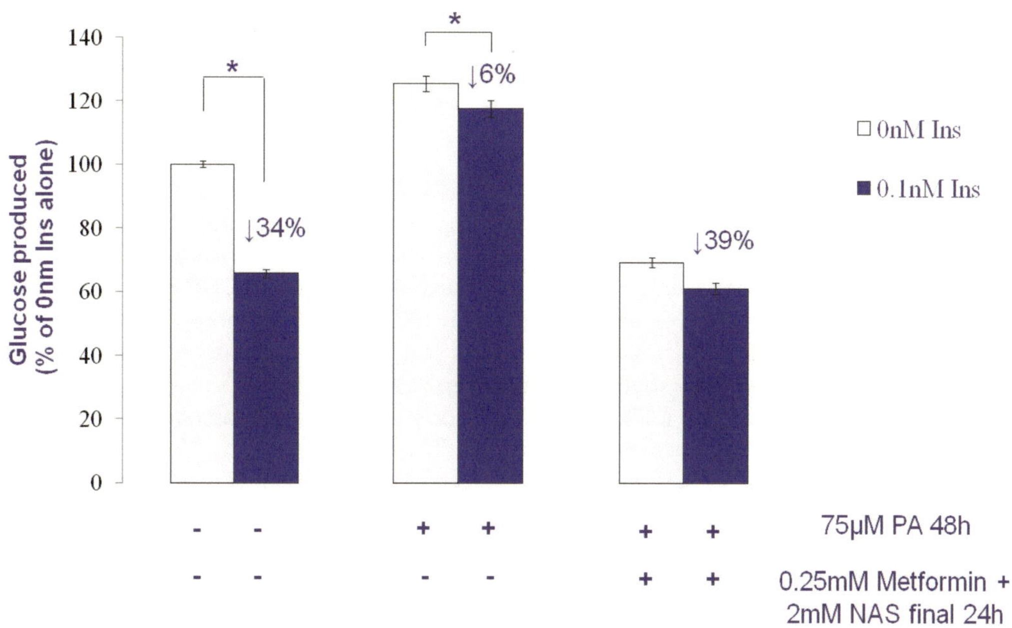

Fig. 6. PA induced insulin resistance in FAO liver cells. Insulin stimulation of FAO hepatocytes decreased glucose production by 34 ± 1% (*, p≤0.005 compared with basal cells, n=8). Exposure of FAO hepatocytes to 75μM PA for 48h decreased insulin-induced suppression of glucose production to only 6 ± 3% (*, p≤0.005 compared with PA-treated, basal hepatocytes, n=8). Addition of 0.25mM metformin and 2mM NAS in the final 24h of the 48h PA treatment reversed this increase in glucose production, reducing insulin-stimulated glucose release to the same levels as observed in vehicle treated cells.

The PA derived GES will be used for the stratification of patient cohorts as described above. We anticipate that the PA derived GES will identify an insulin resistant subpopulation from the cohorts we test it in. A key comparison with the different GES models will be the identity of the subgroups identified, and the degree of overlap (if any) observed in the groups. Drug screening, as well as investigation of the GES genes will also be performed for the PA derived GES.

7. Conclusion

The use of 'omics' style approaches to disease states such as T2D are becoming increasingly accepted as one way research should investigate these diseases in the 21st century. The success of GES technology in the cancer field as both a diagnostic tool and a drug discovery tool is becoming increasingly apparent, and we have shown this technology is equally applicable to the study of T2D. As disease research is progressing towards the development of personalised medicine as the 'holy grail' for treatment regimes, we foresee a future where personalised medicine is seen as the gold standard for patient care. We believe GES technology will provide a platform for the development of novel, personalised treatments for patients with T2D.

8. Acknowledgement

The authors wish to thank Juan Molero for his advice and assistance in the development of the hepatic model of PA induced insulin resistance.

9. References

Alizadeh, A.A., Eisen, M.B., Davis, R.E., Ma, C., Lossos, I.S., Rosenwald, A., Boldrick, J.C., Sabet, H., Tran, T., Yu, X., *et al.* (2000). Distinct types of diffuse large B-cell lymphoma identified by gene expression profiling. Nature *403*, 503-511.

Baudry, A., Leroux, L., Jackerott, M., and Joshi, R.L. (2002). Genetic manipulation of insulin signaling, action and secretion in mice. Insights into glucose homeostasis and pathogenesis of type 2 diabetes. EMBO Rep *3*, 323-328.

Bergman, R.N., and Ader, M. (2000). Free fatty acids and pathogenesis of type 2 diabetes mellitus. Trends Endocrinol Metab *11*, 351-356.

Bilan, P.J., Samokhvalov, V., Koshkina, A., Schertzer, J.D., Samaan, M.C., and Klip, A. (2009). Direct and macrophage-mediated actions of fatty acids causing insulin resistance in muscle cells. Arch Physiol Biochem *115*, 176-190.

CDC (2011). National diabetes fact sheet: national estimates and general information on diabetes and prediabetes in the United States, C.f.D.C.a.P. U.S. Department of Health and Human Services, ed. (Atlanta).

Chavez, J.A., and Summers, S.A. (2003). Characterizing the effects of saturated fatty acids on insulin signaling and ceramide and diacylglycerol accumulation in 3T3-L1 adipocytes and C2C12 myotubes. Arch Biochem Biophys *419*, 101-109.

Cohen, A., and Horton, E.S. (2007). Progress in the treatment of type 2 diabetes: new pharmacologic approaches to improve glycemic control. Curr Med Res Opin *23*, 905-917.

Cui, J., Li, F., Wang, G., Fang, X., Puett, J.D., and Xu, Y. (2011). Gene-expression signatures can distinguish gastric cancer grades and stages. PLoS ONE *6*, e17819.

Cummings, D.E., and Schwartz, M.W. (2003). Genetics and pathophysiology of human obesity. Annu Rev Med *54*, 453-471.

Davies, M.J., Raymond, N.T., Day, J.L., Hales, C.N., and Burden, A.C. (2000). Impaired glucose tolerance and fasting hyperglycaemia have different characteristics. Diabetic Medicine *17*, 433-440.

DeFronzo, R.A. (2004). Pathogenesis of type 2 diabetes mellitus. Med Clin North Am *88*, 787-835, ix.

Drucker, D.J. (2003). Glucagon-like peptide-1 and the islet beta-cell: Augmentation of cell proliferation and inhibition of apoptosis. Endocrinology *144*, 5145-5148.

Drucker, D.J. (2005). Biologic actions and therapeutic potential of the proglucagon-derived peptides. Nat Clin Pract Endocrinol Metab *1*, 22-31.

Dunstan, D.W., Zimmet, P.Z., Welborn, T.A., De Courten, M.P., Cameron, A.J., Sicree, R.A., Dwyer, T., Colagiuri, S., Jolley, D., Knuiman, M., *et al.* (2002). The rising prevalence of diabetes and impaired glucose tolerance: the Australian Diabetes, Obesity and Lifestyle Study. Diabetes Care *25*, 829-834.

Gavin, J.R., Alberti, K.G., Davidson, M.B., DeFronzo, R.A., Drash, A., Gabbe, S.G., Genuth, S., Harris, M., Kahn, R., Keen, H., *et al.* (2003). Report of the expert committee on the diagnosis and classification of diabetes mellitus. Diabetes Care *26 Suppl 1*, S5-20.

GlaxoSmithKline (2010). GlaxoSmithKline Annual Report 2010 (Brentford, United Kingdom, GlaxoSmithKline).

Goring, H.H.H., Curran, J.E., Johnson, M.P., Dyer, T.D., Charlesworth, J., Cole, S.A., Jowett, J.B.M., Abraham, L.J., Rainwater, D.L., Comuzzie, A.G., *et al.* (2007). Discovery of expression QTLs using large-scale transcriptional profiling in human lymphocytes. Nature Genetics *39*, 1208-1216.

Granberry, M.C., and Fonseca, V.A. (1999). Insulin resistance syndrome: options for treatment. South Med J *92*, 2-15.

Groop, L.C. (1992). Sulfonylureas in NIDDM. Diabetes Care *15*, 737-754.

Hanke, S., and Mann, M. (2009). The phosphotyrosine interactome of the insulin receptor family and its substrates IRS-1 and IRS-2. Mol Cell Proteomics *8*, 519-534.

Houstis, N., Rosen, E.D., and Lander, E.S. (2006). Reactive oxygen species have a causal role in multiple forms of insulin resistance. Nature *440*, 944-948.

Iglesias, M.A., Ye, J.M., Frangioudakis, G., Saha, A.K., Tomas, E., Ruderman, N.B., Cooney, G.J., and Kraegen, E.W. (2002). AICAR administration causes an apparent enhancement of muscle and liver insulin action in insulin-resistant high-fat-fed rats. Diabetes *51*, 2886-2894.

Iida, S., Sato, Y., Nakaya, A., Shinohara, Y., Hayashi, Y., Sawada, A., Nagata, H., Kaji, N., Kamiya, H., Baba, Y., *et al.* (2006). Genome wide expression analysis of white blood cells and liver of pre-diabetic Otsuka Long-Evans Tokushima Fatty (OLETF) rats using a cDNA microarray. Biological & Pharmaceutical Bulletin *29*, 2451-2459.

Itani, S.I., Ruderman, N.B., Schmieder, F., and Boden, G. (2002). Lipid-Induced Insulin Resistance in Human Muscle Is Associated With Changes in Diacylglycerol, Protein Kinase C, and IÎºB-Î±. Diabetes *51*, 2005-2011.

Jayapal, M., and Melendez, A.J. (2006). DNA microarray technology for target identification and validation. Clin Exp Pharmacol Physiol *33*, 496-503.

Jove, M., Planavila, A., Sanchez, R.M., Merlos, M., Laguna, J.C., and Vazquez-Carrera, M. (2006). Palmitate induces tumor necrosis factor-alpha expression in C2C12 skeletal muscle cells by a mechanism involving protein kinase C and nuclear factor-kappaB activation. Endocrinology *147*, 552-561.

Kauffmann, A., and Huber, W. (2010). Microarray data quality control improves the detection of differentially expressed genes. Genomics.

Kendall, D.M., Riddle, M.C., Rosenstock, J., Zhuang, D.L., Kim, D.D., Fineman, M.S., and Baron, A.D. (2005). Effects of exenatide (exendin-4) on glycemic control over 30 weeks in patients with type 2 diabetes treated with metformin and a sulfonylurea. Diabetes Care *28*, 1083-1091.

Knowler, W.C., Barrett-Connor, E., Fowler, S.E., Hamman, R.F., Lachin, J.M., Walker, E.A., and Nathan, D.M. (2002). Reduction in the incidence of type 2 diabetes with lifestyle intervention or metformin. N Engl J Med *346*, 393-403.

Konstantopoulos, N., Foletta, V.C., Segal, D.H., Shields, K.A., Sanigorski, A., Windmill, K., Swinton, C., Connor, T., Wanyonyi, S., Dyer, T.D., *et al.* (2011). A Gene Expression Signature for Insulin Resistance. Physiol Genomics *43*, 110-120.

Kristensen, J.S., Frandsen, K.B., Bayer, T., and Muller, P.G. (2000). Compared with repaglinide sulfonylurea treatment in type 2 diabetes is associated with a 2.5-fold increase in symptomatic hypoglycemia with blood glucose levels < 45 mg/dl. Diabetes *49*, A131-A131.

Langeveld, M., and Aerts, J.M. (2009). Glycosphingolipids and insulin resistance. Prog Lipid Res *48*, 196-205.

Lee, J.K., Havaleshko, D.M., Cho, H., Weinstein, J.N., Kaldjian, E.P., Karpovich, J., Grimshaw, A., and Theodorescu, D. (2007). A strategy for predicting the chemosensitivity of human cancers and its application to drug discovery. Proc Natl Acad Sci U S A *104*, 13086-13091.

Lillioja, S., Mott, D.M., Spraul, M., Ferraro, R., Foley, J.E., Ravussin, E., Knowler, W.C., Bennett, P.H., and Bogardus, C. (1993). Insulin-Resistance and Insulin Secretory Dysfunction as Precursors of Non-Insulin-Dependent Diabetes-Mellitus - Prospective Studies of Pima-Indians. New England Journal of Medicine *329*, 1988-1992.

Matthews, D.R., Hosker, J.P., Rudenski, A.S., Naylor, B.A., Treacher, D.F., and Turner, R.C. (1985). Homeostasis model assessment: insulin resistance and beta-cell function from fasting plasma glucose and insulin concentrations in man. Diabetologia *28*, 412-419.

Mayer, C., Popanda, O., Greve, B., Fritz, E., Illig, T., Eckardt-Schupp, F., Gomolka, M., Benner, A., and Schmezer, P. (2011). A radiation-induced gene expression signature as a tool to predict acute radiotherapy-induced adverse side effects. Cancer Letters *302*, 20-28.

McKinlay, J., and Marceau, L. (2000). US public health and the 21st century: diabetes mellitus. Lancet *356*, 757-761.

Meikle, P.J., and Christopher, M.J. (2011). Lipidomics is providing new insight into the metabolic syndrome and its sequelae. Curr Opin Lipidol.

Mettu, R.K.R., Wan, Y.W., Habermann, J.K., Ried, T., and Guo, N.L. (2010). A 12-gene genomic instability signature predicts clinical outcomes in multiple cancer types. Int J Biol Marker *25*, 219-228.

Mitchell, B.D., Kammerer, C.M., Blangero, J., Mahaney, M.C., Rainwater, D.L., Dyke, B., Hixson, J.E., Henkel, R.D., Sharp, R.M., Comuzzie, A.G., *et al.* (1996). Genetic and environmental contributions to cardiovascular risk factors in Mexican Americans. The San Antonio Family Heart Study. Circulation *94*, 2159-2170.

Mlinar, B., Marc, J., Janez, A., and Pfeifer, M. (2007). Molecular mechanisms of insulin resistance and associated diseases. Clin Chim Acta *375*, 20-35.

Nathan, D.M., Buse, J.B., Davidson, M.B., Heine, R.J., Holman, R.R., Sherwin, R., and Zinman, B. (2006). Management of hyperglycemia in type 2 diabetes: A consensus algorithm for the initiation and adjustment of therapy: a consensus statement from the American Diabetes Association and the European Association for the Study of Diabetes. Diabetes Care *29*, 1963-1972.

NCHS (2008). Prevalence of overweight, obesity and extreme obesity among adults: United States, trends 1976-80 through 2005-2006 N.C.f.H.S. (US), ed.

NIDDK (2009). National Diabetes Information Clearinghouse (NDIC).

Nissen, S.E., and Wolski, K. (2010). Rosiglitazone Revisited: An Updated Meta-analysis of Risk for Myocardial Infarction and Cardiovascular Mortality. Arch Intern Med.

Nuyten, D.S., Hastie, T., Chi, J.T., Chang, H.Y., and van de Vijver, M.J. (2008). Combining biological gene expression signatures in predicting outcome in breast cancer: An alternative to supervised classification. Eur J Cancer *44*, 2319-2329.

Oron, A.P., Jiang, Z., and Gentleman, R. (2008). Gene set enrichment analysis using linear models and diagnostics. Bioinformatics *24*, 2586-2591.

Potes, C.S., and Lutz, T.A. (2010). Brainstem mechanisms of amylin-induced anorexia. Physiology & Behavior *100*, 511-518.

Ruan, H., and Lodish, H.F. (2003). Insulin resistance in adipose tissue: direct and indirect effects of tumor necrosis factor-alpha. Cytokine Growth Factor Rev *14*, 447-455.

Salpeter, S., Greyber, E., Pasternak, G., and Salpeter, E. (2006). Risk of fatal and nonfatal lactic acidosis with metformin use in type 2 diabetes mellitus. Cochrane Database of Systematic Reviews, -.

Saltiel, A.R., and Pessin, J.E. (2002). Insulin signaling pathways in time and space. Trends Cell Biol *12*, 65-71.

Schena, M., Shalon, D., Davis, R.W., and Brown, P.O. (1995). Quantitative monitoring of gene expression patterns with a complementary DNA microarray. Science *270*, 467-470.

Schmitz, O., Brock, B., and Rungby, J. (2004). Amylin agonists: a novel approach in the treatment of diabetes. Diabetes *53 Suppl 3*, S233-238.

Sharma, A.M. (2006). The obese patient with diabetes mellitus: from research targets to treatment options. Am J Med *119*, S17-23.

Sinha, S., Perdomo, G., Brown, N.F., and O'Doherty, R.M. (2004). Fatty acid-induced insulin resistance in L6 myotubes is prevented by inhibition of activation and nuclear localization of nuclear factor kappa B. J Biol Chem *279*, 41294-41301.

Smyth, G.K. (2004). Linear models and empirical bayes methods for assessing differential expression in microarray experiments. Stat Appl Genet Mol Biol *3*, Article3.

Stegmaier, K., Ross, K.N., Colavito, S.A., O'Malley, S., Stockwell, B.R., and Golub, T.R. (2004). Gene expression-based high-throughput screening (GE-HTS) and application to leukemia differentiation. Nature Genetics *36*, 257-263.

Stegmaier, K., Wong, J.S., Ross, K.N., Chow, K.T., Peck, D., Wright, R.D., Lessnick, S.L., Kung, A.L., and Golub, T.R. (2007). Signature-based small molecule screening identifies cytosine arabinoside as an EWS/FLI modulator in Ewing sarcoma. Plos Med *4*, 702-714.

Subramanian, A., Tamayo, P., Mootha, V.K., Mukherjee, S., Ebert, B.L., Gillette, M.A., Paulovich, A., Pomeroy, S.L., Golub, T.R., Lander, E.S., *et al.* (2005). Gene set enrichment analysis: a knowledge-based approach for interpreting genome-wide expression profiles. Proc Natl Acad Sci U S A *102*, 15545-15550.

Taylor, S.I. (1999). Deconstructing type 2 diabetes. Cell *97*, 9-12.

Tisch, R., and McDevitt, H. (1996). Insulin-dependent diabetes mellitus. Cell *85*, 291-297.

Unwin, N., Shaw, J., Zimmet, P., and Alberti, K.G.M.M. (2002). Impaired glucose tolerance and impaired fasting glycaemia: the current status on definition and intervention. Diabetic Medicine *19*, 708-723.

van de Vijver, M.J., He, Y.D., van 't Veer, L.J., Dai, H., Hart, A.A.M., Voskuil, D.W., Schreiber, G.J., Peterse, J.L., Roberts, C., Marton, M.J., *et al.* (2002). A gene-expression signature as a predictor of survival in breast cancer. New England Journal of Medicine *347*, 1999-2009.

Watkins, P.B. (2005). Idiosyncratic liver injury: challenges and approaches. Toxicol Pathol *33*, 1-5.

Wellen, K.E., Fucho, R., Gregor, M.F., Furuhashi, M., Morgan, C., Lindstad, T., Vaillancourt, E., Gorgun, C.Z., Saatcioglu, F., and Hotamisligil, G.S. (2007). Coordinated regulation of nutrient and inflammatory responses by STAMP2 is essential for metabolic homeostasis. Cell *129*, 537-548.

WHO (2006). Obesity and Overweight: Fact Sheet # 311 (World Health Organisation).

WHO/IDF (2006). Definition and diagnosis of diabetes mellitus and intermediate hyperglycemia (WHO/IDF).

Yki-Jarvinen, H. (2004). Thiazolidinediones. N Engl J Med *351*, 1106-1118.

Yuan, M., Konstantopoulos, N., Lee, J., Hansen, L., Li, Z.W., Karin, M., and Shoelson, S.E. (2001). Reversal of obesity- and diet-induced insulin resistance with salicylates or targeted disruption of Ikkbeta. Science *293*, 1673-1677.

9

The Role of Single Nucleotide Polymorphisms of Untranslated Regions (Utrs) in Insulin Resistance Pathogenesis in Patients with Type 2 Diabetes

Małgorzata Małodobra
Molecular Techniques Unit, Wroclaw Medical University
Poland

1. Introduction

Insulin resistance (IR) is defined as a condition, in which regular amount of insulin is insufficient to develop physiological respond of the cell. For this reason there is constantly great need for increased level of this hormone within insulin resistant body. Very important factors leading to insulin resistance development are environmental components such as inappropriate diet and sedentary life style. A great important role in insulin resistance pathogenesis plays genetic background, as IR develops more frequently in families with positive history of metabolic disorders. There are severe anomalies in expression level of genes playing role in regulation of insulin action detected in patients with impaired insulin sensitivity. Regulation of gene expression can be exerted at either transcriptional level or post-transcriptional level. The former is related to the primary gene sequence located in the promoter region and it is responsible for controlling whether a gene is transcribed or not. The later utilizes regions of transcript not being translated, located at 5′ and 3′ end of the mRNA named the Untranslated Regions (UTRs). The main roles of UTRs are transcript stability control, initiation or inhibition of translation and sub-cellular localization in the cytoplasm. Regulation by UTRs is mediated in several ways, mainly by interaction of regulatory motifs in UTRs with numerous proteins as well as regulation by microRNA.

1.1 IR: Insulin resistance

The main tissues affected by IR are adipose tissue, skeletal muscle and liver (Hernandez-Morante et al., 2008; Karlsson & Zierath, 2007). Insulin resistance also affects lymphocytes and other peripheral blood leucocytes (Maratou et al, 2007; Piątkiewicz et al. 2007). The first diagnosed symptom of insulin resistance development is the decrease in glucose utilization by skeletal muscles (Patti, 2004), what is mediated by decrease in glycogen synthase (GYS) activity. Furthermore the expression rate and the phosphorylation state of numerous kinases (mainly PI-3K) of insulin pathway is decreased. The phosphorylation of serine residues of IRS-1 and IRS-2 is increased (Boura-Halfon & Zick, 2002). Impaired activity of GYS leads to insulin resistance in liver. Next, the number and metabolism of mitochondria decline (Morino, 2006). At this stage, the glucose utilization becomes impaired in adipose tissue. In parallel, the lipids metabolism deregulation, with increased FFA and TG levels, further impair insulin sensitivity in adipose tissue. Insulin resistance is characterized by dysfunction in GLUT4 translocation and glucose uptake in all cells, where insulin is essential. Despite long and intense studies, the origin and pathomechanism of insulin resistance remain unknown. It is believed that both environmental and genetic factors play role in its pathogenesis. IR causes increase in insulin production and secretion as a compensatory mechanism. The prolong demand for insulin results in decreased in pancreatic β-cells efficiency and insulin secretion. This is a theoretical pathomechanism of type 2 diabetes (T2DM) development.

1.1.1 Insulin resistance, mutations and genes expression

The body of literature reports that at insulin resistant state, severe anomalies in gene expressions encoded proteins involved in insulin pathway are diagnosed. In subjects with insulin resistance the decreased levels of *INSR* gene expression have been reported (Stentz & Kitabchi, 2007). Mutations in *INSR* gene are very rare and their presences result in a severe insulin resistance attendant by *acanthosis nigricans* (Hansen & Shafrir, 2002). Most of described so far changes in *INSR* gene sequence were localized mainly in coding region (Højlund et al., 2006; Kusari et al., 1991). Depending on the place of nucleotide variance the effects might influence diverse INSR function. If the change is placed in α chain, the decrease in affinity to insulin might be observed. On the other hand, nucleotide changes localized in β chain influence the activity of tyrosine kinase and thus the rate of tyrosine domain phosphorylation. Only for few nucleotide changes the relationship with insulin resistance has been confirmed.

The downstream kinases such as IRS proteins, PI-3K, Akt have been also shown to be decreased in insulin resistant patients. (Hansen & Shafrir, 2002). Numerous studies provide data for impairments in *IRS-1, IRS-2* or *PIK3R1* gene expression in all tissues affected by insulin resistance (Boura-Halfon & Zick, 2002; Stentz & Kitabchi, 2007; Andreelli et al., 2000). There are some reports suggesting association between SNPs in *PIK3R1* gene with resistance to insulin, such as Met326Ile (Barroso et al, 2003), however other reports negate this findings (Almind et al., 2002).

The last part of insulin pathway is GLUT4 activation and translocation into cell membrane what is essential for insulin-dependent glucose uptake. There are few polymorphisms in *SLC2A4* gene, mostly located in coding region of *SLC2A4* gene, that have been correlated with insulin resistance (Kusari et al, 1991). However, their presence is relatively rare, so it is unlikely they are responsible for insulin resistance by itself, taking into account the prevalence of this disorder. The mRNA analyses have revealed dysfunction in *SLC2A4* gene expression as well as GLUT4 activation and translocation to the cell membrane in adipose tissue (Shephard & Khan, 1999) and in skeletal muscles (Garvey et al, 1998) after insulin stimulation in insulin resistant subjects. The *SLC2A4* gene expression as well as expression rate of genes encoding others GLUT members, are also decreased in lymphocytes, what is correlated with dysfunction of these cells and very severe and long lasting infections in insulin resistant patients (Maratou et al, 2007; Piątkiewicz et al. 2007).

1.1.2 Insulin resistance and active kinases dephosphorylation – Protein Tyrosine Phosphatases (PTPs)

The initial animal models experiments performed during last decade allowed for accurate assessment of the PTPs role in insulin action and glucose metabolism. Further evaluation of PTPs action in humans correlated their activity with obesity, metabolism dysfunction and impairment in insulin action (LeRoith et al, 1996). Several PTPs have been implicated in insulin signal regulation. The most important in insulin signaling is Protein Tyrosine Phosphatase 1B (PTP1B) encoded by *PTPN1* gene. The PTP1B has been for the first time associated with insulin resistance after improving insulin sensitivity in mice injected with antibodies against PTP1B (Ahmad et al, 1995). Further experiments performed on cell lines confirmed the role of PTP1B in insulin sensitivity regulation (Venable et al., 2000). Increased PTP1B level as well as increased *PTPN1* gene expression rate have been diagnosed in skeletal muscles of obese subject comparing to lean, correlated with decrease in glucose uptake by muscle cells in those patients (Ahmad et al., 1997). On the other hand analyses performed in adipose tissue revealed significantly higher PTP1B level in obese subjects while decreased activity (Cheung et al., 1999). The explanation of this phenomenon might be fact, that PTP1B is activated by INSR. Furthermore, *PTPN1* gene expression is induced by inflammation.

Another phosphatase that has been correlated with insulin resistance is Leukocyte Antigen-Related Phosphatase (LAR). Main data suggesting role of this phosphatase in insulin resistance pathogenesis came from knockout animal model studies that demonstrated severe insulin resistance in animals with decreased glucose uptake rate by skeletal muscles and decreased PI-3K activity (Zabolotny et al., 1999). Studies in humans showed similar pattern, that is significantly higher abundant of mRNA and protein in skeletal muscles and adipose tissue in obese subject, that positively correlated with obesity and insulin resistant state (Worm et al., 1995).

1.1.3 Insulin resistance and obesity

The average human body contains from 10 to 15 kg of adipose tissue that performs diverse functions ranging from energy storage to endocrine secretion. The excess accumulation of adipose tissue impairs insulin sensitivity by (1) excessive secretion of FFA into blood stream and its oxidation, (2) secretion of numerous cytokines that modulate insulin sensitivity, (3) chronic inflammatory state induction (George, 1996).

Abundant FFA level and the metabolite of its oxidation (Acylo-CoA) impair insulin action mainly by IRS-1 and IRS-2 serine/threoine residues phosphorylation, what is mediated through NF-κB pathway (Ragheb et al., 2009). Furthermore, NF-κB pathway activation is associated with increased rate of proinflammatory cytokines production.

Adipose tissue is known as an active endocrine organ producing and secreting into blood stream various cytokines like lepin, adiponectin, RBP4, resistin. Thanks to adipocytokines, adipose tissue connects with the central nervous system (CNS) and regulates energy balance. Some cytokines are implicated in insulin sensitivity regulation (George, 1996). Dysregulation in adipocytokines production, what has place in obesity, causes impairment in phosphorylation rate of numerous important kinases involved in insulin signal transduction (Cohen et al., 2002; Greenspan & Baxter, 1994). Adipose tissue in obese subjects is highly infiltrated by macrophages that change their phenotype into pro-inflammatory cells, secreting pro-inflammatory cytokines like IL -1, 6, 10 (Interleukin 1, 6, 10), TNF-α (Tumor Necrosis Factor-α), MCP-1 (Monocyte Chemotactic Protein-1). Mentioned cytokines are well known factors leading to JNK kinase activation, serine residues phophorylation and insulin sensitivity impairment (Müssig et al., 2005).

Macrophages are not the only cells causing inflammatory state. Some reports provide information that adipocytes hypertrophy is associated with preadipocytes differentiation deregulation and changing their phenotypes into pro-inflammatory cells secreting, similar to macrophages, various cytokines. These cells become typical pro-inflammatory cells with markers expression characteristic for immune cells like CD68 (Gustafson et al., 2009).

1.2 UTRs: Localization, structure and function in post-transcriptional regulation of gene expression

The UTRs are localized at both ends of transcript (mRNA), but are not transcribed to proteins (do not encode proteins). The 5′UTR is localized upstream the start codon AUG (Met), on the other hand 3′UTR is placed downstream the stop codons UAA, UAG, UGA. The average size of 5′UTR in humans is 210,2 nt (nucleotides) with maximal size 2803 nt and minimal size equal 18 nt. The average size for 3′UTR is 1027 nt with maximal size 8555 nt and minimal size equal 21 nt (Mignone et al., 2002). The characteristic feature of those regions is GC content with higher amount of GC in 5′UTR about 60%, on the other hand in 3′UTR GC contents is about 45% (Pesole et al., 1999). Very interesting feature has been seen by Pesole (Pesole et al., 1999), who observed that the higher amount of GC the shorter 3′UTR.

UTRs make numerous conformational structures and tridimensional loops that interact with proteins and other functional and regulatory compounds like ribosomes or microRNA. Within the UTRs a specific functional motifs can be observed, that play important role in function and transcription control (Carmody & Wente, 2009). The most important 5′UTR motif is 5′7-methylguanin (5′7mG), which is added to the transcript just after the transcription initiation, before the whole transcript synthesis is completed (Mignone et al., 2002). Within 5′UTR other motifs can be distinguished like region IRES (Internal Ribosomal Entry Site), which stands for the 5′UTR region that interact with ribosome during translation initiation, numerous hairpins that interact with various proteins controlling transcripts stabilization and ORF (Open Reading Frames). Furthermore others motifs like IRE (Iron Respons Element) that is composed of about 30 nucleotides and has a stem-loop structure (Pickering & Willis, 2005) can be found. The most important motifs localized in 3′UTR are CPE (Cytoplasmic Polyadenylation Element), MRE (microRNA Regulatory Element) and poli(A) tail (Mignone et al., 2002; Carmody & Wente, 2009; Conne et al., 2000).

UTRs play their role thanks to many motifs, conformational loops and hairpins that interact with numerous proteins and others factors like microRNA or ribosomes. The main role of 5′UTR is controlling of translation initialization as well as transcript stabilization, on the other hand 3′UTR is mostly implicated in regulation of transcript stabilization and its localization in cytoplasm (Carmody & Wente, 2009; Pickering & Willis, 2005). Furthermore 3′UTR is the place of microRNA action via MRE. Depending on the cell type various mechanisms and regulatory motifs might regulate transcript stability. For example, IRE element regulates iron homeostasis. On the other hand regulatory proteins, growth factors as well as proto-oncogenes posses long 5′UTRs, what inhibits translation initiation and as a consequence, protein synthesis (Pickering & Willis, 2005).

1.2.1 Regulation of translation initiation

The main regulatory element of translation regulation is the regulation of translation initiation. This process requires interaction of ribosomal 40 S subunit with 5′7-methylguanin (5′7mG). The resulting complex (so called 43 S) further interacts with translation initiation factors like eIF2, eIF4F, eIF4G, eIF3. Next, eIF1A and eIF3 facilitate binding the 43 S subunit with eIF2-GTP-Met-tRNA, what begins the mRNA scanning process and searching for the initiation (start) codon (AUG) in 5′→3′ direction (Carmody & Wente, 2009; Meijer &

Thomas, 2002). Once the start codon has been achieved, the eIF5 facilitates the 40 S and 60 S subunits joining resulting in 80 S ribosomal subunit. The 80 S subunit initiates the protein synthesis and elongation. In the regulation of efficiency of translation initiation and 5'UTR scanning the secondary structures of 5'UTR play a great role. However, the effect on translation initiation has been shown for structures posses the bounding energy higher $\Delta R <$ -50 kcal/mol (Svitkin et al., 2001). In the initiation translation process the most important is 5'7mG and its interaction with 40 S ribosomal subunit as well as with translation initiation factors. The mRNA binding with 40 S subunit is facilitated also by the IRES motif and this process dominates in situation when the translation initiation by 5'7mG is impaired by stress, apoptosis or suppressed by cell-cycle stage (Pickering & Willis, 2005; Meijer & Thomas, 2002). This mechanism is common for mRNA encoding growth factors or transcription factors. IRES is localized close to AUG codon and the IRES-mediated translation regulation depends on the secondary and tertiary structure (Peng et al., 1996) as well as on the complementarity to 18 S rRNA (Chappell et al., 2000). Many genes posses the IRES in 5'UTR e.g. genes involved in apoptosis like *c-myc* (Stoneley et al., 2000), *Apaf-1* (Coldwell et al., 2000), *XIAP* (Holcik & Korneluk, 2000). The *VEGF* gene contains two IRESs in 5'UTR (Meiron et al., 2001).

Very important role in translation initiation plays the nucleotide sequence flanking start codon with following sequence: GCC**R**CC**AUGG**. The **R** stands for purine, usually adenine. The purine in -3 position and **G** in +4 position is the rule of start codon determination and is strong consensus sequence present in animals and plants (Svitkin et al., 2001). The presence of AUG in 5'UTR and false determination of the main ORF decrease the translation initiation process via assignment of upstream open reading frames (uORF). The uORF results in translation initiation and synthesis of false proteins (Mignone et al., 2002; Svitkin et al., 2001). The fate of 40 S subunit that recognized the wrong ORF depends on the size of uORF. The 40 S subunit might dissociate and restart scanning, however, if the uORF is greater than 30 codons, the rescanning is not possible (Peng et al., 1996).

The mechanisms mediated translation initiation vary depending mostly on environmental condition and, in situation, when one mechanism is inhibited, the second is active. For example when the cap-dependent mechanism of translation initiation is inhibited by hypoxia or apoptosis, the translation is initiated by IRES-dependent mechanism. The same changeable mechanisms might be seen for translation regulation via uORF. It is believed that this switch hypothesis is an adaptive mechanism of gene expression regulation in various cellular conditions (Meijer & Thomas, 2002).

1.2.2 Transcript stability

The mRNA stability is mostly regulated via 3'UTR, especially by elements rich in AU repeats - ARE (AU - Rich Elements) (Griffin et al., 2004). AREs are classified into 3 groups depending on AUUUA repetitive units, regulation mechanisms and degradation efficiency. However, the result of its action is fast deadenylation and mRNA degradation (Peng et al., 1996). mRNA degradation is also regulated by numerous endonuclease enzymes, that hydrolyze the poli(A) tail of transcript with following fast degradation of the whole mRNA (Mignone et al., 2002). In the transcript stability regulation important role play hnRNPs (ribonucleoproteins) that stabilize the mRNA and is responsible for its localization in the cells. The recognition site for hnRNPs is located in the 3'UTR (Mignone et al., 2002).

The 5'UTR also plays role in the regulation of transcript stability by process named Nonsense-Mediated mRNA Decay (NMD) (Nicholson et al., 2010). The mechanism of regulation is connected with the proper identification of uORF as the false reading frame and its degradation. It is also responsible for accurate identification of stop codon and the translation termination in a proper position. In physiological conditions the premature translation termination codons (PTCs) are produced in variety of organisms. To prevent from the production of protein lacking C-terminal domains, those transcripts are recognized and subsequently degraded by NMD (Nicholson et al., 2010). The NMD mechanisms are also responsible for controlling the abundance of physiological full length transcripts (Mendell et al., 2004; Rehwinkel et al., 2005).

1.2.3 Regulation of transcript localization in cytoplasm

Subcelluar transcripts localization depends mainly on the type of protein encoded by gene and its demand in the cell. The mRNAs in cytoplasm are connected with ribonucleoproteins (Mignone et al., 2002). Three main mechanisms regulating subcellular localization of mRNA in the cell are known. The prevalent mechanism relies on the active transcript transport into the particular compartments of the cell by cytoskeleton elements and specific proteins interacting with mRNA (in particular with the 3'UTR). The second mechanism is connected with interaction of various proteins with motifs located in 3'UTR thus influencing the transcript localization. The third mechanism relies on the diffusion of mRNA (Mignone et al., 2002).

1.2.4 Post-transcriptional regulation via microRNA

MicroRNAs are short, single stranded classes of RNAs of 19-25 nucleotides (nt) in length. MiRNAs are produced from longer precursors containing hairpin structure (pre-miRNAs) that are generated from pri-miRNAs by nuclear RNase III Drosha. Pre-miRNAs are then transported into the cytoplasm and processed by Dicer RNase III complex to produce about 22 nt mature miRNAs (Kim, 2005). Mature miRNAs appear in the cell as complexes with proteins known as miRNP (miRNA containing ribonucleoprotins complex), or mirgonaute or miRISC (miRNA containing RNA induced silencing complex) (Kim, 2005). Generally one strand of miRNA is cleaved whilst one strand stands for active strand of mature miRNA. In animals including humans miRNAs act by imperfect pairing to the MRE (MiRNA Regulatory Element) in 3'UTR of target transcripts. Because of the mismatch between miRNA and target site in mRNA, one miRNA might target numerous different mRNAs, on the other hand one transcript might be regulated by various miRNAs (Jackson & Standart, 2007). There are several mechanisms of miRNA-dependent gene expression regulation, mainly through translation repression or mRNA decay (Jackson & Standart, 2007; Shuang & Fang, 2009; Zhao & Liu, 2009).

Translation repression might occur at initiation stage or after initiation stage. Three distinct mechanisms mediate translation repression by miRNA. First mechanism relies on blocking translation initiation by repression the assembly of ribosome that is the 60 S subunit to form complete 80 S translation active form (Thermann & Hentze, 2007). Second mechanism targets the translation initiation by repression the translation complex formation, mainly by blocking the eIF4E assembly to 5'7mG (Shuang & Fang, 2009). Third mechanism by which miRNA modulated translation initiation is connected with PolyA Binding Proteins (PABPs) action, or rather with the PolyA tail deadenylation (Wakiyama et al., 2007). There are

various post-initiation mechanisms that influence translation initiation mediated by miRNA. It has been shown that microRNA represses the IRES depended translation initiation, inhibits the LIN4 protein synthesis or causes timely ribosome drop-off and early translation termination (Shuang & Fang, 2009).
Numerous studies provide data reported mRNA degradation as a main aspect of gene expression repression mediated by miRNAs. MiRNA acts, in contrary to siRNA not by endonucleolytic cleavage, but rather by deadenylation and decapping of target mRNA and its subsequent degradation (Wu et al., 2005). The process of mRNA decay by miRNA has place in a cytoplasms foci named P-bodies (Processing bodies) that contain miRNAs, target mRNAs and enzymes required for mRNA decay (Jackson & Standart, 2007).

1.2.5 UTRs data bases

In order to classify the knowledge and to comprehensively understand the mechanisms of post-transcriptional regulation of gene expression mediated by UTRs, various data bases were created. Data bases provide information about functions and regulation mechanisms on the basis of primary and secondary structure of regulatory motifs. All data assembled in UTRs data bases have been determined by experimental studies and published (Mignone et al., 2005; Huang et al., 2006). Data bases contain information about sequence and structure of regulatory motifs like IRES, IRE, MRE, ARE, indicating the region of transcript that the particular motif appears. Furthermore, data bases provide information about regulatory factors interacting with particular motif (transcription factor, regulatory protein, miRNA). All data bases stand for useful tool for therapeutic possibility anticipating and searching. Examples of the most common UTRs data bases with short characterization are presented in table 1.

<table>
<tr><th>Name</th><th>Web site</th><th>Description</th></tr>
<tr><td>ERPIN (Easy RNA Profile IdentificatioN)</td><td>http://tagc.univ.mrs.fr/erpin/</td><td>Identification of a wide range of secondary structure, orientation and regulatory motifs in mRNA sequence.</td></tr>
<tr><td>MicroInspector</td><td>http://bioinfo.uni-plovdiv.bg/microinspector/</td><td rowspan="3">Tools for miRNA target site prediction as well as for searching miRNAs of analyzed mRNA.</td></tr>
<tr><td>miRanda</td><td>http://www.microrna.org/microrna/home.do</td></tr>
<tr><td>miRBase</td><td>http://www.mirbase.org/</td></tr>
<tr><td>RegRNA</td><td>http://regrna/mbc.nctu.edu.tw/</td><td rowspan="2">Identification of regulatory motifs and elements in mRNA sequence with functional effects.</td></tr>
<tr><td>RNA Analyzer</td><td>http://rnaanalyzer.bioapps.biozentrum.uni-wuerzburg.de/</td></tr>
<tr><td>UTRdb, UTRsite</td><td>http://utrdb.ba.itb.cnr.it/tool/utrscan</td><td>Identification regulatory motifs in 3′ and 5′UTRs important in post-transcriptional regulation.</td></tr>
</table>

Table 1. Characterization of main UTRs data bases.

1.3 Single nucleotide polymorphisms in UTRs and insulin resistance

5′ and 3′ UTRs are highly rich in polymorphisms like Alu elements or long polymorphisms LINE. In UTRs are present also mini and microSTRs as well as SNPs in a high abundance. The heterogeneity regions of UTRs for human are approximately 36% for 3′UTR and 12% for 5′UTR (Mignone et al., 2002). Single Nucleotide Polymorphism (SNP) is the replacement, deletion or insertion of a single base in genome sequence and is the most common change in human genome. The effects of nucleotide replacement vary, depend on the place, where the nucleotides have been changed. In most cases, SNPs do not have the phenotypic effects, and stand for the genomic heterogeneity within or between distinct populations. On the other hand SNPs in coding region of the genome (cSNPs - coding SNPs) might result in amino acids replacement and finally changes in protein structure and function. SNPs located in introns might influence the splicing process with effect on ensuing transcript. The great influence on mRNA and proteins synthesis possess SNPs located in regulatory regions like promoter region of the gene or in UTRs. Changes in those regions are associated with deregulation in gene expression at transcriptional and post-transcriptional levels (Doss et al., 2008).
The body of literature associate SNPs located in UTRs with gene expression regulation (Mendell et al., 2005; Chen et al., 2006). The proper nucleotide sequence in motifs described above ensures accurate function of these regions and gene expression regulation (Mendell & Dietz, 2001). Nucleotide changes in the functional transcripts regions influence the mRNA synthesis, splicing, transcripts stabilization and decay. Other mechanisms that SNPs might influence post-transcriptional gene expression regulation are the translation initiation or uORF generation. Nucleotide changes cause conformation changes in UTRs, especially in 5′UTR what notably influence the efficiency of translation initiation, the 5′UTR scanning and start codon searching. Furthermore changes in motifs that interact with 40 S ribosomal subunit, proteins, transcription factors or miRNA abolish the binding sites for these factors thus impair regulatory mechanisms.
So far, majority of investigators have focused mainly on genetic variants located in coding region. In recent decade polymorphisms in functional region have been emphasized. The growing interest dues to the fact that most diseases have been associated with abnormalities in gene expression rate as the main cause, thus the regulatory mechanisms have been widely investigated. Initially, investigators focused on genetic variants in regulatory regions as the cause of abnormities in gene expression during carcinogenesis. Next, more diseases have been correlated with changes in those regions (Conne et al., 2000; Pickering & Willis, 2005; Chen et al., 2006; Sethupathy & Collins, 2008; Halvorsen et al., 2010).

1.3.1 SNP in 5' and 3'UTRs and insulin resistance

The correlations between insulin resistance and genetic variants in UTRs have been reported previously by many investigators (Xia et al., 1999; Chen et al., 2006; Nelsøe et al, 2006). The associations linking genetic variations in UTRs of such genes as *PPP1R3A, PTPN1, KCNJ9, RETN, SOCS1, INSR,PIK3R1* or *FASL* with insulin resistance have been shown previously. In *PPP1R3A* gene the polymorphism has been connected with ARE and the nucleotide change (5bp deletion) impaired gene expression rate by increased mRNA degradation (Xia et al., 1999). Dinucleotide GT microSTR polymorphism in *FASL* gene has been correlated with insulin resistance in type 2 diabetes by affecting the mRNA stability (Nelsøe et al, 2006). The SNP in *PTPN1* gene, where change relyed on additional guanine insertion in 3′UTR, increased transcript stability, thus protein abundance and its activity. Increased PTP1B activity on the other hand impaired phophorylation rate of INSR and IRSs and insulin sensitivity (Di Paola et al., 2002). The A allele of SNP located in 3'UTR of resistin gene showed decreased risk of type 2 diabetes and hypertension comparing to G allele (Tan et al., 2003). In independent study the same SNP showed association with obesity and insulin-related phenotype (Duman et al., 2007). Wolford et al. have shown the association of SNPs including the SNPs located in 3'UTR of *KCNJ9* gene with insulin resistance and type 2 diabetes in Pima Indians, however, the associations was not strong. It is believed that investigated SNPs are in linkage disequilibrium with others functional SNPs (Wolford et al., 2001). Zhang et al. demonstrated allele dependent gene expression rate of *GFPT2* gene. The SNP located in 3'UTR of this gene positively correlated with mRNA abundance. The lower mRNA amount has been diagnosed in C allele carries, on the other hand significantly higher amount of mRNA has been diagnosed in T allele carriers (Zhang et al., 2004). Furthermore the T allele correlated with higher risk of type 2 diabetes development and its complications. Further examples of polymorphism in UTRs implicated in insulin resistance provided Villuendas et al. that revealed association between ACAA insertion/deletion polymorphism in *IGFIIR* gene with type 2 diabetes. The ACAA deletion variant played protective role. What's more authors suggested that this polymorphism might be a good surrogate insulin resistance marker (Villuendas et al., 2006). Bennet et al. in their work performed computational analysis in order to assess the influence of SNPs in insulin resistance syndrome development. Using bioinformatics and experimental approaches they revealed the association of nineteen SNPs located in 3'UTR with IR and T2DM. Nine SNPs were located in UTRs of genes implicated in insulin function and regulation pathway, nine SNPs were placed in UTRs of genes regulating cytokines synthesis and inflammation processes and one SNP in 3'UTR of gene classified into regulation of glucose metabolism and glucose transport (Bennet et al., 2001).

1.3.2 SNPs in microRNA genes/ microRNA target sites and insulin resistance

Gene expression regulation via microRNAs is crucial for maintaining body homeostasis. Dysregulation of this process might be a reason for various metabolic diseases (Sethupathy & Collins, 2008). Numerous factors affect miRNA translation regulation such as mutations in the proteins involved in miRNA processing and maturation (*trans factors*) as well as mutations in miRNA target sites (*cis factors*). Many SNPs located in target sites for miRNA action are correlated with miRNA mediated metabolic disorders like Tourette's Syndrome, Spastic Paraplegia, Hypertension, Parcinson Disease and various types of cancers (Sethupathy & Collins, 2008). MiRNA dysfunction is also correlated with obesity, insulin resistance and type 2 diabetes pathogenesis (Ferland-McCollough et al., 2010; Poy et al., 2007). Genome wide association studies (GWA) as well as meta-analysis studies demonstrated several SNPs correlated with higher risk of type 2 diabetes (Salonen et al., 2007; Zeggini et al., 2008; Dupuis et al., 2010). Among all SNPs with the highest significant association for type 2 diabetes, Glinsky selected twelve SNPs that possessed homology sequence to 8 microRNAs (Glinsky, 2008). Furthermore ten of twelve SNPs exhibited sequence homology to microRNAs targeting mRNA of *KPNA1* gene. According to authors SNPs that demonstrated sequence homology to following miRNAs: let-7, miR-548, miR-519, miR-520, miR-181, miR-541 act as phenocode of type 2 diabetes risk. These data suggested that SNPs in non coding but functional genome regions play important role in common human systemic diseases.

In our previous study we have shown difference in genotype distribution of two SNPs located in 3'UTR of *INSR* gene and *PIK3R1* gene and its correlation with insulin resistant phenotype (Malodobra et al., 2011). It has been shown that G/G genotypes of two SNPs (rs3756668 of *PIK3R1* gene and rs3745551 of *INSR* gene) correlated with BMI, insulin resistant ratios (HOMA-IR and QUICKI) and increased risk of IR .

INSR (Insulin Receptor) is a transmembrane glycoprotein formed by four chains: 2 α and 2 β subunits. The α subunit is responsible for ligand (insulin) binding, whilst the β subunit possesses the activity of tyrosine kinase that autophosphorylate tyrosine residues of β subunit and further kinases (IRS proteins) (Hubbard et al., 1994).

PIK3R1 gene encodes the p85α regulatory subunit of phosphatydylinositol 3-kinase that plays important role in insulin signal transduction, GLUT4 activation and substantially glucose uptake by the cell. Both kinases are extremely important for insulin action (Boura-Halfon & Zick, 2009).

The present work is devoted to evaluation of the influence of two investigated SNPs (rs3756668 of *PIK3R1* gene and rs3745551 of *INSR* gene) on gene expression rate and insulin resistance and type 2 diabetes risk. In presented study the relationships between genotypes and the mRNA levels of interest genes were elucidated.

2. Material and methods

The experimental protocols were approved by ethical review boards at Wroclaw Medical University, No. KB – 556/2008, November 30, 2008.

2.1 Peripheral lymphocytes and adipose tissue collection

Visceral adipose tissue biopsies were taken during abdominal surgery after receiving written agreement. Samples were immediately preserved in RNA*Later* (Ambion), incubated in 4°C for 24 h and then stored at -70°C until analysis. Lymphocytes were isolated from the whole blood taken on anticoagulant by centrifugation on Gradisol G (AquaLab). The 5 ml of the whole blood were placed on 2 ml of Gradisol and centrifuged 2000 rpm for 30 min in 4°C. The lymphocytes ring was collected and washed twice with PBS, the red blood cells were removed by lysis buffer (NH_4Cl, $KHCO_3$, EDTA-Na_2). Then lymphocytes were suspended in PBS, counted and portioned for $3x10^6$ cells per one tube, next centrifuged at max speed for 2 min in 4°C. PBS was discarded and lymphocytes pellet was frozen in -75°C till analysis.

Adipose tissue biopsies were collected from 15 patients with T2DM (6 men and 9 women) and from 24 controls (11 men and 13 women) in similar age (56±8 years for patients and 49±10 years for healthy subjects). Adipose tissue donors were inpatients of First Department and Clinic of General, Gastroenterological and Endocrinological Surgery, Wroclaw Medical University and of Provincial Specialist Hospital, Kamieńskiego in Wroclaw. The aims of abdominal surgeries were mainly cholecystectomy, surgery of abdominal hernia or gastric surgery. Lymphocytes were collected from 34 type 2 diabetic patients (21 men and 13 women) and from equal number of control subjects (17 men and 17 women) in similar age (mean age of diabetic patients was 58±7 years, controls 52±8 years). T2DM patients were inpatients of Department of Angiology, Hypertension and Diabetology, Wroclaw Medical University. Control subjects were selected based on fast glucose level below 106 mg/dl, lack of diabetes in family history, additionally for women no gestational diabetes in the past. Diabetic patients were divided into two subgroups depending on the insulin sensitivity: *IS* – insulin sensitive and *IR* – insulin resistant.

2.2 BMI and insulin resistance ratios

BMI was assessed dividing weight in kilograms by square of height in meters [kg/m^2]. Overweight was assigned with BMI > 25 kg/m^2, obesity with BMI > 30 kg/m^2.
Insulin resistance rate was estimated by insulin resistance ratios, calculated using following formulas:

1. HOMA-IR – [(glucose [mmol/l] * insulin [μU/ml])/22.5],
2. QUICKI – [(log glucose [mg/dl] + log insulin [μU/ml])].

Insulin resistance state was diagnosed with HOMA-IR > 2.5 and QUICKI < 0.321 (Ruano et al., 2006).

2.3 Bioinformatics analysis of investigated SNPs

The bioinformatical analyses of investigated SNPs were done with the use of bioinformatics tools available on-line: http://utrdb.ba.itb.cnr.it/tool/utrscan. The analyses were done to assess the localization of investigated SNPs in functional motifs of *INSR* and *PIK3R1* genes 3'UTRs.

2.4 RNA isolation and gene expression level

RNA from peripheral lymphocytes was isolated with the use of mirVana™ miRNA Isolation Kit (Ambion) according to manufactures protocol dedicated for total RNA isolation. RNA from visceral adipose tissues was isolated using TriPure Isolation Reagent (Roche) according to manufactured protocol. The tissues were homogenized using 2,0 mm Zirconia Beads (BioSpec Products, Inc). After homogenization tissues were centrifuged at max speed for 5 min in 4°C in order to collect the fat depot at the top of tube. The fat was discarded and the homogenate was extracted with 200 μl of chloroform, briefly vortexed and centrifuged for 15 min at max speed in 4°C. The aqueous phase was collected and RNA was precipitated with 500 μl of isopropanol, centrifuged for 10 min at max speed and washed with 1 ml of 70% ethanol in DEPC-treated water. RNA pellet was suspended in RNase-Free water and stored in -75°C.
Reverse transcription was performed with the use of High Capacity cDNA Reverse Transcription Kit (Applied Biosystems) according to manufactured protocol. The *PIK3R1* and *INSR* genes expression levels were analyzed in real-time PCR with the use of TaqMan Gene Expression Assay (Applied Biosystems) and Real-Time PCR Universal MasterMix (Applied Biosystems). The quantitative analysis was done as relative gene expression level normalized to two housekeeping genes: *β-actin* and *GUS-β* utilizing delta-delta (ΔΔCt) mathematical model (Pfaffl, 2001).

2.5 Statistical analysis

Statistical analysis was done using STATISTICA8 software. Statistical significance was considered with $p < 0.05$. The association of investigated SNPs with clinical parameters and *PIK3R1* and *INSR* gene expression levels were done with use of one way variance analysis ANOVA. Correlation between gene expression and biochemical parameters were assessed by Pearson's coefficient of correlation.

3. Results

3.1 Anthropometrical and biochemical characterization of analyzed groups

67.5% of all diabetic patients were insulin resistant (*IR*). 32.5% diabetic patients displayed proper insulin sensitivity (*IS*). *IR* patients were characterized by increased BMI value (*p=0.0203*) and fasting insulin level (*p=0.0000*) as well as insulin resistance ratios (*p=2.1E-06* and *p=1.6E-13* for HOMA-IR and QUICKI, respectively) in comparison to *IS* patients. Glucose level did not show statistical difference between groups of patients with slight increase in *IR* group (*p=0.0538*). Furthermore, *IR* patients manifested higher hypertension and increased TG level. Moreover insulin resistance rate correlated positively with BMI value (HOMA-IR: R=0.44, *p=0.000;* QUICKI R=-0.53. *p=0.000*). Type 2 diabetic patients displayed higher TG (p=0.0316) and lower HDL (0.0006) level.

In previous study the correlation between genotype and insulin resistant phenotype has been presented (Malodobra et al., 2011). Furthermore we have noticed higher frequency of G/G genotypes of both SNPs in *INSR* and *PIK3R1* genes higher risk of this disorders (OR = 1.83 (0.21-0.84) of rs3756668; OR = 2.27 (0.13-0.69) of rs3745551 and OR = 3.14 (0.11-0.28) of G/G_G/G haplotype). Increasing the number of investigated subjects we have revealed the association of rs3756668 G/G_rs3745551 G/G haplotype with insulin resistant phenotype. Carriers of both G/G genotypes were more insulin resistant and were characterized with higher BMI, glucose and insulin level. Results are presented in figure 1.

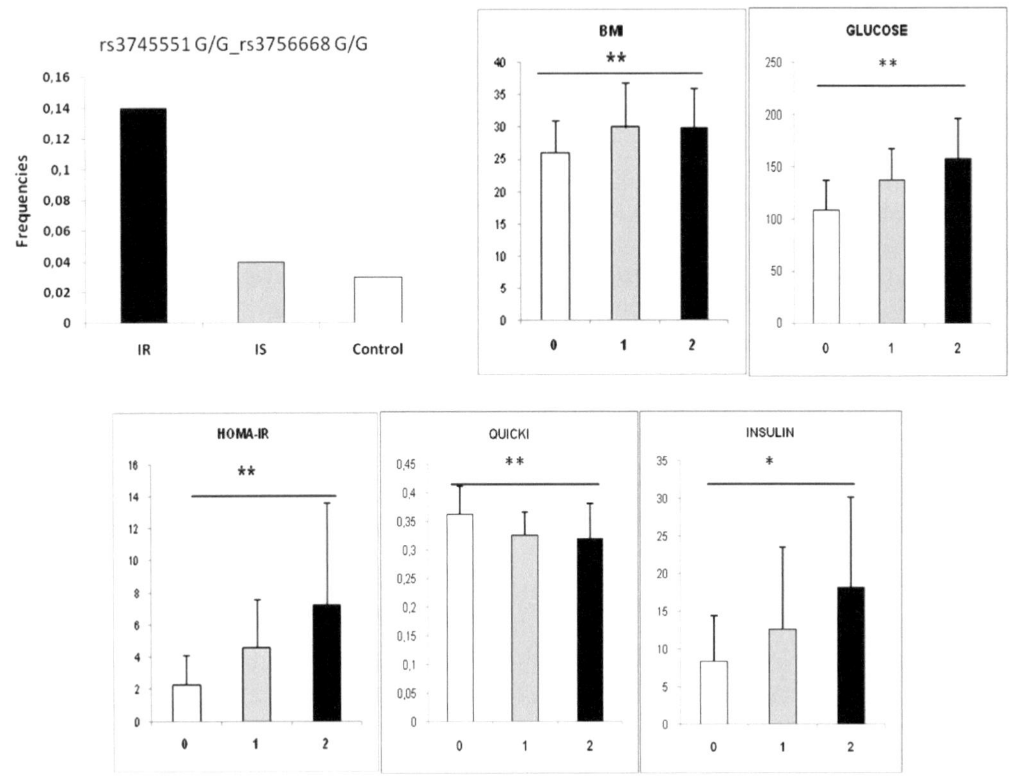

Fig. 1. The relationship between clinical features and number of G/G genotype (**0** - lack, **1** – one G/G genotype either rs3745551 or rs3756668, **2** – carriers of both genotypes; ** < 0.001, * <0.05).

3.2 Bioinformatics analysis of investigated SNPs

The bioinformatics analysis was done in order to evaluate the localization of investigated SNPs in regulatory motifs of *INSR* and *PIK3R1* genes UTRs as well as to determine how the nucleotide change influence the regulatory elements structure and potentially their function. The analysis has been done for all isoforms of *PIK3R1* and *INSR* genes. The analysis revealed that all investigated SNPs were located in uORF of 3'UTR of examined genes. However, uORF in 3'UTR did not posses functional importance. What's more, the range of regulatory motifs reading frame did not change with the nucleotide substitution. The results of bioinformatics analysis are presented in table 2.

Gene name	rs ID	Type of change	Region	Position in mRNA	Regulatory Element	The wild type reading frame	The mutation type reading frame
INSR (NM_000208.2)	rs1052371 rs3745551	C>T A>G	3' UTR 3' UTR	8739 7034	uORF[1] uORF	8735÷9004 7030÷7174	8735÷9004 7030÷7174
INSR (NM_001079817.1)	rs1052371 rs3745551	C>T A>G	3' UTR 3' UTR	8696 7001	uORF	8669÷8968 ———	8669÷8968 ———
PIK3R1 (NM_181523.1)	rs3756668	A>G	3' UTR	4876	uORF	4853÷5038	4853÷5038
PIK3R1 (NM_181504.2)	rs3756668	A>G	3' UTR	4086	uORF	4063÷4248	4063÷4248
PIK3R1 (NM_181524.1)	rs3756668	A>G	3' UTR	4246	uORF	4223÷4408	4223÷4408

Table 2. The bioinformatics analysis of investigated SNPs.

3.3 *INSR* and *PIK3R1* genes expression rate measurements

The *INSR* and *PIK3R1* genes expression levels were measured in peripheral lymphocytes and visceral adipose tissues in both groups. There was no significant difference in *INSR* and *PIK3R1* genes expression levels performed in lymphocytes between analyzed groups. Similar results were obtained normalized to both housekeeping genes (data not shown). On the other hand there were a significant differences in investigated genes expression levels measured in visceral adipose tissues. Both, the *IR* and *IS* diabetic patients displayed significantly lower mRNA abundance of both analyzed genes comparing to healthy subjects. The differences in genes expression level were statistically significant when normalized to *β-actin* (($p=0.004$ and $p=0.0159$ for *PIK3R1*gene and *INSR* gene respectively). The relative analyses of genes expression rate normalized to *GUS-β* were close to be significant.

3.4 Genotype association with the *INSR* and *PIK3R1* genes expression levels

In order to analyze whether the genotype of investigated SNPs located in 3'UTRs of *INSR* and *PIK3R1* gene might influence gene expression rate the genotyping results (described previously, Malodobra et al., 2011), and gene expression analyses results were analyzed

using ANOVA. There was no significant relationship between genotype of analyzed SNPs and gene expression rates in peripheral lymphocytes (data not shown). There was no relationship between genotypes of SNP located in 3'UTR of *PIK3R1* gene and *PIK3R1* gene expression in adipose tissue. Despite the fact, that *PIK3R1* gene showed decreased expression level in adipose tissue in diabetic patients and the rs3756668 of *PIK3R1* showed higher frequency in G/G genotype in those patients, the decreased *PIK3R1* gene expression did not correlate with genotype.
On the other hand there was statistically significant relationship between rs3745551 located in 3'UTR of *INSR* gene and *INSR* gene expression rate. The G/G genotype carriers displayed considerably lower mRNA abundance in visceral adipose tissue comparing to homozygotes A/A and heterozygotes A/G. However the relationship was seen for healthy subjects only. In type 2 diabetic patients, both in *IR* and *IS* the *INSR* gene expression level was low and with no substantially differences between genotype carriers. The relationship between gene expression rate of investigated genes in adipose tissue and genotype of analyzed SNPs is presented in figure 2.

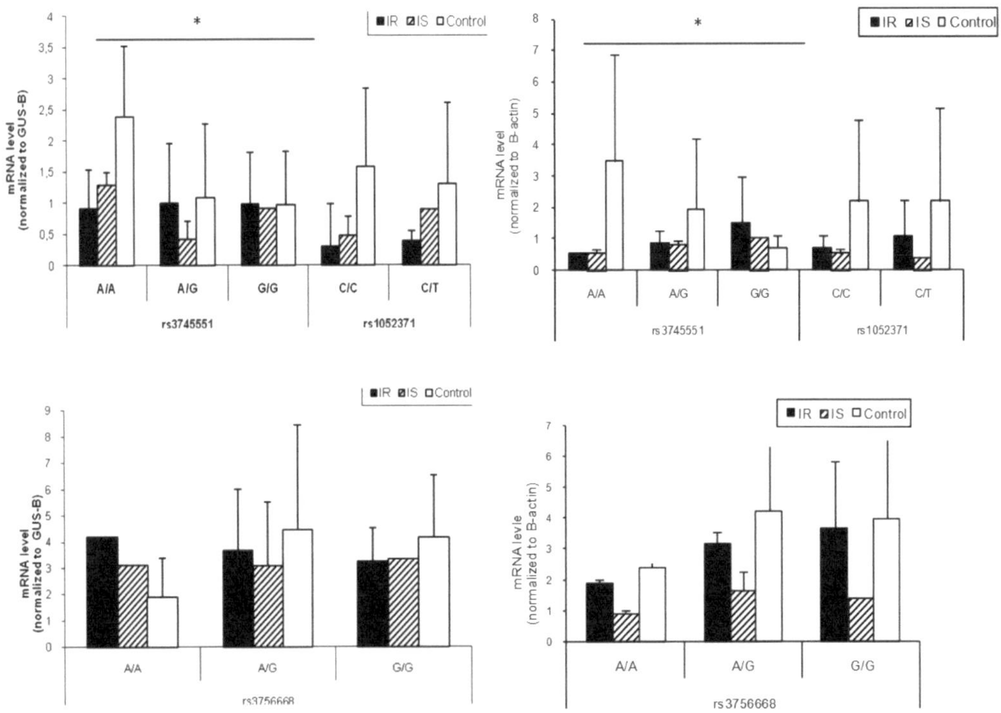

Fig. 2. Relationship between *INSR* and *PIK3R1* genes expression level and genotypes of investigated SNPs (* $p<0.05$).

3.5 Correlation between *INSR* and *PIK3R1* genes expression levels, biochemical parameters and insulin resistant phenotype

The *INSR* and *PIK3R1* genes expression rates measured in lymphocytes showed correlation with insulin resistance ratios. There was negative correlation between *INSR* and *PIK3R1* mRNA level and fasting insulin concentration and HOMA-IR as well as positive correlation

between mRNA level and QUICKI. In addition *INSR* gene expression rate showed negative correlation with TG and CHOL. Similar results were seen for gene expression normalization to both housekeeping genes. The correlation between investigated gene expression rate and clinical parameters is presented in table 3.
The *INSR* and *PIK3R1* genes expression rates measured in adipose tissue correlated neither with analyzed clinical feature nor with insulin resistance ratios (data not shown). However, *PIK3R1* gene expression rate showed negative correlation with TNF-α concentration (R = (-0.82), p=0.026 normalized to *β-actin* and R = (-0.70), p=0.08 normalized to *GUS-β*). The relationship between *PIK3R1* mRNA level and TNF-α concentration presents figure 3.

	Glucose [R(p)]	Insulin [R(p)]	HOMA [R(p)]	QUICKI [R(p)]	TG [R(p)]	CHOL [R(p)]	HDL [R(p)]	LDL [R(p)]	BMI [R(p)]
PIK3R1_B	n.s.	-0.42 (0.02)	-0.44 (0.022)	0.46 (0.015)	n.s.	n.s.	n.s.	n.s.	n.s.
PIK3R1_G	n.s.	n.s.	n.s.	n.s.	n.s.	n.s.	n.s.	n.s.	n.s.
INSR_B	-0.33 (0.02)	-0.48 (0.02)	-0.53 (0.01)	0.53 (0.01)	-0.31 (0.09)	-0.35 (0.06)	n.s.	n.s.	n.s.
INSR_G	n.s.	-0.57 (0.006)	-0.59 (0.004)	0.66 (0.001)	-0.32 (0.06)	-0.54 (0.005)	n.s.	-0.37 (0.05)	n.s.

Table 3. The correlation between genes expression and clinical parameters (_B - normalized to *β-actin*; _G - normalized to *GUS-β*; n.s. - not significant).

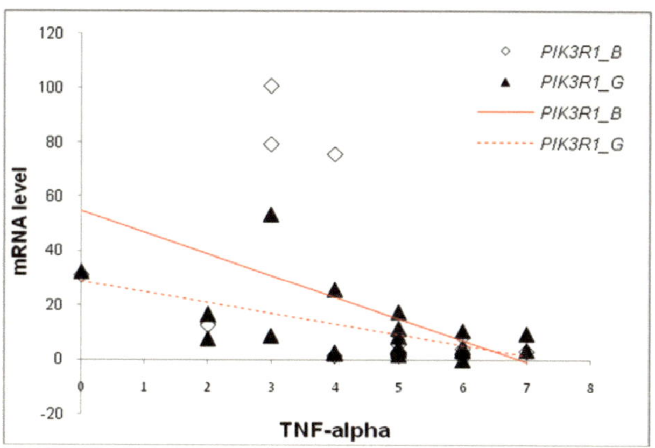

PIK3R1_B R = (-0.82), p = 0.026
PIK3R1_G R = (-0.70), p = 0.08

Fig. 3. The correlation between *PIK3R1* mRNA and TNF-α (_B - normalized to *β-actin*; _G - normalized to *GUS-β*).

4. Discussion

The genetic predispositions are large components that trigger the IR and T2DM risk and pathogenesis. SNPs in functional region are in great interests of numerous investigators and are associated with variety of diseases pathogenesis. The relationships between IR and SNPs in UTRs have been reported by many investigators (Xia et al., 1999; Chen et al., 2006; Nelsøe et al et al., 2006). Especially 3'UTR is considered as a "hot spot" of pathology and polymorphic sites located within 3'UTR are associated with increased risk of numerous diseases (Conne et al., 2000). Taking into consideration the fact that IR is characterized by deregulations in numerous genes expression rates encoding important for insulin signaling kinases, the SNPs located in UTRs of these genes were particularly under investigation. Numerous SNPs located in *INSR, PIK3R1, PTPN1* and *SLC2A4* genes were genotyped and correlated with insulin resistant phenotype (Malodobra et al., 2011). Overwhelmingly two out of seven genotyped SNPs showed the association with insulin resistant phenotype (BMI, HOMA-IR, QUICKI) as well as with increased risk of IR development (assessed based on OR (95%Cl)). The G/G genotypes of rs3756668 located in 3'UTR of *PIK3R1* gene and rs3745551 located in 3'UTR of *INSR* gene positively correlated with higher BMI value, fasting glucose and insulin level, as well as G/G carriers were more insulin resistant (based on HOMA-IR and QUICKI ratios). It is worth to mention that in logistic regression analysis we displayed additional interaction between G/G genotypes of those two SNPs with increased OR value (Malodobra et al., 2011).

In present work, the *PIK3R1* and *INSR* genes expression analyses in peripheral lymphocytes and adipose tissue were presented. The main aim of this paper was to evaluate the role of those two SNPs in gene expression regulation at post-transcriptional level and how the nucleotide changes influence mRNA level in the cell.

The present work contains as well the influence the G/G haplotype of rs3745551 (*INSR*) and rs3756668 (*PIK3R1*) on insulin and glucose metabolism and insulin resistant phenotype.

Previously described results (Malodobra et al., 2011) demonstrated that two out of seven genotyped SNPs showed the association with insulin resistant phenotype. Those two SNPs displayed as well increased risk of IR development. Thus in present work thanks to increasing the number of analyzed subjects we were able to evaluate the relationship between two SNPs haplotype (rs3756668 G/G and rs3745551 G/G) and insulin resistant phenotype. Very interesting correlation has been observed with progressively increased insulin resistance state (assessed by clinical parameters: fasting glucose and insulin concentrations, HOMA-IR and QUICKI ratios) depending on number of G/G genotypes. The higher insulin resistant state has been seen for carriers of both G/G genotype, moderate values of measured parameters have been seen for carriers one of at risk genotypes. The lowest values of measured parameters possessed subject not affected by at risk G/G genotype.

In contradictory to results described by others investigators (Maratou et al., 2007; Piatkiewicz et al., 2007), we did not detect impairments in insulin signaling in patients with T2DM both in *IS* (insulin sensitive) and *IR* (insulin resistant) measured in lymphocytes. There was no difference in *INSR* and *PIK3R1* genes expression rates between investigated groups. In type 2 diabetic patients, both *IS* and *IR*, the mRNA levels of investigated genes were similar to those measured in healthy controls. Piatkiewicz et al. suggested that peripheral lymphocytes might stand for perfect cellular model for insulin signaling investigation in type 2 diabetes (Piatkiewicz et al., 2007). Obtained results did not confirm that statement, there was no evidence for defects in insulin signal transduction and GLUT4 activation (at mRNA level). However, presented results ought to be evaluated on protein level. On the other hand, expression rates of analyzed genes measured in lymphocytes negatively correlated with fasting glucose and insulin concentrations as well as with HOMA-IR values, whilst positively with QUICKI ratio. These results suggest that peripheral lymphocytes are very sensitive for environmental changes in glucose and insulin level.

The pathomechanism of impairment in insulin sensitivity in adipose tissue is quite different than in other tissues (skeletal muscles, liver) (George, 1996). In adipose tissue the main dysfunction leading to insulin resistance is the adipogenesis deregulation favoring differentiation towards pro-inflammatory cells (Gustafson et al., 2009). In addition hypertrophy and hyperplasia of adypocytes further lead to insulin sensitivity impairment. The visceral adipose tissue is especially implicated in metabolic syndrome pathogenesis including IR (Preis et al., 2010), for that reason this type of adipose tissue has been collected for analysis. Adipose tissue is characterized by deregulation in expression as well as phosphorylation rate of numerous genes and kinases (Ahmad et al., 1995; Andreelli et al., 2000; Patti, 2004; Rasouli & Kern, 2008).

In presented study in type 2 diabetics adipose tissues, *IR* as well as *IS* patients, the mRNA levels of *INSR* and *PIK3R1* genes were significantly lower comparing to healthy controls. These data stand for the fact, that insulin signaling in adipocytes in type 2 diabetic patients is impaired by decrease in gene expression. Similar results have been observed and described by others authors, who also diagnosed lower mRNA as well as protein abundance of INSR and p85 α in T2DM patients (George, 1996; Hansen & Shafrir, 2002; Rasche et al., 2008).

It has been proved by many investigators that SNPs in UTRs might affect mRNA stability and translation initiation processes (Mendell et al., 2005; Chen et al., 2006). In order to assess whether investigated SNPs in *INSR* and *PIK3R1* genes might influence the mRNA abundance in the cells we analyzed genotyping and expression rates results. First of all, however, the bioinformatical tools were utilized in order to evaluate the exact localization of SNPs in regulatory elements of 3′UTRs and whether the nucleotide change might reorganize the frames of regulatory motifs in UTRs. The investigated SNPs were localized in uORFs of 3′UTR and the changes in nucleotide sequence did not influence the reading frames of those regulatory elements.

Despite the fact we performed evaluation how particular genotype of investigated SNPs affects the gene expression rate. We did not notice significant changes in *INSR* and *PIK3R1* genes expression rates measured in peripheral lymphocytes. There was no difference in mRNA abundance in relation to genotypes. Similar results were received for all groups and for genes expression analyses normalized to both housekeeping genes. Obtained results negate the possible role of investigated SNPs in genes expression regulation at post-transcriptional level.

Similar analysis has been done for *INSR* and *PIK3R1* genes expression measurements in adipose tissues and for genotypes of investigated SNPs (rs3745551 and rs1052371). One of the investigated SNP displayed relationship with mRNA abundance with difference statistically significant. The G/G carriers were characterized by the lowest mRNA level comparing to A/A and A/G carriers. It is worth to mention that G/G genotype of this SNP in previous study showed association with IR risk and with insulin resistant phenotype. However, the difference reached significance only in healthy subjects. In type 2 diabetic patients the mRNA level was very low and did not differ depending on genotype. Probably some others factors (genetic of environmental) strongly influenced *INSR* gene expression in those subjects thus, noticed in healthy controls relationship between mRNA level and

genotype, in groups exposed to those factors, has been abolished. Second polymorphism investigated in *INSR* gene (rs1052371) did not display relationship between mRNA abundant in relation to genotype.
The rs3756668 located in 3'UTR of *PIK3R1* gene in previous study, similar to rs3745551 of *INSR* gene, showed association with increased IR risk and with insulin resistant phenotype. However, when genotyping results were compared with *PIK3R1* gene expression rate, there was no relationship between genotypes of this SNP and mRNA level. Lack of correlation might be due to the low number of analyzed samples. Further experiments must be done in order to evaluate how this SNP influence increased risk to IR and T2DM.
Described in present study results provide the first evidence for association of SNPs in UTRs of *INSR* and *PIKR1* genes with genes expression rates. So far, all investigated in these genes SNPs were localized mainly in coding regions (Kusari et al., 1991; Baynes et al., 2000; Almind et al., 2002; Jamshidi et al., 2006; Højlund et al., 2006). Presented results stand for the first report where evaluation of SNPs in UTRs of *INSR* and *PIK3R1* genes with gene expression levels was performed in peripheral lymphocytes and adipose tissues.

5. Conclusion

Concluding genes expression measurements, presenting results negate the dysfunction in insulin signaling in peripheral lymphocytes, at least at mRNA level. On the other hand the expression rate of genes implicated in insulin action is decreased in adipose tissue of patients with T2DM. The rs3745551, that in previous study showed correlation with insulin resistance, in present work, displayed relationship with *ISNR* gene mRNA level in adipose tissue. The relationship however was seen for healthy controls only. The second SNP that in previous study showed association with insulin resistance, in present work we did not show the relationship between genotype and mRNA level. Further study must be done in order to evaluate how this SNP is implicated in increased risk to IR.
The present study also showed the effect of two SNPs haplotype influence on insulin resistant phenotype.

6. Acknowledgments

This project was supported by Ministry of Science and Higher Education of Poland, Grant No: N N401 009436.

7. References

Ahmad, F.; Azevedo, J.L.; Cortright, R.Jr.; Dohm, G..L; Goldstein, B.J. (1997). Alteration in skeletal muscle protein-tyrosine phosphatase activity and expression in insulin-resistance human obesity and diabetes. *J. Clin. Invest.*, Vol.100, No.2, pp. 449-458, ISSN 0021-9738

Ahmad, F.; Li, P.M.; Meyerovitch, J. & Goldstein, B.J. (1995). Osmotic loading of neutralizing antibodies defines a role for protein-tyrosine phosphatase 1B in negative regulation of the insulin action pathway. *J. Biol. Chem.*, Vol.270, No.35, pp. 20503-20508, ISSN 0021-9258

Almind, K.; Delahaye, L.; Hansen, T.; van Obberghen, E.; Pedersen, O. & Kahn, C.R. (2002). Characterization of the Met326Ile variant of phosphatidylinositol 3-kinase p85α. *PNAS*, Vol.99, No.4, pp. 2124-2128, ISSN 0027-8424

Andreelli, F.; Laville, M.; Vega, N.; Riou, J-P. & Vidal, H. (2000). Regulation of gene expression during severe caloric restriction: lack of induction of p85alpha phosphatidylinositol 3-kinase mRNA in skeletal muscle of patients with type 2 (non-insulin-dependent) diabetes mellitus. *Diabetologia*, Vol.43, No.3, pp. 356-363, ISSN 0012-186X

Barroso I, Luan J, Middelberg R P S Harding A-H, Franks P W, Jakes R W, Clayton D, Schafer A J, O'Rahilly S, Wareham, N. (2003). Candidate gene associated study in type 2 diabetes indicates a role for genes involved in β-cell function as well as insulin action. *Plos Biology*, Vol.1, No.1, pp. 41-55, ISSN 1545-7885

Baynes, K.; Beeton, C.A.; Panayotou, G.; Stein, R.; Soos, M.; Hansen, T.; Simpson, H.; O'Rahilly, S.; Shepherd, R.P. & Whitehead, J.P. (2000). Natural variants of human p85 alpha phosphoinositide 3-kinase in severe insulin resistance: a novel variant with impaired insulin stimulated lipid kinase activity. *Diabetologia*, Vol.43, No3, pp. 690-693, ISSN 0012-186X

Bennet, .AM.; Näslung, T.I.; Morgenstern, R. & De Faire, U. (2001). Bioinformatic and experimental tool for identification of single nucleotide polymorphisms in genes with a potential for the development of the insulin resistance syndrome. *Journal of Internal Medicine*, Vol.249, No.2, pp. 127-136, ISSN 0954-6820

Boura-Halfon, S. & Zick, Y. (2009). Phosphorylation of IRS protein, insulin action and insulin resistance. *Am. J. Physiol. Endocrinol. Metab.*, Vol.296, pp. 581-591, ISSN 0193-1849

Carmody, S.R. & Wente, S.R. (2009). mRNA nuclear export at a glance. *J. Cell. Sci.*, Vol.122, No.12, pp. 1933-1937, ISSN 0021-9533

Chappell, S.A.; Edelman, G.M. & Mauro, V.P. (2000). A 9-nt segment of a cellular mRNA can function as an internal ribosome entry site (IRES) and when present in linked multiple copies greatly enhances IRES activity. *Proc. Natl. Acad. Sci.*, Vol.97, No.4, pp. 1536-1541, ISSN 0027-8424

Chen, J-M.; Férec, C. & Cooper, D.N. (2006). A systematic analysis of disease-associated variants in the 3′ regulatory regions of human protein-coding genes II: the importance of mRNA secondary structure in assessing the functionality of 3′ UTR variants. *Hum. Genet.*, Vol.120, No.3, pp. 301-333, ISSN 0340-6717

Cheung A, Kusari J, Jansen D, Bandyopadhyay D, Kusari A, Bryer-Ash M. (1999): Marked impairment of protein tyrosine phosphatase 1B activity in adipose tissue of obese subjects with and without type 2 diabetes mellitus. *J. Lab. Clin. Med.*, Vol.134, No.2, pp. 115-123, ISSN 0022-2143

Cohen, B.; Novick, D. & Rubinstein, M. (1996). Modulation of insulin activities by leptin. *Science*, Vol.274, No.5290, pp. 1185-1188, ISSN 0036-8075

Coldwell, M.J.; Mitchell, S.A.; Stoneley, M.; MacFarlane, M. & Willis, A.E. (2000). Initiation of Apaf-1 translation by ribosome entry. *Oncogene*, Vol.19, No.7, pp. 899-905, ISSN 0950-9232

Conne, B.; Stutz, A. & Vassalli, J-D. (2000). The 3′ untranslated region of messenger RNA: A molecular "hotspot" for pathology? *Nat. Med.*, Vol.6, No.6, pp. 637-641, ISSN 1078-8956

Di Paola, R.; Frittitta, L.; Miscio, G.; Bozzali, M.; Baratta, R.; Centra, M.; Spampinato, D.; Santagati, M.G.; Ercolino, T.; Cisternino, C.; Soccio, T.; Mastroianno, S.; Tassi, V.; Almgren, P.; Pizzuti, A.; Vigneri, R. & Trischitta, V. (2002). A variation in 3′ UTR of *hPTPN1B* increases specific gene expression and associated with insulin resistance. *Am. J. Hum. Genet.*, Vol.70, No.3, pp. 806-812, ISSN 0002-9297

Doss, C.G.P.; Sudandiradoss, C.; Rajasekaran, R.; Choudhury, P.; Sinha, P.; Hota, P.; Batra, U.P. & Rao, S. (2008). Application of computational algorithm tools to identify functional SNPs. *Funct Integr Genomics*, Vol.8, No.4, pp. 309-316, ISSN 1438-793X

Duman, B.S.; Cagatay, P.; Hatemi, H. & Öztürk, M. (2007). Association of resistin gene 3′-Untranslated region EX4-44 G→A polymorphism with obesity- and insulin-related phonotypes in Turkish type 2 diabetes patients. *Rev Diabet Stud*, Vol.4, No.1, pp. 49-55, ISSN 1614-0575

Dupuis, J.; Langenberg, C.; Prokopenko, I. et al. (2010). New genetic loci implicated in fasting glucose homeostasis and their impact on type 2 diabetes risk. *Nature Genetics*, Vol.42, No.2, pp. 105-120, ISSN 1546-1718

Ferland-McCollough, D.; Ozanne, S.E.; Siddle, K.; Willis, A.E. & Bushell, M. (2010). The involvement of microRNAs in Type 2 Diabetes. *Biochem. Soc.*, Trans. Vol.38, No.6, pp. 1565-1570, ISSN 1470-8752

Garvey, W.T.; Maianu, L.; Zhu, J-H.; Brechtel-Hook, G.; Wallace, P. & Baron. A.D. (1998). Evidence for defects in the trafficking and translocation of GLUT4 glucose transporters in skeletal muscle as a cause of human insulin resistance. *J. Clin. Invest.*, Vol.101, No.11, pp. 2377-2386, ISSN 0021-9738

George, A.B. (1996). Endocrinology and metabolism clinics of North America. Obesity. In: *W B Saunders Company*, 25 (4).

Glinsky, G.V. (2008). An SNP-guided microRNA map of fifteen common human disorders identifies a consensus disease phenocode aiming at principal components of the nuclear import pathway. *Cell Cycle*, Vol.7, No.16, pp. 2570-2583, ISSN 1551-4005

Greenspan, F.S. & Baxter, J.D. (1994). Basic & Clinical Endocrinology. In: *Appletin & Lange*, Fourth edition, Norwalk, Connecticut, USA.

Griffin, M.E.; Hamilton, B.J.; Roy, K.M.; Du, M.; Willson, A.M.; Deenan, B.J.; Wang, X.W. & Nichols, R.C. (2004). Post-transcriptional regulation of glucose transporter-1 by an AU-rich element in the 3′UTR and by hnRNP A2. *Biochem Biophys Res Commun*, Vol.318, No.4, pp. 977-982, ISSN 0006-291X

Gustafson, B.; Gogg, S.; Hedjazifar, S.; Jenndahl, L.; Hammarstedt, A. & Smith, U. (2009). Inflammation and impaired adipogenesis in hypertrophic obesity in man. *Am. J. Physiol. Endocrinol. Metab.*, Vol.297, Doi:10.1152.00377.2009, ISSN 1522-1555

Halvorsen, M.; Martin, J.S.; Broadaway, S.; Laederach, A. (2010). Disease-associated mutations that alter the RNA structural ensemble. *Plos Genetics*, Vol.6, No.8, pp. e1001074, ISSN 1553-7404

Hansen, B. & Shafrir, E. (2002). Insulin resistance and insulin resistance syndrome. In: *Taylor & Francis*, New York, NY, USA

Hernandez-Morante, J.J.; Milagrot, F.I.; Lujan, J.A.; Martinez, J.A.; Zamora, S. & Garaulet, M. (2008). Insulin effect on adipose tissue (AT) adiponectin expression is regulated by the insulin resistance status of the patients. *Clin. Endocrinol.*, Vol.69, No.3, pp. 412-417, ISSN 1365-2265

Højlund, K.; Wojtaszewski, J.F.P.; Birk, J.; Hansen, B.F.; Vestergaard, H. & Beck-Nielsen H. (2006). Partial rescue of in vivo insulin signalling in skeletal muscle by impaired insulin clearance in heterozygous carriers of a mutation in the insulin receptor gene. *Diabetologia*, Vol.49, No.8, pp. 1827-1837, ISSN 0012-186X

Holcik, M. & Korneluk, R.G. (2000). Functional characterization of the X-linked inhibitor of apoptosis (XIAP) internal ribosome entry site element: role of La autoantigen in XIAP translation. *Mol. Cell. Biol.*, Vol.20, No.13, pp. 4648-4657, ISSN 0270-7306

Huang, H-Y.; Chien, C-H.; Jen, K-H. & Huang, H-D. (2006). RegRNA: an integrated web server for identifying regulatory RNA motifs and elements. *Nucleic Acids Res.*, Vol.34, pp. 429-434, ISSN 1362-4962

Hubbard, S.R.; Wei, L.; Ellis, L. & Hendrickson, W.A. (1994). Crystal structure of the tyrosine kinase domain of the human insulin receptor. *Nature*, Vol.372, No.6508, pp. 746-754, ISSN 0028-0836

Jackson, R.J. & Standart, N. (2007). How do microRNA regulated gene expression? *Sci STKE*, Vol.367, pp. 1-13, ISSN 1525-8882

Jamshidi, Y.; Snieder, H.; Wang, X.; Pavitt, M,J.; Spector, T.D.; Carter, N.D. & O'Dell, S.D. (2006). Phosphatidylinositol 3-kinase p85α subunit gene *PIK3R1* haplotype is associated with body fat and serum leptin in a female twin population. *Diabetologia*, Vol.49, No.11, pp. 2659-2667, ISSN 0012-186X

Karlsson, H.K.R. & Zierath, J.R. (2007). Insulin signaling and glucose transport in insulin resistant human skeletal muscle. *Cell Biochem. Biophys.*, Vol.48, No.2, pp. 103-113, ISSN 1085-9195

Kim, V.N. (2005). MicroRNA biogenesis: coordinated cropping and dicing. *Nature*, Vol.6, No.5, pp. 376-385, ISSN 1471-0072

Kusari, J.; Verma, F.B.; Henry, R.R. & Olefsky, J.M. (1991). Analysis of the gene sequences of the insulin receptor and the insulin sensitive glucose transporter (GLUT4) in patients with common type non-dependent diabetes mellitus. *J. Clin. Invest.*, Vol.88, No.4, pp. 1323-1330, ISSN 0021-9738

LeRoith, D.; Taylor, S.I. & Olefsky, J.M. (1996). Diabetes Mellitus. A fundamental and clinical text. In: *Lippincott-Raven Publishers*, Philadelphia, PA

Malodobra, M.; Pileckam A.; Gworys, B. & Adamiec, R. (2011). Single nucleotide polymorphisms within functional regions of genes implicated in insulin action and association with the insulin resistance phenotype. *Mol Cell Biochem*, Vol.349, No.1-2, pp. 187-193, ISSN 1573-4919

Maratou, E.; Dimitriadis, G.; Kollias, A.; Boutati, E.; Lambadiri, V.; Mitrou, P & Raptis, S.A. (2007). Glucose transporter expression on the plasma membrane of resting and activated white blood cells. *Eur. J. Clin. Invest.*, Vol. 37, No.4, pp. 282-290, ISSN 0014-2972

Meijer, H.A. & Thomas, A.A.M. (2002). Control of eukaryotic protein synthesis by upstream open reading frames in the 5'-untranslated region of an mRNA. *Biochem. J.*,Vol.367, pp. 1-11, ISSN 0264-6021

Meiron, M.; Anunu, R.; Scheinman, E.J.; Hashmueli, S. & Levi, B.Z. (2001). New isoforms of VEGF are translated from alternative initiation CUG codons located in its 5'UTR. *Biochem. Biophys. Res. Commun.*, Vol.282, No.4, pp. 1053-1060, ISSN 0006-291X

Mendell, J.T. & Dietz, H.C. (2001). When the message goes awry: Disease-producing mutations that influence mRNA content and performance. *Cell*, Vol.107, No.4, pp. 411-414, ISSN 0092-8674

Mendell, J.T.; Sharifi, N.A.; Meyers, J.L.; Martinez-Murillo, F. & Dietz, H.C. (2004). Nonsense surveillance regulates expression of diverse classes of mammalian transcripts and mutes genomic noise. *Nat Genet*, Vol.36, No.10, pp. 1073-1078, ISSN 1061-4036

Mignone, F.; Gissi, C.; Liuni, S. & Pesole, G. (2002). Untranslated regions of mRNAs. *Genome Biol.*, Vol.3, No.3, pp. 1-10, ISSN 1465-6906

Mignone, F.; Grillo, G.; Licciulli, F.; Iacono, M.; Liuni, S.; Kersey, P.J.; Duarte, J.; Saccone, C. & Pesole, G. (2005). UTRdb and UTRsite: a collection of sequences and regulatory motifs of the untranslated regions of eukaryotic mRNAs. *Nucleic Acids Res.*, Vol.33, pp. 141-146, ISSN 1362-4962

Morino, K.; Petersen, K.F. & Shulman G I. (2006). Molecular mechanisms of insulin resistance in humans and their potential links with mitochondrial dysfunction. *Diabetes,* Vol.55, No.2, pp. 9-15, ISSN 0012-1797

Müssig, K.; Fiedler, H.; Staiger, H.; Weigert, C.; Lahmann, R.; Schleicher, E.D. & Haring, H.U. (2005). Insulin-induced stimulation of JNK and the PI 3-kinase/mTOR pathway leads to phosphorylation of serine 318 of IRS-1 in C2C12 myotubes. *Biochem Biophys Res Commun*, Vol.335, No.3, pp. 819-825, ISSN 0006-291X

Nelsøe, R.L.; Hamid, Y.H.; Pociot, F.; Paulsen, S.; Andersen, K.M.; Borch-Johnsen, K.; Drivsholm, T.; Hansen, T.; Pedersen, O. & Mandrup-Poulsen, T. (2006). Association of a microsatellite in FASL to type 2 diabetes and of the FAS-670G>A genotype in insulin resistance. *Genes Immun.*, Vol.7, No.4, pp. 316-321, ISSN 1466-4879

Nicholson, P.; Yepiskoposyan, H.; Metze, S.; Orozco, R.Z.; Kleinschmidt, N. & Mühlemann, O. (2010). Nonsense-mediated mRNA decay in human cells: mechanistic insights, functions beyond quality control and the double-life of NMD factors. *Cell. Mol. Life Sci.*, Vol.67, pp. 677-700, ISSN 1420-9071

Patti, M.E. (2004). Gene expression in human with diabetes and prediabetes: what have we learned about diabetes pathophysiology. *Curr Opin Clin Nutr Metab Care,* Vol.7, No.4, pp. 383-390, ISSN 1363-1950

Peng, S.S.; Chen, C.Y. & Shyu, A.B. (1996). Functional characterization of a non-AUUUA AU-rich element from the c-jun proto-oncogene mRNA: evidence for a novel class of AU-rich elements. *Mol Cell Biol*, Vol.16, No.4, pp. 1490-1499, ISSN 0270-7306

Pesole G, Bernardi G & Saccone C. (1999). Isochore specificity of AUG initiator context of human genes. *FEBS, Lett*, Vol.464, No.1-2, pp. 60-62

Pfaffl, M.W. (2001). A new mathematical model for relative quantification in real-time RT-PCR. *Nucleic Acids Res*, Vol.29, No.9, pp. 2002-2007, ISSN 1362-4962

Piątkiewicz, P.; Czech, A. & Tatoń, J. (2007). Glucose transport in human peripheral blood lymphocytes influenced by type 2 diabetes. *Arch. Immunol. Ther. Exp.*, Vol.55, No.2. pp. 119-126, ISSN 0004-069X

Pickering, B.M. & Willis, A.E. (2005). The implications of structured 5′ untranslated regions on translation and disease. *Semin. Cell Dev. Biol.*, Vol.16, pp. 39-47, ISSN 1084-9521

Poy, M.N.; Spranger, M. & Stoffel, M. (2007). microRNAs and the regulation of glucose and lipids metabolism. *Diabetes, Obesity and Metabolism*, Vol.9, No.2, pp. 67-73, ISSN 1462-8902

Preis, S.R.; Massaro, J.M.; Robins, S.J.; Hoffmann, U.; Vasan, R.S.; Irlbeck, T.; Meigs, J.B.; Sutherland, P.; D'Agostino, R.B. Sr; O'Donnell, C.J. & Fox,, C.S. (2010). Abdominal subcutaneous and visceral adipose tissue and insulin resistance in the Framingham heart study. *Nature*, Vol.18, No.11, pp. 2192-2198, ISSN 1930-7381

Ragheb, R.; Shanab, G.M.L.; Medhat, A.M.; Seoudi, D.M.; Adeli, K. & Fantus, I.G. (2009). Free fatty acid-induced muscle insulin resistance and glucose uptake dysfunction: Evidence for PKC activation and oxidative stress-activated signaling pathways. *Biochem. Biophys. Res. Commun.*, Vol.3589, No.2, pp. 211-216, ISSN 1090-2104

Rasche, A.; Al-Hasami, H. & Herwig, R. (2008). Meta-analysis approach identifies candidate genes and associated molecular networks for type 2 diabetes mellitus. *BMC Genomics*, Vol.9, pp. 310-327, ISSN 1471-2164

Rasouli, N. & Kern, P.A. (2008). Adipocytokines and the metabolic complications of obesity. *J Clin Endocrinol Metab*, Vol.93, No.11, pp. 64-73, ISSN 0021-972X

Rehwinkel, J.; Lutenic, I.; Raes, J.; Bork, P. & Izaurralde, E. (2005). Nonsense-mediated mRNA decay factors act in concert to regulate common mRNA targets. *RNA*, Vol.11, No.10, pp. 1530-1544, ISSN 1355-8382

Ruano, M.; Silvestre, V.; Castro, R.; Garcia-Lescun, M.C.G.; Aguirregoicoa, E.; Marco, A.; Rodriguez, A. & Garcia-Blanch, G. (2006). HOMA, QUICKI and MFfm to measure insulin resistance in morbid obesity. *Obes Surg*, Vol.16, No.5, pp. 549-553, ISSN 0960-8923

Salonen, J.T.; Uimari, P.; Aalto, J.M. et al. (2007). Type 2 diabetes whole genome association study in four population. The DiaGen Consortium, *Am J Med Genet*, Vol.81, No.2, pp. 338-345, ISSN 0002-9297

Sethupathy, P. & Collins, F.S. (2008), MicroRNA target site polymorphisms and human disease. Trends. Genet., Vol.24, No.10, pp. 489-497, ISSN 0168-9525

Shepherd, P.R. & Khan, B.B. (1999). Glucose transporters and insulin action. Implications for insulin resistance and diabetes mellitus. *N. Engl. J. Med.*, Vol.341, No.4, pp. 248-257, ISSN 0028-4793

Shuang, Z.; Fang, L. (2009). Mechanisms of microRNA-mediated gene regulation. *Sci. China, C, Life Sci.*, Vol.52, No.12, pp. 1111-1116, ISSN 1862-2798

Stentz, F.B. & Kitabchi, A.E. (2007). Transcriptome and proteome expressions involved in insulin resistance in muscle and activated T-lymphocytes of patients with type 2 diabetes. *Geno. Prot. Bioinfo.*, Vol.5, No.3-4, pp. 216-235, ISSN 1672-0229

Stoneley, M.; Chappell, S.A.; Jopling, C.K.; Dickens, M.; MacFarlene, M. & Willis, A.E. (2000). c-Myc protein synthesis in initiated from the internal ribosome entry segment during apoptosis. *Mol. Cell. Biol.*, Vol.20, No.4. pp. 1162-1169, ISSN 0270-7306

Svitkin, Y.V.; Pause, A.; Haghighat, A.; Pyronnet, S.; Witherall, S.; Belsham, G.J. & Sonenberg, N. (2001). The requirement for eukaryotic initiation factor 4A (eIF4A) in translation is in direct proportion to the degree of mRNA 5′ secondary structure. *RNA*, Vol.7, No.3, pp. 382-394, ISSN 1355-8382

Tan, M.S.; Chang, S.Y.; Chang, D.M.; Tsai, J.C.R. & Lee, J.Y. (2003). Association of resistin gene 3′Untranslated Region +64G→A polymorphisms with type 2 diabetes and hypertension in a Chinese population. J Clin Endocrinol Metab., Vol.88, No.3, pp. 1258-1263, ISSN 0021-972X

Thermann, R. & Hentze, M.W. (2007). Drosophila miR-2 induces pseudo-polysomes and inhibits translation initiation. *Nature*, Vol.447, No.7146, pp. 875-878, ISSN 1476-4687

Venable, C.L.; Frevert, E.U.; Kim, Y.B.; Fischer, B.M.; Kamatkar, S.; Neel, B.G. & Kahn, B.B. (2000). Overexpression of protein-tyrosine phosphatase-1B in adipocytes inhibits insulin-stimulated phosphoinositide 3-kinase activity without altering glucose transport or Akt/protein kinase B activation. *J. Biol. Chem.*, Vol.275, No.24, pp. 18318-18326, ISSN 0021-9258

Villuendas, G.; Botella-Carretero, J.I.; López-Bermejo, A.; Gubern, C.; Ricart, W.; Fernández-Real, J.M.; San Millán, J.L. & Escobar-Morreale, H.F. (2006). The ACAA-insertion/deletion polymorphism at the 3' UTR of the IGF-II receptor gene is associated with type 2 diabetes and surrogate markers of insulin resistance. *Eur J Endocrinol.*, Vol. 155, No.2, pp. 331-336, ISSN 0804-4643

Wakiyama, M.; Takimoto, K.; Ohara, O. et al. (2007). Let-7 microRNA –mediated mRNA deadenylation and translation repression in a mammalian cell-free system. *Genes Dev.*, vol.21, pp. 1857-1862, ISSN 0890-9369

Wolford, J.K.; Hanson, R.L.; Kobes, S.; Bogardus, C. & Prochazka, M. (2001). Analysis of linkage disequilibrium between polymorphisms in the *KCNJ9* gene with type 2 diabetes mellitus in Pima Indians. *Mol Genet Metab*, Vol.73, No.1, pp. 97-103, ISSN 1096-7192

Worm, D.; Vinten, J.; Staehr, P.; Henriksen, J.E.l; Handberh, A. & Beck-Nielsen, H. (1995). Altered basal and insulin-stimulated phophotyrosine phosphatase (PTPase) activity in skeletal muscle form NIDDM patients compared with control subjects. *Diabetologia*, vol.39, No.10, pp. 1208-1214, ISSN 0012-186X

Wu, L.; Fan, J. & Belasco, J.G. (2005). MicroRNAs direct rapid deadenylation of mRNA. *Proc. Natl. Acad. Sci.*, Vol.103, No.11, pp. 4034-4039, ISSN 0027-8424

Xia, J.; Bogardus, C. & Prochazka, M. (1999). A type 2 diabetes associated polymorphic ARE motif affecting expression of *PPP1R3* is involved in RNA-protein interaction. *Mol. Genet. Metab.*, Vol.68, No.1, pp. 48-55, ISSN 1096-7192

Zabolotny, J.M.; Kim, Y.B.; Peroni, O.D.; Kim, J.K.; Pani, M.A.; Boss, O.; Klaman, L.D.; Kamatkar, S.; Shulman, G.I.; Kahn, B.B. & Neel, B.G. (2001). Overexpression of the LAR (Leukocyte Antigen Related) protein-tyrosine phosphatase in muscle causes insulin resistance. *PNAS*, Vol.98, No.9, pp. 5187-5192, ISSN 0027-8424

Zeggini, E.; Scott, L.J.; Saxena, R. & Voight, B.F. (2008). Meta-analysis of genome wide association data and large scale replication identifies additional susceptible loci for type 2 diabetes. Nature Genetics, Vol.40, No.5, pp. 634-645, ISSN 1546-1718

Zhang, H.; Jia, Y.; Cooper, J.J.; Hale, T.; Zhang, Z. & Elbein, S.C. (2004). Common variants in Glutamine Fructose-6-Phosphate Amidotransferase 2 (GFPT2) gene are associated with type 2 diabetes, diabetic nephropathy and increased GFPT2 mRNA levels. *J Clin Endocrinol Metab.*, Vol.89, No.2, pp. 748-755, ISSN 0021-972X

Zhao, S. & Liu, M.F. (2009). Mechanisms of microRNA mediated gene regulation. *Sci China Ser C-Life Sci*, Vol.52, No.12, pp. 1111-1116, ISSN 1862-2798

10

Genetics of Endothelial Damage Associated to Diabetes Mellitus Type 2

Lorena García[1], Carlos Wolff[2], Verónica Araya[3], Gloria López[3], Sergio Lobos[1], Pilar Durruty[2] and Daniela Seelenfreund[1]
[1]Department of Biochemistry, Faculty of Chemical and Pharmaceutical Sciences, University of Chile
[2]Diabetes Unit, Department of Medicine, Faculty of Medicine, University of Chile,
[3]Endocrinology Section, Clinical Hospital of the University of Chile
Chile

1. Introduction

Diabetes mellitus (DM) is a serious worldwide public health problem due to its frequency, chronic complications and their high associated costs. This disease is considered a multifactorial pathology that involves insulin resistance and is associated to obesity, dyslipidemia, endothelial dysfunction, inflammation and hypertension (Petersen & Shulman, 2006). Type 2 diabetes (DM2) is one of the most common diseases in the developed world and is recognized now as a global burden (van Dieren et al., 2010). Released in 2000, the initial edition of the Diabetes Atlas estimated the global prevalence of this disease at 4.6%, representing 151 million people, and projected an increase to 333 million people by 2025. On the basis of the most recent evidence, the current Diabetes Atlas has predicted that the number of people with diabetes will have risen to a staggering 438 million or 7.8% of the world`s population in 2030 (Colagiuri, 2010; www.diabetesatlas.org).
The development of DM2 requires the involvement of genetic and environmental factors such as android obesity and sedentary lifestyle that determine hyposecretion of insulin in response to glucose stimulation and a decreased insulin action in peripheral tissues. Most of the complications associated to DM2 are related to pathophysiological alterations of the vascular endothelium, and are the main cause of morbidity and mortality among DM patients. Endothelial dysfunction is the initial event that predisposes the vascular wall to diverse alterations leading to the establishment of so-called cardiovascular complications of diabetes. Known risk factors of diabetic complications such as hyperglycemia, hypertension and dyslipidemia stimulate the production of reactive oxygen species (ROS) in the vascular wall. Hyperglycemia is now considered a key causal factor in the development of chronic complications of diabetes (Giuliano et al., 2008).
The vascular endothelium consists of endothelial cells and is a type of monostratified squamous epithelium that lines the inner surface of all blood vessels including the heart. Its crucial role is to regulate the vascular tone and it also has a structural function. In addition, the vascular endothelium normally inhibits platelet and leukocyte adhesion to the vascular surface and maintains a balance between profibrinolytic and prothrombotic activities

(Sandoo et al., 2010). Under physiological conditions a balance between endothelium-derived relaxing and contracting factors exists, which is altered in diabetes and atherosclerosis, contributing to the progression of vascular damage (Tabit et al., 2010). Endothelial cells, such as capillaries in the glomerulus and renal mesangial cells are more vulnerable to sustained hyperglycemia since they lack the ability to rapidly reduce glucose transport into the cell (Kaiser et al., 1993).

Several routes have been described that are related to vascular damage induced by unregulated blood glucose, such as i) the increased activity of the polyol pathway, causing accumulation of sorbitol and fructose in endothelial cells, ii) the formation of advanced glycation end products (AGE), activation of protein kinase C (PKC) and of the transcription factor NFκB, iii) an increased hexosamine pathway flux, iv) increased oxidative stress, mainly due to an overproduction of superoxide anions by the mitochondrial electron transport chain and v) the increase of inflammatory processes through induction of cytokine secretion by monocytes and adipocytes (Giugliano et al., 2008; Aronson, 2008).

In several cases, vascular damage due to oxidative stress induced by hyperglycemia and / or inadequate metabolic control is not sufficient to explain the severity of micro- and macroangiopathic complications and mortality observed in DM2 patients. Here we review the pathophysiology of diabetic macro- and microangiopathic complications and the impact of genetic variants of several candidate genes that may explain the higher morbility and mortality of these patients.

2. Diabetic complications

Chronic complications of DM type 1 (DM1) and DM2 are basically the same. Many studies indicate that there are genetic factors associated to the development of chronic complications of DM and that these factors differ from those involved in the development of diabetes. In this work we will analyze the importance of genetic variants of genes associated to an increased risk of vascular damage in DM.

In both DM1 and DM2 the most common macrovascular complications are cardiovascular disease (CVD), cerebral vascular and peripheral vascular disease. In diabetic microangiopathy, hyperglycemia induces biochemical and molecular changes in microvascular cells that ultimately progress to retinal, renal and neural complications and extends to other complications, including advanced periodontal disease (Roy et al., 2010). It is known that already from initial stages (glucose intolerance) the patient is under an important risk of chronic complications, mainly macrovascular coronary damage and also microvascular complications, where retinopathies, neuropathies and diabetic nephropathy (DN) are the most frequent and devastating.

2.1 The genetic factor in the chronic complications of DM

Factors involved in the etiology of DM2 are different from those that lead to chronic complications. Not all diabetic patients will develop complications or with the same severity. Prospective studies suggest that hyperglycemia and hypertension are important, but not sufficient for the development of chronic complications, requiring genetic susceptibility. As has been suggested, genetic variants exist that could explain these differences. We will analyze the importance of genetic variants of genes associated to an increased risk of vascular damage in DM, with a special emphasis on the endothelial isoform of nitric oxide synthase (NOS) superoxide dismutase (SOD), catalase and aldose reductase, among others.

Single nucleotide polymorphisms (SNPs) are small genetic changes or variations of a single base found in the sequence of DNA and are defined as polymorphisms when they are present at 1% or more within a population. Most of these are not in coding sequences, since only 3 to 5% of the human DNA sequence encodes proteins. Within a gene, SNPs can be located in promoter regions, exons, introns or untranslated (5'UTR and 3'UTR) regions (Figure 1). The frequency of each SNP is highly variable between different populations within a single species. There are an estimated 5 to 10 million SNPs in the human genome and each SNP is named with a specific code (NCBI, http://www.ncbi.nlm.nih.gov/snp). The discovery of relevant polymorphisms is complicated by the sheer number of SNPs encountered in genes and in non-coding sequences. During the first years, association studies usually started tackling non-synonymous SNPs, i.e. SNPs that change one amino acid to a different one. Later, polymorphisms that modulate mRNA processing started gaining importance, since at least 15% of point mutations are related to human genetic disease caused by RNA splicing defects (Wang et al., 2005). The disproportionate effort invested in studying SNPs which turned out to be neutral or irrelevant to the disease, lead to the development of specialized algorithms designed to select significant SNPs (bioinformatic analysis). Although there are millions of SNPs deposited in public SNP databases, only a small proportion of these are functional polymorphisms that contribute to disease phenotypes. Thus, prioritizing SNPs based on their phenotypic risks is essential for association studies. Yuan et al. (2006) designed a decision tree for prioritizing a SNP based on its functional effects, according to 13 phenotypic risks and putative functional effects, such as changes at the transcriptional level, pre-mRNA splicing and protein structure.

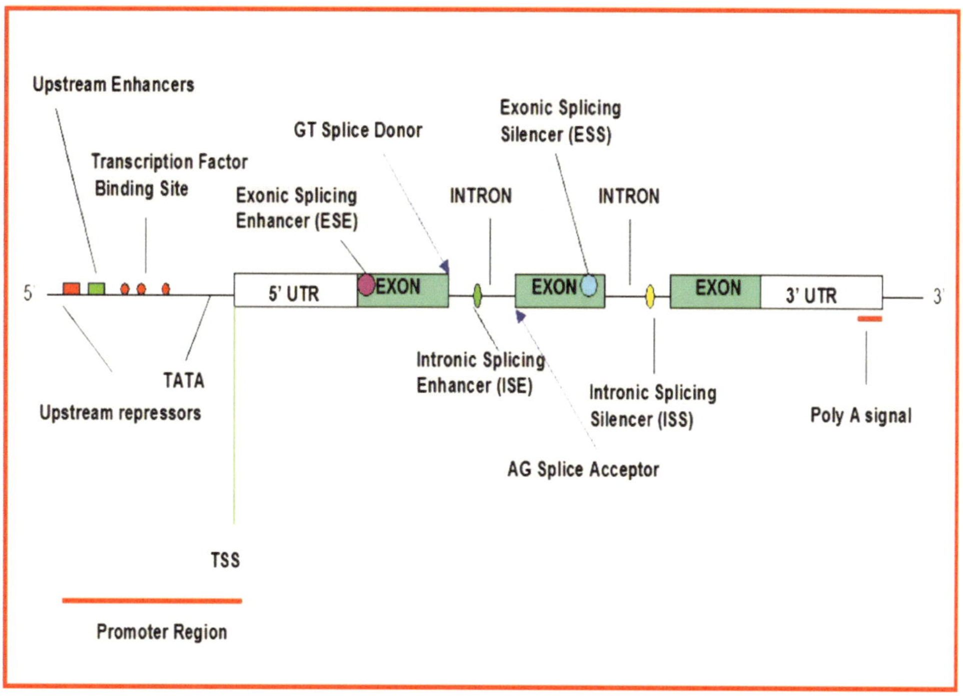

Fig. 1. General structure of a prototype mammalian gene (taken from A. Chattopadhyay, Ph.D., Genetic Variation Resources, Health Science Library System, U. of Pittsburgh, USA).

Missense mutations or non-synonymous polymorphisms may alter protein structure, however apparently silent polymorphisms and point mutations in introns or untranslated regions that do not seem to affect protein structure, can also alter gene function (Kimchi-Sarfaty et al., 2007). For instance, mutations affecting mRNA processing can be located in introns (but also in exons), resulting in exon skipping or creating new splice sites (Baralle & Baralle, 2005). Therefore it is clearly of interest to examine polymorphisms that might appear neutral for translation, but which may alter sequences inactivating regulatory elements that participate in mRNA processing.

2.2 Macroangiopathic complications

DM is preceded by glucose intolerance (pre-diabetes), in which there are already pronounced macrovascular complications. The increase in cardiovascular risk includes coronary heart disease (CHD), stroke and peripheral artery disease. The severity of these complications is significantly greater than the risk observed in the non-diabetic population and corresponds to the first cause of mortality in diabetic patients. In the past 40 years coronary mortality in the general population has decreased, but to a lesser extent in diabetic patients.

The frequency of CHD in diabetics is directly related to the prevalence of the disease in the general population, high in certain ethnic groups and low in others (Japan and China), which relates to its genetic basis. Environmental influences are also important, since the frequency of the disease increases when low-risk individuals are transferred to areas of high prevalence.

Coronary artery disease is the leading cause of death in both DM1 and DM2, hyperglycemia being directly a risk factor for mortality. There is evidence of a direct positive correlation between plasma glucose levels expressed as glycated hemoglobin (HbA1c) and the prevalence and incidence of CVD (Stettler et al., 2006). In DM2 patients the risk is increased even before the appearance of diabetes, in the pre-diabetic state and during the prior period of insulin resistance. These stages are characterized by the presence of a number of other cardiovascular risk factors, such as hypertension, central obesity, atherogenic dyslipidemia, pro-inflammatory and pro-thrombotic states, along with an increase of oxidative stress. All these elements are part of the Metabolic Syndrome (Hunt et al., 2004) and may contribute to the frequent presence of macroangiopathy in DM2 at diagnosis (Stratter et al., 2000). Most studies report a frequency of CHD between 2 and 4 times higher than the general population. The famous Framingham study found that diabetes doubled the risk of CHD in men and tripled in women. Even after correction for age, the risk remained significantly higher after adjusting for all other classical factors such as hypertension, smoking, dyslipidemia and left ventricular hypertrophy (Kannel & McGee, 1979). All the above have led to the inclusion of DM as an independent risk factor. Diabetes and myocardial infarction are similarly strong predictors of total mortality in men. Higher mortality from noncardiovascular causes is observed in those with diabetes only, whereas prior myocardial infarction is more strongly predictive of coronary mortality than diabetes at any age and level of cardiovascular risk factors. The difference in coronary mortality is most evident in the first 10 years of follow-up (Vaccaro et al., 2004). DM in women eliminates the relative protection compared with men before the onset of CHD. Also, high risk determinants occur 15 years earlier in the life of DM individuals compared to control subjects without DM. All the above data and results of prospective studies, such as the San Antonio Heart Study that compared non-DM individuals who had suffered a myocardial infarction and DM patients without previous myocardial infarction, showed that mortality from CHD and non-fatal heart attacks in DM patients without CHD was similar to that of non-DM individuals with a previous myocardial infarction (Haffner et al., 1998). This led to consider DM as a CHD equivalent. Further data have weakened this statement and have considered that the diagnosis of DM is not equivalent to coronary disease, unless when added to other cardiovascular risk factors (Pignone et al., 2010; ADA, 2011). In DM1, the situation is even more serious, as mortality from CHD at age 55 is between 4 to 8 times higher than for the non-diabetic population (Nathan et al., 2009). In time overall CVD mortality has declined between 24-28% since 1975 in the USA, and has stabilized since 1990, but remains the leading cause of death. There is still an unfavourable difference in black males compared to white males and women, and also in diabetics *versus* non-DM individuals (López et al., 2006). This can be attributed in part to genetic factors.

The influence of cardiovascular risk factors can also be assessed by measuring the effect of treatment of the each particular risk factor and its impact on cardiovascular morbidity and mortality. In this regard, the increased and continued control of glycemia has shown to reduce these parameters in the long term, with strong evidence in DM1 (Nathan et al., 2009) and less evidently in DM2 (Patel et al., 2008; Turnbull et al., 2009).

To summarize, diabetes is an independent risk factor for (CVD), which in some cases is similar to the risk of a previous myocardial infarct. Also, diabetic women suffer loss of their natural gender pre- menopausal protection. Treatment of diabetes and its associated risks improves morbidity and mortality, but is unable to reach normal population levels. Incidence of myocardial infarction and mortality for this cause is decreasing for the general population, but to a lesser extent for diabetic patients.

New biochemical markers of endothelial damage are being investigated as early signals indicating appearance of this macroangiopathic damage, such as cystatin C, high sensitive C-reactive protein (hsCRP), adiponectin and IL-6. Cystatin C is a non-glycosylated protein produced by nucleated cells and functions as an endogenous inhibitor of cysteine proteases and lysosomal proteinases. Patients with increased cystatin C are at a higher risk of developing both CVD and chronic kidney disease and increased concentrations of cystatin C appear to be indicative of preclinical kidney disease associated with adverse outcomes (Taglieri et al., 2009). There is consensus that serum cystatin C is a good marker of impaired renal function. It has been shown that serum levels of cystatin C are a better indicator of incipient DN in patients with DM2 than serum creatinine and creatinine clearance. Cystatin C would provide more information than other parameters of renal function in risk stratification of morbidity and mortality in patients with acute coronary syndrome (García, 2009).

The association of cystatin C with long-term mortality appears stronger than would be expected for the glomerular filtration rate, so a hypothesis has emerged that it could be linked to mortality, independently of renal function (Stevens & Levey, 2005). It has also been postulated to have a predictor character of cardiovascular damage in diabetic patients (Shlipak et al., 2006). We have shown that cystatin C levels are significantly higher in DM2 patients with cardiovascular damage; coronary condition was assessed using extensive MIBI-dipyridamole procedures (Table 1). Diabetics with coronary artery disease have higher levels of cystatin C, which are closely correlated with serum creatinine levels (Wolff et al., 2009). Studies in progress have found that cystatin C levels are significantly different in groups of low and medium risk according to the cardiovascular Framingham scale adapted to the Chilean population (Villalón, 2011).

Cystatin C (mg/ml)			
Patients	**Media**	**Range**	
Controls	0.68	0.55 - 0.75	$p < 0.0001$
DM2-non coronary	0.81	0.71 - 1.08	
DM2-coronary	1.50	0.89 - 2.19	$p < 0.0001$

Table 1. Serum cystatin C values per group (Wolff et al., 2009).

hsCRP is an acute phase protein synthesized by the liver and also by macrophages, and is usually not found in plasma. It is deposited at inflammatory processes, such as at the intima of arteries, at sites of atherogenesis. For several years hsCRP has been used as a marker of inflammation, since it is useful for detecting acute inflammatory processes. More sensitive methods can detect low levels of hsCRP which are needed for the prediction of cardiovascular risk. Blood hsCRP levels may be decreased due to anti-inflammatory treatment or the use of statins and increase in patients with chronic inflammation (Shlipak et al., 2006).

Adiponectin corresponds to 0.01% of total plasma proteins. Its concentration varies between 5 and 10 mg/ml, and women have higher levels than men (Waki et al., 2003). Adiponectin is a protein hormone of 247 amino acids (30 kDa), synthesized in adipocytes (Scherer et al., 1995). Circulating levels of adiponectin are inversely proportional to body mass index (BMI) and the percentage of body fat; its levels are reduced in obesity, DM2 and coronary disease (Weyer et al., 2001). Adiponectin is a hormone with antiatherogenic, anti-inflammatory and anti-diabetic functions. Low adiponectin levels constitute a marker of insulin resistance and increased risk of DM2 (Lorensatti et al., 1999). Adiponectin has been proposed as a marker in the prevention and evolution of vascular disease (Weyer et al., 2001), however adiponectin values show a high degree of dispersion, making the measurement of adiponectin unreliable for individual evaluation of the cardiovascular risk in DM2 patients (Wolff et al., 2009).

Variants in the adiponectin gene have been suggested to contribute to the risk of DM2 and circulating levels of adiponectin In fact, genome-wide scans have mapped a susceptibility locus of the metabolic syndrome and DM2 to chromosome 3q27, where the adiponectin gene is located. Subsequently, several SNPs and haplotypes of the adiponectin gene have been associated with insulin resistance, DM2 and hypoadiponectinemia. No association of the SNP 45 or SNP 276 of the adiponectin gene with adiponectin level or other metabolic variables was found (Salmenniemi et al., 2005), although other authors suggest a significant role of adiponectin gene variants at the same positions in the development of insulin resistance in healthy Greek women (Melistas et al., 2009). Adiponectin levels are high in cases of DN (Jaziri et al., 2010). In two recent studies (DIABHYCAR and SURDIAGENE), the −11391A and +45G alleles were associated with a higher incidence of renal events (Jaziri et al., 2010). Medium- (MMW) and low-molecular weight (LMW) isoforms of adiponectin were more abundant in cases with renal events, indicating that in subjects with DM2 and early renal dysfunction, adiponectin gene variants are determinants of renal risk. The −11391A and +45G alleles may affect renal risk by leading to high circulating adiponectin concentrations, at least those of MMW and LMW isoforms (Jaziri et al., 2010). Also, a promoter polymorphism (-11377C/G) of the adiponectin gene is associated with DN in female DM1 patients (Zhang et al., 2010).

Adiponectin (μg/ml)			
Patients	Media	Range	
Controls	9.5	5.5 - 14.1	NS
DM2-non coronary	8.4	1.4 - 15.1	
DM2-coronary	6.7	2.6 - 15.4	NS

Table 2. Serum adiponectin values per group. (Wolff et al., 2009). NS: Not significant.

IL-6 is relevant to many disease processes such as diabetes (Kristiansen & Mandrup-Poulsen et al., 2005). IL-6 is an interleukin that acts both as a pro-inflammatory and anti-inflammatory cytokine. It is secreted by T cells and macrophages to stimulate the immune response to tissue damage leading to inflammation. Smooth muscle cells in the tunica media of many blood vessels also produce IL-6 as a pro-inflammatory cytokine. IL-6's role as an anti-inflammatory cytokine is mediated through its inhibitory effects on TNF-alpha and IL-1, and activation of IL-1 and IL-10. Elevated plasma IL-6 concentrations are observed in obese, as opposed to non-obese, DM2 patients. Elevated plasma IL-6 concentrations are attributed to the prevalence of obesity and not necessarily associated with DM2 (Hansen et al., 2010).

2.3 Microangiophatic complications

2.3.1 Diabetic Retinopathy (DR)

DR is the leading cause of blindness worldwide. The Wisconsin Epidemiological Study of Diabetic Retinopathy (WESDR))(Klein et al., 1989) showed that DR prevalence is over 70% in DM1 patients (with diagnosis of DM under 30 years of age) and 39% in patients diagnosed when over 30 years of age (mainly DM2). The frequency of DR is of 82% in patients with 20 or more years of DM. A variable percentage of DR is already present at DM2 diagnosis (Stratton et al., 2000). It is the most glycemic-control-related diabetic complication, and therefore the diagnosis of DR and glucose levels are the criteria used for diagnosis of diabetes. Both in DM1 and DM2 it has been proved that intensified glycemic control can prevent the development and progression of DR (LeClaire et al., 2006). The general use of more intensive treatment in recent decades has been associated with better prognosis in developed countries like Sweden, Finland and the USA, with a range of 32 - 59% prevalence of DR at 10 years of DM1 debut and a decrease of the extreme forms of DR (Vallance et al., 2008). A similar behavior has occurred in DM2 (Humphrey et al., 1994). Readers are referred to recent reviews on this topic (Jackson & Barber, 2010; Ockrim & Yorston, 2010).

2.3.2 Diabetic neuropathy

Diabetic microvascular pathology comprises a variety of debilitating neuropathies; all of them seem related to the hyperglycemic state (Nassar et al., 2007) for extended periods. This complication is present in 8% of patients at the time of diagnosis and increases to 50% after 20 years of DM; the total prevalence of diabetic neuropathy is between 28 and 34% (Jadzinsky, 2003). This neuropathy can be very painful and is invalidating, as it causes diabetic foot. It develops as a consequence of vascular and metabolic factors which lead to endoneural hypoxia and decreased blood circulation. An association of diabetic neuropathy with glucose control in both DM1 and DM2 has been proved, as well as the beneficial effect of intensified treatment, as shown in the Diabetes Control Complications Trial (DCCT) and United Kingdom Prospective Diabetes Study (UKPDS) (Nathan et al., 2009; Stratton et al., 2000). The trend of recent years has been favorable, despite the fact that the risk of amputation of lower extremities remains significantly higher than in the general population (11% at 25 years after diagnosis) (Bojstig et al., 1994). The neuropathies developing in patients with diabetes are known to be heterogeneous by their symptoms, pattern of neurologic involvement, course, risk covariates, pathologic alterations and underlying mechanisms. An update on classification, definitions, diagnostic criteria, and treatments of diabetic neuropathies has been published recently (Tesfaye et al., 2010).

2.3.3 Diabetic Nephropathy (DN)

This complication is also a frequent microangiopathic complication of DM, occurring in 20-40% of patients after 10 years of natural evolution. Despite current treatments, 20% of DM2 patients develop renal failure. DN is the leading cause of End Stage Renal Disease (ESRD), chronic hemodialysis and renal transplantation worldwide. Before the intensified treatment approach, 25 to 45% of DM1 patients had diabetic kidney disease (DKD) and the majority of them progressed to ESRD. This situation has improved significantly in recent decades, as the cumulative incidence of DKD at 20 years of diagnosis has dropped to 8.9% and 2% of ESRD, according to the monitoring studies of the Diabetes Control and Complications Trial/Epidemiology of Diabetes Interventions and Complications (DCCT/EDIC) studies. In DM2 patients a significant decrease in the incident of DKD in the Caucasian population in the USA has been recently observed, with a decrease from 32 to 15 x1000 patient /year in the cohorts of 1991-1994 and 1999-2002, respectively (Nathan et al., 2009). This improvement may be explained by the intensified glucose control (DCCT, UKPDS) (Adler et al., 2003) and by early screening, more aggressive management of other risk factors such as hypertension, the use of inhibitors of the angiotensin converting enzyme (IACE) and of hypolipidemic drugs. However, disparities still exist despite these improvements, as African-Americans, Mexican-Americans and Pima Indians present 3-6 times higher frequencies of DKD and ESRD than Caucasian populations. Specifically, Pima Indians have a very high prevalence of DKD (50%) and ESRD (15%) at 20 years of follow-up (Pavkov et al., 2006). Some of the differences may be attributed to social and economic factors, but genetic and ethnic factors cannot be out ruled (Cowie et al., 1989; Adler, 2004; Brancati et al., 1992).

2.3.4 Periodontal Disease (PD)

PD is a chronic infection of the gums which is characterized by a loss of attachment between the tooth and the jawbone. PD affects the general population; however it is more frequent in obese, pre-diabetic and diabetic individuals. Its treatment might permit better metabolic control and should be implemented in the routine care of diabetic patients. Chronic periodontitis is a highly prevalent inflammatory disease, associated with bacterial infection and characterized by attachment loss, alveolar bone loss, periodontal pockets and gingival inflammation, all of which can lead to tooth loss, without the proper treatment.

Reports from populations in the USA indicate that subjects with DM present increased prevalence, extent, severity and progression of PD with increased risk of alveolar bone loss and are positively associated with attachment loss (Grossi et al., 1994). Conversely, periodontitis predicts the development of both overt nephropathy and ESRD in an American-Indian population with DM2 (Shultis et al., 2007). PD in Central and South

America exhibits a prevalence of nearly 35% (Gjermo et al., 2002). In Chile, a recent study showed that the adult population showed a high prevalence and extension of clinical attachment loss (>6 mm) in adult populations (69% in seniors and 38% in younger subjects). Age, sex (male), education level and smoking were the main risk indicators of severe clinical attachment loss in this population (Gamonal et al., 2010). In a sample of 66 DM2 subjects (55.6±9.3 years of age from Santiago, Chile), we found a frequency of periodontitis of 92%, compared with 75% in a sample of 91 non-diabetic subjects (43.0±14.3 years of age) (V. Araya, et al., manuscript submitted).

Periodontitis is a complex disease and both genetic and environmental factors are involved. Environmental factors play an important role in the expression of periodontitis. These factors include oral hygiene / bacterial plaque, smoking and stress that may exacerbate the inflammatory pathology associated with periodontitis. Since diabetes is a proinflammatory state, increased levels of circulating cytokines suggest a causal role for inflammation in its etiology (López et al., 2009). The activation of the broad axis of innate immunity through up-regulation of proinflammatory cytokines from monocytes and polymorphonuclear leucocytes includes IL-1β, IL-6, IL-8, tumour necrosis factor alpha (TNF-α) and prostaglandin E_2. In diabetic subjects, inappropriate secretion of these cytokines, in terms of either type or quantity, characterizes a dysregulated immune response that leads to the destruction of periodontal tissues in the presence of some Gram-negative bacteria that form biofilm complexes adhering to the tooth surface (Araya et al., 2003; Nassar et al., 2007; Nishimura et al., 2007). The formation of AGEs that bind to AGE receptors on critical target cell surfaces lead to over-secretion of these inflammatory mediators (Mealey, 2006).

As for other inflammatory diseases, nitric oxide (NO) could play a role in the pathophysiology of periodontitis and the presence of inducible NOS (iNOS) in healthy and inflamed human gingival tissue has been demonstrated. On the other hand, the expression of iNOS in gingival tissues and its increase following some dental proceedings have been demonstrated. Moreover, it has been stated that lipopolysaccharide induced macrophages express iNOS (Pan et al., 2010). eNOS mediated NO production is also involved in critical processes relevant to periodontal disease pathogenesis, including inhibition of cyclooxygenase, regulation of osteoblast activity, prevention of the leukocyte adhesion and superoxide anion release from leukocytes, and suppressing T-cell proliferation (Uğar-Cankal & Ozmeric, 2006).

Several studies indicate that different SNPs of specific genes could be associated with diverse forms of periodontitis in different populations. These include the genes that affect the expression of IL-1, IL-6, TNF-α, IL-10, and eNOS; some of these have been evaluated in diabetic subjects. In Chilean type 1 diabetic subjects with and without aggressive periodontitis the TNF-α SNP at position -308 was assessed, but no association between this SNP and periodontitis was found (Pérez et al., 2004). In a different Chilean population, no significant differences in IL-1A -899, -1B +3954, or -1RN genotype frequencies were found between patients with diabetes and patients without diabetes (López et al., 2009). Interestingly, however, periodontitis was significantly associated with some specific IL-1 gene polymorphisms, such as the IL-1A -889 TT, IL-1B +3954 TT and IL-1B -511 CC genotypes (López et al., 2009).

Periodontitis is also a known risk factor for CVD. One study in Pima Indians with DM2, periodontitis was a strong predictor of mortality, isquemic heart disease and DN. The effect of PD is another factor in addition to traditional risk factors for these diseases (Saremi et al.,

2005). There is also emerging evidence of an independent association between periodontitis and the development of DKD (Shultis et al., 2007).

The inflammatory nature of periodontitis can affect metabolic control of diabetes. Several studies in diabetic subjects with periodontitis have shown an improvement of HbA1c (0.9 – 1% decrease) after conventional periodontal treatment with or without the addition of antibiotics; however, many of these changes were not statistically significant (Darre et al., 2008; Taylor & Borgnakke, 2008). In our study, 12 DM2 subjects with severe periodontitis were selected for periodontal treatment. These patients continued without modifications in their antidiabetic therapy. A non-significant decrease in the mean HbAlc (from 8.8±0.7% to 8.0±0.6%) after 6 months of periodontal treatment was found (Araya et al., manuscript submitted). These results are comparable to those described by other authors. Nevertheless, periodontal treatment could have a similar effect of decreasing HbA1c as other glucose lowering therapies. Therefore, although periodontal treatment appears to be less important in improving metabolic control of DM, a significant improvement of periodontitis in these clinical aspects determines a better quality of life in these patients.

To summarize, microangiopathic complications of diabetes lead to various associated complex and invalidating diseases, which severely compromise the specific tissues. Traditionally, diabetic nephropathy, neuropathy and retinopathy were considered the main complications, but recently, PD is being considered an additional diabetic complication, which determines a decreased quality of life of diabetic patients.

2.4 The contribution of specific genes to diabetic complications

2.4.1 Nephrin

The gene for nephrin was initially identified as the gene responsible for congenital nephrotic syndrome of Finnish type, in which individuals suffer massive proteinuria *in utero* and nephrosis at birth severe (Beltcheva et al., 2001). The protein (nephrin) has 1241 amino acids and is a cell adhesion protein of the immunoglobulin family that is expressed in the kidney, but also in the pancreas and the central nervous system (Beltcheva et al., 2003). Nephrin is the central structural and signaling molecule in the slit diaphragm of the kidney (Hauser et al., 2009). Conditions of endothelial injury, such as preeclampsia, hypertension, diabetes and high fat diet were found to induce a loss of nephrin (Hauser et al., 2009). Its extracellular domain plays a fundamental structural role in podocytes, interacting with various proteins such as podocin (Kestilä et al., 1998). These findings indicate that podocyte physiology is strongly linked to vascular endothelial cells via molecular signaling. As podocytes are non-proliferating terminally differentiated cells, apoptosis of podocytes leads to a reduction in nephrin (Hauser et al., 2009). Nephrin in the pancreas is found at the plasma membrane and on insulin vesicles and its expression is decreased in islets from diabetic patients when compared with nondiabetic control subjects (Fornoni et al., 2010). These results suggest that nephrin is an active component of the insulin vesicle machinery that may affect vesicle-actin interaction and mobilization to the plasma membrane (Fornoni et al., 2010).

Nephrin is a good indicator of both of genetic and acquired renal disease and animal studies have shown that nephrin loss causes proteinuria (Pätäri-Sampo et al., 2006). In fact, a decrease in nephrin mRNA correlates with the presence of proteinuria in renal biopsies of patients with DM2 (Toyoda et al., 2004). More important still, in DM1 patients with DN, nephrin appears in the urine, proving an association between the presence of this protein in the urine (nefrinuria) and kidney damage. Normal controls have no nefrinuria (Pätäri et al., 2003).

Over 300 polymorphisms in the nephrin gene *(NPHS1)* gene have been described. The Finn-Diane Study 3 examined non-synonymous SNPs (E117K, R408Q and N1077) in the *NPHS1* gene in Finnish patients with DM1 without finding association between these variants and DN (Pettersson-Fernholm et al., 2003). Another study found several polymorphisms in a Japanese population, specifically in exon 3 (C294T), exon 17 (C2289T) and intron 5 (-61C/G) of the nephrin gene to be associated with DM2 (Daimon et al., 2006).

We analyzed Chilean patients with diabetes type 1 and type 2, to determine if the frequency of an intronic SNP (rs466452, located in intron 24) of the nephrin gene differs in diabetic patients and control individuals, since bioinformatic analysis suggested that this genetic variant could produce alterations in the processing of the nephrin transcript. No association was found with the degree of renal damage (normo, micro and macroalbuminuric diabetic patients), either in DM1 or DM2 patients, as the distribution of genotypes was not significantly different between these groups. The molecular analysis of nephrin transcripts obtained from a renal biopsy of a patient with DM2 however indicated that no change in splicing of this gene had occurred (González et al., 2009). Results of this study strongly advocate the importance of validating results obtained from bioinformatic analysis.

In another study we identified purine-rich GAGA boxes in the nephrin gene promoter, which Kennedy and Rutter (1992) described as important transcriptional regulation elements of insulin expression. We conducted a genomic study of 100 individuals in Chile, in search of the presence of polymorphisms in this element and its possible association with DN in DM2 patients. Sequence analysis of 20 healthy individuals, 20 patients with non-diabetic nephropathies, 20 non-diabetic subjects with coronary disease, 20 normoalbuminuric DM2 patients without coronary disease and 19 macroalbuminuric DM2 patients with coronary disease, indicated that the GAGA elements did not present polymorphisms, suggesting a lower level of heterogeneity than surrounding regions (González et al., 2007).

To summarize, in association to chronic diabetic complications, polymorphisms studied in the nephrin gene include genetic variants present in the promoter (GAGA boxes), coding (E117K, C294T, R408Q and N1077) and non-coding regions (intron 24), do not differ in the frequency found in control subjects and diabetic patients with nephropathy.

2.4.2 eNOS

NO is a major mediator in vascular biology, regulating regional blood flow and blood pressure. Changes in NO production and of the enzymes that synthesize NO may contribute contribute to the aetiology of vascular pathologies (Bruckdorfer, 2005). NO is an important cellular signaling molecule and in DM, over-production of NO might play a role in the development of DN, while reduced NO production may be related to the development of DR and diabetic neuropathy, where VEGF (vascular endothelial growth factor) levels are increased in a counter-regulatory manner. NO is an endogenous vasodilator involved in inflammatory and autoimmune response, and in the pathophysiology of diabetic vascular disease. There are three isoenzymes of NOS that catalyze the production of NO from L-arginine: endothelial NOS (eNOS encoded by the gene *NOS3*), neuronal NOS (nNOS, gene *NOS1*) and the inducible isoform (iNOS encoded by *NOS2*). In this section, greater attention will be focused on eNOS, considering its relevance to angiopathies. Studies have provided evidence for altered NO metabolism and impaired endothelial function in diabetes, probably due to polymorphisms in the eNOS gene (Channon & Guzik, 2002).

The enzyme eNOS is essential for the vasodilation control in physiological conditions, producing NO which reacts with free radicals. Any anomalies in the function of this enzyme will alter physiological levels of vascular NO. It is known that vascular damage has a genetic component, and the search of polymorphisms of the gene that codifies for eNOS and its metabolites (nitrite, nitrate and oxidized proteins) would allow identifying individuals with a greater risk of presenting vascular damage.

Several eNOS polymorphisms have been studied in different populations, analyzing their association to vascular damage, such as Glu298Asp and T-786C in the regulatory region of the *NOS3* gene. We analyzed two eNOS polymorphisms in groups of DM2 patients and nondiabetic controls, one SNP corresponding to rs6947833 which changes Cysteine 991 to Serine and the SNP rs891512 in intron 23 which changes G at position 24943 to A. Our results suggest that these SNPs are not associated with DM2 (Seelenfreund et al., unpublished results).

eNOS genotype	type 2 diabetic patients	control subjects
Number	93.0	76.0
GG (%)	74.2	75.0
GA (%)	22.5	18.4
AA (%)	3.3	6.6
Allele frequency		
G (%)	85.5	84.2
A (%)	14.5	15.8

Table 3. Genotype frequencies (%) and allele distribution at the rs891512 polymorphism according to study groups. Differences in genotype and allelic frequencies were not significant for any group.

2.4.3 Antioxidant enzymes: Superoxide dismutase (SOD) and catalase

Chronic extracelular hyperglycemia in diabetes stimulates ROS production and increased oxidative stress plays an important role in the development of diabetic complications (Brownlee, 2005). Hyperglycemia-induced ROS activate many pathways of diabetic tissue damage, including production of superoxide anions by the mitochondrial electron transport chain. As a result of the high glucose levels inside diabetic cells, more donors (NADPH and $FADH_2$) are produced and increases in electron transfer occur, thereby generating superoxide. The excess of ROS production in the diabetic cell (superoxide, hydrogen peroxide and reactive nitrogen species such as NO) oxidize proteins, nucleic acids and membrane lipids and thereby damage cellular structure and function (Shi et al., 2009).

SOD, catalase and glutathione-S-transferases are enzymes that protect against the damage caused by oxidative stress by scavenging free radicals. SOD and catalase directly eliminate ROS. SOD, which catalyzes the dismutation of the superoxide anion into hydrogen peroxide and molecular oxygen, is one of the most important antioxidant enzymes. SOD enzymes are classified into three groups: cytosolic CuZn-SOD, mitochondrial Mn-SOD, and extracellular Ec-SOD (Zelko et al., 2002). Catalase is present as a dumbbell-shaped tetramer of four identical subunits in peroxisomes and removes hydrogen peroxide molecules that are by-products of the SOD reaction (Goyal & Basak, 2010).

Most enzymes involved in defense mechanisms against oxidative stress are polymorphic (Wang et al., 2007). Studies evaluating the association of polymorphic markers in genes encoding antioxidant enzymes regulate the production of ROS. A case-control study indicated that homozygosity for the SOD2 rs4880 Val allele is associated with an increased risk of DN, thus supporting the hypothesis that oxidative stress contributes to this severe long-term complication in diabetic patients (Môllsten et al., 2007). Other studies showed that oxidative stress in DM1 and DM2 can be accelerated not only due to increased ROS production caused by hyperglycemia, but also by the reduced ability of the antioxidant defense system caused at least partly by deleterious SNPs of some scavenger enzymes (Flekac et al., 2008). The presence of the TT (Val/Val) homozygous genotype of the SOD2 gene was associated with poorer diabetes control in comparison with CT (Ala/Val) and CC (Ala/Ala) genotypes. Observed macroangiopathy was associated with significantly lower frequency of the C (Ala) allele of Ala16Val SNP of the SOD2 gene. No differences in genotype frequencies were associated with microangiopathy (Flekac et al., 2008). However, Lee et al. (2006) suggest that this Ala16Val SNP of the SOD2 gene is not related to the pathogenesis of diabetes, but correlates with microangiophathy expressed as microalbuminuria. Other authors found a statistically significant association of the MnSOD Ala16Val polymorphism with DR in a Finnish population (Kangas-Kontio et al., 2010).

Several polymorphisms of the gene coding for catalase have been studied, however in alleles of SNPs located in the promoter region (-21A/T) no statistically significant differences between DM2 patients and controls were found (Flekac et al., 2008). The -262C/T polymorphism in the promoter of catalase gene has also been analyzed in Caucasian-Brazilians with DM2, but no association with DR, DN and ischemic heart disease was found (dos Santos, 2006). Only a weak association was detected between the C111T SNP in exon 9 and a decrease in catalase activity in blood of DM2 patients (Tarnai et al., 2007). These results suggest that genetic variants of the catalase gene do not seem to be involved in the development of vascular complications of DM2.

2.4.4 Aldose reductase

The aldose reductase gene (ALR2) codes for an enzyme involved in glucose-induced pathways and catalyzes the reduction of carbonyl-containing compounds to their respective alcohols. In a two-step metabolic process, the polyol-pathway reduces excess glucose to sorbitol and fructose in insulin-independent tissues (Alexiou et al., 2009). ALR2 is a key regulator, as it is the first and rate-limiting enzyme of the polyol pathway catalyzing the NADPH-dependent reduction of glucose to sorbitol, which is subsequently converted to fructose by sorbitol deshidrogenase, using NAD+ as a co-factor. Both ALR2 and sorbitol deshidrogenase are expressed in human tissues that are sites of diabetic complications and are active when intracelular glucose concentration is elevated. The activation of the polyol pathway produces osmotic stress and oxidative stress, from the accumulation of sorbitol and leads to diabetic lesions in these tissues (Chung et al., 2003; Ramasamy & Goldberg, 2010).

The functional ALR2 gene consists of 10 exons and is located on chromosome 7q35 (Wang et al., 1993). In a 8-year prospective case-control study the association of the z-2 allele of the 5'-(CA)(n) microsatellite and C-106T promoter polymorphisms of the aldose reductase gene with DN in Chinese DM2 patients was assessed. In this cohort, these polymorphisms independently predicted new onset of renal and cardiorenal end points, with the latter being largely mediated through renal disease. Compared with noncarriers, patients with two risk-confering genotypes had a twofold increased risk of renal and cardiorenal end points (So et al., 2008).

In other studies, the association of these polymorphisms with the risk of albuminuria and retinopathy were analyzed in a Finish population. The C-106T polymorphism of the ALR2 gene was related to the early development of microalbuminuria, but not DR (Sivenius et al., 2004a). However, it has also been reported that the C-106T polymorphism may contribute to an early development of neurophysiologic deterioration in DM2 patients (Sivenius et al., 2004b). In Japanese DM2 patients, the C-106T variant was also associated with diabetic macroangiopathy, were the CT or TT genotype showed association with increased risk of stroke (Watarai et al., 2006).

2.4.5 Other genes

Polymorphisms of several other candidate genes may also be related to the susceptibility of patients to develop complications. For example, cyclooxigenase, which has an important role mediating inflammatory processes in periodontal tissues, appears as a candidate gene related to the development of PD. Two polymorphisms (rs20417 and rs689466) of the COX-2 gene, which codes for the cyclooxygenase enzyme, have been reported to be associated with periodontitis (Schaefer et al., 2010).

Polymorphisms in adhesion molecules have also been reported, such as the K469E polymorphism of the intracellular adhesion molecule 1 (ICAM-1) gene, which is associated with proliferative DR in Caucasian DM2 patients (Petrovic et al., 2008), while the 469KK genotype could be a genetic risk factor for DR (Kamiuchi et al., 2002). ICAM-1 is mainly expressed in endothelial cells and is implicated in the recruitment of leukocytes, especially macrophages in inflammatory situations (Muller, 2011). In spite of the fact that ICAM-1 has a fundamental role in the inflammatory process, is not clear whether this molecule is simply a marker of the inflammatory process or might actually play a causative role in the resultant organ dysfunction.

VEGF appears to play a central role, since it mediates microvascular pathology of DR. VEGF induces early alterations of DR, such as leucotaxis and may be operative in the pathogenesis of diabetic blood-retinal barrier breakdown. At the cellular level, blood-retinal barrier breakdown is associated with endocytic vesicle formation and, to a lesser extent, degenerative endothelial changes (Qaum et al., 2001). In DM1 or DM2 patients with DR, diabetic controls without DR and non-diabetic controls, VEGF SNPs rs699947, rs2010963, rs2146232, rs3025033, rs3025039 gene were genotyped, but no association was found (Kangas-Kontio et al., 2009). Other studies on the -634C/G SNP of the VEGF gene found no association with DR (Yang et al., 2010), however these results are controversial (Zhao & Zhao, 2010). A study of the 936 C/T polymorphism of the VEGF gene in a Korean population suggested that this genetic variant may be an important factor determining plasma VEGF levels and is related with DR, since a higher frequency of the TT genotype was observed in patients with proliferative DR. Additionally, plasma levels of VEGF were significantly higher in the TT genotype. There was no difference in VEGF genotype distribution between the control and diabetic patients based on the state of diabetic neuropathy and DN (Kim et al., 2009).

2.4.6 Genome wide association studies

The classical methods of linkage analysis have been useful to identify loci with strong effects; however they are of limited use for discovering genetic variants with a modest impact on complex diseases. Association studies of candidate genes have also been useful, but they are necessarily biased, since they are based on prior knowledge. In addition, they only rely on coding regions and disregard the possible effect of intergenic sequences.

During the last decade, the completion of the Human Genome Project and the development of high throughput technologies have spurted novel strategies termed Genome Wide Association Studies (GWAS), which allow the unbiased analysis of millions of SNPs in very large cohorts. GWAS of DM2 have lead already to the discovery of over 30 SNPs associated with the development of this disease and more than 20 SNPs associated with glycemic traits (Billings & Florez, 2010; Bonnefond et al., 2010). Until recently, the search for genetic determinants of diabetic complications was also constrained to a small number of candidate genes selected on the basis of their postulated role in cellular pathways linking glucose to tissue damage (Doria, 2010). Current initiatives have centered on kidney disease and cardiovascular disease, but not specifically associated to diabetes (Doria, 2010). Recent reports promise the first results of GWA studies of macroangiopathic diabetic complications (Bowden et al., 2010). To date no GWAS data are available for diabetic retinopathy (Doria, 2010). In the near future, GWAS will generate a large output of valuable information of many novel genetic variants related to the development of micro- and macroangiopathic complications. It is expected that this knowledge will provide unprecedented insights on the pathogenesis of diabetic complications (Doria, 2010).

3. Conclusion

Diabetic complications are an important factor contributing to the high morbility and mortality among diabetic patients. It is well known that genetic factors contribute to the appearance and development of these chronic micro- and macroangiopathic complications, but environmental factors usually trigger their appearance. Among these factors, as a product of hyperglicemia, ROS generate endothelial damage. Several genes have been identified, however research related to the contribution of each gene remains controversial and the importance of different genetic variants to the development of diabetic complications is a field of active research were definite conclusions have not yet been established. Figure 2 shows the main genes contributing to the development of diabetic complications. Although there is a prolific literature on polymorphisms of genes involved in vascular damage, clear results are still lacking and more research is needed in order to define the importance of genetic variants and their incidence in disease outcome. In the next years, most probably the use of GWA studies will identify new susceptibility markers related to diabetic complications.

4. Acknowledgment

Part of the work described in this chapter was financed by the grant "Domeyko-Salud, Obesidad y Diabetes" from the University of Chile, Santiago, Chile.

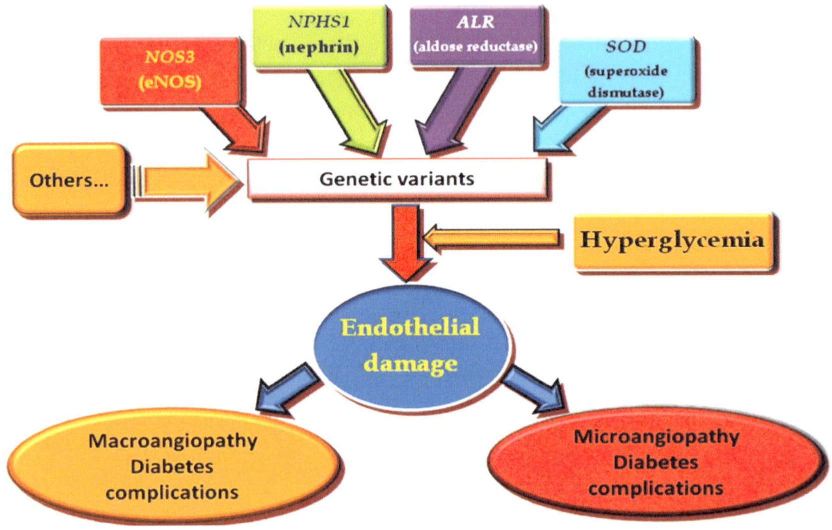

Fig. 2. General overview of genes involved in the development of diabetes complications.

5. References

ADA (American Diabetes Association). (2011). Standards of medical care in diabetes--2011. *Diabetes Care*. Vol. 34, No. Suppl 1, (January 2011), pp. S11-S61.

Adler, A.I., Stevens, R.J., Manley, S.E., Bilous, R.W., Cull, C.A., & Holman, R.R. UKPDS GROUP. (2003). Development and progression of nephropathy in type 2 diabetes: The United Kingdom Study Prospective Diabetes Study (UKPDS64). *Kidney International*, Vol. 63, No. 1, (January 2003), pp. 225-232.

Adler, S. (2004). Diabetic Nephropathy: linking histology, cell biology and genetics. *Kidney International*, Vol. 66, No. 5, (November 2004), pp. 2095-2106.

Alexiou, P., Pegklidou, K., Chatzopoulou, M., Nicolaou, I. & Demopoulos, V.J. (2009). Aldose reductase enzyme and its implication to major health problems of the 21(st) century. *Current Medicinal Chemistry*. Vol. 16, No 6, pp. 734-752.

Araya, A.V., Pavéz, V., Pérez, C., González, F., Colombo, A., Aguirre, A., Schiattino, I. & Aguillón, J.C. (2003). *Ex vivo* lipopolysaccharide (LPS)-induced TNF-α, IL-1β, IL-6 and PGE2 secretion in whole blood from type 1 diabetes mellitus patients with or without periodontitis. *European Cytokine Network* 14, No. 3 (July-September 2003), pp. 128-133.

Aronson, D. (2008). Hyperglycemia and the pathobiology of diabetic complications. *Advances in Cardiology*. Vol 45, pp. 1-16.

Baralle, D. & Baralle, M. (2005). Splicing in action: assessing disease causing sequence changes. *Journal of Medical Genetics*, Vol. 42, No. 10 (October 2005), pp. 737-748.

Beltcheva, O., Martin, P., Lenkkeri, U. & Tryggvason, K. (2001). Mutation spectrum in the nephrin gene (NPHS1) in congenital nephrotic syndrome. *Human Mutation*. Vol. 17, No. 5, (May 2001), pp. 368-373.

Beltcheva, O., Kontusaari, S., Fetissov, S., Putaala, H., Kilpeläinen, P., Hökfelt, T. & Tryggvason, K. (2003). Alternatively used promoters and distinct elements direct tissue-specific expression of nephrin. *Journal of the American Society of Nephrology*. Vol. 14, No. 2, (February 2003), pp. 352-358.

Billings, L.K. & Florez, J.C. (2010). The genetics of type 2 diabetes: what have we learned from GWAS? *Annals of the New York Academy of Sciences*, Vol. 1212, (November 2010), pp. 59-77

Bojstig, M., Arnquist, H.J, Hermansson, G., Karlberg, B.E. & Ludvigsson, J. (1994). Declining incidence of nephropathy in insulin-dependent diabetes mellitus. *New England Journal of Medicine*, Vol. 330, No. 1, (January 1994), pp. 15-18.

Bonnefond, A., Froguel, P. & Vaxillaire M. (2010). The emerging genetics of type 2 diabetes. *Trends in Molecular Medicine*, Vol. 16, No. 9, (September 2010), pp. 407-416.

Bowden, D.W., Cox, A.J., Freedman, B.I., Hugenschimdt, C.E., Wagenknecht, L.E., Herrington, D., Agarwal, S., Register, T.D., Maldjian, J.A., Ng, M.C., Hsu, F.C., Langefeld, C.D., Williamson, J.D. & Carr, J.J. (2010). Review of the Diabetes Heart Study (DHS) Family of Studies: A Comprehensively Examined Sample for Genetic and Epidemiological Studies of Type 2 Diabetes and its Complications. *Review of Diabetes Studies*, Vol. 7, No. 3 (Fall 2010), pp. 188-201.

Brancati, F.L., Whittle, J.C., Whelton, P.K., Seidler, A.J. & Klag, M.J. (1992). The excess incidence of diabetic end-stage renal disease among blacks. A population-based study of potencial explanatory factors. *The Journal of the American Medical Association*, Vol. 268, No. 21, (December 1992), pp. 3079-3084.

Brownlee, M. (2005). The pathobiology of diabetic complications: a unifying mechanism. *Diabetes*, Vol. 54, No. 6, (June 2005), pp. 1615-1625.

Bruckdorfer, R. (2005). The basics about nitric oxide. *Molecular Aspects of Medicine*, Vol. 26, No. 1-2, (Feb-Apr 2005), pp. 3-31.

Channon, K.M. & Guzik, T.J. (2002). Mechanisms of superoxide production in human blood vessels: relationship to endothelial dysfunction, clinical and genetic risk factors. *Journal of Physiology and Pharmacology*, Vol. 53, No. 4 Pt 1, (December 2002), pp. 515-524.

Chung, S.S., Ho, E.C., Lam, K.S., & Chung, S.K. (2003). Contribution of polyol pathway to diabetes-induced oxidative stress. *Journal of the American Society of Nephrology*, Vol. 15, No. 8 Suppl 3, (August 2003), pp. S233-S236.

Colagiuri, R. (2010) Diabetes: a pandemic, a development issue or both? . *Expert Review of Cardiovascular Therapy*, Vol. 8, No. 3, (March 2010), pp 305-309.

Cowie, C.C., Port, F.K., Wolfe, R.A., Savage, P.J., Moll, P.P. & Hawthorne, V.M. (1989). Disparities in incidence of diabetic end-stage renal disease according to race and type of diabetes. *New England Journal of Medicine*, Vol. 321, No. 16 (October 1989), pp. 1074-1079.

Daimon, M., Ji, G., Oizumi, T., Kido, T., Baba, M., Jimbu, Y., Kameda, W., Susa, S., Yamaguchi, H., Ohnuma, H., Muramatsu, M. & Kato, T. (2006). Association of nephrin gene polymorphisms with type 2 diabetes in a Japanese population: The Funagata study. *Diabetes Care*, Vol. 29, No. 5 (May 2006), pp. 1117-1119.

Darre, L., Vergnes, J.N., Gourdy, P. & Sixou, M. (2008). Efficacy of periodontal treatment on glycaemic control on diabetic patients: A meta-analysis of interventional studies. *Diabetes & Metabolism*, Vol. 34, No. 5 (November 2008), pp. 497-506.

Doria, A. (2010). Genetics of Diabetes Complications. *Current Diabetes Reports*. Vol. 10, No. 6, (December 2010), pp. 467–475.

dos Santos, K.G., Canani, L.H., Gross, J.L., Tschiedel, B., Souto, K.E. & Roisenberg, I. (2006). The catalase -262C/T promoter polymorphism and diabetic complications in Caucasians with type 2 diabetes. *Disease Markers*. Vol. 22, No. 5-6, pp. 355-359.

Flekac, M., Skrha, J., Hilgertova, J., Lacinova, Z. & Jarolimkova, M. (2008). Gene polymorphisms of superoxide dismutases and catalase in diabetes mellitus. *BMC Medical Genetics*, Vol. 9, (April 2008), pp. 30-39.

Fornoni, A., Jeon, J., Varona Santos, J., Cobianchi, L., Jauregui, A., Inverardi, L., Mandic, S.A., Bark, C., Johnson, K., McNamara, G., Pileggi, A., Molano, R.D., Reiser, J., Tryggvason, K., Kerjaschki, D., Berggren, P.O., Mundel, P. & Ricordi, C. (2010). Nephrin is expressed on the surface of insulin vesicles and facilitates glucose-stimulated insulin release. *Diabetes*, Vol. 59, No. 1, (January 2010), pp. 1990-1999.

Gamonal, J., Mendoza, C., Espinoza, I., Muñoz, A., Urzúa, I., Aranda, W., Carvajal, P. & Arteaga, O. (2010). Clinical Attachment Loss in Chilean Adult Population: First Chilean National Dental Examination Survey. *Journal of Periodontology*, Vol. 81, No. 10 (October 2010), pp. 1403-1410.

García, J.M. (2009). La cistatina C aporta más información que otros parámetros de función renal en la estratificación del riesgo de los pacientes con síndrome coronario agudo. *Revista Española de Cardiología*.Vol. 62, pp. 519-519.

Giugliano, D., Ceriello, A. & Esposito, K. (2008). Glucose metabolism and hyperglycemia. *The American Journal of Clinical Nutrition*. Vol. 87, No. 1 (January 2008), pp. 217S-222S.

Gjermo, P., Rösing, C.K., Susin, C. & Oppermann, R. (2002). Periodontal diseases in Central and South America. *Periodontology 2000*, Vol. 29, No. 1, (April 2002), pp. 70–78.

González, R., Tirado, A., Balanda, M., Alvo, M., Barquín, I., Durruty, P., Lobos, S. & Seelenfreund, D. (2007). A pilot study on genetic variation in purine-rich elements in the nephrin gene promoter in type 2 diabetic patients. *Biological Research*, Vol. 40, No. 3 (April 2007), pp. 357-364. ISSN 0716-9760

González, R., Tirado, A., Rojas, L.A., Ossandón, F., Alvo, M., Wolff, C., Seelenfreund, D., Durruty, P. & Lobos, S. (2009). Analysis of the intronic single nucleotide polymorphism rs#466452 of the nephrin gene in patients with diabetic nephropathy. *Biological Research*, Vol. 42, No. 2 (August 2009), pp. 189-198.

Goyal, M.M., & Basak, A. Human catalase: looking for complete identity. (2010). *Protein Cell*. Vol. 1, No. 10 (October 2010), pp. 888-897.

Grossi, S.G., Zambon, J.J., Ho, A.W., Koch, G., Dunford, R.G., Machtei, E.E., Norderyd, O.M. & Genco, R.J. (1994). Assessment of risk for periodontal disease. I. Risk indicators for attachment loss. *Journal of Periodontology*, Vol. 65, No. 3, (March 1994), pp. 65: 260–267.

Haffner, S.M., Lehto, S., Ronnemaa, T., Pyörälä, K. & Laakso, M. (1998). Mortality from coronary heart disease in subjects with type 2 diabetes and in nondiabetic subjects with and without a prior myocardial infarction. *New England Journal of Medicine*, Vol. 339, No. 4, (July 1998), pp. 229-234.

Hansen, D., Dendale, P., Beelen, M., Jonkers, R.A., Mullens, A., Corluy, L., Meeusen, R. & van Loon, L.J. (2010). Plasma adipokine and inflammatory marker concentrations are altered in obese, as opposed to non-obese, type 2 diabetes patients. *European Journal of Applied Physiology*. Vol. 109, No. 3, (June 2010), pp. 397-404.

Hauser, P.V., Collino, F., Bussolati, B. & Camussi, G. (2009). Nephrin and endothelial injury. *Current Opinion in Nephrology & Hypertension*, Vol. 18, No. 1, (January 2009), pp. 3-8.

Humphrey, L.L., Palumbo, P.J., Butters, M.A., Hallett, J.W. Jr., Chu, C.P., O'Fallon, W.M. & Ballard, D.J. (1994). The contribution of non insulin- dependent diabetes to lower-extremity amputation in the community. *Archives of Internal Medicine*, Vol. 154, No. 8, (April 1994), pp. 885-892.

Hunt, K.J., Resendez, R.G., Haffner, S.M., Stern, M.P. & San Antonio Heart Study. (2004). National Cholesterol Education Program versus World Health Organization Metabolic Sindrome in relation to all-cause and cardiovascular mortality in the San Antonio Heart Study. *Circulation,* Vol. 110, No. 10, (September 2004), pp. 1251-1277.

Jackson, G.R. & Barber, A.J. (2010). Visual dysfunction associated with diabetic retinopathy. *Current Diabetes Report,* Vol. 10, No. 5, (October 2010), pp. 380-384.

Jadzinsky, M.N. (2003). Neuropatía diabética periférica y autonómica, In: *Diabetes Mellitus,* M. García de los Ríos & P. Durruty, pp. 243- 259, 2nd edition, Published by "Fundación de Investigación y Perfeccionamiento Médico", ISBN 96, Santiago, Chile.

Jaziri, R., Aubert, R., Roussel, R., Emery, N., Maimaitiming, S., Bellili, N., Miot, A., Saulnier, .PJ., Travert, F., Hadjadj, S., Marre, M., Fumeron, F., DIABHYCAR and SURDIAGENE Study Groups. (2010). Association of ADIPOQ genetic variants and plasma adiponectin isoforms with the risk of incident renal events in type 2 diabetes. *Nephrology Dialisis Transplantation.* Vol. 25, No. 7, (July 2010), pp. 2231-2237.

Kaiser, N., Sasson, S., Feener, E.P., Boukobza-Vardi, N., Higashi, S., Moller, D.E., Davidheiser, S., Przybylski, R.J. & King, G.L. (1993). Differential regulation of glucose transport and transporters by glucose in vascular endothelial and smooth muscle cells. *Diabetes,* Vol. 42, No. 1, (January 1993), pp. 80-89.

Kamiuchi, K., Hasegawa, G., Obayashi, H., Kitamura, A., Ishii, M., Yano, M., Kanatsuna, T., Yoshikawa, T. & Nakamura, N. (2002). Intercellular adhesion molecule-1 (ICAM-1) polymorphism is associated with diabetic retinopathy in Type 2 diabetes mellitus. *Diabetes Medicine,* Vol. 19, No. 5, (May 2002) pp. 371-376.

Kangas-Kontio, T., Vavuli, S., Kakko, S.J., Penna, J., Savolainen, E.R., Savolainen, M.J. & Liinamaa, M.J. (2009). Polymorphism of the manganese superoxide dismutase gene but not of vascular endothelial growth factor gene is a risk factor for diabetic retinopathy. *British Journal of Ophthalmology,* Vol. 93, No. 10, (October 2009), pp. 1401-1414.

Kannel, W. & McGee, D. (1979). Diabetes and glucose tolerance as risk factors for cardiovascular disease: the Framingham study. *Diabetes Care,* Vol. 2, No. 2 (March-April 1979), pp. 120-126.

Kennedy, G.C. & Rutter, W.J. (1992). Pur-1, a zinc-finger protein that binds to purine-rich sequences, transactivates an insulin promoter in heterologous cells. *Proceedings of the National Academic Sciences U S A.* Vol. 89, No. 23, (December 1992), pp. 11498-11502.

Kestilä, M., Lenkkeri, U., Männikkö, M., Lamerdin, J., Mccready, P., Putaala, H., Ruotsalainen, V., Morita, T., Nissinen, M., Herva, R., Kashtan, C.E., Peltonen, L., Holmberg, C., Olsen, A. & Tryggvason, K. (1998). Positionally cloned gene for a novel glomerular protein - nephrin - is mutated in congenital nephrotic syndrome. *Molecular Cell,* Vol. 1, No. 4, (March 1998), pp. 575-582.

Kim, H.W., Ko, G.J., Kang, Y.S., Lee, M.H., Song, H.K., Kim, H.K. & Cha, D.R. (2009). Role of the VEGF 936 C/T polymorphism in diabetic microvascular complications in type 2 diabetic patients. *Nephrology (Carlton).* Vol. 14, No. 7, (October 2009), pp. 681-688.

Kimchi-Sarfaty, C., Oh, J.M., Kim, I.W., Sauna, Z.E., Calcagno, A.M., Ambudkar, S.V. & Gottesman, M.M. (2007). A "silent" polymorphism in the MDR1 gene changes substrate specificity. *Science,* Vol. 315, No. 5811, (January 2007), pp. 525-528.

Klein, R., Klein, B.E., Moss, S.E., Davis, M.D. & DeMets, D.L. (1989). The Wisconsin Epidemiologic Study of Diabetic Retinopathy. X. Four-year incidence and progression of diabetic retinopathy when age at diagnosis is 30 years or more. *Archives of Ophthalmology*, Vol. 107, No. 2, (February 1989), pp. 244-249.

Kristiansen, O.P. & Mandrup-Poulsen, T. (2005). "Interleukin-6 and diabetes: the good, the bad, or the indifferent?". *Diabetes*. Vol. 54, No. Suppl 2, (December 2005), pp. S114–124

Lecaire, T., Palta, M., Zhang, H., Allen, C., Klein, R. & D'Alessio, D. (2006). Lower-than-expected prevalence and severity of retinopathy in an incident cohort followed during the first 4-14 years of type 1 diabetes: the Wisconsin Diabetes Registry Study. *American Journal of Epidemiology*, Vol. 164, No. 2 (July 2006), pp. 143-150.

Lee, S.J. & Choi, M.G. (2006). Association of manganese superoxide dismutase gene polymorphism (V16A) with diabetic macular edema in Korean type 2 diabetic patients. *Metabolism*, Vol. 5, No. 12, (December 2006), pp. 1681-1688.

López, A.D., Mathers, C.D., & Ezzati, M, Jamison, D.T. & Murray, C.J. (2006). Global and regional burden of disease and risk factors, 2001: systematic analysis of population health data. *Lancet*, Vol. 367, No. 9524, (May 2006), pp. 1747-1757.

López, N.J., Valenzuela, C.Y. & Jara, L. (2009). Interleukin-1 gene cluster polymorphisms associated with periodontal disease in type 2 diabetes. *Journal of Periodontology*, Vol. 80, No. 10, (October 2009), pp. 1590-1598.

Mealey, B.L. (2006). Periodontal disease and diabetes: A two-way street. *Journal of the American Dental Association*, Vol. 137, No. 10 suppl., (October 2006), pp. 26S–31S.

Melistas, L., Mantzoros, C.S., Kontogianni, M., Antonopoulou, S., Ordovas, J.M. & Yiannakouris, N. (2009). Association of the +45T>G and +276G>T polymorphisms in the adiponectin gene with insulin resistance in nondiabetic Greek women. *European Journal of Endocrinology*. Vol. 161, No. 6, (December 2009), pp. 845-852.

Möllsten, A., Marklund, S.L., Wessman, M., Svensson, M., Forsblom, C., Parkkonen, M., Brismar , K., Groop, P.H. & Dahlquist, G. (2007). A functional polymorphism in the manganese superoxide dismutase gene and diabetic nephropathy. *Diabetes*, Vol. 56, No. 1, (January 2007), pp. 265-269.

Muller, W.A. (2011). Mechanisms of leukocyte transendothelial migration. *Annual Review of Pathology*, Vol. 28, No. 6, (February 2011), pp. 323-344.

Nassar, H., Kantarci, A. & Van Dyke, T.E. (2007). Diabetic periodontitis: a model for activated innate immunity and impaired resolution of Inflammation. *Periodontology 2000*, Vol. 43, No. 1, (February 2007), pp. 233–244.

Nathan, D.M., Zinman, B., Cleary, P.A., Backlund, J.Y., Genuth, S., Miller, R. & Orchard, T.J. (351 colaborators). Diabetes Control and Complications Trial/Epidemiology of Diabetes Interventions and Complications (DCCT/EDIC) Research Group. (2009). Modern-day clinical course of type 1 diabetes mellitus alter 30 year's duration: the Diabetes Control and Complications Trial/ Epidemiology of Diabetes Interventions and Complications and Pittsburgh epidemiology of diabetes complications experience (1983-2005). *Archives of Internal Medicine*, Vol. 169, No. 14 (July 2009), pp. 1307-1316.

Nishimura, F., Iwamoto, Y. & Soga, Y. (2007). The periodontal host response with diabetes. *Periodontology*, Vol. 43, No. 1, (February 2007), pp. 245–253.

Ockrim, Z. & Yorston, D. (2010). Managing diabetic retinopathy. *British Medical Journal*, Vol. 341, (October 2010), pp. c5400.

Pan, Z., Guzeldemir, E., Toygar, H.U., Bal, N. & Bulut, S. (2010). Nitric oxide synthase in gingival tissues of patients with chronic periodontitis and with and without diabetes *Journal of Periodontology*. Vol. 81, No. 1, (January 2010), pp. 109-120.

Pätäri, A., Forsblom, C., Havana, M., Taipale, H., Groop, P.H., & Holthöfer, H. (2003). Nephrinuria in diabetic nephropathy of type 1 diabetes. *Diabetes,* Vol.52, No. 12, (December 2003), pp. 2969-2974.

Pätäri-Sampo, A., Ihalmo, P. & Holthöfer, H. (2006). Molecular basis of the glomerular filtration: nephrin and the emerging protein complex at the podocyte slit diaphragm. *Annals of Medicine*. Vol. 38, No. 7, pp. 483-492.

Patel, A., MacMahon, S., Chalmers, J., Neal, B., Billot, L., Woodward, M., Marre, M., Cooper, M., Glasziou, P., Grobbee, D., Hamet, P., Harrap, S., Heller, S., Liu, L., Mancia, G., Mogensen, C.E., Pan, C., Poulter, N., Rodgers, A., Williams, B., Bompoint, S., de Galan, B.E., Joshi, R. & Travert, F. Advance Collaborative Group. (2008). Intensive blood glucose control and vascular outcomes in patients with type 2 diabetes. *New England Journal of Medicine,* Vol. 358, No. 24, (June 2008), pp. 2560-2572.

Pavkov, M.E., Knowler, W.C., Bennett, P.H., Looker, H.C., Krakoff, J. & Nelson, R.G. (2006). Increasing incidence of proteinuria and declining incidence of end-stage renal disease in diabetic Pima Indians. *Kidney International,* Vol. 70, No. 10, (November 2006), pp. 1840- 1846.

Pérez, C., González, F.E., Pavéz, V., Araya, A.V., Aguirre, A., Cruzat, A., Contreras-Levicoy, J., Dotte, A., Aravena, O., Salazar, L., Catalán, D., Cuenca, J., Ferreira, A., Schiattino, I. & Aguillón, J.C. (2004). The –308 polymorphism in the promoter region of the tumor necrosis factor-alpha (TNF-a) gene and *ex vivo* lipopolysaccharide-induced TNF-α expression in patients with aggressive periodontitis and/or type 1 diabetes mellitus. *European Cytokine Network,* Vol. 15, No. 4, (October-December 2004), pp. 364-370.

Petersen, K.F. & Shulman, G.I. (2006). Etiology of insulin resistance. *American Journal of Medicine,* Vol. 119, No. 5 Suppl 1, (May 2006), pp. S10-S16.

Petrovic, M.G., Osredkar, J., Saraga-Babić, M. & Petrovic, D. (2008). K469E polymorphism of the intracellular adhesion molecule 1 gene is associated with proliferative diabetic retinopathy in Caucasians with type 2 diabetes. *Clinical and Experimental Ophthalmology*. Vol. 36, No. 5, (July 2008), pp. 468-472.

Pignone, M., Alberts, M.J., Colwell, A., Cushman, M., Inzucchi, S.E., Mukherjee, D., Rosenson, R.S., Williams, C.D., Wilson, P.W. & Kirkman, M.S.; American Diabetes Association; American Heart Association; & American College of Cardiology Foundation. (2010). Aspirin use for primary prevention of cardiovascular events in people with diabetes. A Position Statement of the American Diabetes Association, a Scientific Statement of the American Heart Association and an Expert Consensus of the American College of Cardiology Foundation. *Diabetes Care,* Vol. 33, No. 6, (June 2010), pp. 1395-1402.

Qaum, T., Xu, Q., Joussen, A.M., Clemens, M.W., Qin, W., Miyamoto, K., Hassessian, H., Wiegand, S.J., Rudge, J., Yancopoulos, G.D. & Adamis AP. (2001). VEGF-initiated blood-retinal barrier breakdown in early diabetes. *Investigative Ophthalmoly and Visual Science,* Vol. 42, No. 10, (September 2001), pp. 2408-2413.

Ramasamy, R. & Goldberg, I.J. (2010). Aldose reductase and cardiovascular diseases, creating human-like diabetic complications in an experimental model. *Circulation Research,* Vol. 106, No. 9, (May 2010), pp. 1449-1458.

Roy, S., Trudeau, K., Roy, S., Behl, Y., Dhar, S. & Chronopoulos, A. (2010). New insights into hyperglycemia-induced molecular changes in microvascular cells. *Journal of Dental Research*. Vol. 89, No. 2, (February 2010), pp. 116-127.

Salmenniemi, U., Zacharova, J., Ruotsalainen, E., Vauhkonen, I., Pihlajamäki, J., Kainulainen, S., Punnonen, K. & Laakso, M. (2005). Association of adiponectin level and variants in the adiponectin gene with glucose metabolism, energy expenditure, and cytokines in offspring of type 2 diabetic patients. *Journal of Clinical Endocrinology Metababolism,* Vol. 90, No. 7, (July 2005), pp. 4216-4223.

Sandoo, A., van Zanten, J.J., Metsios, G.S., Carroll, D. & Kitas, G.D. (2010). The endothelium and its role in regulating vascular tone. (2010). *Open Cardiovascular Medical Journal,* Vol. 23, No. 4, (December 2010), pp. 302-312.

Saremi, A., Nelson, R.G., Tulloch-Reid, M., Hanson, R.L., Sievers, M.L., Taylor, G.W., Shlossman, M., Bennett, P.H., Genco, R. & Knowler, W.C. (2005). Periodontal Disease and Mortality in Type 2 Diabetes. *Diabetes Care,* Vol. 28, No. 1, (January 2005), pp. 27-32.

Schaefer, A.S., Richter, G.M., Nothnagel, M., Laine, M.L., Noack, B., Glas, J., Schrezenmeir, J., Groessner-Schreiber, B., Jepsen, S., Loos, B.G. & Schreiber, S. (2010). COX-2 is associated with periodontitis in Europeans. *Journal of Dental Research,* Vol. 89, No. 4, (April 2010), pp. 384-388.

Scherer, P.E., Williams, S., Fogliano, M., Baldini, G. & Lodish, H.F. (1995). A novel serum protein similar to C1q, produced exclusively in adipocytes. *Journal of Biological Chemistry,* Vol. 270, No. 45, (November 10), pp. 26746-26749.

Shi, Y. & Vanhoutte, P.M. (2009). Reactive oxygen-derived free radicals are key to the endothelial dysfunction of diabetes. *Journal of Diabetes.* Vol. 1, No. 3, (September 2005), pp. 151-162.

Shlipak, M.G., Katz, R., Sarnak, M.J., Fried, L.F., Newman, A.B., Stehman-Breen, C., Seliger, S.L., Kestenbaum, B., Psaty, B., Tracy, R.P. & Siscovick, D.S. (2006). Cystatin C and prognosis for cardiovascular and kidney outcomes in elderly persons without chronic kidney disease. *Annals of Internal Medicine,* Vol. 145, No. 4, (August, 15), pp. 237-246.

Shultis, W.A., Weil, E.J., Looker, H.C., Curtis, J.M., Shlossman, M., Genco, R.J., Knowler, W.C. & Nelson, R.G. (2007). Effect of periodontitis on overt nephropathy and end-stage renal disease in type 2 diabetes. *Diabetes Care,* Vol. 30, No. 2, (February 2007), pp. 306-311.

Sivenius K, Pihlajamäki J, Partanen J, Niskanen L, Laakso M, Uusitupa M. (2004a). Aldose reductase gene polymorphisms and peripheral nerve function in patients with type 2 diabetes. *Diabetes Care.* Vol. 27, No. 8, (August 2004) pp. 2021-2026.

Sivenius, K., Niskanen, L., Voutilainen-Kaunisto, R., Laakso, M. & Uusitupa, M. (2004b). Aldose reductase gene polymorphisms and susceptibility to microvascular complications in Type 2 diabetes. *Diabetes Medicine,* Vol. 21, No. 12, (December 2004), pp. 1325-1233.

So, W.Y., Wang, Y., Ng, M.C., Yang, X., Ma, R.C., Lam, V., Kong, A.P., Tong, P.C. & Chan J.C. (2008). Aldose reductase genotypes and cardiorenal complications: an 8-year prospective analysis of 1,074 type 2 diabetic patients. *Diabetes Care.* Vol. 31, No. 11, (November 2008), pp. 2148-2153.

Stettler, C., Allemann, S., Jüni, P., Cull, C.A., Holman, R.R., Egger, M., Krähenbühl. S. & Diem, P. (2006). Glycemic control and macrovascular disease in type 1 and 2 diabetes mellitus: Meta-analysis of randomized trials. *American Heart Journal*, Vol. 152, No. 1, (July 2006), pp. 27-38.

Stevens, L. & Levey, A. (2005). Chronic kidney disease in the elderly how to assess risk. *New England Journal of Medicine*. Vol. 352, No. 20, (May 19), pp. 2122-2124.

Stratton, I.M., Adler, A.I., Neil, H.A., Matthews, D.R., Manley, S.E., Cull, C.A., Hadden, D., Turner, R.C. & Holman, R.R. (2000). Association of glycaemia with macrovascular and microvascular complications of type 2 diabetes. (UKPDS35): prospective observational study. *British Medical Journal*, Vol. 321, No. 7258, (August 2000), pp. 405-412.

Tabit, C.E., Chung, W.B., Hamburg, N.M. & Vita, J.A. (2010). Endothelial dysfunction in diabetes mellitus: molecular mechanisms and clinical implications. *Review Endocrinology Metabolic Disorders*, Vol. 11, pp. 61-74.

Taglieri, N., Koenig, W. & Kaski, J.C. (2009). Cystatin C and cardiovascular risk. *Clinical Chemistry*. Vol. 55, No. 11, (November 2009), pp. 1932-1943.

Tarnai, I., Csordás, M., Sükei, E., Shemirani, A.H., Káplár, M. & Góth, L. (2007). *Free Radical Research*. Vol. 41, No. 7, (July 2007), pp. 806-811.

Taylor, G.W. & Borgnakke, W.S. (2008). Periodontal disease: associations with diabetes, glycemic control and complications. *Oral Diseases*, Vol. 14, No. 3, (April 2008), pp. 191–203.

Tesfaye, S., Boulton, A.J., Dyck, P.J., Freeman, R., Horowitz, M., Kempler, P., Lauria, G., Malik, R.A., Spallone, V., Vinik, A., Bernardi, L., Valensi, P.; & Toronto Diabetic Neuropathy Expert Group. (2010). Diabetic neuropathies: update on definitions, diagnostic criteria, estimation of severity, and treatments. *Diabetes Care, Vol.* 33, No. 10, (October 2010), pp. 2285-2293.

Toyoda, M., Suzuki, D., Umezono, T., Uehara, G., Maruyama, M., Honma, M., Sakai, T., & Sakai, H. (2004). Expression of human nephrin mRNA in diabetic nephropathy. *Nephrology Dialysis Transplantation*, Vol. 19, No. 2, (February 2004), pp. 380-385.

Turnbull, F.M., Abraira, C., Anderson, R.J., Byinton, R.P., Chalmers, J.P., Duckworth, W.C., Evans, G.W., Gerstein, H.C., Holman, R.R., Moritz, T.E., Neal, B.C, Ninomiya, T., Patel, A.A., Paul, S.K,, Travert, F. & Woodward, M. Control Group, (2009). Intensive glucose control and macrovascular outcomes in type2 diabetes. *Diabetologia*, Vol. 52, No. 11, (November 2009), pp. 2288-2298.

Uğar-Cankal, D. & Ozmeric, N. (2006). A multifaceted molecule, nitric oxide in oral and periodontal diseases. *Clinica Chimica Acta*, Vol. 366, No. 1-2, (April 2006), pp. 90-100.

Vaccaro, O., Eberly, L.E., Neaton, J.D., Yang, L., Riccardi, G., Stamler, J.; & Multiple Risk Factor Intervention Trial Research Group. (2004). Impact of diabetes and previous myocardial infarction on long-term survival: 25-year mortality follow-up of primary screenees of the Multiple Risk Factor Intervention Trial. *Archives of Internal Medicine*, Vol. 164, No. 13, (July 2004), pp. 1438-1443.

Vallance, J.H., Wilson, P.J., Leese, G.P., McAlpine, R., MacEwen, C.J. & Ellis, J.D. (2008). Diabetic retinophaty: more patients, less laser: a longitudinal population-based study in Tayside, Scotland. *Diabetes Care*, Vol. 31, No. 6, (June 2008), pp. 1126-1131.

Van Dieren, S., Beulens, J.W., van der Schouw, Y.T., Grobbee, D.E. & Neal, B. (2010). The global burden of diabetes and its complications: an emerging pandemic. *European Journal of Cardiovascular Prevention and Rehabilitatio*, Vol. 17, Suppl 1, (May 2010); pp .S3-S8.

Villalón, P. (2011). Relación entre niveles séricos de cistatina-C y riesgo cardiovascular estimado por las tablas de Framingham adaptadas a la población chilena. Tesis para optar al grado de Magíster en Nutrición. Faculty of Medicine, University of Chile. Santiago, Chile.

Waki, H., Yamauchi, T., Kamon, J., Ito, Y., Uchida, S., Kita, S., Hara, K., Hada, Y., Vasseur, F., Froguel, P., Kimura, S., Nagai, R. & Kadowaki, T. (2003). Impaired multimerization of human adiponectin mutants associated with diabetes. Molecular structure and multimer formation of adiponectin. *Journal of Biological Chemistry*. Vol. 278, No. 41, (October 2003), pp. 40352-40363.

Wang, K., Bohren, K.M. & Gabbay KH. (1993). Characterization of the human aldose reductase gene promoter. *Journal of Biological Chemistry*. Vol. 268, No.21, (July 25), pp.16052-16058.

Wang, J., Smith, P.J., Krainer, A.R. & Zhang, M.Q. (2005). Distribution of SR protein exonic splicing enhancer motifs in human protein-coding genes. *Nucleic Acids Research*, Vol. 33, No. 16, (September 2005), pp. 5053-5062.

Wang, X., Tomso, D.J., Chorley, B.N., Cho, H.Y., Cheung, V.G., Kleeberger, S.R. and Bell, D.A. (2007). Identification of polymorphic antioxidant response elements in the human genome. *Human Molecular Genetics*. Vol. 16, No. 10, (May 15), pp. 1188-2200.

Watarai, A., Nakashima, E., Hamada, Y., Watanabe, G., Naruse, K., Miwa, K., Kobayashi, Y., Kamiya, H., Nakae, M., Hamajima, N., Sekido, Y., Niwa, T., Oiso, Y. & Nakamura, J. (2006). Aldose reductase gene is associated with diabetic macroangiopathy in Japanese Type 2 diabetic patients. *Diabetic Medicine*, Vol. 23, No. 8, (August 2006), pp. 894-899.

Weyer, C., Funahashi, T., Tanaka, S., Hotta, K., Matsuzawa, Y., Pratley, R.E., Tataranni, P.A. (2001). Hypoadiponectinemia in obesity and type 2 diabetes: close association with insulin resistance and hyperinsulinemia. *Journal of Clinical Endocrinology & Metabolism*. Vol. 86, No. 5, (May 2001), pp. 1930-1935.

Wolff, C., Durruty, P., Espinoza, J., Ripamonti, S. & Díaz, J. (2009). Cistatina C y adiponectina en pacientes diabéticos tipo 2 coronarios y no coronarios. *Revista Médica de Chile*. Vol. 137, No. 6, (June 2009), pp. 729-736.

Yang, Y., Andresen, B.T., Yang, K., Zhang, Y., Li, X., Li, X. & Wang, H.. (2010). Association of vascular endothelial growth factor -634C/G polymorphism and diabetic retinopathy in type 2 diabetic Han Chinese. *Experimental Biology & Medicine (Maywood)*. Vol. 235, No. 10, (October 2010), pp. 1204-1211.

Yuan, H.Y., Chiou, J.J., Tseng, W.H., Liu, C.H., Liu, C.K., Lin, Y.J., Wang, H.H., Yao, A., Chen, Y.T. & Hsu, C.N. (2006). FASTSNP: an always up-to date and extendable service for SNP function analysis and prioritization. *Nucleic Acids Research*. Vol. 34, (July 2006), pp. W635-W641.

Zelko, I.N., Mariani, T.J. & Folz, R.J. (2002). Superoxide dismutase multigene family: a comparison of the CuZn-SOD (SOD1), Mn-SOD (SOD2), and EC-SOD (SOD3) gene structures, evolution, and expression. *Free Radical Biology & Medicine*, Vol. 33, No. 3, (August 2002), pp. 337-349.

Zhang, D., Efendic, S., Brismar, K. & Gu. H.F. (2010). Effects of MCF2L2, ADIPOQ and SOX2 genetic polymorphisms on the development of nephropathy in type 1 Diabetes Mellitus *BMC Medical Genet*ics, Vol. 28, No. 11, (July 2010), pp. 116-123.

Zhao, T. & Zhao, J. (2010). Association between the -634C/G polymorphisms of the vascular endothelial growth factor and retinopathy in type 2 diabetes: a meta-analysis. *Diabetes Research and Clinical Practice*. Vol. 90, No. 1, (October 2010), pp. 45-53.

11

Functional Context Network of T2DM

Anja Thormann and Axel Rasche
Max-Planck-Institute for Molecular Genetics, Department of Vertebrate Genomics
Germany

1. Introduction

Type-2 diabetes mellitus (T2DM) is a complex disease with multiple causes covering several functional entities of the metabolism. Environmental factors contribute to the pathogenesis of the disease - most notably nutrition and weight of the organism. The identification of disease genes is the driving power of many research projects. In a previous paper (Rasche et al. 2008) we presented a method that integrates results from different T2DM related studies and identifies candidate genes with high disease relevance. This chapter is designated to elaborate on our work from a network based perspective. Network biology is a promising field that can shed light on interrelations between disease genes and from disease genes to their functional neighborhood. We use network-based tools to advance from a single-gene analysis towards a subnet, a functional module, of disease genes.

Proteins are gene products that are associated with particular molecular functions. Molecular functions are interpreted as activities that can be performed by individual proteins following the definitions introduced by the Gene Ontology Consortium (Ashburner et al. 2000). Examples of molecular functions are catalytic activity, transporter activity or binding. Additionally, a biological process is accomplished by one or more ordered assemblies of molecular functions (Ashburner et al. 2000).

Proteins physically interact with each other in order to carry out a biological function. A biological function is related to the term *biological process*. A signal transduction cascade whose biological function is to transmit information from a receptor to a transcription factor is a succession of protein-protein interactions (PPIs). Both the molecular function of a protein and the biological function in which it is involved are best deduced by studying the environment where it operates in.

To this end, scientists pursue the ambitious goal of assembling all PPIs in an organism - the *interactome* - to elucidate how proteins work together and promote individual biological processes and eventually the complete cellular machinery. Today, mainly two methods are used to detect PPIs: Yeast two-hybrid screens (Fields & Sternglanz 1994) and affinity purification (Pandey & Mann 2000). These large-scale technologies provide vast numbers of interactions but have high false positive rates. Additionally, such experiments only reflect one environmental condition and not the dynamics of interactions between different phyiological states leading to high false negative rates.

Regarding the current size of the human interactome, we have only a draft of the complete set of interactions. However, looking at the course of construction (fig. 1) so far and bearing in mind new quality standards we are continuously moving towards the completion of a comprehensive human PPI network. For now we have to take into account that the network is incomplete and noisy.

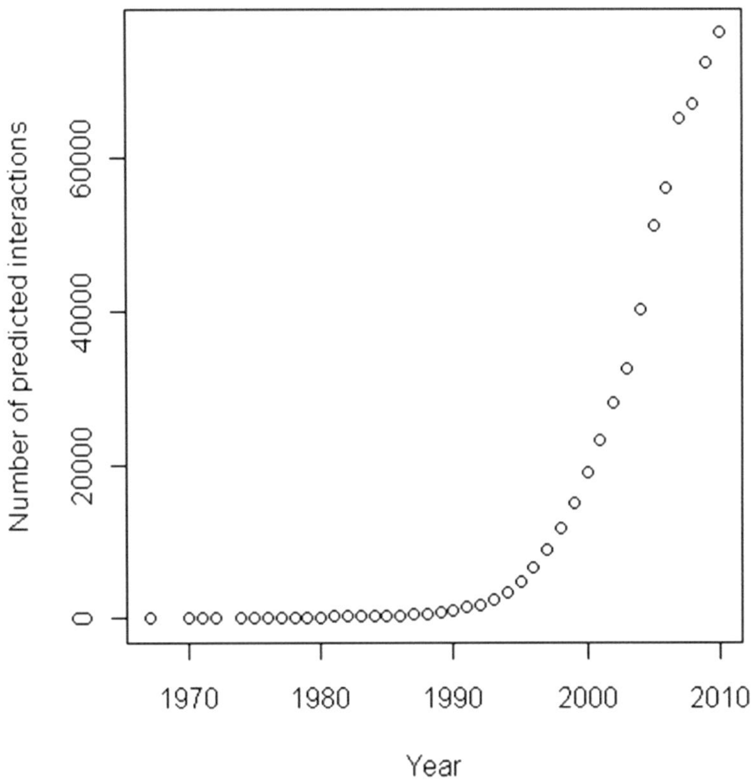

Fig. 1. Cumulative number of detected PPIs of the last years. The data is taken from the ConsensusPathDB website. The data may contain false positive interactions.

Interactions are consolidated in many different databases. For further analysis we take advantage of ConsensusPathDB (Kamburov et al. 2009; Kamburov et al. 2011), a resource joining various human molecular interaction networks including protein-protein, metabolic, signaling and gene regulatory interaction networks. ConsensusPathDB integrates interaction data from many interaction databases, consequently providing us with a comprehensive resource of the currently known interactome.

2. Meta-analysis

T2DM is a polygenic disease subject approached by diverse studies using a variety of experimental methods to dissect the molecular basis of T2DM. In Rasche et al. (2008) we conducted a meta-analysis approach merging different heterogeneous data sources for the identification of disease candidate genes. The analysis included transcriptome studies from multiple tissues in mouse and human, genetic information using knock-out mice, text mining as well as signaling protein data.

We computed scores for all genes in each individual study and summarized the scores across the different studies. Thus a basic disease relevance score was established.

Comparing the aggregated scores against a bootstrap background sample defined a cut-off score. Using this threshold, a list of 213 candidate genes was identified. The set of candidate genes was related to different T2DM gene predictions, monogenic mouse models for T2DM and major association studies with considerable overlap. These overlaps showed clearly that gene lists can be generated relying on a single aspect or technology but our meta-analysis rather encompasses a broad range of biomolecular aspects of T2DM. Functional enrichment analyses for KEGG pathways revealed a tight connection with diabetes-specific pathways. However, some genes exhibit a higher interconnection and contribute to an extensive crosstalk between *Insulin signaling, Type II diabetes mellitus* and *PPAR signaling*. Several candidate genes in particular are hubs in the protein interaction networks with many interactions and linking several of the pathways.

With the set of candidate genes we identified biological networks on different layers of cellular information: Signaling and metabolic pathways, gene regulatory networks and protein-protein interaction networks. However, we only provided parts of different networks as separated results. In this study the 213 candidate genes and their respective gene scores are used to identify a subnetwork of the human interactome provided over several functional levels by the ConsensusPathDB.

3. PPI networks

From a mathematical point of view proteins can be described as nodes (vertices) and interactions can be described as undirected links (edges) between interacting proteins. This abstraction allows us to characterize PPI networks by mathematical means. It helps to uncover underlying organizing principles of biological networks, describing the role of proteins in terms of topological parameters. Although computational methods are impaired by incomplete data sets they could be used to point out crucial proteins and structures.

Local topological properties characterize single proteins in a PPI network and may be averaged over all proteins. We give short definitions for the most common topological properties. More detailed descriptions can be found on the website introducing the Network Analyzer plug-in (Assenov et al. 2008). The defined topological parameters are computed in the Cytoscape (Cline et al. 2007) environment using the Network Analyzer plug-in and summary distributions are visualized in fig. 2 and 3.

Degree: The node degree of a node n is equal to the number of nodes that interact with node n.

Neighborhood connectivity: The connectivity of a node n is equal to its node degree. The neighborhood connectivity of a node n is defined as the average node degree of all neighbors of n.

Clustering coefficient: The clustering coefficient is a ratio between the number of edges between the neighbors of n, and the maximum number of edges that could possibly exist between the neighbors of n.

Betweenness centrality: The betweenness centrality of a node n equals the fraction of shortest paths (excluding paths starting or finishing in n) in a network that pass through the node n. A shortest path between two nodes corresponds to the minimal number of edges that has to be traversed in the graph to get from one node to the other.

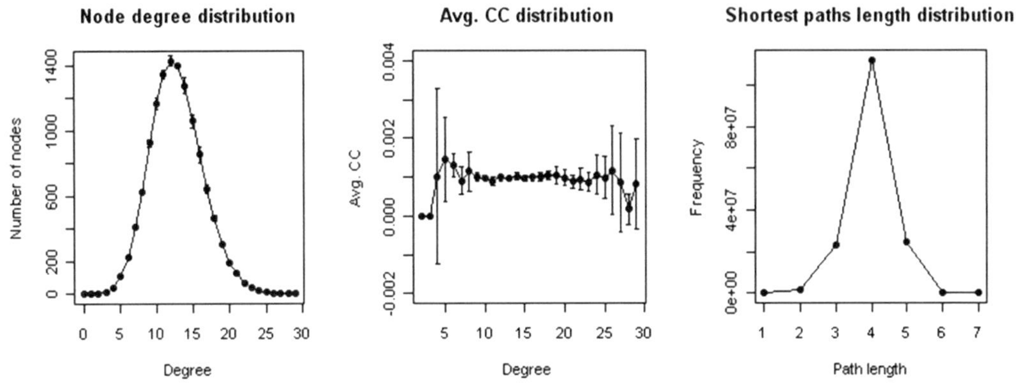

Fig. 2. Topological parameters are computed for five random PPI networks. Initial number of nodes is 12733. The probability for a node being part of the network is 0.01. The computation was done with igraph (Csardi & Nepusz 2006). Abbrv.: CC, clustering coefficient.

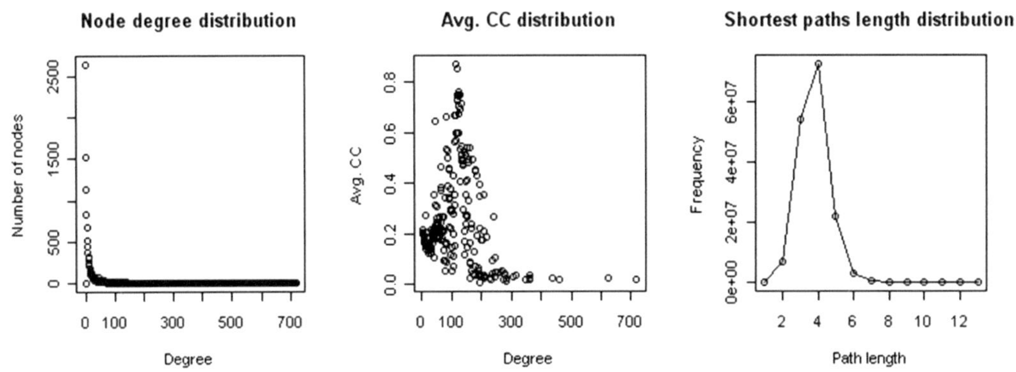

Fig. 3. Topological parameters for the ConsensusPathDB PPI network with 12733 nodes and 101613 undirected interactions

Global network properties emerge from the sum of all local topological properties and follow well-defined organizing principles (Barabási & Oltvai 2004):

Degree distribution: The degree distribution returns the probability that a randomly selected node is connected to *k* other nodes.

Average clustering coefficient distribution: The average clustering coefficient distribution returns the average over the clustering coefficients of all nodes with the same node degree *k*.

Shortest paths distribution: Considering all possible shortest paths in the network, the shortest paths distribution gives for each attained shortest path length the number of node pairs having such a path length.

These graph-theoretical criteria are important to show that biological networks are not comparable with random graphs following the well established Erdős–Rényi model (Erdős & Rényi 1960) since it does not sufficiently capture the wiring principles of PPI networks. In random graphs most nodes have approximately the same number of neighbors. In PPI networks there are only a few highly connected nodes called hubs. Most nodes only have a few neighbors. This property is described by scale-free networks (Barabasi & Albert 1999) whose node degree distribution follows a power-law. Additionally, PPI networks have properties of "small-world" networks (Watts & Strogatz 1998): PPI networks exhibit a high degree of clustering and small path lengths between nodes. Modularity, a high degree of clustering and a degree distribution following a power law account for a hierarchical organization of the PPI network (Ravasz & Barabási 2003).

We build a PPI network from the set of PPIs in the ConsensusPathDB. We map genes to their respective protein identifiers and draw the parameter distributions for all candidate genes as well as for the total set of genes which are part of the PPI network (control). We want to quantify to which extent candidate genes separate from the whole network. Following Xu & Li (2006) we computed:

1N index: The 1N index is the ratio between the number of interactions with candidate genes and the number of all interactions for a given node *n*.

2N index: The 2N index is the average over all 1N indexes for interaction partners of node *n*.

Average distance to candidate genes: The average distance to candidate genes is the average over the shortest paths from a given node *n* to all candidate genes.

Positive topological coefficient: The positive topological coefficient is the average over the number of shared neighbors with any candidate genes.

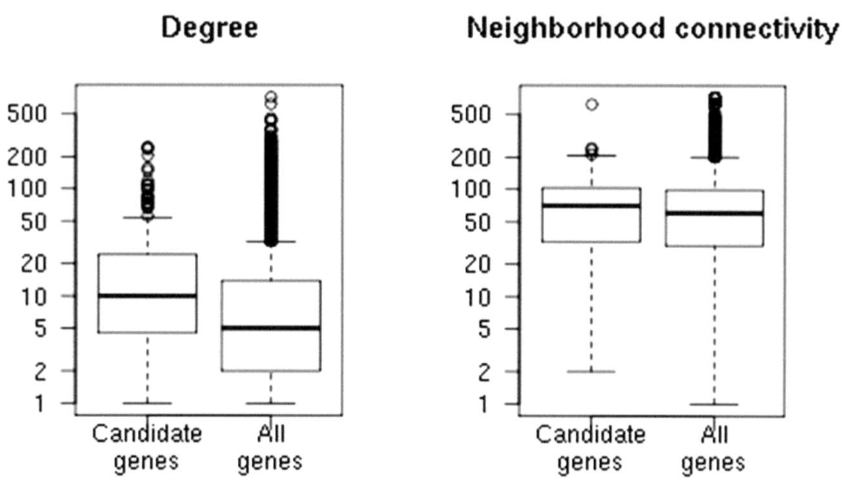

Fig. 4. Degree distributions and neighborhood connectivity distributions for candidate genes and all genes displayed on a log scale.

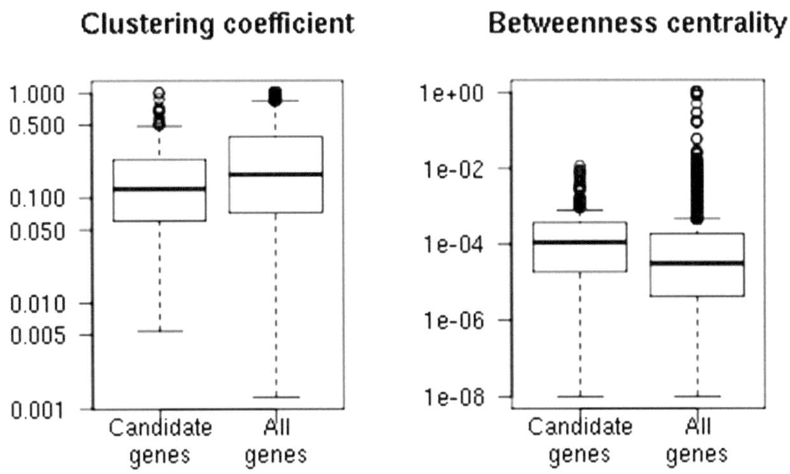

Fig. 5. Clustering coefficient distributions and betweenness centrality distributions for candidate genes and all genes displayed on a log scale.

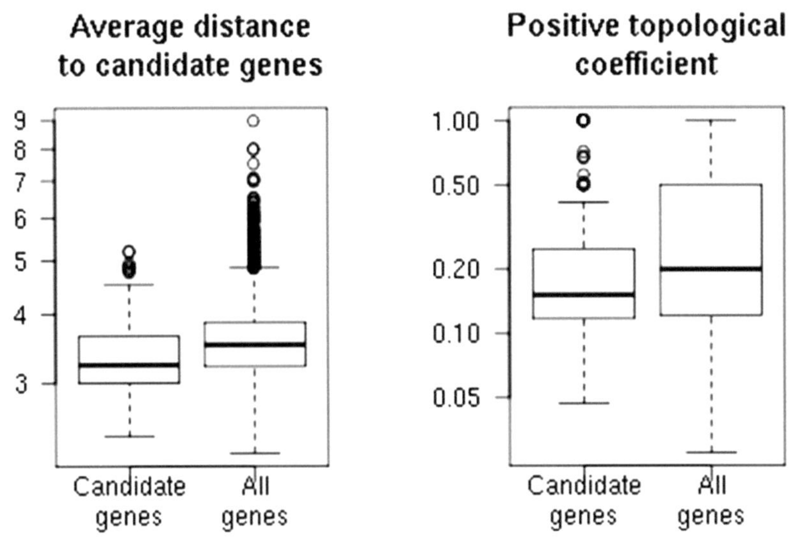

Fig. 6. Average distance to candidate genes distributions and positive topological coefficient distributions for candidate genes and all genes displayed on a log scale.

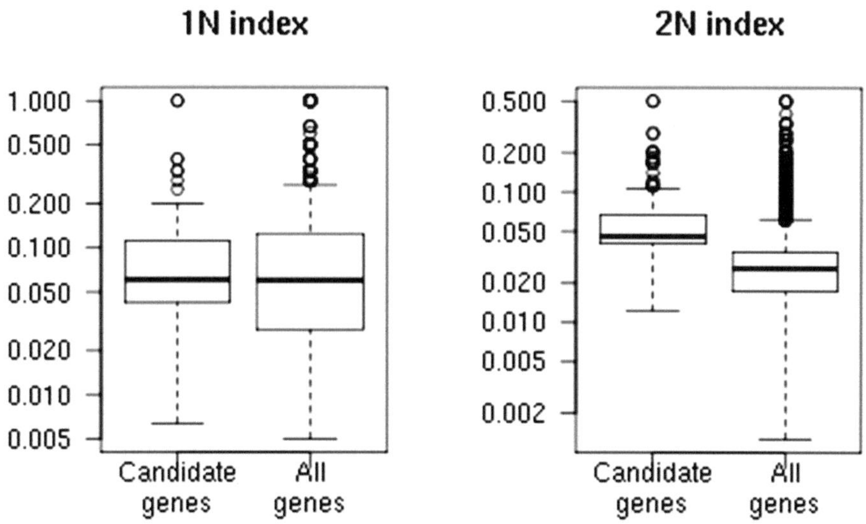

Fig. 7. 1N index distributions and 2N index distributions for candidate genes and all genes displayed on a log scale.

Distributions of the parameters are on display in fig. 4-7. In order to assess the significance of the distributions difference in the means parameter distributions for candidate genes and control we use the Wilcoxon rank sum test; resulting *p*-values are listed in table 1. For the degree, betweenness centrality, 2N index and average distance to candidate genes a significant deviation from the complete PPI network is ascertained.

Parameter	**H0**	**H1**	***p*-value**
Degree	A = B	A > B	2.038e-10
Neighborhood Connectivity	A = B	A > B	0.1103
Clustering coefficient	A = B	A > B	1
Betweenness Centrality	A = B	A > B	2.563e-08
1N index	A = B	A > B	0.1439
2N index	A = B	A > B	< 2.2e-16
Positive topological coefficient	A = B	A > B	0.9999
Average distance to candidate genes	A = B	A < B	3.038e-12

Table 1. Results for Wilcoxon rank sum test: A – distribution for candidate genes, B – distribution for all genes, H0 – null hypothesis, H1 – alternative hypothesis.

4. Functional modules

Proteins that form a local neighbourhood, topological module, and share a biological function can be summarized in a functional module. Following the interpretation that a disease results as a consequence of a disrupted or disturbed functional module, such a module represents the fingerprint of a disease - the disease module (Barabási et al. 2011). The close relationship between topology, functionality and disease relevance demands for algorithms which can decompose the PPI network into distinct subnetworks. We want to identify a subnetwork (module) with high disease relevance.

As interaction data encodes only topological information we need to incorporate biological data which provides information on genes that are for example differentially expressed in the course of a disease and points to irregularities in biological function. Additionally, expression data provides temporal and spatial information. With the set of measured genes or proteins we build a node induced network containing the measured proteins and their interactions.

Finding a subnetwork of high disease relevance was first addressed by Ideker et al. (2002). The solution to the raised problem involves the following two steps: First, nodes in the network are weighted according to some criteria, usually according to their degree of differential expression. Highly differentially expressed nodes are assigned a positive value. Remaining nodes are assigned a negative value. Second, a maximally scoring network is computed.

Mathematically this is equivalent to finding a maximum-weight connected subnetwork. If the graph contains positive and negative weighted nodes finding such MWCS is an NP-hard problem (cannot be computed efficiently) (Ideker et al. 2002). NP-hard problems are often solved with heuristic algorithms. However, heuristic methods cannot guarantee optimal solutions and are highly sensitive to parameter settings. A review over the progress in computational methods for finding functional modules is given by Wu et al. (2009). A major progress was introduced with an algorithm (Dittrich et al. 2008) that computes exact solutions for the MWCS problem in reasonable time. They reformulate the MWCS problem and solve it with techniques from linear programming. Beforehand, a scoring function allows to aggregate *p*-values from several studies. The *p*-value distribution is decomposed into signal and noise modeled by different distributions. A likelihood ratio test computes positive values for highly differentially expressed genes and negative values for moderately or not differentially expressed genes belonging to the background noise. The score functions are provided as an R package (Beisser et al. 2010).

Here, we deviate from the presented approach. Our main objective is to present a functional module whose computation is based on the knowledge from the meta-analysis. Therefore we consider the complete PPI network and assign all candidate genes its scores from the meta-analysis. Non-candidate genes are assigned a negative value. With the algorithm introduced by Dittrich et al. (2008) we compute a functional module. The method reduces the complexity of large networks to biologically relevant modules of interpretable size. Induced by the weighted candidate genes we compute a functional module which points to biological functions that are impaired in T2DM.

The relevance of a module can be checked with gene set enrichments. Here we use an overrepresentation analysis (ORA) with the hypergeometric test as provided for all gene sets in the ConsensusPathDB (Kamburov et al. 2011). Reducing the list to Reactome pathways results in table 2 with an emphasis on inflammation and pyruvate metabolism pathways. Table 2 also shows nicely how candidate genes are complemented by closely related but non-significant genes. This modified set of module genes dissects the Reactome root pathways to closer defined metabolic or signaling entities. The ORA is also applied to the gene ontology (GO) database in table 3. GO is only analysed on level 3 of its hierarchical biological process structure and highlights links between the functional module and several regulatory elements in metabolism. In fig.8 selected overrepresented pathways are highlighted in the functional module.

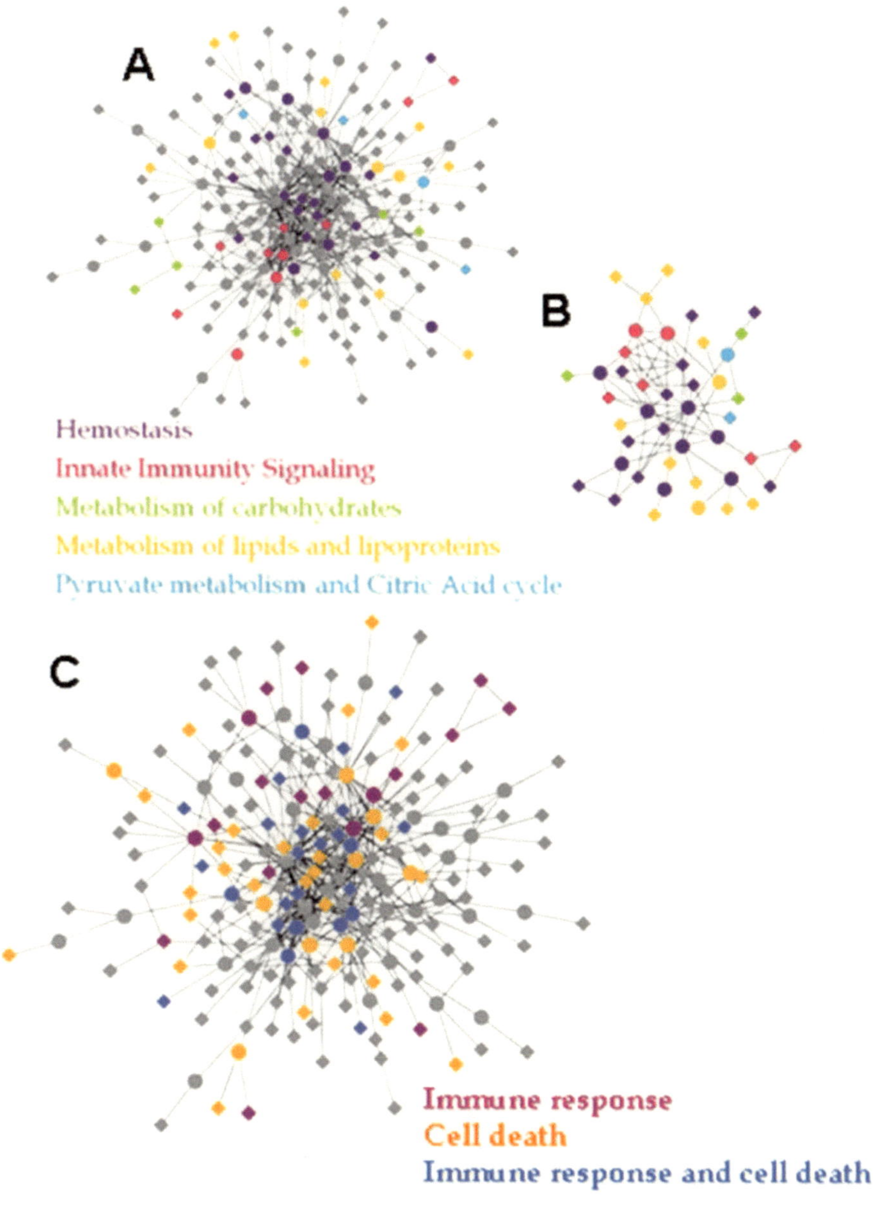

Fig. 8. Reactome interaction network. The concept of a reaction where reactant A is transformed to product B in reaction r1 and reactant B is transformed to product C in reaction r2 is reformulated into a relation where reaction r1 interacts with reaction r2. The relation is directed towards r2 because r2 precedes r1. The resulting reaction network consists of several sub-networks.

In the following we reinterpret the Reactome (Matthews et al. 2009) pathway information and characterize the module by impairment of reactions. Reactome is an expert-authored, peer-reviewed knowledge base. Reactome contains metabolic and signaling pathways. In metabolic pathways, proteins act as enzymes and in signaling pathways proteins are the main components that transfer information through interactions. We identify all reactions whose reactants, products or modifiers (enzymes) are part of the functional module and address them as covered. With the pathway information from Reactome we built a network (fig.9) where nodes represent reactions and edges represent relations between reactions: There is a directed out-going edge from a reaction to all its following reactions annotated in Reactome and there are directed in-coming edges to a reaction from all its preceding reactions. This interpretation may in mathematical terms be seen as a dual graph of the Reactome network. We compute shortest paths between all covered reactions and visualize the results in fig. 10. Nodes (covered reactions and non-covered) lying on these paths are included in the final set of reactions. The initial Reactome network is reduced to those reactions which are impaired in the course of T2DM and those reactions that link impaired reactions. Such a network can guide future research: Which pathways interfere with the proper functioning of other pathways? What is the link between proteins that interact with each other but are involved in different pathways?

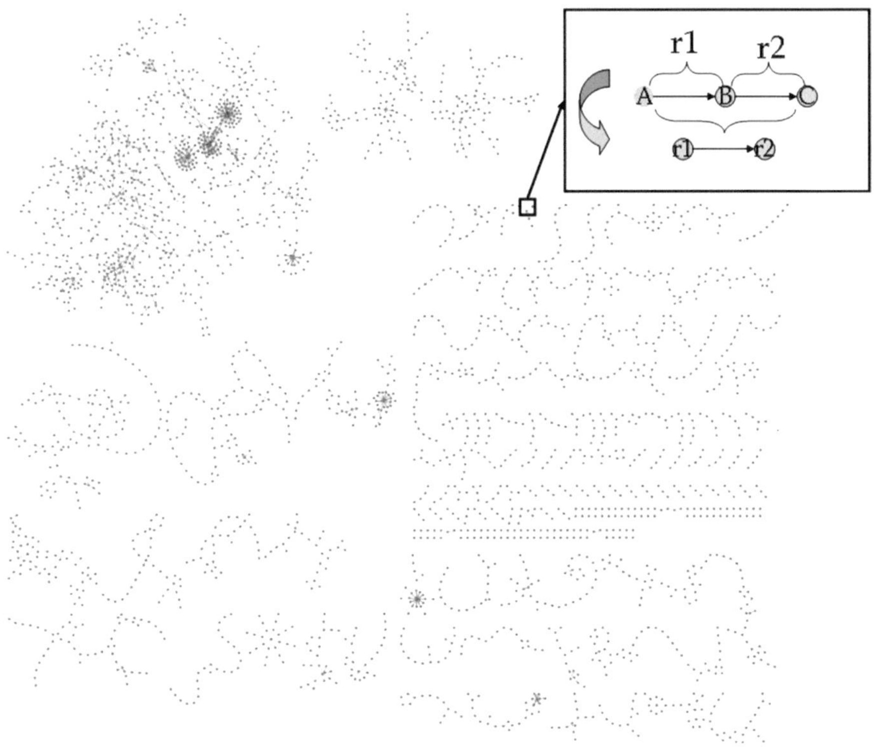

Fig. 9. A) The network shows the functional module where candidate genes are marked with diamonds and over-represented (OR) pathways are colored. B) Nodes in functional module involved in OR pathways tend to interact with each other. (C) Similarly OR GO-terms are colored in the functional module.

p-value	*q*-value	Pathway	Root	All	FM	Gene set
3.3e-5	0.0022	Alternative complement activation	IIS	3	3	C3*, CFB*, CFD*
2.0e-4	0.0087	TRAF6 Mediated Induction of proinflammatory cytokines	IIS	64	9	APP, ATF1, IKBKG, MAPK1*, MAPK9*, NFKB2, NFKBIA*, PPP2R1B, RELA*
3.0e-4	0.0087	NFkB and MAP kinases activation mediated by TLR4 signaling repertoire	IIS	67	9	
4.0e-4	0.0089	TLR3 Cascade	IIS	70	9	APP, ATF1, IKBKG, MAPK1*, MAPK9*, NFKB2, NFKBIA*, PPP2R1B, RELA*
5.0e-4	0.0089	MyD88-independent cascade initiated on plasma membrane	IIS	71	9	
6.0e-4	0.0089	TRAF6 mediated NF-kB activation	IIS	22	5	APP, IKBKG, NFKB2, NFKBIA*, RELA*
6.0e-4	0.0089	TRAF6 mediated induction of NFkB and MAP kinases upon TLR7/8 or 9 activation	IIS	74	9	APP, ATF1, IKBKG, MAPK1*, MAPK9*, NFKB2, NFKBIA*, PPP2R1B, RELA*
7.0e-4	0.0089	MyD88 dependent cascade initiated on endosome	IIS	75	9	APP, ATF1, IKBKG, MAPK1*, MAPK9*, NFKB2, NFKBIA*, PPP2R1B, RELA*
7.0e-4	0.0089	TLR7/8 Cascade	IIS	75	9	
8.0e-4	0.0091	TLR4 Cascade	IIS	90	10	APP, ATF1, CD14*, IKBKG, MAPK1*, MAPK9*, NFKB2, NFKBIA*, PPP2R1B, RELA*
9.0e-4	0.0091	Mitochondrial Fatty Acid Beta-Oxidation	MLL	14	4	ACADL*, HADHB, MCEE*, PCCB
9.0e-4	0.0091	human TAK1 activates NFkB by phosphorylation and activation of IKKs complex	IIS	24	5	APP, IKBKG, NFKB2, NFKBIA*, RELA*
0.0010	0.0091	TLR1, 2, 6, 9 Cascade	IIS	79	9	APP, ATF1, IKBKG, MAPK1*, MAPK9*, NFKB2, NFKBIA*, PPP2R1B, RELA*
0.0018	0.0129	TLR Cascades	IIS	100	10	APP, ATF1, CD14*, IKBKG, MAPK1*, MAPK9*, NFKB2, NFKBIA*, PPP2R1B, RELA*
0.0019	0.0129	Viral dsRNA:TLR3:TRIF Complex Activates RIP1	IIS	28	5	APP, IKBKG, NFKB2, NFKBIA*, RELA*
0.0019	0.0129	Chylomicron-mediated lipid transport	MLL	17	4	APOA1, LDLR*, LPL*, P4HB

p-value	q-value	Pathway	Root	All	FM	Gene set
0.0021	0.0141	Activated TLR4 signalling	IIS	86	9	APP, ATF1, IKBKG, MAPK1*, MAPK9*, NFKB2, NFKBIA*, PPP2R1B, RELA*
0.0022	0.0141	Lipoprotein metabolism	MLL	29	5	APOA1, LDLR*, LPL*, P4HB, PLTP*
0.0043	0.0253	Lipid digestion, mobilization, and transport	MLL	48	6	APOA1, FABP4*, LDLR*, LPL*, P4HB, PLTP*
0.0049	0.0277	Fatty acid, triacylglycerol, and ketone body metabolism	MLL	82	8	ACADL*, ACLY*, ACSL1*, FASN*, HADHB, MCEE*, MED1*, PCCB
0.0060	0.0327	Propionyl-CoA catabolism	MLL	4	2	MCEE*, PCCB
0.0075	0.0377	Advanced glycosylation endproduct receptor signaling	IIS	13	3	APP, LGALS3*, MAPK1*
0.0089	0.0434	Pyruvate metabolism and Citric Acid cycle	PM	40	5	BSG*, DLD, FH*, NNT*, PDK4*
0.0098	0.0458	Beta oxidation of lauroyl-CoA to decanoyl-CoA-CoA	MLL	5	2	ACADL*, HADHB

Table 2. Pathway over-representation analysis for proteins contained in the functional module, restricted to root level pathways IIS, MLL and PM. The table lists Reactome pathways in which proteins of our functional module are enriched. All: Number of proteins represented in the specified pathway. FM: Number of proteins represented in the specified pathway and contained in the functional module. Root: Specifies the root pathway as defined by Reactome for the given pathway (IIS – Innate Immunity Signaling, MLL – Metabolism of lipids and lipoproteins and PM – Pyruvate metabolism and Citric Acid (TCA) cycle). Candidate genes are succeded by a star in the last column.

5. Discussion

Many applications have been developed based on the analyses of topological network properties which provide insights into the evolution, function, stability and dynamic responses of PPI networks (Albert 2005). Deciphering the wiring scheme and determining topological properties of individual nodes could help to derive protein function and formulate predictions about disease involvement. Special attention is drawn towards highly connected nodes whose removal has serious, or even lethal, consequence for the network. Highly connected nodes are probably evolutionarily conserved or encoded by essential genes (Goh et al. 2007). There is evidence that in literature-curated PPI networks disease genes share common topological characteristics which differ from non-disease genes: Hereditary disease genes selected from OMIM (Hamosh et al. 2005) have a larger degree, the tendency to interact with each other, more common neighbors and fast communication to other disease genes (Xu & Li 2006).

The tendency of proteins involved in the same disease to interact with each other can be traced to the chromosome level (Oti et al. 2006). Genes that interact with known disease genes have a higher likelihood of being also disease relevant. In summary, network analysis reveals properties of potential disease genes. There are good reasons to assume that disease genes are not randomly placed in the interactome.

The meta-analysis is a valuable method for ranking genes according to their disease relevance. In a follow-up step we put the candidate genes from Rasche et al. into a functional context. We took advantage of PPI data in two ways: First, we characterized disease genes with respect to their topological parameters. Second, we applied an algorithm that channels all available PPIs into a sub-network. This subnetwork seems to contain relevant information about the underlying biological functions impaired in T2DM. The topological characterization of candidate genes reveals properties which distinguish them from the complete set genes: Compared to the complete set of candidate genes have higher node degrees (fig. 4), higher betweenness centrality coefficients (fig. 5), higher 2N indices (fig. 7) and shorter average distances to other candidate genes (fig. 6). The ten candidate genes with highest degree are: PIK3R1 (246), ACTB (244), RELA (236), MAPK1 (206), EIF4A2 (157), YBX1 (148), NFKBIA (119), TNFRSF1B (110) and B2M (108). These genes are well described in the literature. They are associated with different diseases. Although there is a relation between node degree and disease relevance we have to consider a bias towards genes where disease relevance and connectivity is established. The meta-analysis also identifies genes with a small node degree as relevant for T2DM: ACSL1, AKR1B10, AOX1, CCNI, GATM, GPD2, GPX2, LGMN, LRP10, NNT, P4HA1, RETN, SLC38A2, TMSB4X, YIPF5 and ZSCAN21 (all with node degree of one).

Candidate genes exhibit higher betweenness centrality coefficients. Candidate genes with highest betweenness centrality coefficients are: ACTB (0.011), PIK3R1 (0.009), MAPK1 (0.008), RELA (0.007), B2M (0.005), HSPA5 (0.004), DYNLL1 (0.003), C1QBP (0.003), TNFRSF1B (0.003) and NFKBIA (0.003). Nodes with a high betweenness centrality coefficient are termed bottlenecks (Yu et al. 2007). Many shortest paths pass through a node with high betweenness centrality coefficient; a perturbation in a node with high betweenness centrality coefficient easily deranges the rest of the network. Betweenness centrality better accounts for the prediction of node's essentiality in the network than the node degree. A perturbation in a node with a high degree which lies in the outer part of the network probably has less severe consequences than a node which lies more central in the network. Candidate genes do not differ in clustering coefficient and neighbourhood connectivity from the set of all genes. Direct neighbors of candidate genes are not more likely also candidate genes (1N index). However, the 2N index for candidate genes is higher than for non-candidate genes: Neighbors of neighbors of candidate genes are more likely also candidate genes. These results indicate that T2DM involves several impaired biological functions. A higher 1N index for candidate genes would suggest that a single biological function is perturbed. Related to the higher 2N index for candidate genes is the smaller average shortest paths length from a candidate gene to all other candidate genes. Topological parameters may not isolate disease genes if they are individually considered. But in this study they indicate that candidate genes link several biological processes as shown by the high betweenness centrality and the high 2N index.

p-value	*q*-value	Term name	All	FM
1.7e-39	1.1e-36	response to organic substance	1072	65
5.4e-30	1.7e-27	regulation of cell death	1115	49
3.2e-29	6.7e-27	positive regulation of biological process	2465	79
9.4e-29	1.5e-26	regulation of response to stimulus	648	40
1.4e-27	1.7e-25	regulation of immune system process	545	38
3.0e-27	3.1e-25	regulation of immune response	319	30
2.1e-26	1.9e-24	response to inorganic substance	316	33
3.3e-24	2.6e-22	programmed cell death	1321	59
4.8e-24	3.3e-22	response to drug	341	33
1.7e-23	1.1e-21	positive regulation of immune response	214	22
2.7e-23	1.6e-21	response to molecule of bacterial origin	187	22
7.9e-23	4.1e-21	response to hormone stimulus	580	43
2.5e-22	1.2e-20	negative regulation of cell death	548	39
4.4e-22	2.0e-20	cell differentiation	1899	67
1.7e-21	7.0 e-20	positive regulation of macromolecule metabolic process	1109	45
1.8e-21	7.0e-20	negative regulation of biological process	2193	76
2.5e-21	9.2e-20	regulation of developmental process	942	44
3.4e-21	1.2e-19	organ development	2026	71
7.2e-21	2.4e-19	system development	2622	81
1.0e-20	3.2e-19	antigen processing and presentation via MHC class Ib	16	3
1.9e-20	5.7e-19	adaptive immune response	166	20
4.7e-19	1.3e-17	antigen processing and presentation of exogenous antigen	19	4
8.3e-19	2.3e-17	regulation of cellular process	5922	126
1.2e-18	3.2e-17	positive regulation of cell death	613	27
3.1e-18	7.7e-17	positive regulation of cellular metabolic process	1141	44
1.8e-17	4.4e-16	protein complex assembly	681	42
2.0e-17	4.7e-16	T cell mediated cytotoxicity	29	7
2.7e-17	5.9e-16	immune effector process	269	27
3.4e-16	7.4e-15	positive regulation of biosynthetic process	875	35
3.9e-16	8.0e-15	cellular response to chemical stimulus	547	36
5.0e-16	9.8e-15	macromolecular complex assembly	853	45
5.0e-16	9.8e-15	positive regulation of immune effector process	72	14

Table 3. GO term over-representation analysis (terms downstream to term *biological process* level 3) for genes in the functional module.

Next, we identified a sub-network in the complete PPI network with enrichment in candidate genes. The algorithm used was proposed by Dittrich et al. for the computation of functional modules. Candidate genes were weighted with their meta-analysis score and the remaining nodes in the network with a negative score. A pathway over-representation analysis points to the pathways *Hemostasis, Innate immunity signaling, Pyruvate metabolism and citric acid cycle, Metabolism of lipids and lipoproteins and Metabolism of carbohydrates.* Our results confirm a known relation between inflammation and metabolic disorders (Hotamisligil 2006). The link between metabolism and immune response pathways can be retraced to common ancestral structures (Hotamisligil 2006). The Toll-like receptor (TLR) pathway comprises elements which regulate metabolic and immune functions. TLR4, receptor for bacterial LPS and component of innate immune system acts as a sensor for free fatty acids (Shi et al. 2006). Free fatty acids are increased in obesity and are a probable link to lipid-induced insulin resistance. The functional module contains genes (RELA, NFKBIA, NFKB2, ATF1, MAPK1, IKBKG, MAPK9) which are activated downstream to TLR4 (Akira & Takeda 2004). Analysis of the functional module also reveals a link to platelet dysfunction (Vinik et al. 2001).

Over-representation analysis for GO terms with root node biological function reveals terms lying downstream to cell death and immune response. Pathway and GO terms analysis suggests and supports the strong link between inflammation and T2DM. We extended this knowledge by annotated pathways, e.g. by introducing the notion of covered reactions. A covered reaction involves a protein from the functional module, either as enzyme, reactant or product. We suppose that an impaired covered reaction may have a negative influence on the network.

Using the PPI network, a list of candidate genes could be characterized according to distributions of topological parameters, especially in comparison to the full set of PPI. At the current stage of knowledge we can only use a static PPI graph, since the complete graph is unknown. We assume that we already have a representative subset of PPIs in the databases. We pointed out that known PPIs reflect only static, sometimes artificial, settings. In these settings interactions depend on many factors and thus proteins may only interact under certain circumstances. To overcome some of these constraints the candidate genes are extended to a functional module using the MWCS method. Genes lacking interaction information are skipped and only non-candidate genes which are directly linked and are in direct proximity to candidates are included in the module. The functional module genes are related to functional entities by applying ORA to Reactome and GO gene sets. These databases cover far less genes than PPI networks but with much more detailed descriptions about the purpose of the genes within a biological context. Module genes are related to the discussed functional entities which shows that current knowledge is well incorporated in the functional module. Furthermore, Reactome was also the basis for a modified description of its functional content with the notation of covered reactions. This is a possible way of identifying several pathways which interact in a direct or indirect manner. In the case of the functional module it elucidates how over-represented pathways are linked in T2DM and which module genes possibly modulate this link.

6. Conclusion

Results of a single-gene meta-analysis are combined with methods from network biology. We have to keep in mind that PPI networks are not static but are modified for changing cellular states. In the long term it does not suffice to consider topological properties alone. We have to elaborate on an understanding of the dynamics of PPIs. Different conditions influence structural rearrangements in the cell which we need to measure and depict. Computation of functional modules is an attempt of including additional levels to the interaction data. We see overlapping functions rather than a clear division in single biological sections.

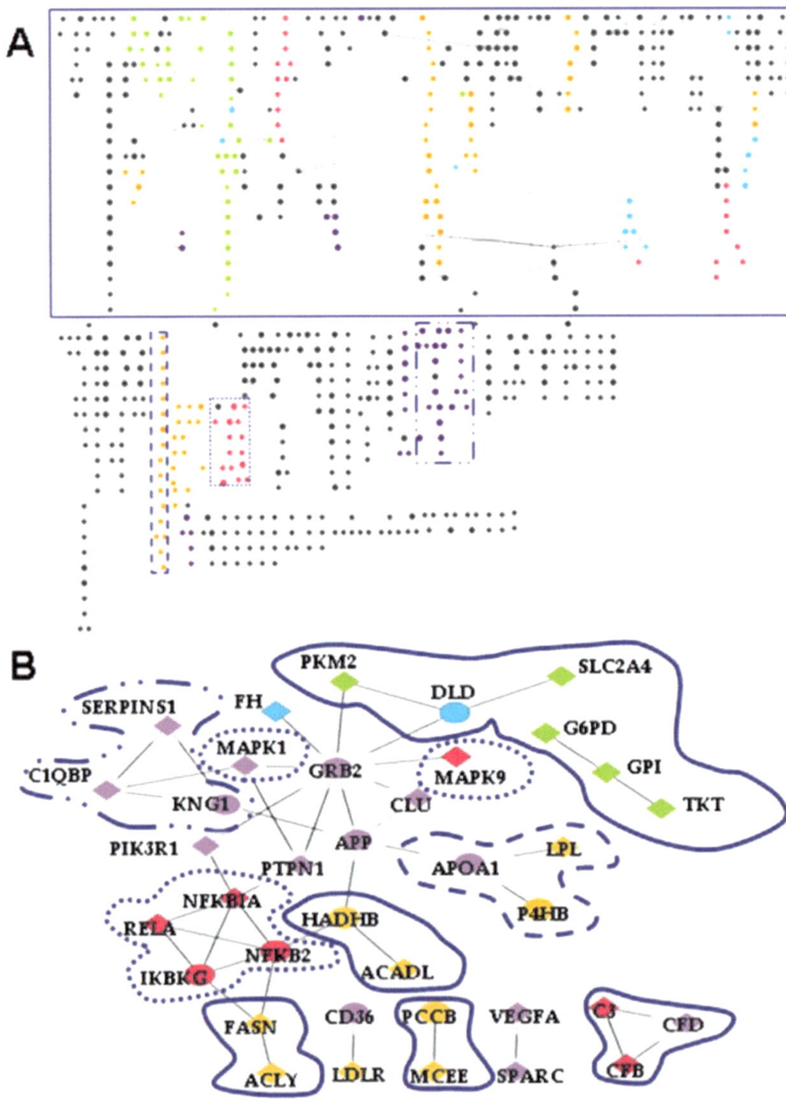

Fig. 10. A) Hierarchical view of shortest paths between all covered reactions. A covered reaction is shown as diamond, non-covered reaction as circle, non-covered reactions connect covered reactions. Over-represented pathways in the functional module are highlighted according to the color scheme in fig. 9. B) Genes from the functional module which are involved in a covered reaction. Frames with different line types in A) and B) elucidate how the functional module connects different pathways.

7. Acknowledgements

We want to acknowledge Atanas Kamburov who is the lead developer of the Consensus-PathDB and Dr. Ralf Herwig for initiating the topic, study design and funding. The work was partly funded by the European Union under its 6th Framework Programme with the grant SysProt (LSHG-CT-2006-037457) and the BMBF NGFN-transfer project (01GR0809).

8. References

Akira, S. & K. Takeda (2004). Toll-like receptor signalling. Nat Rev Immunol 4(7): 499-511.

Albert, R. (2005). Scale-free networks in cell biology. J Cell Sci 118(Pt 21): 4947-4957.

Ashburner, M., C. A. Ball, J. A. Blake, et al. (2000). Gene ontology: tool for the unification of biology. The Gene Ontology Consortium. Nat Genet 25(1): 25-29.

Assenov, Y., F. Ramírez, S.-E. Schelhorn, et al. (2008). Computing topological parameters of biological networks. Bioinformatics 24(2): 282-284.

Barabasi & Albert (1999). Emergence of scaling in random networks. Science 286(5439): 509-512.

Barabási, A.-L., N. Gulbahce & J. Loscalzo (2011). Network medicine: a network-based approach to human disease. Nat Rev Genet 12(1): 56-68.

Barabási, A.-L. & Z. N. Oltvai (2004). Network biology: understanding the cell's functional organization. Nat Rev Genet 5(2): 101-113.

Beisser, D., G. W. Klau, T. Dandekar, et al. (2010). BioNet: an R-Package for the functional analysis of biological networks. Bioinformatics 26(8): 1129-1130.

Cline, M. S., M. Smoot, E. Cerami, et al. (2007). Integration of biological networks and gene expression data using Cytoscape. Nat Protoc 2(10): 2366-2382.

Csardi, G. & T. Nepusz (2006). The igraph Software Package for Complex Network Research. InterJournal Complex Systems: 1695.

Dittrich, M. T., G. W. Klau, A. Rosenwald, et al. (2008). Identifying functional modules in protein-protein interaction networks: an integrated exact approach. Bioinformatics 24(13): i223-i231.

Erdos, P. & A. Renyi (1960). On the evolution of random graphs. Publ. Math. Inst. Hung. Acad. Sci 5: 17-61.

Fields, S. & R. Sternglanz (1994). The two-hybrid system: an assay for protein-protein interactions. Trends Genet 10(8): 286-292.

Goh, K.-I., M. E. Cusick, D. Valle, et al. (2007). The human disease network. Proc Natl Acad Sci U S A 104(21): 8685-8690.

Hamosh, A., A. F. Scott, J. S. Amberger, et al. (2005). Online Mendelian Inheritance in Man (OMIM), a knowledgebase of human genes and genetic disorders. Nucleic Acids Res 33(Database issue): D514-D517.

Hotamisligil, G. S. (2006). Inflammation and metabolic disorders. Nature 444(7121): 860-867.

Ideker, T., O. Ozier, B. Schwikowski, et al. (2002). Discovering regulatory and signalling circuits in molecular interaction networks. Bioinformatics 18 Suppl 1: S233-S240.

Kamburov, A., K. Pentchev, H. Galicka, et al. (2011). ConsensusPathDB: toward a more complete picture of cell biology. Nucleic Acids Res 39(Database issue): D712-D717.

Kamburov, A., C. Wierling, H. Lehrach, et al. (2009). ConsensusPathDB--a database for integrating human functional interaction networks. Nucleic Acids Res 37(Database issue): D623-D628.

Matthews, L., G. Gopinath, M. Gillespie, et al. (2009). Reactome knowledgebase of human biological pathways and processes. Nucleic Acids Res 37(Database issue): D619-D622.

Oti, M., B. Snel, M. A. Huynen, et al. (2006). Predicting disease genes using protein-protein interactions. J Med Genet 43(8): 691-698.

Pandey, A. & M. Mann (2000). Proteomics to study genes and genomes. Nature 405(6788): 837-846.

Rasche, A., H. Al-Hasani & R. Herwig (2008). Meta-analysis approach identifies candidate genes and associated molecular networks for type-2 diabetes mellitus. BMC Genomics 9: 310.

Ravasz, E. & A.-L. Barabási (2003). Hierarchical organization in complex networks. Phys Rev E Stat Nonlin Soft Matter Phys 67(2 Pt 2): 026112.

Shi, H., M. V. Kokoeva, K. Inouye, et al. (2006). TLR4 links innate immunity and fatty acid-induced insulin resistance. J Clin Invest 116(11): 3015-3025.

Vinik, A. I., T. Erbas, T. S. Park, et al. (2001). Platelet dysfunction in type 2 diabetes. Diabetes Care 24(8): 1476-1485.

Watts, D. J. & S. H. Strogatz (1998). Collective dynamics of 'small-world' networks. Nature 393(6684): 440-442.

Wu, Z., X. Zhao & L. Chen (2009). Identifying responsive functional modules from protein-protein interaction network. Molecules and Cells 27(3): 271-277.

Xu, J. & Y. Li (2006). Discovering disease-genes by topological features in human protein-protein interaction network. Bioinformatics 22(22): 2800-2805.

Yu, H., P. M. Kim, E. Sprecher, et al. (2007). The importance of bottlenecks in protein networks: correlation with gene essentiality and expression dynamics. PLoS Comput Biol 3(4): e59.

Part 4

Complications of Type 2 Diabetes

12

Sarcopenia, Sarcopenic Obesity and Insulin Resistance

John A. Batsis[1] and Silvio Buscemi[2]
[1]*Dartmouth Medical School, Dartmouth-Hitchcock Medical Center*
[2]*University of Palermo, Departmentof Internal Medicine, Cardiovascular and Kidney Diseases*
[1]*United States*
[2]*Italy*

1. Introduction

The number of people greater than 65 years old will increase from 35.9 million in 2003 (12.4%) to 71.5 million (20%) by the year 2030. Current estimates in the United States demonstrate that this population is numbered at 39.6million, representing 12.6% of the population, or one in every eight Americans. Women tend to outnumber men and their life expectancy is undoubtedly longer. These numbers reflect predominantly the influx of baby boomers into this age group (Spillman and Lubitz 2000).

Since the early part of 1900, the elderly age group has nearly tripled from 4.1% in 1900 to 12.9% in 2009, and the number of individuals has increased over thirteen times (from 3.1 to 39.6 million). The 'old old', persons aged >80 are one of the fastest growing segments of the population (A Profile of Older Americans 2010). In addition, life expectancy in the elderly has been increasing in the past few decades and continues to do so (Lubitz et al. 2003). For instance, those reaching the age of 65 years, had a mean life expectancy of 19.9 and 17.2 years, respectively, for females and males. Framed alternatively, life expectancy at birth in 2007 was 77.9 years, approximately 30 years longer than a child born in 1900. Compounded with a reduced death rate due to medical advances, patients are living longer than they previously were, much of this due to improved survival from cardiovascular and cerebrovascular diseases (Ford et al. 2007). Figure #1 demonstrates data on the aging population in the United States, and Figure #2 demonstrates estimates from worldwide figures.

In a report published by the Organisation for Economic Co-operation and Development (OECD) in 2007, these trends observed in the United States are paralleled elsewhere. In certain countries, specifically Italy and Japan, one out of every five people is aged 65+ (Trends in Severe Disability Among Elderly People: Assessing the Evidence in 12 OECD Countries and the Future Implications 2007). As in the United States, Table #1 illustrates the proportion of people that will be 85+, which is the fastest growing segment of the population. Understandably these are worrisome trends as these individuals are, from a public health standpoint, the ones with the most number of chronic conditions, disabilities and greatest long-term care needs. It is believed that unless there are significant improvements in functional awareness and improvement, this group poses the largest burden on existing healthcare resources.

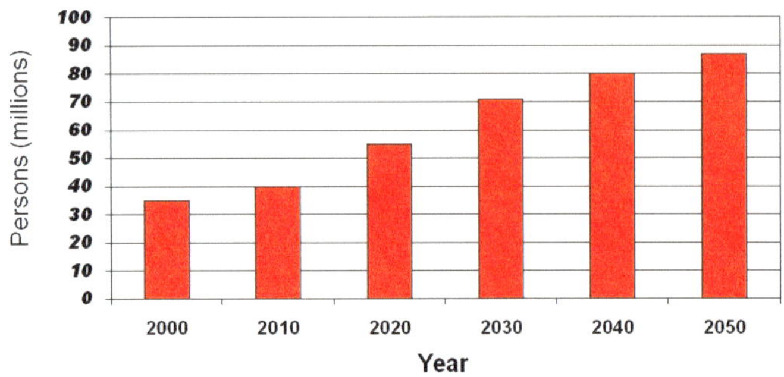

Data obtained from the US Census Bureau from the year 2000. *www.census.gov*

Fig. 1. Projected Elderly Population of the United States: 2000-2050

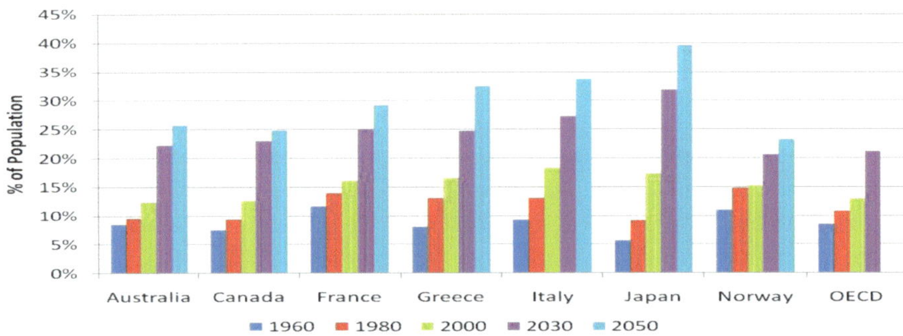

Fig. 2. Population in OECD Countries of Elderly >65 years old. Proportion of People >65 years old in a sample of Organisation for Economic Co-operation and Development (OECD) countries from 1960 to projects at 2050. Lafortune, G. and G. Balestat (2007), "Trends in Severe Disability Among Elderly People: Assessing the Evidence in 12 OECD Countries and the Future Implications", OECD Health Working Papers, No. 26, http://dx.doi.org/10.1787/217072070078

Country	1960	1980	2000	2030	2050
Australia	0.4	0.7	1.3	3.2	5.7
Canada	0.4	0.8	1.3	2.7	5.8
France	0.7	1.1	2.1	3.8	7.6
Greece	0.4	0.9	1.3	2.9	4.9
Italy	0.5	0.8	2.1	4.7	7.9
Japan	0.2	0.5	1.8	7.4	10.2
Norway	0.7	1.1	1.9	2.6	4.5
OECD	0.4	0.7	1.4	3.0	5.2

Table 1. Proportion of Patients Aged >85 years in OECD Countries. All numbers in the table above are percentages Lafortune, G. and G. Balestat (2007), "Trends in Severe Disability Among Elderly People: Assessing the Evidence in 12 OECD Countries and the Future Implications", OECD Health Working Papers, No. 26, http://dx.doi.org/10.1787/217072070078

2. Health needs as one gets older

As patients age, health needs escalate, resulting in disproportionate consumption of health care resources (Lakdawalla, Goldman, and Shang 2005). According to a 1995 US Bureau of Census publication, approximately 80% of >65 year olds will have a minimum of one chronic medical illness, with many suffering multiple. A number of elderly subjects report a type of disability, including hearing impairment, visual impairment, cognitive impairment, self-care troubles, or needing higher level of care. A number of studies have demonstrated the impact of aging on disability. An early study by Vita et al (Vita et al. 1998) studied 1,741 university alumni, first surveyed in 1962 (mean age 43 years) and then annually in 1986. Cumulative disability was determined using a health-assessment questionnaire. Those with high health risks at baseline had earlier onset of disability and had a lower follow-up disability index. The onset of disability was postponed by more than 5 years in the low-risk subject group than those with high risk behaviors. Predictors of subsequent disability included smoking, body mass index and exercise patterns in midlife and late-adulthood. These authors concluded that although disability is inevitable, the time frame was compressed into fewer years at the end of life.

In one study the number of geriatric conditions was related to dependency in activities of daily living (Cigolle et al. 2007). These authors used data from the Health and Retirement study survey administered in 2000 on subjects >65 years (n=11,093) residing either in the community or in nursing homes, and assessed the number of geriatric syndromes and dependency of activities of daily living (ADL)s. Of those >65 years, ~49.9% had at least one geriatric syndrome, prevalence rates that were as common as heart disease and diabetes. After adjusting for demographic characteristics and chronic diseases, the risk ratio for dependence on ADLs were 2.1 [95%CI: 1.9-2.4] for one geriatric condition, 3.6 [3.1-4.1] for two conditions, and 6.6 [5.6-7.6] for greater than 3 conditions. This important study highlights the similar prevalences of geriatric conditions to chronic diseases in elderly adults and their strong association to disability. As the authors note, these are often overlooked in the care of older adults. One's reported disability increases with age. In a study by the Administration on Aging in the United States, approximately 56% of persons >80years reported a severe disability and 29% reported the need for some type of assistance (A Profile of Older Americans 2010). This is of course impairs one self-reported health status and may lead to institutionalization.

3. Muscle changes with aging – Sarcopenia

As one ages, there are changes in body composition. As patients age, there is a reduction in lean mass and a progressive increase in fat mass. This normally occurs after the age of 20-30 years and can be extensive, involving up to 40% of a population (Baumgartner et al. 1995; Flynn et al. 1989; Gallagher et al. 1997; Muller et al. 1996). As is demonstrated in Figure #3, maximal fat free mass (muscle mass) is usually reached at about 20 years of age and fat mass peaks at the ages between 60 and 70 years (Baumgartner et al. 1995; Gallagher et al. 1997). Particularly after the age of 70 years, there is a redistribution of body fat and fat free mass, with reductions in peripheral skeletal muscle (Beaufrere and Morio 2000), increases in intramuscular and intrahepatic fat, both of which are associated with insulin resistance (Cree et al. 2004).

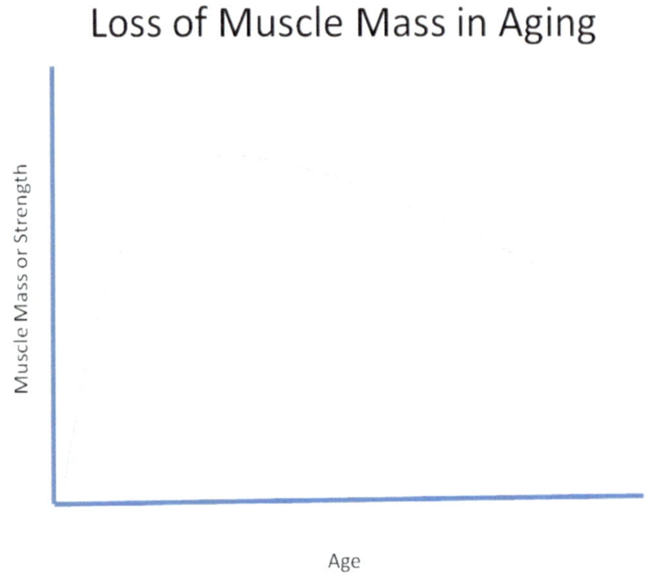

Fig. 3. Muscle Mass Changes with Aging.
Peak muscle mass occurs between the ages of 20 and 30 years, and naturally declines as one ages.

Declining function parallels the concept of sarcopenia. Sarcopenia comes from the Greek word, "Sarcos" meaning flesh, and 'penia' meaning lack of. This age-related decline in lean body mass can affect ambulation, mobility, and functional independence (Morley et al. 2001). An analogy often used is the age-related decline in bone mass, where, once it reaches a critical level, one's risk of fracture is increased. Sarcopenia can be conceptualized on the spectrum of frailty and disability and has been shown to be increasingly prevalent with age. More recently, the concept of declining strength has been incorporated into the definition, although, a widely accepted definition of sarcopenia has yet to be established (Cruz-Jentoft et al. 2010)). Sarcopenia indeed can be considered a geriatric syndrome. These are common, complex and costly entities of impaired health in elderly individuals which involve multiple systems, have a myriad of interactions, and have varied phenotypes. Falls, urinary incontinence and delirium are but some examples of such. Sarcopenia has also been associated with malnutrition and diminished physical function, both of which are associated with geriatric functional decline and mortality. The loss of muscle mass during the aging process is important clinically as it reduces strength and exercise capacity, both which are needed to perform one's activity of daily living. It is hypothesized that subjects reach a given threshold at which impairment in function occurs. Absolute loss of muscle mass leads to reduced muscle function and hence physical performance measures are increasingly being used in the definition and identification of sarcopenia. There are a number of definitions outlined in the literature making standardization, particularly in clinical practice, rather difficult (Baumgartner et al. 1998; Bouchard, Dionne, and Brochu 2009; Davison et al. 2002; Zoico et al. 2004) . Prevalence rates can vary dramatically and is the subject of current investigation. This syndrome has a number of risk factors, a number that are modifiable over the course of one's life span, but can have profound impact on one's overall state of health and quality of life.

The trajectory of one's muscle loss can be altered by physical exercise and/or the environment. Muscle mass develops up to the age of 20 and 30 years, and is relatively maintained throughout adult life. As one ages, muscle mass decreases and one reaches a threshold whereby low muscle mass will inevitably lead to disability and future complications (Sayer et al. 2008).

Assessing sarcopenia has been a challenge in the research literature. There are a number of definitions that have been proposed, yet they have been developed on different populations and ethnicities, factors which are known to affect body composition. Additionally, muscle quality and strength have yet to be incorporated into such definitions. Recently, there was a European consensus on the definition and diagnosis on Sarcopenia (Cruz-Jentoft et al. 2011). This taskforce suggested the use of both low muscle mass and low muscle function (strength or performance) for the diagnosis of sarcopenia. The rationale for using these criteria include that muscle mass and muscle strength are not directly correlated to each other (Goodpaster et al. 2006; Janssen et al. 2004). DEXA scanning is unique in that it not only allows ascertainment of muscle mass but can be used concurrently to assess bone density as well. Bioelectrical impedance on the other hand is inexpensive, and easily reproducible with prediction equations available to calculate various measures of body composition (Chumlea et al. 2002) and has been considered as a portable alternative to DEXA. Body water can affect these results, though, and elders' changes in body composition, both in health and disease, may affect such estimates. Unfortunately, the relative availability and cost of DEXA in particular can be prohibitively expensive, not portable, and would be impractical to use for routine use in an office setting (Chien, Kuo, and Wu 2010). Other measures, including grip strength, knee strength, or gait speed have been proposed but no studies have validated such measures.

Figure #4 (Cruz-Jentoft et al. 2011) illustrates the proposed mechanisms of sarcopenia. These vary over one's lifespan and are impacted by each other, with interactions that are poorly understood.

4. Aging and obesity

Along with the rise in the number of elderly patients, the number of patients diagnosed with overweight and obesity are increasing. Obesity is defined by the World Health Organization (WHO) as a body mass index (BMI) greater than or equal to over 30kg/m^2, calculated as the body weight in kilograms divided by the height in meters squared (Quetelet 1871). Little attention has been given to the obese elder, largely due to a paucity of studies including elderly (>65 years old) patients. Yet, current estimates, specifically in the United States population, indicate that the prevalence of obesity continues to rise, and exceeds 35% of the general population, a trend that is also observed in elderly subjects. The prevalence of obesity has increased almost three-fold from 1960-2008, and continues to rise at a frightening rate (Flegal et al. 2011). Latest estimates illustrate by using body mass index as a surrogate for obesity estimates, that 33.6% of women and 37.1% of males are classified as having obesity over the age of 60years (Flegal et al. 2010). These numbers are remarkably higher than estimates in 1999 whereby 31.8% of males were obese, yet prevalence estimates seem to be similar in females. However, trends demonstrate rises in prevalence rates, in particular subjects with morbid obesity (BMI >40kg/m^2). Figure #5 illustrates these trends.

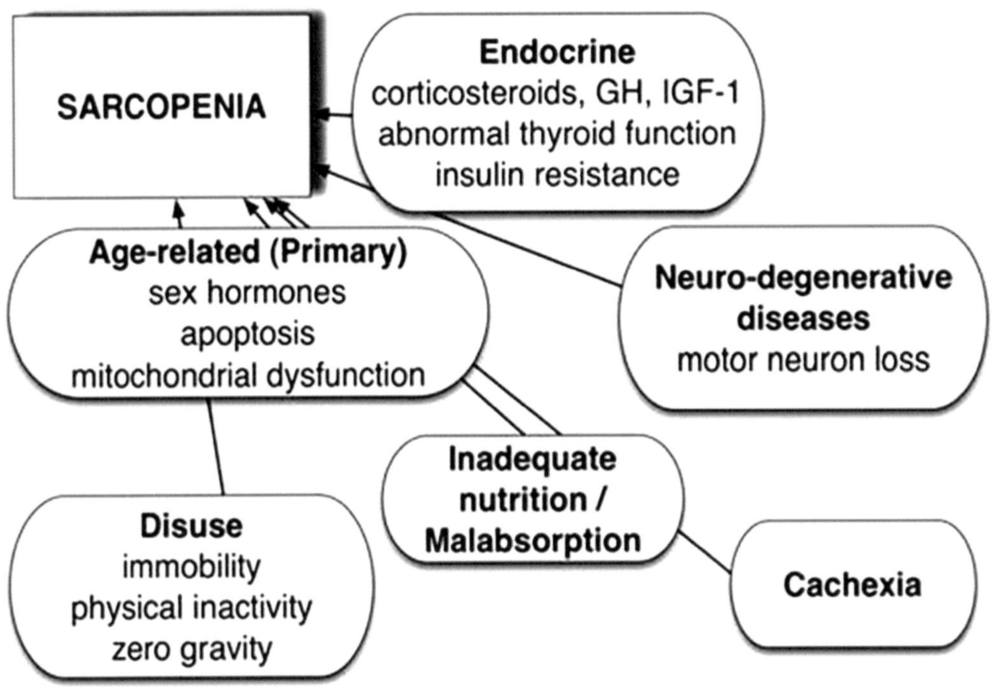

Fig. 4. Mechanisms of Sarcopenia. The Sarcopenia taskforce did conclude the importance of identifying such mechanisms to better understand the underlying pathophysiology, and to allow the identifications of interventions these targets.

Obesity is associated with an increased number of medical conditions and complications, and is a recognized independent cardiovascular risk factor. Obesity is associated with an increased risk of both physical and cognitive disability (Beydoun, Beydoun, and Wang 2008; Jensen 2005). Houston et al used data from the Health, Aging and Body Composition Study in looking the association between overweight and/or obesity in young, middle, and late adulthood and its cumulative effect on incident mobility limitation in 2,845 community dwelling US adults (Houston et al. 2009). The authors identified mobility limitations as difficulty walking ¼ mile or climbing 10 steps over a 7-year of follow-up. Men and women who were overweight or obese at all three time points had increased risk of mobility limitations compared to normal weights (HR 1.61 [1.25-2.06], and 2.85 [2.15-3.78]. There appeared to be a graded response ($P<0.001$) on risk of mobility limitations on the cumulative effect of obesity in men and women. Earlier onset of obesity in life contributed to increased mobility limitations of old age (Houston et al. 2009). This is also observed in Figure #6.

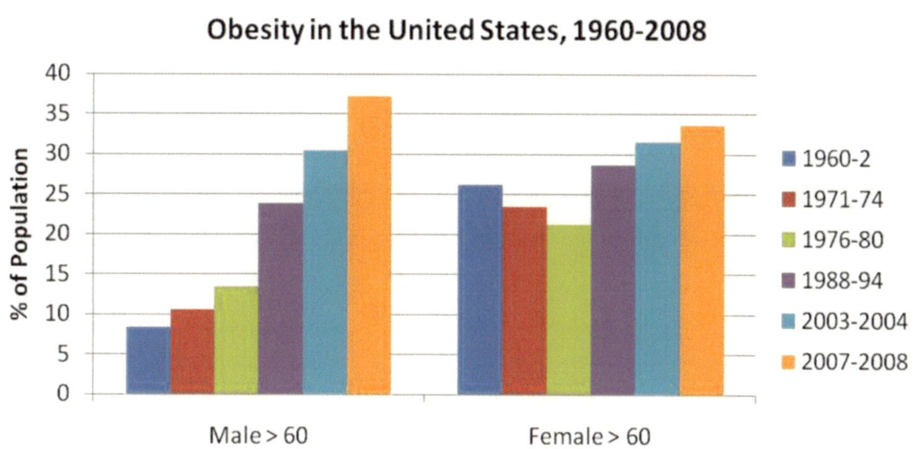

Fig. 5. Obesity in the United States, 1960-2008.Trends in the obesity epidemic in the United States in both males and females over the age of 60 years. In males, the trajectory of multiple epidemiological surveys is that of an increase. In females, there was an initial drop, but subsequent, yet steady increase

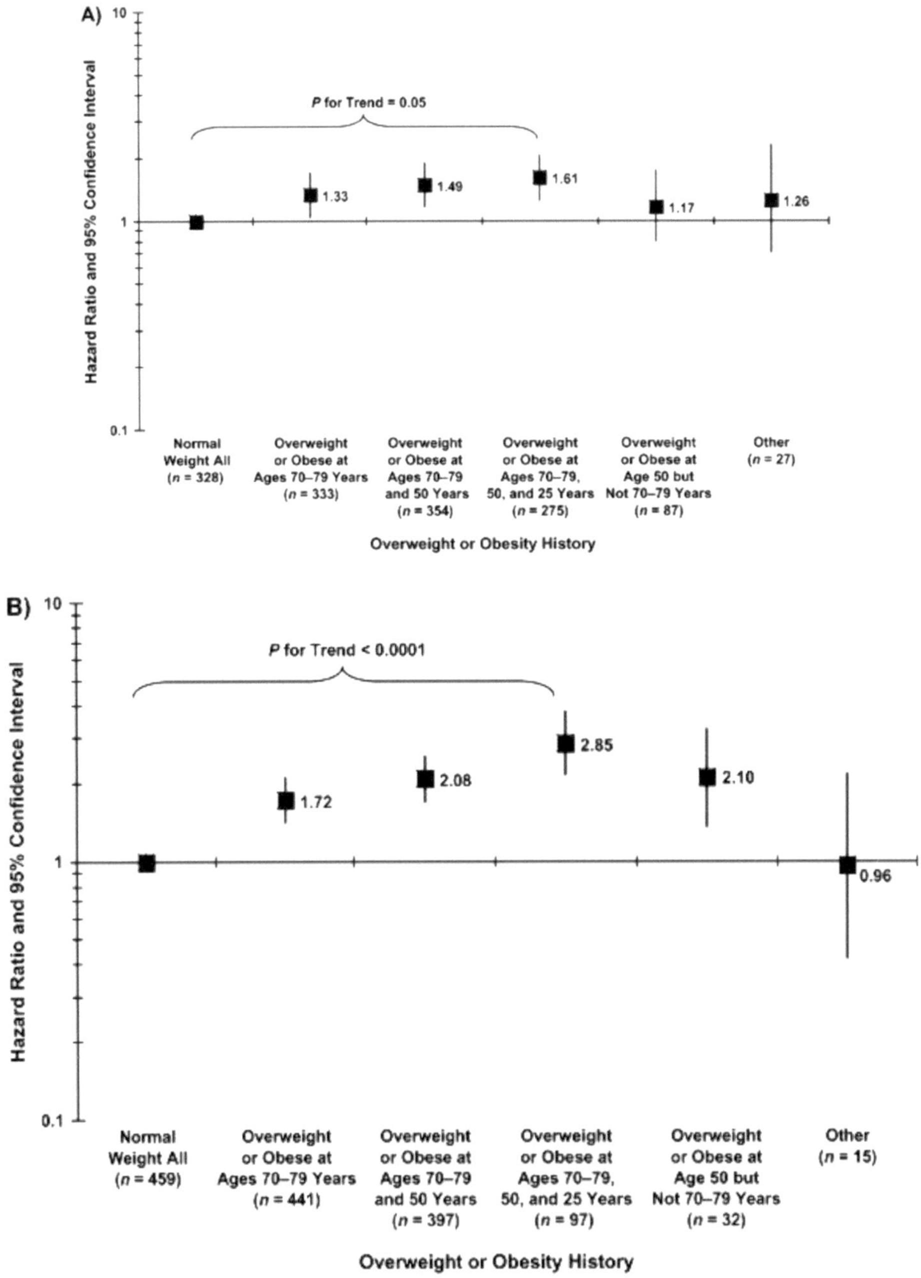

Caption: Hazard ratios and 95% confidence intervals for incident mobility limitation among Men (A) and women (B) by history of overweight or obesity (BMI >25kg/m^2), the Health, Aging and Body Composition Study, 7 years of followup. Models were adjusted for age, race, field center, education, smoking status, alcohol consumption, and physical activity at study baseline. (Houston et al. 2009)

Fig. 6. Mobility Limitations and Body Size

A recent study using NHANES data demonstrated a J or U-shaped association between overweight/obesity and years of life lost, with the study authors concluding that obesity appears to decrease life expectancy (Figure #7) (Flegal et al. 2005). In addition, recent meta-analyses using body mass index as a surrogate for obesity have demonstrated that regardless of age, mortality is increased in patients with a BMI <22kg/m^2 and those who are morbidly obese (BMI>35kg/m^2) [Figure #8] (Whitlock et al. 2009). Continued debate in the literature with regard to associations of mortality with BMIs between 25 and 35 continue and will not be reviewed here. Obesity has also been demonstrated to be associated with disability, lower quality of life, and increased resource utilization, particularly in elderly subjects (Guralnik, Fried, and Salive 1996). **O**besity is associated with nursing home admissions and increasing one's risk to be homebound (Jensen et al. 2006; Valiyeva et al. 2006; Zizza et al. 2002). These issues all create a worrisome public health concern in that, in one study, 9% of all total excess healthcare costs may be attributable to overweight or obesity (Finkelstein, Fiebelkorn, and Wang 2003).

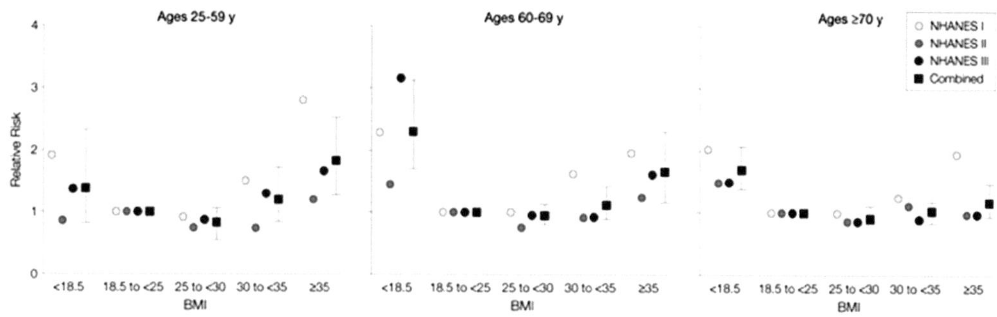

Caption: BMI indicates body mass index, measured as weight in kilograms divided by the square of height in meters. The reference category with relative risk 1.0 is BMI 18 to <25. Error bars indicate 95% confidence intervals. Copyright © American medical Association, JAMA 2005;293:1861-1867, All Rights Reserved. (Flegal et al. 2005)

Fig. 7. Relative Risks of Mortality by Body Mass Index Category by Epidemiological Survey Data

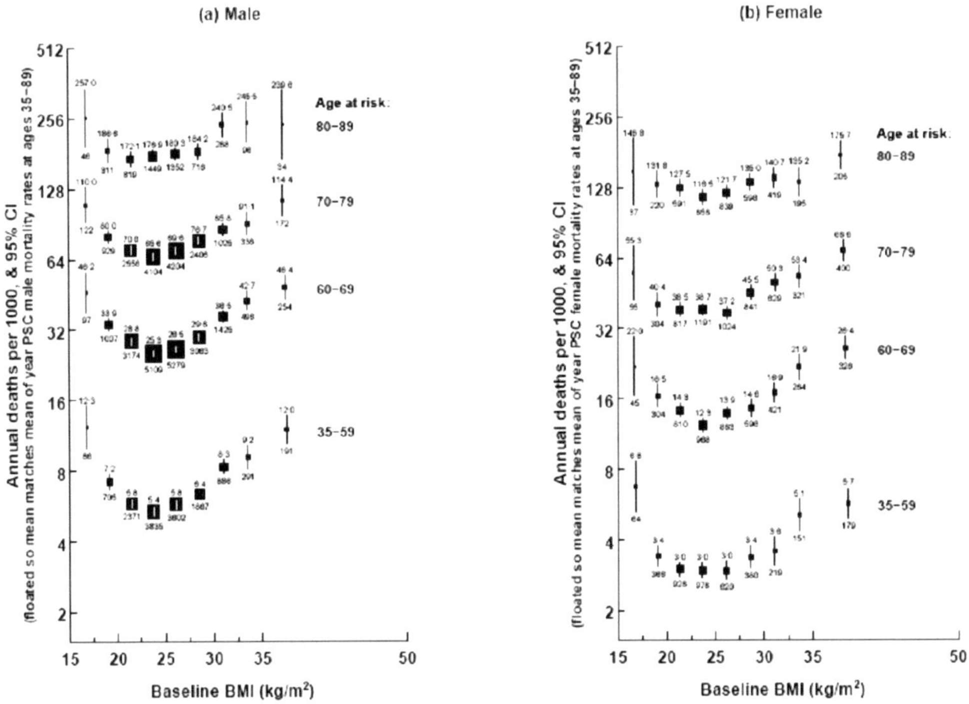

Fig. 8. All-cause mortality vs. Body Mass Index.
These studies demonatrate J-shaped curves in all age groups, in the range 15-50kg/m^2 by age at risks (excluding the first 5 years of followup) (Whitlock et al. 2009)

5. Sarcopenic obesity – A subset of sarcopenia and obesity

Often times, we consider sarcopenia in the context of weight loss and cachexia; but sarcopenia can occur with obesity. The impact of obesity on sarcopenia continues to be a subject of investigation and emerging as a public health problem. In subjects who gain weight, there is proportionally an increase in fat mass as compared to lean mass. As described above, both entities lead to disability and the synergistic effects lead to worsening disability. These subjects can also be considered 'fat frail' who suffer from increased weakness from sarcopenia and the requirement to carry additional weight from obesity (Launer et al. 1994).

Common inflammatory pathways have linked sarcopenia and obesity yet the interplay between these two entities is poorly understood. One author hypothesized that both sarcopenia and obesity are similar behaviorally and biologically (Roubenoff 2000). One of the most trophic effects on muscle is physical activity, which normally falls as people age. Concurrently, there is a positive energy balance and weight gain, predominantly fat in nature. Additionally, this loss of fat-free mass (muscle) lowers the amount of tissues that can respond to insulin targeting, thereby promoting insulin resistance, metabolic syndrome and obesity (Reaven 1988). Muscle and fat are both metabolically active, the latter producing TNF-a, IL-6 and adipokines all of which have a direct catabolic effect on the former, and promote insulin resistance. Leptin and low adiponectin concentrations have been found to negatively impact muscle mass and lead to a decline in muscle quality (Hamrick et al. 2010). On a biological level, macrophages in adipocytes or in adipose tissue, produce such proinflammatory cytokines (Fantuzzi 2005) which can upregulate the inflammatory response. Cesari et al. evaluated the relationship between body-composition measures and inflammatory markers, using data from the Trial of Angiotensin Converting Enzyme Inhibition and Novel Cardiovascular Risk Factors study (Cesari et al. 2005). These authors demonstrated the positive association of CRP and IL-6 with BMI ($p=0.03$ and $p<0.001$) and total fat mass (<0.001 and <0.001), and inverse association with fat-adjusted appendicular lean mass ($p<0.002$ and $p=0.02$). Using data from the INChianti study, global and central obesity directly affect inflammation, negatively affects muscle strength and can contribute to the development and progression of sarcopenic obesity (Schrager et al. 2007).

This cycle continues until the development of disability and medical illnesses. Furthermore, compounding the decline in neuronal and hormonal signals that occur with aging, malnutrition, and loss of a-motor units and changes in gene expression, further increase the risk of this entity in occurring (Doherty et al. 1993; Marcell 2003; Morley et al. 2001). This pro-inflammatory state leads to a perpetuating cycle of reduced muscle strength among obese subjects inevitably further contributing to functional decline. The aging process also itself leads to elevated IL-6 levels, TNF-α and CRP as well. While a number of chronic medical conditions prevalent in elders, including cancer, COPD and heart failure are associated with elevated pro-inflammatory levels and can lead to loss of muscle mass, the process of age-related sarcopenia is a natural phenomenon and differs from such.

Baumgartner et al. defined sarcopenic obesity as a muscle mass index less than two standard deviations below the sex-specific reference for a young healthy population (Baumgartner 2000). Alternative definitions have been used by other authors (Bouchard, Dionne, and Brochu 2009; Davison et al. 2002; Zoico et al. 2004), yet a harmonious definition has yet to be solidified at this time. More recently, the incorporation of muscle quality into these definitions has been proposed (Cruz-Jentoft et al. 2010). The debate is outside the scope of this chapter.

A number of studies have outlined the differences between those with and without sarcopenia or obesity. In one of the pivotal studies, 52 subjects matched obese elderly, non-obese frail, and non-obese, non-frail were evaluated on objective measures of functional status and health-related quality of life and differences in body composition (Villareal et al. 2004). They discovered that obese and non-obese frail groups had lower and similar scores in physical function, functional status and impairments in strength and walking speed. They concluded that physical frailty in obese elders was associated with lower fat free mass (lean mass), poor muscle quality and worsening quality of life.

One of the more pivotal studies by Baumgartner's group demonstrated the combined effect of obesity and muscle mass or strength on physical functioning or disability (Baumgartner 2000). Baumgartner's group examined the impact of sarcopenic obesity and incident instrumental ADL disability in the New Mexico elder health survey and New Mexico aging process study (Baumgartner et al.). This study ascertained ADLs in patients longitudinally and assigned points (0-2) depending on whether someone could not perform an instrumental activities of daily living, could do it with difficulty, or could do it independently. Their primary outcome was time to a drop in ADL, defined as a drop in 2 points. As can be seen in the Figure #9 below, only those with sarcopenic obesity had a markedly shorter time to drop in ADLs. The other three groups were no different from each other (sarcopenic non-obese, obese non-sarcopenic, and non-obese non-sarcopenic).

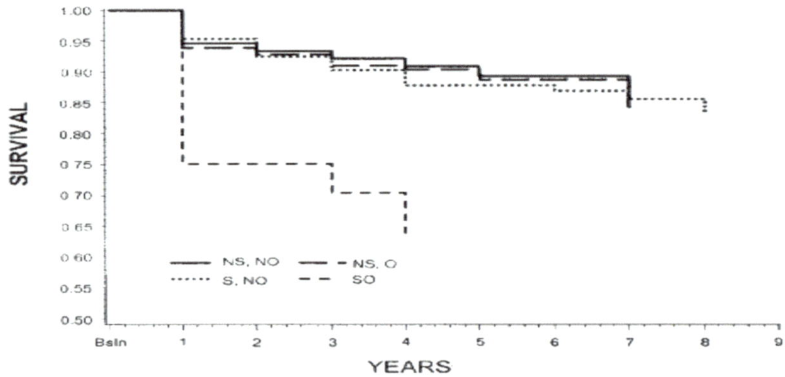

SO - sarcopenic obesity; S - sarcopenia; O - obesity; NS - non-sarcopenic; NO - non-obese

Fig. 9. Incident Disabilty over Time.
The data demonstrate that subjects with Sarcopenic Obesity have worsened disability, than subjects with sarcopenia alone, obesity alone, or neither sarcopenia nor obesity(Baumgartner et al. 2004).

Other cross-sectional studies have demonstrated conflicting results based on NHANES III (Davison et al. 2002) and a sample of elder females in Verona (Zoico et al. 2004). Davison's study looked at 1,526 females and 1,391 males who were 70 years and older. These authors observed that women in the highest quintile for percent body fat were twice as likely to report functional limitations than in the other comparison groups, and weaker but similar relationships were observed in men. Low muscle mass and sarcopenia with obesity, in this study were not associated with additional limitations. In Zoico's cross-sectional study of 167 females, aged 67-78, those in the highest quintile of body fat demonstrated a significantly higher prevalence of functional limitation, but 40% of sarcopenic elderly women and 50% of elderly women with high body fat and normal muscle mass were functionally limited (Figure #10). Functional limitation increased in those with a higher degree of sarcopenia. They demonstrated that isometric leg strength was significantly lower in subjects with sarcopenia and sarcopenic obesity. These two studies used the same categorization to define these entities. It was felt that using muscle mass instead of a functional measure such as strength as an indicator of sarcopenia may have explained the lack of results.

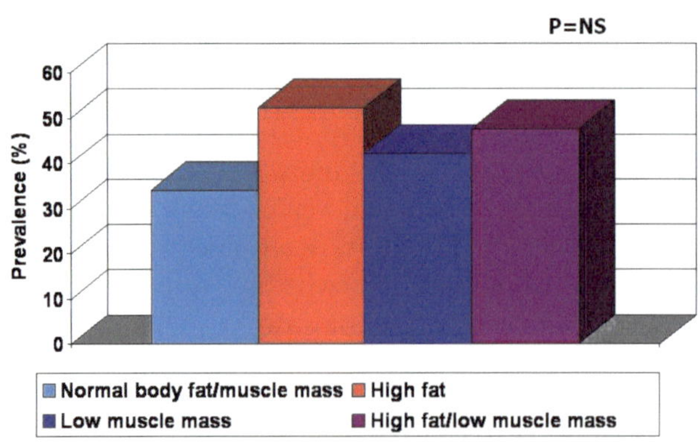

Fig. 10. Self-Reported Functional Limitations

There were no differences between subjects in this cohort on self-reported functional limitations with regard to body composition measures (Zoico et al. 2004).
There are other studies that have demonstrated the relationship between sarcopenic obesity and higher degrees of functional limitations. Stenholm et al (Stenholm et al. 2008) examined the association between different obesity indicators and walking limitations in examining the role of C-reactive protein and handgrip strength. This cross-sectional study of a Finnish population looked at subjects >55 years, and demonstrated that the highest two quartiles of body fat percent and C-reactive protein and the lowest two quartiles of handgrip strength were significantly associated with greater risk of walking limitations after adjusting for chronic diseases and other pertinent co-variates. The prevalence of walking limitations were higher in persons who had high fat and low handgrip (61%) than in those with low fat and high handgrip (7%). Their results are better observed in the figure below:

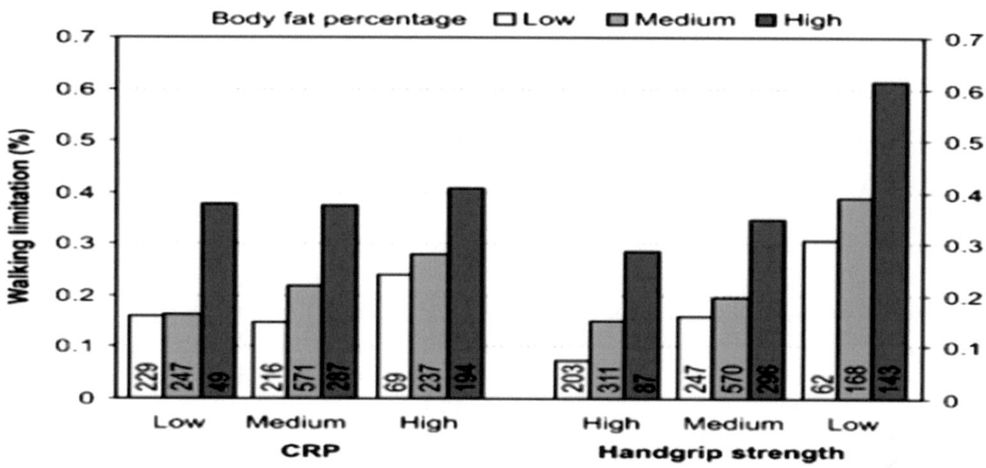

Fig. 11. Walking Limitations, C-reactive Protein and Handgrip Strength.
Age- and sex-adjusted prevalence of walking limitations according to body fat percentage levels according to C-reactive protein (CRP) and handgrip strength. Low, medium and high levels of body fat percentage, CRP and handgrip strength were defined by recoding quartiles of each variable in to three categories by combining quartiles II and III. Numbers inside the bars indicate the number of subjects in each category (Stenholm et al. 2008).

Finally, Cesari's group (Cesari et al. 2009), using the InCHIANTI study, analyzed data from 934 participants aged 65 years and older with at least 6 years of follow-up. In unadjusted analyzes, muscle density (HR 0.78 [0.69-0.88]), muscle area (HR 0.75 [0.66-0.86]) and fat area (HR 0.82 [0.73-0.92) were associated with mortality. However, adjusting for confounders, these associations were no longer significant. Walking speed was associated with mortality risk (HR 0.73 [0.60-0.88]). The relationship with mortality, though, has been examined by other others. Rantanen (Rantanen et al. 2000). Those who were overweight in the lowest grip strength tertile had 1.4 times higher mortality risk compared to normal weight persons in the highest grip strength. Muscle strength has been previously examined as a predictor of mortality (Gale et al. 2007; Newman et al. 2006; Rantanen et al. 2003) and that of obesity has been fully described previously.

6. Aging, sarcopenia, insulin and insulin resistance

There are hormonal changes linking age-related decline in muscle strength and mass, which include insulin, growth hormone, and catecholamines as a few examples. On a cellular level, animal studies have demonstrated a relationship between obesity-related insulin resistance and insulin receptor signaling pathway. A low grade inflammation often is present in most obese patients which is a result of chronic activation of the innate immune system, leading to insulin resistance, impaired fasting glucose and diabetes. The involvement of cytokines and inflammation in obesity in relation to glucose metabolism continues to be controversial. Both IL-6 and TNF-α alter insulin sensitivity by impacting given steps in the insulin signaling pathway. In animal models, resistin induces insulin resistance, but whether this occurs in humans is unclear. Subjects with obesity-related insulin resistance, type 2 diabetes and coronary heart disease have low levels of adiponectin. This hormone is known to inhibit liver gluconeogenesis and can promote fatty acid oxidation in skeletal muscle. These cytokines also are known to impact NF-kB and JNK systems (Zamboni et al. 2007).

With aging, muscle can be infiltrated with fat, and this may eventually perpetuate insulin resistance. In a large study of 2,964 elderly subjects with a mean age of 73.6 years, despite similar amounts of subcutaneous thigh fat, intermuscular fat was higher in subjects with type 2 diabetes and impaired glucose tolerance than in subjects with normal glucose tolerance ($p<0.001$) (Goodpaster et al. 2003). As expected higher rates of intermuscular fat and visceral abdominal fat were associated with higher fasting insulin levels. This study concluded that elderly men and women with normal body weight may be at risk for metabolic abnormalities, including type 2 diabetes if they possess an inordinate amount of muscle fat or visceral abdominal fat. A smaller study by the same group elucidated whether thigh fat was a determinant of insulin resistance. They compared a small number of subjects and confirmed that muscle composition reflected increased fat content was associated with insulin resistance (Goodpaster, Thaete, and Kelley 2000).

Furthermore, insulin is well known to be an anabolic hormone which may have a pleiotrophic effect on muscle tissue and protein metabolism. Lower protein synthesis and higher insulin levels occur in elderly subjects compared to younger subjects after food intake. Previous studies have shown that subjects with insulin resistance can negatively predict muscle strength, often seen in elderly subjects with diabetes. The correlation between insulin resistance and muscle strength is quite poor and accelerates the loss of leg muscle strength and quality. In a pilot study examining this relationship examined the homeostasis model assessment (HOMA-IR) in type 2 diabetes, demonstrated that knee extension, adjusted for body weight was significantly correlated with HOMA-IR in both sexes and that this relationship persisted as an independent determinant in a stepwise regression model (Nomura et al. 2007). In another study, the degree of insulin resistance was evaluated using HOMA-IR and muscle strength using handgrip strength. BMI-adjusted handgrip strength correlated positively with physical activity, muscle area, and muscle density (Abbatecola et al. 2005). Physical activity has a positive effect on muscle mass and quality specifically with resistance training (Goodpaster and Brown 2005). This latter activity is also known to improve insulin sensitivity and glycemic control.

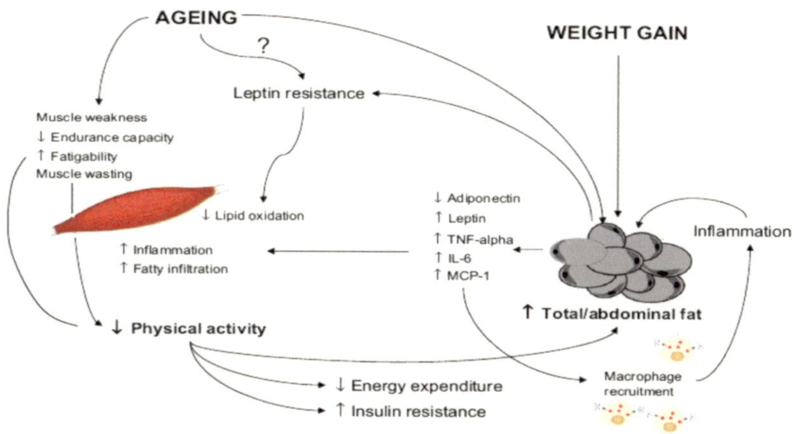

Fig. 12. Possible Mechanisms linking Ageing, Obesity, Sarcopenia and Insulin resistance (Zamboni et al. 2008)

7. Growth hormone and insulin-like growth factor 1

Additional contributors to sarcopenia include insulin-like growth factor-1 (IGF-1) and growth hormone (GH), both of which decline with age. Growth hormone is associated with low fat mass, increased lean body mass and ideal metabolic profile, while IGF-1 can increase protein synthesis in existing muscles. One study partially described the relationship of the hypothalamic pituitary axis in subjects with sarcopenia and sarcopenic obesity. Using DEXA, they ascertained 45 subjects with varying degrees of adiposity and lean mass and measured pituitary function (Waters et al. 2008). They demonstrated that appendicular skeletal muscle mass was independently and negatively correlated with leptin in all groups, even after adjusting for body fat, and that subjects with sarcopenic obesity had lowered and blunted GH responses. Low levels of this anabolic hormone has been proposed to be positively associated with low muscle strength (Ceda et al. 2005). Using data from the Longitudinal Ageing Study Amsterdam (LASA), among subjects aged 65-88 years, serum testosterone levels were positively associated with muscle strength and physical performance (Schaap et al. 2005). With respect to IGF-1 levels, physiologically one would expect that the age-associated decline in IGF-1 levels would be associated with poorer muscle strength and mobility. Data from 617 women from Women's Health and Aging Study were examined and demonstrated a positive association between IGF-1 levels and knee extensor strength ($p=0.004$) and walking speed ($P<0.001$). A decline in IGF-1 levels was associated with difficulty self-reported mobility tasks. It is hypothesized that the aging muscle loses the capability of secreting GH and the responsiveness to IGF-1 is also likely attenuated. Evidence suggests that exercise can reverse the latter. These may be molecular targets in the future to promote muscle building and prevent sarcopenia.

8. Diabetes and geriatric syndromes

Diabetes is associated with an increased incidence of many geriatric syndromes. Many studies have demonstrated the impact of diabetes on functional impairment, including inability to ambulate and perform instrumental ADLs (Volpato et al. 2002; Gregg et al. 2002).

Diabetes itself, on a microvascular level can lead to functional impairment, but notably, complications of diabetes have also been implicated. Diabetes has been implicated in fall risk (Volpato et al. 2005), fractures (Schwartz et al. 2001), urinary incontinence (Ebbesen et al. 2007) and depression (Anderson et al. 2001).

9. Diabetes and sarcopenia

There are a number of similarities between diabetes and sarcopenia. It is known that persons with diabetes have an accelerated aging process leading to disability and frailty. Diabetes is known to lead to each of the components of the operationalized definition of frailty and insulin resistance appears to be a core factor in this pathophysiology (Morley 2008). In the Health, Aging and Body Composition study, type 2 diabetes was associated with lower skeletal muscle strength and quality, as well as excessive skeletal muscle mass loss (Park et al. 2006; Park et al. 2009). Loss of muscle mass has also been associated with type 2 diabetes in elderly subjects. Low grip strength as a surrogate for sarcopenia is associated with features of metabolic syndrome as well, post-prandial glucose levels and HOMA index/ insulin-resistance. It is believed that hyperglycemia directly impairs skeletal muscle contractility and force (Sayer et al. 2005) ; whether this is due to excessive toxicity of sugar alcohols on muscles remains elusive at this time. Other hypotheses include the accumulation of lipids which may affect insulin signaling (Janssen and Ross 2005; Furler et al. 2001; Shulman 2000), impaired rate of synthesis of muscular proteins, seen in both ageing and insulin resistance (Nair 2005; Rasmussen et al. 2006). Diabetics are at high risk for sarcopenia as there is a 1.5-2.0 fold increased rate of skeletal muscle mass and strength loss (Park et al. 2007). There are a number of similarities between metabolic syndrome and insulin resistance and one study by Sayer examined the relationship between these entities and sarcopenia (Sayer et al. 2007). Their findings suggested that impaired grip strength was associated, not only with individual constructs of the metabolic syndrome but also the composite definition itself. Although the authors acknowledge that further investigation is required to understand the underlying mechanisms, the potential for using grip strength and interventions tested thereof to improve muscle strength, could also potentially improve insulin resistance. The following figure (Figure #13) demonstrates some of the potentiating cellular mechanisms observed in diabetes.

There are a number of emerging studies observing the relationship between sarcopenia, obesity, sarcopenic obesity and diabetes. The Korean Sarcopenic Obesity Study examined the prevalence of sarcopenia in Korean subjects with and without type 2 diabetes (Kim et al. 2000). The study included 810 subjects, of which 414 had diabetes and 396 were controls, and demonstrated that the prevalence of sarcopenia was 15.7% and 6.9% in subjects with and without diabetes. Skeletal muscle index (muscle mass adjusted for height squared), as a measure of sarcopenia, was significantly lower in patients with diabetes compared to subjects without diabetes. In their multiple logistic regression model, type 2 diabetes was independently associated with sarcopenia (OR 3.06 [1.42-6.6.62)] than subjects without diabetes after adjusting for age, sex, BMI, smoking, alcohol consumption, physical activity, medications, blood pressure and lipid profiles. Quite interestingly, though, the prevalence of type 2 diabetes was highest in Mexican Americans using NHANES III data with the lowest prevalence of obesity and sarcopenia, while Whites had the highest prevalence of sarcopenic obesity (Castaneda and Janssen 2005). This study challenges whether there indeed is a relationship between sarcopenia and obesity. Whether ethnicities need to be accounted for due to differences in body composition is a matter of further investigation.

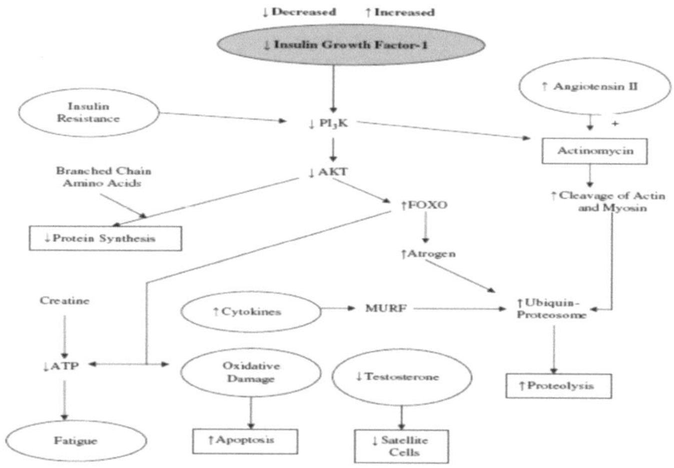

↓, decreased, ↑ increased; KT, active human protein kinase (protein kinase-B); FOXO, forkhead protein; MURF, muscle ring finger protein; P13K, phosphatidyl inositol-3-kinase (Morley 2008).

Fig. 13. Biochemical Changes in Muscle in Diabetes

In other population, specifically, dialysis subjects, diabetes is thought to be a risk factor for losing lean mass (Pupim et al. 2005). Muscle mass, particularly in dialysis patients, are known to decline continuously and hence this study suggested that controlling a risk factor for incipient sarcopenia (diabetes), would reduce this declining process. Many of the changes suggested, in one editorial, were due to systemic inflammatory cytokines previously described, often which are implicated in diabetes and insulin resistance (Kaysen 2005). This was echoed in another small study looking at changes in inflammatory cytokines implicated in losing lean mass (Pedersen et al. 2003).

Subjects with diabetes are at higher risk of developing peripheral neuropathy, which leads to a decrease in one's motor end plates. This entity is important in maintaining muscle homeostasis and coordination of muscle contraction, therefore their loss can perpetuate and accelerate age-related decline in muscle mass. Diabetics also have impaired levels of growth hormone and pro-inflammatory cytokines. Additionally, the microvascular damage from hypoxia not only affects nerves, renal glomeruli and optic nerves, but also can lead to muscle hypoxia. Macrovascularly, atherosclerosis can lead to diminished peripheral blood flow to leg muscles leading to impaired strength. Other cellular entities are implicated, as well as other endocrine changes as illustrated in the figure below. Undoubtedly there is a relationship between the underlying pathophysiology of sarcopenia, insulin resistance and diabetes.

10. Conclusion

A number of studies are increasingly confirming the relationship between sarcopenia and reduced functional activities and disability. Sarcopenia and obesity are often thought as a preludes to frailty, known to adversely predict hospitalizations, morbidity, institutionalization and mortality (Figure #14). Reduced physical activity and a sedentary lifestyle are important risk factors for developing sarcopenia, which subsequently leads to physical disability and reduced physical performance (Figure #15). More importantly, those with elevated fat mass with sarcopenia are at even high risk. The relationship between sarcopenia, sarcopenic obesity and insulin resistance requires further investigation. The clinical implications are not insignificance in that globally, sedentary lifestyles are becoming the norm and the potential implications on utilization are not significant.

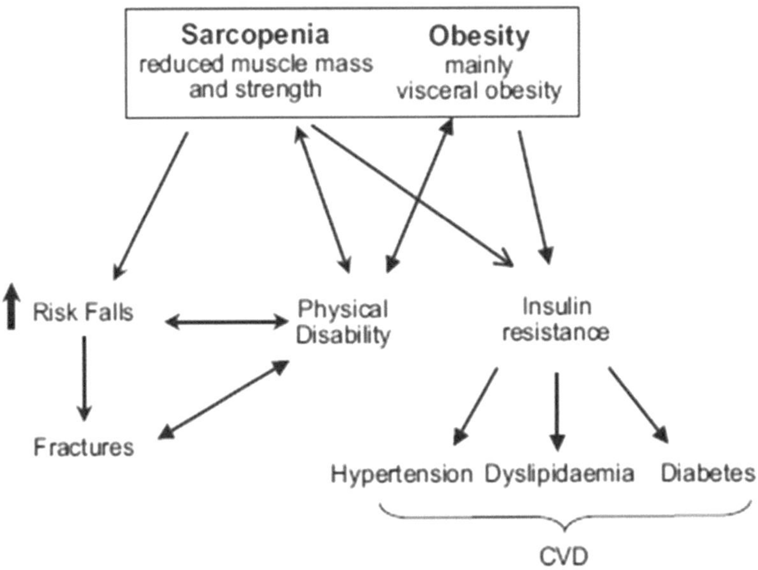

Fig. 14. Possible Consequence of sarcopenic obesity in the Elderly (Zamboni et al. 2008)

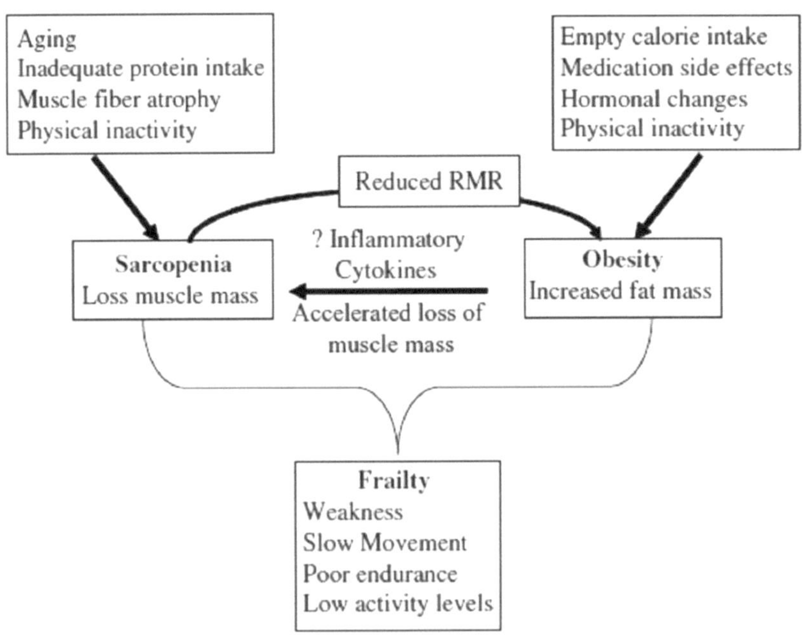

Fig. 15. Body Composition Changes Leading to Sarcopenic Obesity (Jarosz and Bellar 2009)

11. Abbreviations

ADL - Activities of Daily Living
BMI - body mass index
BIA - bioelectrical impedance analysis;
DEXA - Dual Energy X-Ray Absorptiometry
HOMA - homeostatic model assessment
HOMA-IR - homeostasis model of assessment - insulin resistance
OECD - Organisation of Economic Cooperation and Development
US - United States
TNF-α - tumor necrosis factor α
IL-6 - interleukine 6
GH - growth hormone
NK-kB - nuclear factor-kappa B
JNK - Jun N-terminal kinases
IGF-1 - insuline-like growth factor 1

12. References

Abbatecola, A. M., L. Ferrucci, G. Ceda, C. R. Russo, F. Lauretani, S. Bandinelli, M. Barbieri, G. Valenti, and G. Paolisso. 2005. Insulin resistance and muscle strength in older persons. *J Gerontol A Biol Sci Med Sci* 60 (10):1278-82.

Anderson, R. J., K. E. Freedland, R. E. Clouse, and P. J. Lustman. 2001. The prevalence of comorbid depression in adults with diabetes: a meta-analysis. *Diabetes Care* 24 (6):1069-78.

Baumgartner, R. N. 2000. Body composition in healthy aging. *Ann N Y Acad Sci* 904:437-48.

Baumgartner, R. N., K. M. Koehler, D. Gallagher, L. Romero, S. B. Heymsfield, R. R. Ross, P. J. Garry, and R. D. Lindeman. 1998. Epidemiology of sarcopenia among the elderly in New Mexico. *Am J Epidemiol* 147 (8):755-63.

Baumgartner, R. N., P. M. Stauber, D. McHugh, K. M. Koehler, and P. J. Garry. 1995. Cross-sectional age differences in body composition in persons 60+ years of age. *J Gerontol A Biol Sci Med Sci* 50 (6):M307-16.

Baumgartner, R. N., S. J. Wayne, D. L. Waters, I. Janssen, D. Gallagher, and J. E. Morley. 2004. Sarcopenic obesity predicts instrumental activities of daily living disability in the elderly. *Obes Res* 12 (12):1995-2004.

Beaufrere, B., and B. Morio. 2000. Fat and protein redistribution with aging: metabolic considerations. *Eur J Clin Nutr* 54 Suppl 3:S48-53.

Beydoun, M. A., H. A. Beydoun, and Y. Wang. 2008. Obesity and central obesity as risk factors for incident dementia and its subtypes: a systematic review and meta-analysis. *Obes Rev* 9 (3):204-18.

Bouchard, D. R., I. J. Dionne, and M. Brochu. 2009. Sarcopenic/obesity and physical capacity in older men and women: data from the Nutrition as a Determinant of Successful Aging (NuAge)-the Quebec longitudinal Study. *Obesity (Silver Spring)* 17 (11):2082-8.

Castaneda, C., and I. Janssen. 2005. Ethnic comparisons of sarcopenia and obesity in diabetes. *Ethn Dis* 15 (4):664-70.

Ceda, G. P., E. Dall'Aglio, M. Maggio, F. Lauretani, S. Bandinelli, C. Falzoi, W. Grimaldi, G. Ceresini, F. Corradi, L. Ferrucci, G. Valenti, and A. R. Hoffman. 2005. Clinical implications of the reduced activity of the GH-IGF-I axis in older men. *J Endocrinol Invest* 28 (11 Suppl Proceedings):96-100.

Cesari, M., S. B. Kritchevsky, R. N. Baumgartner, H. H. Atkinson, B. W. Penninx, L. Lenchik, S. L. Palla, W. T. Ambrosius, R. P. Tracy, and M. Pahor. 2005. Sarcopenia, obesity, and inflammation--results from the Trial of Angiotensin Converting Enzyme Inhibition and Novel Cardiovascular Risk Factors study. *Am J Clin Nutr* 82 (2):428-34.

Cesari, M., M. Pahor, F. Lauretani, V. Zamboni, S. Bandinelli, R. Bernabei, J. M. Guralnik, and L. Ferrucci. 2009. Skeletal muscle and mortality results from the InCHIANTI Study. *J Gerontol A Biol Sci Med Sci* 64 (3):377-84.

Chien, M. Y., H. K. Kuo, and Y. T. Wu. (2010) Sarcopenia, cardiopulmonary fitness, and physical disability in community-dwelling elderly people. *Phys Ther* 90 (9):1277-87.

Chumlea, W. C., S. S. Guo, R. J. Kuczmarski, K. M. Flegal, C. L. Johnson, S. B. Heymsfield, H. C. Lukaski, K. Friedl, and V. S. Hubbard. 2002. Body composition estimates from NHANES III bioelectrical impedance data. *Int J Obes Relat Metab Disord* 26 (12):1596-609.

Cigolle, C. T., K. M. Langa, M. U. Kabeto, Z. Tian, and C. S. Blaum. 2007. Geriatric conditions and disability: the Health and Retirement Study. *Ann Intern Med* 147 (3):156-64.

Cree, M. G., B. R. Newcomer, C. S. Katsanos, M. Sheffield-Moore, D. Chinkes, A. Aarsland, R. Urban, and R. R. Wolfe. 2004. Intramuscular and liver triglycerides are increased in the elderly. *J Clin Endocrinol Metab* 89 (8):3864-71.

Cruz-Jentoft, A. J., J. P. Baeyens, J. M. Bauer, Y. Boirie, T. Cederholm, F. Landi, F. C. Martin, J. P. Michel, Y. Rolland, S. M. Schneider, E. Topinkova, M. Vandewoude, and M. Zamboni. 2010. Sarcopenia: European consensus on definition and diagnosis: Report of the European Working Group on Sarcopenia in Older People. *Age Ageing* 39 (4):412-23.

Davison, K. K., E. S. Ford, M. E. Cogswell, and W. H. Dietz. 2002. Percentage of body fat and body mass index are associated with mobility limitations in people aged 70 and older from NHANES III. *J Am Geriatr Soc* 50 (11):1802-9.

Doherty, C, PN Benotti, MB Butler, MW Clare, EP Dillinger, GN Goodman, DS EHess, LM Howel, EE Mason, DK Millre, AZ Newhoff, D Popoola, DM Van Nostrand, EC Woerz, and R Zemel. 1993. Rationale for the Surgical Treatment of Severe Obesity. *Obesity Surgery* 3:430-433.

Ebbesen, M. H., Y. S. Hannestad, K. Midthjell, and S. Hunskaar. 2007. Diabetes and urinary incontinence - prevalence data from Norway. *Acta Obstet Gynecol Scand*:1-7.

Fantuzzi, G. 2005. Adipose tissue, adipokines, and inflammation. *J Allergy Clin Immunol* 115 (5):911-9; quiz 920.

Finkelstein, E. A., I. C. Fiebelkorn, and G. Wang. 2003. National medical spending attributable to overweight and obesity: how much, and who's paying? *Health Aff (Millwood)* Suppl Web Exclusives:W3-219-26.

Flegal, K. M., M. D. Carroll, C. L. Ogden, and L. R. Curtin. 2010. Prevalence and trends in obesity among US adults, 1999-2008. *Jama* 303 (3):235-41.

Flegal, K. M., B. I. Graubard, D. F. Williamson, and M. H. Gail. 2005. Excess deaths associated with underweight, overweight, and obesity. *Jama* 293 (15):1861-7.

Flynn, M. A., G. B. Nolph, A. S. Baker, W. M. Martin, and G. Krause. 1989. Total body potassium in aging humans: a longitudinal study. *Am J Clin Nutr* 50 (4):713-7.

Fontaine, KR, DT Redden, C Wang, AO Westfall, and DB Allison. 2003. Years of Life Lost due to Obesity. *JAMA* 289 (2):187-193.

Ford, E. S., U. A. Ajani, J. B. Croft, J. A. Critchley, D. R. Labarthe, T. E. Kottke, W. H. Giles, and S. Capewell. 2007. Explaining the decrease in U.S. deaths from coronary disease, 1980-2000. *N Engl J Med* 356 (23):2388-98.

Furler, S. M., A. M. Poynten, A. D. Kriketos, A. J. Lowy, B. A. Ellis, E. L. Maclean, B. G. Courtenay, E. W. Kraegen, L. V. Campbell, and D. J. Chisholm. 2001. Independent influences of central fat and skeletal muscle lipids on insulin sensitivity. *Obes Res* 9 (9):535-43.

Gale, C. R., C. N. Martyn, C. Cooper, and A. A. Sayer. 2007. Grip strength, body composition, and mortality. *Int J Epidemiol* 36 (1):228-35.

Gallagher, D., M. Visser, R. E. De Meersman, D. Sepulveda, R. N. Baumgartner, R. N. Pierson, T. Harris, and S. B. Heymsfield. 1997. Appendicular skeletal muscle mass: effects of age, gender, and ethnicity. *J Appl Physiol* 83 (1):229-39.

Goodpaster, B. H., and N. F. Brown. 2005. Skeletal muscle lipid and its association with insulin resistance: what is the role for exercise? *Exerc Sport Sci Rev* 33 (3):150-4.

Goodpaster, B. H., S. Krishnaswami, H. Resnick, D. E. Kelley, C. Haggerty, T. B. Harris, A. V. Schwartz, S. Kritchevsky, and A. B. Newman. 2003. Association between regional adipose tissue distribution and both type 2 diabetes and impaired glucose tolerance in elderly men and women. *Diabetes Care* 26 (2):372-9.

Goodpaster, B. H., S. W. Park, T. B. Harris, S. B. Kritchevsky, M. Nevitt, A. V. Schwartz, E. M. Simonsick, F. A. Tylavsky, M. Visser, and A. B. Newman. 2006. The loss of skeletal muscle strength, mass, and quality in older adults: the health, aging and body composition study. *J Gerontol A Biol Sci Med Sci* 61 (10):1059-64.

Goodpaster, B. H., F. L. Thaete, and D. E. Kelley. 2000. Thigh adipose tissue distribution is associated with insulin resistance in obesity and in type 2 diabetes mellitus. *Am J Clin Nutr* 71 (4):885-92.

Gregg, E. W., C. M. Mangione, J. A. Cauley, T. J. Thompson, A. V. Schwartz, K. E. Ensrud, and M. C. Nevitt. 2002. Diabetes and incidence of functional disability in older women. *Diabetes Care* 25 (1):61-7.

Guralnik, J. M., L. P. Fried, and M. E. Salive. 1996. Disability as a public health outcome in the aging population. *Annu Rev Public Health* 17:25-46.

Hamrick, M. W., S. Herberg, P. Arounleut, H. Z. He, A. Shiver, R. Q. Qi, L. Zhou, C. M. Isales, and Q. S. Mi. (2010) The adipokine leptin increases skeletal muscle mass and significantly alters skeletal muscle miRNA expression profile in aged mice. *Biochem Biophys Res Commun* 400 (3):379-83.

Houston, D. K., J. Ding, B. J. Nicklas, T. B. Harris, J. S. Lee, M. C. Nevitt, S. M. Rubin, F. A. Tylavsky, and S. B. Kritchevsky. 2009. Overweight and obesity over the adult life course and incident mobility limitation in older adults: the health, aging and body composition study. *Am J Epidemiol* 169 (8):927-36.

Janssen, I., R. N. Baumgartner, R. Ross, I. H. Rosenberg, and R. Roubenoff. 2004. Skeletal muscle cutpoints associated with elevated physical disability risk in older men and women. *Am J Epidemiol* 159 (4):413-21.

Janssen, I., and R. Ross. 2005. Linking age-related changes in skeletal muscle mass and composition with metabolism and disease. *J Nutr Health Aging* 9 (6):408-19.

Jarosz, P. A., and A. Bellar. 2009. Sarcopenic obesity: an emerging cause of frailty in older adults. *Geriatr Nurs* 30 (1):64-70.

Jensen, G. L. 2005. Obesity and functional decline: epidemiology and geriatric consequences. *Clin Geriatr Med* 21 (4):677-87, v.

Jensen, G. L., H. J. Silver, M. A. Roy, E. Callahan, C. Still, and W. Dupont. 2006. Obesity is a risk factor for reporting homebound status among community-dwelling older persons. *Obesity (Silver Spring)* 14 (3):509-17.

Kaysen, G. A. 2005. Diabetes, a cause of progressive sarcopenia in dialysis patients? *Kidney Int* 68 (5):2396-7.

Kim, T. N., M. S. Park, S. J. Yang, H. J. Yoo, H. J. Kang, W. Song, J. A. Seo, S. G. Kim, N. H. Kim, S. H. Baik, D. S. Choi, and K. M. Choi. (2010) Prevalence and determinant factors of sarcopenia in patients with type 2 diabetes: the Korean Sarcopenic Obesity Study (KSOS). *Diabetes Care* 33 (7):1497-9.

Lakdawalla, D. N., D. P. Goldman, and B. Shang. 2005. The health and cost consequences of obesity among the future elderly. *Health Aff (Millwood)* 24 Suppl 2:W5R30-41.

Launer, L. J., T. Harris, C. Rumpel, and J. Madans. 1994. Body mass index, weight change, and risk of mobility disability in middle-aged and older women. The epidemiologic follow-up study of NHANES I. *Jama* 271 (14):1093-8.

Lubitz, J., L. Cai, E. Kramarow, and H. Lentzner. 2003. Health, life expectancy, and health care spending among the elderly. *N Engl J Med* 349 (11):1048-55.

Marcell, T. J. 2003. Sarcopenia: causes, consequences, and preventions. *J Gerontol A Biol Sci Med Sci* 58 (10):M911-6.

Morley, J. E. 2008. Diabetes, sarcopenia, and frailty. *Clin Geriatr Med* 24 (3):455-69, vi.

Morley, J. E., R. N. Baumgartner, R. Roubenoff, J. Mayer, and K. S. Nair. 2001. Sarcopenia. *J Lab Clin Med* 137 (4):231-43.

Muller, D. C., D. Elahi, J. D. Tobin, and R. Andres. 1996. The effect of age on insulin resistance and secretion: a review. *Semin Nephrol* 16 (4):289-98.

Nair, K. S. 2005. Aging muscle. *Am J Clin Nutr* 81 (5):953-63.

Newman, A. B., V. Kupelian, M. Visser, E. M. Simonsick, B. H. Goodpaster, S. B. Kritchevsky, F. A. Tylavsky, S. M. Rubin, and T. B. Harris. 2006. Strength, but not muscle mass, is associated with mortality in the health, aging and body composition study cohort. *J Gerontol A Biol Sci Med Sci* 61 (1):72-7.

Nomura, T., Y. Ikeda, S. Nakao, K. Ito, K. Ishida, T. Suehiro, and K. Hashimoto. 2007. Muscle strength is a marker of insulin resistance in patients with type 2 diabetes: a pilot study. *Endocr J* 54 (5):791-6.

Park, S. W., B. H. Goodpaster, J. S. Lee, L. H. Kuller, R. Boudreau, N. de Rekeneire, T. B. Harris, S. Kritchevsky, F. A. Tylavsky, M. Nevitt, Y. W. Cho, and A. B. Newman. 2009. Excessive loss of skeletal muscle mass in older adults with type 2 diabetes. *Diabetes Care* 32 (11):1993-7.

Park, S. W., B. H. Goodpaster, E. S. Strotmeyer, N. de Rekeneire, T. B. Harris, A. V. Schwartz, F. A. Tylavsky, and A. B. Newman. 2006. Decreased muscle strength and quality in older adults with type 2 diabetes: the health, aging, and body composition study. *Diabetes* 55 (6):1813-8.

Park, S. W., B. H. Goodpaster, E. S. Strotmeyer, L. H. Kuller, R. Broudeau, C. Kammerer, N. de Rekeneire, T. B. Harris, A. V. Schwartz, F. A. Tylavsky, Y. W. Cho, and A. B. Newman. 2007. Accelerated loss of skeletal muscle strength in older adults with type 2 diabetes: the health, aging, and body composition study. *Diabetes Care* 30 (6):1507-12.

Pedersen, M., H. Bruunsgaard, N. Weis, H. W. Hendel, B. U. Andreassen, E. Eldrup, F. Dela, and B. K. Pedersen. 2003. Circulating levels of TNF-alpha and IL-6-relation to truncal fat mass and muscle mass in healthy elderly individuals and in patients with type-2 diabetes. *Mech Ageing Dev* 124 (4):495-502.

A Profile of Older Americans 2010. 2010. US Department of Health and Human Services.

Pupim, L. B., O. Heimburger, A. R. Qureshi, T. A. Ikizler, and P. Stenvinkel. 2005. Accelerated lean body mass loss in incident chronic dialysis patients with diabetes mellitus. *Kidney Int* 68 (5):2368-74.

Quetelet, LAJ. 1871. *Antropometrie ou Mesure des Differences Facultes de l'Homme*. Brussels: Musquardt.

Rantanen, T., T. Harris, S. G. Leveille, M. Visser, D. Foley, K. Masaki, and J. M. Guralnik. 2000. Muscle strength and body mass index as long-term predictors of mortality in initially healthy men. *J Gerontol A Biol Sci Med Sci* 55 (3):M168-73.

Rantanen, T., S. Volpato, L. Ferrucci, E. Heikkinen, L. P. Fried, and J. M. Guralnik. 2003. Handgrip strength and cause-specific and total mortality in older disabled women: exploring the mechanism. *J Am Geriatr Soc* 51 (5):636-41.

Rasmussen, B. B., S. Fujita, R. R. Wolfe, B. Mittendorfer, M. Roy, V. L. Rowe, and E. Volpi. 2006. Insulin resistance of muscle protein metabolism in aging. *Faseb J* 20 (6):768-9.

Reaven, G. M. 1988. Banting lecture 1988. Role of insulin resistance in human disease. *Diabetes* 37 (12):1595-607.

Roubenoff, R. 2000. Sarcopenic obesity: does muscle loss cause fat gain? Lessons from rheumatoid arthritis and osteoarthritis. *Ann N Y Acad Sci* 904:553-7.

Sayer, A. A., E. M. Dennison, H. E. Syddall, H. J. Gilbody, D. I. Phillips, and C. Cooper. 2005. Type 2 diabetes, muscle strength, and impaired physical function: the tip of the iceberg? *Diabetes Care* 28 (10):2541-2.

Sayer, A. A., H. E. Syddall, E. M. Dennison, H. J. Martin, D. I. Phillips, C. Cooper, and C. D. Byrne. 2007. Grip strength and the metabolic syndrome: findings from the Hertfordshire Cohort Study. *Qjm* 100 (11):707-13.

Sayer, A. A., H. Syddall, H. Martin, H. Patel, D. Baylis, and C. Cooper. 2008. The developmental origins of sarcopenia. *J Nutr Health Aging* 12 (7):427-32.

Schaap, L. A., S. M. Pluijm, J. H. Smit, N. M. van Schoor, M. Visser, L. J. Gooren, and P. Lips. 2005. The association of sex hormone levels with poor mobility, low muscle strength and incidence of falls among older men and women. *Clin Endocrinol (Oxf)* 63 (2):152-60.

Schrager, M. A., E. J. Metter, E. Simonsick, A. Ble, S. Bandinelli, F. Lauretani, and L. Ferrucci. 2007. Sarcopenic obesity and inflammation in the InCHIANTI study. *J Appl Physiol* 102 (3):919-25.

Schwartz, A. V., D. E. Sellmeyer, K. E. Ensrud, J. A. Cauley, H. K. Tabor, P. J. Schreiner, S. A. Jamal, D. M. Black, and S. R. Cummings. 2001. Older women with diabetes have an increased risk of fracture: a prospective study. *J Clin Endocrinol Metab* 86 (1):32-8.

Shulman, G. I. 2000. Cellular mechanisms of insulin resistance. *J Clin Invest* 106 (2):171-6.

Spillman, B. C., and J. Lubitz. 2000. The effect of longevity on spending for acute and long-term care. *N Engl J Med* 342 (19):1409-15.

Stenholm, S., T. Rantanen, M. Heliovaara, and S. Koskinen. 2008. The mediating role of C-reactive protein and handgrip strength between obesity and walking limitation. *J Am Geriatr Soc* 56 (3):462-9.

Trends in Severe Disability Among Elderly People: Assessing the Evidence in 12 OECD Countries and the Future Implications. 2007. edited by L. Directorate for Employment, and Social Affairs Health Committee.

Valiyeva, E., L. B. Russell, J. E. Miller, and M. M. Safford. 2006. Lifestyle-related risk factors and risk of future nursing home admission. *Arch Intern Med* 166 (9):985-90.

Villareal, D. T., M. Banks, C. Siener, D. R. Sinacore, and S. Klein. 2004. Physical frailty and body composition in obese elderly men and women. *Obes Res* 12 (6):913-20.

Vita, A. J., R. B. Terry, H. B. Hubert, and J. F. Fries. 1998. Aging, health risks, and cumulative disability. *N Engl J Med* 338 (15):1035-41.

Volpato, S., C. Blaum, H. Resnick, L. Ferrucci, L. P. Fried, and J. M. Guralnik. 2002. Comorbidities and impairments explaining the association between diabetes and lower extremity disability: The Women's Health and Aging Study. *Diabetes Care* 25 (4):678-83.

Volpato, S., S. G. Leveille, C. Blaum, L. P. Fried, and J. M. Guralnik. 2005. Risk factors for falls in older disabled women with diabetes: the women's health and aging study. *J Gerontol A Biol Sci Med Sci* 60 (12):1539-45.

Waters, D. L., C. R. Qualls, R. I. Dorin, J. D. Veldhuis, and R. N. Baumgartner. 2008. Altered growth hormone, cortisol, and leptin secretion in healthy elderly persons with sarcopenia and mixed body composition phenotypes. *J Gerontol A Biol Sci Med Sci* 63 (5):536-41.

Whitlock, G., S. Lewington, P. Sherliker, R. Clarke, J. Emberson, J. Halsey, N. Qizilbash, R. Collins, and R. Peto. 2009. Body-mass index and cause-specific mortality in 900 000 adults: collaborative analyses of 57 prospective studies. *Lancet* 373 (9669):1083-96.

Zamboni, M., V. Di Francesco, U. Garbin, A. Fratta Pasini, G. Mazzali, C. Stranieri, E. Zoico, F. Fantin, O. Bosello, and L. Cominacini. 2007. Adiponectin gene expression and adipocyte NF-kappaB transcriptional activity in elderly overweight and obese women: inter-relationships with fat distribution, hs-CRP, leptin and insulin resistance. *Int J Obes (Lond)* 31 (7):1104-9.

Zamboni, M., G. Mazzali, F. Fantin, A. Rossi, and V. Di Francesco. 2008. Sarcopenic obesity: a new category of obesity in the elderly. *Nutr Metab Cardiovasc Dis* 18 (5):388-95.

Zizza, C. A., A. Herring, J. Stevens, and B. M. Popkin. 2002. Obesity affects nursing-care facility admission among whites but not blacks. *Obes Res* 10 (8):816-23.

Zoico, E., V. Di Francesco, J. M. Guralnik, G. Mazzali, A. Bortolani, S. Guariento, G. Sergi, O. Bosello, and M. Zamboni. 2004. Physical disability and muscular strength in relation to obesity and different body composition indexes in a sample of healthy elderly women. *Int J Obes Relat Metab Disord* 28 (2):234-41.

13

Type 2 Diabetes and Pancreatic Cancer – A Possible Reason

Parviz M Pour
UNMC/Eppley Cancer Center, University of Nebraska Medical Center, Omaha, USA

1. Introduction

Nearly 80% patients of pancreatic cancer (PC) have impaired glucose metabolism, either frank diabetes or impaired glucose tolerance (IGT)[1, 2] and the majority of diabetes associated with PC is diagnosed either concomitantly or during the two years before the diagnosis of PC[3] Karmody and Kyle reported that PC was diagnosed within one year from the onset of the diabetes in 40 out of 51 patients (78.4%)[4] According to Gullo et al.[5], diabetes in patients with PC is frequently (56.1%) of the recent onset type and is presumably caused by the tumor. In this study, in 43.9% of the patients, the diagnosis of diabetes preceeded the diagnosis of PC by three years and in 37.2% it was five or more years. In a more recent study, the diagnosis of PC and diabetes was made concomitantly or shortly before the tumor diagnosis in 65% of the patients [6]. Presently, a number of investigators consider diabetes to be a clinical manifestation of PC rather than a risk factor for the disease. This view is in sharp contrat to views that diabetes is a predisposing factor for PC. In many retrospective case-control and prospective cohort studies, an association between longstanding diabetes and an increased rate of subsequent death from PC was indicated [7-9]. In recent studies, however, when the latency period between the onset of diabetes and PC was considered, the issue became muddled. In some studies, when the patients with short latency periods were excluded from the sample size, the relative risk of diabetes for PC was markedly diminished[3-5]. In another population-based case control study, a significant positive trend in risk for PC was detected (p=0.016) in patients with diabetes diagnosed ten or more years prior to cancer detection[10].The meta-analysis of more than 20 epidemiologic studies indicated the relative risk of PC for diabetics diagnosed at least five years prior to the diagnosis of cancer as 2.0[11]. In two prospective cohort studies with more than 20 years follow-up, an increased risk was found among subjects with high post-load plasma glucose levels [12, 13]. In the latter study, the risk was 2.2-fold higher for participants whose post-load glucose level was at least 200 mg/dl at baseline compared with those with the levels equal or less than 119 mg/dl. These studies evidently show that glucose intolerance may preceed the onset of PC rather than just being a consequence.

The major problem of such epidemiological studies is that the exact onset time of both diabetes and PC is obscure and insidious. The non-insulin-dependent diabetes mellitus may take more than seven years before it is clinically diagnosed [14]. The latency of PC is also unclear, and the development of some cancers seems to take ten years[15] or even longer[16]. Undiagnosed diabetes or PC may have proceeded for many years without diagnosis. For

these reasons, estimation of the exact duration needed to conclude that the diabetes occurred before or after the development of PC is difficult.
The incidental pancreatic cancer detection indicates that this cancer can remain silent for a considerable time or grow very slowly [17]. Nevertheless, the notion that diabetes is a predisposing factor for PC remains questionable. Data gained from experimental pancreatic cancer model unquestionably indicate that the IGT is associated with the development of pancreatic cancer. We performed the following study to understand reasons for the development of diabetes in pancreatic cancer.
Eight-week-old out bred Syrian Golden hamsters (SGH) of the Eppley colony were used. They were housed in the centralized Comparative Medicine Animal Facilities, an AAALAC International accredited animal facility, in plastic cages on corncob bedding (Bed-O-Cobs, The Anderson Cob Co., Maumee, OH) under standard laboratory conditions (temperature, 21 ± 2°C; humidity, 40±5%; light/dark cycle, 12 hr/12 hr; 10x air changes/hr). They were fed a commercial diet (Wayne Lab Blox, Allied Mills, Chicago, IL) and had free access to tap water. The maintenance and humane treatment of the animals followed the guidelines of the UNMC Animal Care and Use Committee.
For the determination of glucose metabolism, five randomly selected 8-week-old male SGH with an average weight of 100 g were treated with the potent pancreatic carcinogen, N-nitrosobis(2-oxopropyl)amine (BOP) at a dose of 10 mg/kg body weight once a weak for four weeks. The same number of animals served as controls. Ten weeks after the last BOP injection, at the time generally proliferative and hyperplastic lesions appears, glucose tolerance was determined in all hamsters as reported [18]. Following the test the pancreas of all hamsters was examined histologically.
The presence of Insulin and glucagon assay in pancreatic juice and plasma was investigated in thirty 8-week-old male SGH with an average weight of 100g, who were treated with BOP as above. Thirty hamsters of the same age and weights were served as controls. In each group, the insulin content of pancreatic juice and plasma were assayed in 10 hamsters each at 12, 16 and 20 weeks after the last BOP injection as reported [19, 20].
From our tumor archieve, the pancreatic tissue of 30 SGH with tumors induced by BOP at a dose of 10 mg/kg body weight weekly for six weeks were examined immunohistochemically using antibodies to insulin, glucagon, somatostatin and PP with a multilabeling technique, developed in our laboratory [21]. Sixty seven surgically removed human pancreatic cancer specimens from our previous study [22] were also subjected to immunohistochemical examination for the expression of insulin, glucagon, somatostatin and PP as above.
The results of these experiments showed that at 10 weeks after BOP treatment plasma insulin level did not change compared to that in untreated control hamsters, whereas the glucose level increased significantly at 120 minutes (Fig. 1). Histologically focal or multi-focal ductal and ductular hyperplasia and in one hamster ductal in situ carcinoma were found. As in our previous studies, intrainsular ductular proliferation were found in all hamsters.
Insulin assay in pancreatic juice and plasma: As summarized in Table 1, although at week 12 the plasma insulin concentration did not differ from the control value, it decreased by one-half at week 16 but was significantly lower at week 20. On the contrary the level of insulin in pancreatic juice increased successively and was significantly decreased significantly and successively while juice insulin level conversely increased significantly by time (Table 1). The glucagon level in plasma did not change significantly at either point, whereas its level increased significantly and successively and was the highest at 20 week (Table 2).

Proliferative and hyperplastic ductal lesions were found at week 12 and 16 and a few in situ carcinomas and a microcarcinoma at week 20. A remarkably large number of endocrine cells (primarily β-cells) were found in hyperplastic ducts and in the microcarcinoma (Fig. 2), as well as some of hybrid type containing endocrine granules and mucin.
Immunohistochemically in all hyperplastic, premalignant and malignant lesions in human tissues, scattered or generally a large number of endocrine cells, composed primarily of insulin and glucagon, and less frequently somatostatin cells were found in the basal layer, but sometimes within the papillary fonts (Fig. 2). Insulin immunoreactivity was also present in the luminal content of hyperplastic ducts and malignant glands.

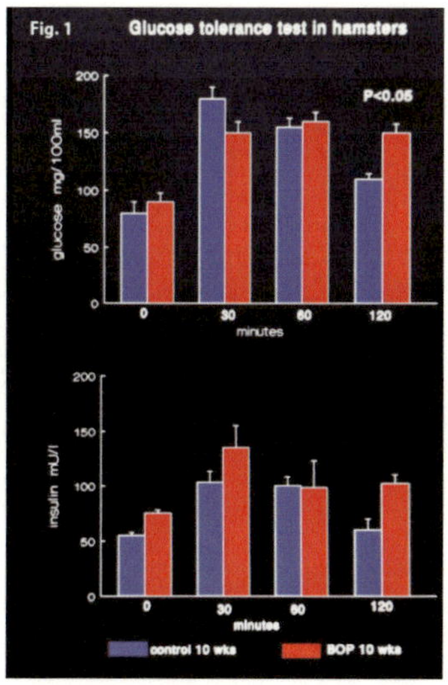

Fig. 1. Glucose tolerance test in SGH treated with BOP weekly for 6 weeks (red) and in untreated controls (blue)

Week	Plasma	Juice
12	6.07±1.96	4.28±1.40
16	3.02±1.67	5.07±2.05
20	2.52±0.12*	8.43±2.40*
*p<0.05 compared to control values		

Table 1. Insulin Levels (µU/ml)

Week	Plasma	Juice
12	0.62±0.07	25.8±4.40*
16	3.02±1.67	35.4±2.19*
20	2.52±0.12	39.4±3.10*
*p<0.001 compared to control values		

Table 2. Levels of Glucagon (ng/ml)

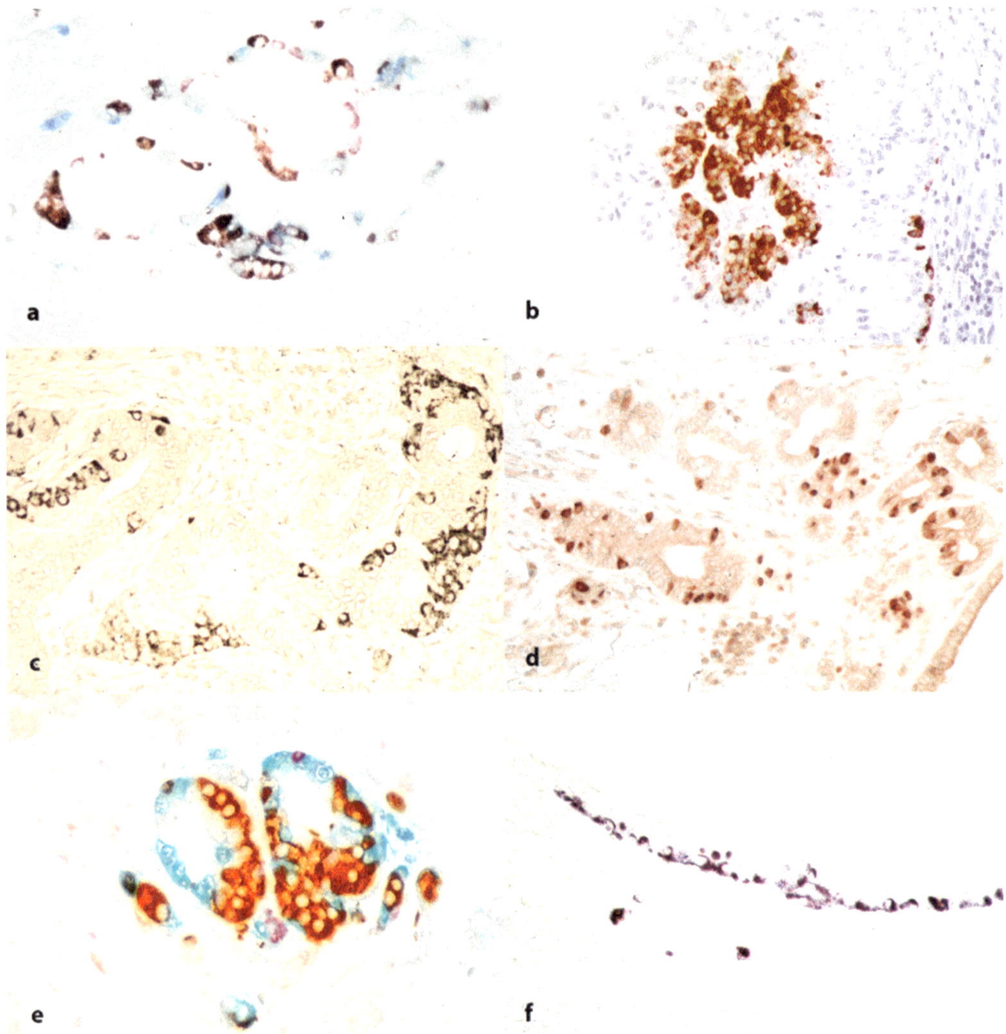

Fig. 2. Endocrine cells in pancreatic cancer. a) hamster adenocarcinoma. Insulin (brown), glucagon (blue), somatostatin (red). Multilabeling technique x65. B) Insulin cells in papillary fond and in the basal layer of the malignant epithelial cells of a human intraductal cancer. x50. c) insulin cells in human pancreatic cancer. x50; d) Insulin cells in proliferative ductal lesion in a hamster. x50; e) a large number of endocrine cells in human pancreatic cancer. insulin (blue); glucagon (brown); somatostatin (red). Multilabeling technique x50), f. endocrine cells covering the whole length of the basal layer of a tumor in a patient. X45.

Similar to the findings in the hamster tissue, insulin, glucagon and, less frequently, somatostatin cells were found in hyperplastic, but in extremely large numbers in well differentiated malignant glandular structures in human PC. In many areas the number of endocrine cells exceeded the number of malignant cells in glandular structures (Fig. 2). Remarkably, in the lumen of several malignant glands, many cells and debris immunoreactive with anti-insulin were identified (Fig. 3).

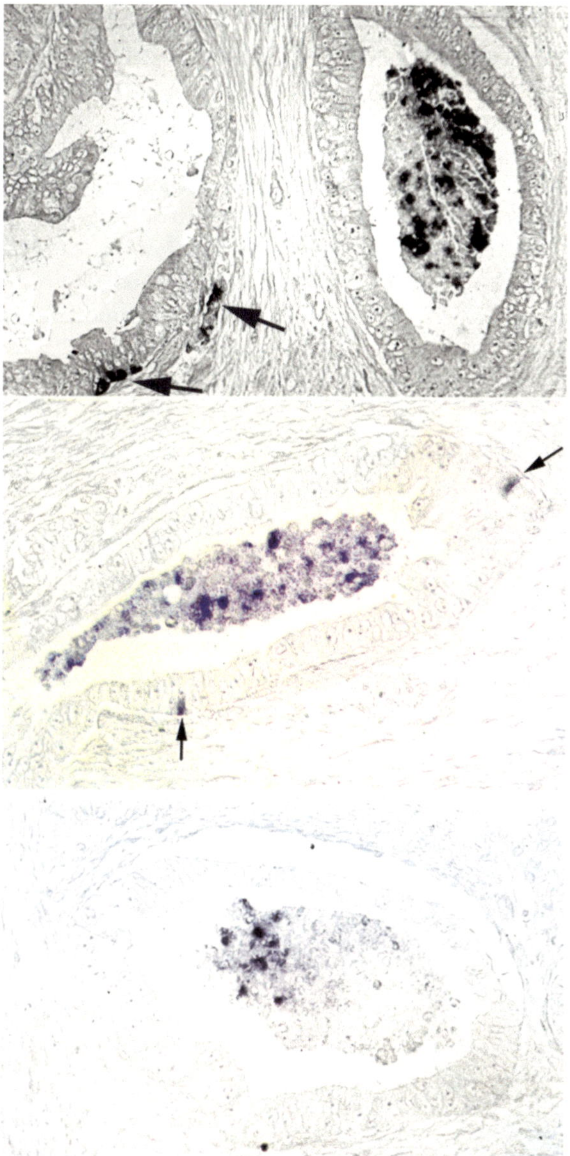

Fig. 3. Cells and debris immunoreactive with anti-insulin in the lumen of malignant gland structures. β cells are also present in the base of the epithelium (arrows). X65

Experimental models have opened avenues for studying areas of research that are impossible to obtain from humans. Among the existing pancreatic cancer model, SGH has provided the most relevant model for translational research. Morphologically, the wide spectrum of human pancreatic cancer, including the rare tumors, is reproducible in this species. Most human pancreatic cancer-associated antigens, including blood group antigens, as well as carbohydrate antigens are also expressed in cancers induced in hamsters. Most genetic mutations, methylation or deletions found in human pancreatic cancer, including the K-*ras*, $p16^{INK4A}$, DPC4/SMAD4, DCC and FHIT are also detected in hamster pancreatic cancer[25]. Remarkably, the deletion of chromosome Y, frequently found in human pancreatic cancer [23, 24] occurs also in the hamster tumor. Moreover, among other existing PC models, including transgenic mouse models, the hamster model is the only model that shows insulin secretion abnormality, occurring in over 80% of PC patients.

Based on these similarities, the model offered a useful tool to understand the existing controversial view on the association between type 2 diabetes and PC. Although SGH are not prone to diabetes, under certain diet they present pre-diabetic condition such as peripheral insulin resistance, which, as in humans, can be controlled by Metformin[26]. Because in this model initial alteration occurs within the islets by formation of intrainsular ductular structures, which progressively leads to the development of cancer that destroys the islet [27], studies were performed to explore the effect of such alteration on glucose metabolism. Ahrén and Andrén-Sandberg, were the first to demonstrate the abnormality in glucose tolerance occurs at the very early stages of carcinogenesis[18]. In their study, where the glucose tolerance and insulin secretion during the development of pancreatic cancer was examined, the glucose tolerance and glucose-stimulated insulin secretion were found to be normal at 6, 12, and 18 weeks after start of carcinogen treatment compared with age-matched saline-injected controls. By contrast, after 24, 30, and 42 weeks, at which time proliferative and neoplastic lesions develop, an exaggerated plasma-glucose response and a concomitant impaired plasma-insulin response occurred during the glucose infusion ($P < 0.05$). Hence, it was conclude that the development of pancreatic cancer in this model is accompanied by glucose intolerance and impaired insulin secretion, and that these effects occur concomitantly with the development of cancer. In the present study using the same experimental protocol confirmed the development of IGT (Fig. 1). At the time of proliferative and hyperplastic ductal lesions.

Reasons for examining the pancreatic juice during pancreatic cancer development was based on our findings of insulin-like and growth hormone-like substances in pancreatic juice of untreated hamsters[19]. Literature search revealed that this discovery was not unique to hamsters and has been reported in pancreatic juice of humans and laboratory species [28-34] supporting the assumption for the existence of an insuloacinar portal system to regulate exocrine pancreatic functions by islet hormones[35]. The question on the mechanism of whether insulin enters into the ductal system by passive or active mechanism has remained illusive. Since CCK is a powerful stimulant for the release of insulin and somatostatin[34], the greater effect of CCK infusion in eliciting a higher concentration of immunoreactive insulin and somatostatin in the pancreatic juice[34] indicated that the hormones in the juice derive directly from the islets to the ductules[29]. This view is further supported by our electron microscopical findings that revealed the likelihood of the direct route of insulin into the ductal lumen, as insulin granules were found in large numbers in peri ductal and peri vascular spaces, suggesting that insulin secretion occurs into both blood vessels and ductal lumen[36]. Hence, It appears that in the normal condition pancreatic hormones is secreted into blood vessels and ductal system possibly in a controlled defined proportion. The physiological importance of insulin secretion via ductal system as a potent growth factor for gastrointestinal epithelium has been discussed by us elsewhere[36].

As stated earlier, the initial development of ductular structures within the islets with gradual proliferation, malignant alteration and gradual replacement of the islets [27]suggested alteration in insulin secretion. The development of mixed ductular-insular structures, suggesting intimate communication between islet cells and ductal cells prompted us to examine the pancreatic juice of hamsters during tumor development. In a study, we measured the concentrations of insulin, glucagon, somatostatin, and islet amyloid polypeptide (IAPP) in plasma and secretin-stimulated pancreatic juice at 12 and 27 weeks after the treatment of hamsters with BOP[20]. At 12 weeks after BOP, plasma glucagon levels were significantly increased. An exaggerated plasma-glucose response were observed at 27 but not at 12 weeks after BOP. Plasma IAPP concentrations, but not glucagon or somatostatin, were elevated at 27 weeks. Tissue concentrations of IAPP were substantially reduced in BOP-treated hamsters at 27 weeks. The study, nevertheless, showed that islet hormone changes accompany the early development of pancreatic tumors in this model. Thus, the hormone changes and apparent insulin resistance resemble the metabolic changes found in humans with pancreatic cancer[20].

In the present study, a dramatic increase of insulin and glucagon levels was found in pancreatic juice of hamsters during pancreatic carcinogenesis indicating an alteration in islet function causing a shift in insulin secretion. Indeed, in both humans and hamsters islet cells during cancer development undergo alterations, including transdifferentiation of hormone producing cells into duct-like elements[23] that could explain the reduction in the level of plasma insulin. The level of insulin in pancreatic juice, however, is maintained and further increased by another event. In the hamster model and in human pancreatic cancer subjects as well, normal ducts, but more often altered ducts and especially malignant glandular structures show a large number of endocrine cells immunoreactive to ani-insulin and anti-glucagon antibodies, embedded within the epithelium ([27], and Fig 2). In some cases, the number of endocrine cells exceeded the number of the malignant epithelial cells (Fig 2). Within the malignant epithelium as well as in the lumen of several malignant glands many cells immunoreactive with anti-insulin were identified (Fig. 3). The finding suggested than insulin-containing cells, produced by malignant glands, are expelled into the glandular lumen, as are malignant cells, and thus into the pancreatic juice. Remarkably, we could not find any study examining the presence of hormones in pancreatic juice of pancreatic cancer patients, although, as stated earlier, endocrine hormones in pancreatic juice has been recognized many years ago in patients without pancreatic cancer.

The above information along with our current results let us conclude that the induction of proliferative and malignant lesions in the pancreas is associated with IGT, which also occurs in the majority of human cases. In fact, a study in Japan has shown that the incidence of IGT in PC patients was dependent on the size of cancer; in patients with tumor size >2.1 cm, the incidence of IGT was 56%, in tumors of 2.0 cm in size, it was 36%, in those with 1.1-2 cm, it was 39% and in 7 patients with tumors <1 cm, it was 28%. In the latter case, the abnormality was the only clinically detectable abnormality [37]. Remarkably, the determination of IGT has not yet been adapted as a routine test in the United States possibly awaiting additional validating data to be presented.

2. Conclusion

In SGH the development of PC is associated with IGT, as has also been suggested in humans. 2) In the normal pancreas, insulin is also secreted into pancreatic juice, both in humans and in animals. 3) The reduced level of insulin in blood but its increased concentration in pancreatic juice during pancreatic carcinogenesis is likely responsible for the IGT and diabetes, and 4) the development of IGT, along with hypersecretion of insulin in pancreatic juice could present early marker for PC.

3. References

[1] Permert J, Ihse I, Jorfeldt L, von Schenck H, Arnqvist HJ, Larsson J. Pancreatic cancer is associated with impaired glucose metabolism. Eur J Surg 1993;159:101-7.

[2] Schwarts SS, Zeidler A, Moossa AR, Kuku SF, Rubenstein AH. A prospective study of glucose tolerance, insulin, C-peptide, and glucagon responses in patients with pancreatic carcinoma. Am J Dig Dis 1978;23:1107-14.

[3] Gullo L, Pezzilli R, Morselli-Labate AM. Diabetes and the risk of pancreatic cancer. N Engl J Med 1994;331:81-4.

[4] Karmody AJ, Kyle J. The association between carcinoma of the pancreas and diabetes mellitus. Br J Surg 1969;56:362-4.

[5] Gullo L. Diabetes and the risk of pancreatic cancer. Ann Oncol 1999;10 Suppl 4:79-81.

[6] Chow WH, Gridley G, Nyren O, Linet MS, Ekbom A, Fraumeni JF, Jr., Adami HO. Risk of pancreatic cancer following diabetes mellitus: a nationwide cohort study in Sweden. J Natl Cancer Inst 1995;87:930-1.

[7] Silverman DT, Swanson CA, Gridley G, Wacholder S, Greenberg RS, Brown LM, Hayes RB, Swanson GM, Schoenberg JB, Pottern LM, Schwartz AG, Fraumeni JF, Jr., Hoover RN. Dietary and nutritional factors and pancreatic cancer: a case-control study based on direct interviews. J Natl Cancer Inst 1998;90:1710-9.

[8] Cuzick J, Babiker AG. Pancreatic cancer, alcohol, diabetes mellitus and gall-bladder disease. Int J Cancer 1989;43:415-21.

[9] Ragozzino M, Melton LJ, 3rd, Chu CP, Palumbo PJ. Subsequent cancer risk in the incidence cohort of Rochester, Minnesota, residents with diabetes mellitus. J Chronic Dis 1982;35:13-9.

[10] Silverman DT. Risk factors for pancreatic cancer: a case-control study based on direct interviews. Teratog Carcinog Mutagen 2001;21:7-25.

[11] Everhart J, Wright D. Diabetes mellitus as a risk factor for pancreatic cancer. A meta-analysis. JAMA 1995;273:1605-9.

[12] Smith GD, Egger M, Shipley MJ, Marmot MG. Post-challenge glucose concentration, impaired glucose tolerance, diabetes, and cancer mortality in men. Am J Epidemiol 1992;136:1110-4.

[13] Gapstur SM, Gann PH, Lowe W, Liu K, Colangelo L, Dyer A. Abnormal glucose metabolism and pancreatic cancer mortality. JAMA 2000;283:2552-8.

[14] Harris MI, Klein R, Welborn TA, Knuiman MW. Onset of NIDDM occurs at least 4-7 yr before clinical diagnosis. Diabetes Care 1992;15:815-9.

[15] Brat DJ, Lillemoe KD, Yeo CJ, Warfield PB, Hruban RH. Progression of pancreatic intraductal neoplasias to infiltrating adenocarcinoma of the pancreas. Am J Surg Pathol 1998;22:163-9.

[16] Michaud DS, Fuchs CS. Obesity and pancreatic cancer: overall evidence and latency period. Cancer Epidemiol Biomarkers Prev 2005;14:2678; author reply 2678-9.

[17] Kimura W, Morikane K, Esaki Y, Chan WC, Pour PM. Histologic and biologic patterns of microscopic pancreatic ductal adenocarcinomas detected incidentally at autopsy. Cancer 1998;82:1839-49.

[18] Ahren B, Andren-Sandberg A. Glucose tolerance and insulin secretion in experimental pancreatic cancer in the Syrian hamster. Res Exp Med (Berl) 1993;193:21-6.

[19] Helgeson AS, Lawson T, Pour P. Exocrine pancreatic secretion in the Syrian golden hamster Mesocricetus auratus--III. Effects of carcinogen administration and development of pancreas cancer. Comp Biochem Physiol C 1984;77:191-7.

[20] Permert J, Herrington M, Kazakoff K, Pour PM, Adrian TE. Early changes in islet hormone secretion in the hamster pancreatic cancer model. Teratog Carcinog Mutagen 2001;21:59-67.

[21] Pour PM, Kazakoff K, Dulaney K. A new multilabeling technique for simultaneous demonstration of different islet cells in permanent slides. Int J Pancreatol 1993;13:139-42.

[22] Pour PM, Schmied BM, Ulrich AB, Friess H, Andren-Sandberg A, Buchler MW. Abnormal differentiation of islet cells in pancreatic cancer. Pancreatology 2001;1:110-6.

[23] Bardi G, Johansson B, Pandis N, Mandahl N, Bak-Jensen E, Andren-Sandberg A, Mitelman F, Heim S. Karyotypic abnormalities in tumours of the pancreas. Br J Cancer 1993;67:1106-12.

[24] Johansson B, Bardi G, Heim S, Mandahl N, Mertens F, Bak-Jensen E, Andren-Sandberg A, Mitelman F. Nonrandom chromosomal rearrangements in pancreatic carcinomas. Cancer 1992;69:1674-81.

[25] Takahashi M HM, Mutoh M, Wakabayashi K, Nakagama H. Experimental Animal Models of Pancreatic Carcinogenesis for Prevention Studies and Their Relevance to Human Disease. Cancers 2011;3:582-602.

[26] Schneider MB, Matsuzaki H, Haorah J, Ulrich A, Standop J, Ding XZ, Adrian TE, Pour PM. Prevention of pancreatic cancer induction in hamsters by metformin. Gastroenterology 2001;120:1263-70.

[27] Pour PM, Standop J, Batra SK. Are islet cells the gatekeepers of the pancreas? Pancreatology 2002;2:440-8.

[28] Bailey CJ, Flatt PR, Atkins TW, Matty AJ. Immunoreactive insulin in bile and pancreatic juice of rat. Endocrinol Exp 1976;10:101-11.

[29] Conlon JM, Rouiller D, Boden G, Unger RH. Characterization of immunoreactive components of insulin and somatostatin in canine pancreatic juice. FEBS Lett 1979;105:23-6.

[30] Ertan A, Taminato T, Akdamar K, Ryan J, Agrawal NM, Schally AV, Arimura A. Immunoreactive somatostatin in human pancreatic secretion. J Clin Endocrinol Metab 1981;52:589-91.

[31] Fischer U, Hommel H, Ziegler M, Nowak W, von Dorsche HH. The mechanism of insulin secretion after oral glucose administration. VIII. Pancreatic juice insulin excretion after glucose loading and meal ingestion in normal and vagotomized dogs. Endokrinologie 1976;68:327-37.

[32] Prinz RA, Kirsteins L, Connick E, Paloyan E, Lawrence AM. Insulin and glucagon in human pancreatic exocrine fluid. Horm Metab Res 1980;12:38-9.

[33] Runzi M, Muller MK, Schimiczek M, von Schonfeld J, Goebell H. Identification of somatostatin-14 and -28 in rat pancreatic juice by a new HPLC method. Int J Pancreatol 1992;11:19-22.

[34] Sarfati PD, Green GM, Brazeau P, Morisset J. Presence of somatostatin-like immunoreactivity in rat pancreatic juice: a physiological phenomenon. Can J Physiol Pharmacol 1986;64:539-44.

[35] Ipp E, Dobbs RE, Harris V, Arimura A, Vale W, Unger RH. The effects of gastrin, gastric inhibitory polypeptide, secretin, and the octapeptide of cholecystokinin upon immunoreactive somatostatin release by the perfused canine pancreas. J Clin Invest 1977;60:1216-9.

[36] Pour PM, Hauser RE. Exocrine secretion of pancreatic hormones: possible mechanisms. Int J Pancreatol 1987;2:277-87.

[37] Ariyama J. Abnormal glucose tolerance in patients with early pancreatic carcinoma. Int J Pancreatol 1994;16:91.

14

Pathophysiology in Type 2 Diabetes – Type 2 Diabetes and Sleep-Disordered Breathing/Sleep Apnea – Role of Adipocytokines

Ken Kishida
Department of Metabolism and Atherosclerosis, Graduate School of Medicine, Osaka University, Japan

1. Introduction

Sleep is a complex behavioral state that occupies one-third of the human life span. Although viewed as a passive condition, sleep is a highly active and dynamic process. Sleep was considered to be primarily important for restoration of brain function. However, to date, there is increasing evidence that sleep also modulates the metabolic, endocrine and cardiovascular systems [Trenell, 2007; Boethel, 2002; Knutson & Van Cauter, 2007; Knutson, 2008]. It is known that if left untreated, sleep disorders can have significant impact on daytime function, including learning, memory, attention, and behavior. The approach to the treatment of these disorders (whether with or without pharmacotherapy) is dependent on a thorough evaluation of the sleep complaint and accurate diagnosis. Previous studies reported a consistent difference between diabetic and non-diabetic subjects in the number of sleep disturbances per hour, indicating possible influence of diabetes on sleep pattern [Resnick, 2003; Kawakami, 2004]. Several studies have shown that patients with T2DM sleep less than the general population [Vgontzas, 2000; Buxton, 2010]. A gradual decrease in self-reported sleep duration seems to have developed over the same period as the dramatic increase in the incidence of obesity and diabetes, including a close relationship between sleep cycle and diabetes [Van Cauter, 1997; Spiegel, 2005; Chasens, 2007; Knutson & Van Cauter, 2008]. Sleeping disorders related to T2DM include insomnia, restless leg syndrome, periodic leg movement disorder, excessive daytime sleepiness, sleepwalking, nightmares, narcolepsy, and SDB, especially SA.

T2DM and SDB/SA are both prevalent diseases that share several risk factors, including advanced age and obesity [Tishler, 2003; Young, 1993]. T2DM is associated with higher incidence of cardiovascular, cerebrovascular, and renal diseases. There is also mounting evidence that SDB/SA is an independent risk factor for cardiovascular and cerebrovascular diseases. Interest in a potential independent link between the two diseases continues to grow.

2. Sleep loss

Chronic sleep loss is increasingly common in industrialized countries. The sleep impairment may result from various common disturbances, such as insomnia and OSA and may lead to

striking changes in metabolic and endocrine functions [Spiegel, 1999]. Chronic sleep loss is a potential risk factor for obesity, insulin resistance, and T2DM.
Previous studies reported that both short (<6 hours) and long (>8 hours) sleepers as well as those with sleep loss, are at greater risk for glucose intolerance and T2DM [Sridhar & Madhu, 1994; Scheen, 1997; Ayas, 2003; Mallon, 2005; Gottlieb, 2005; Mallon, 2005; Yaggi, 2006; Chaput, 2007; Nakajima, 2008].

3. Sleep apnea

SA is a sleep disorder characterized by pauses in breathing during sleep. There are several forms of SA, but the obstructive type is the commonest. In OSA, pauses in breathing are caused by a physical block to airflow, usually in the oropharynx. OSA is usually defined by interruptions of airflow of at least 10-second duration (apneas), or by a decrease in airflow of at least 10 seconds (hypopneas) followed by blood oxygen desaturation and arousal (brief arousal associated with airway opening and resumption of breathing) [Report of American Academy of Sleep Medicine Task Force, 1999; Masood & Phillips, 2000].

3.1 Symptoms

SA is often first noticed by the bed partner who witness episodes of apneas or is suspected based on history of habitual snoring and/or excessive daytime sleepiness, general fatigue or near-miss car accidents. Other symptoms reported by patients with SA include [Bresnitz, 1994; Gupta, 2010; Wickwire & Collop, 2010] 1) irritability, 2) poor memory, 3) morning headache, 4) depression, 5) mood changes, 6) sexual dysfunction, and 7) nocturia.

3.2 Diagnosis

SDB/SA is often diagnosed by an overnight cardiorespiratory test called polysomnography [Jafari & Mohsenin, 2010]; though other simpler methods are currently available, such as type 3 cardiopulmonary monitoring [Collop, 2007]. The recorded signals are analyzed for the numbers of apneas and hypopneas, episodes of oxygen desaturation, as well as lowest oxygen saturation, average oxygen saturation, and time at desaturation <90% in minutes of the total bedtime for the entire night. Apnea is defined as a decrease in the amplitude of the airflow or respiratory effort signal to <10% of the baseline lasting at least 10 seconds. Hypopnea is defined as a decrease in the airflow or respiratory effort to <70% of the baseline for at least 10 seconds accompanied by >4% fall in oxygen saturation. The apnea-hypopnea index (AHI) is defined as the number of apneas/hypopneas per hour of sleep time. The latter is measured from the recorded signals of the electroencephalogram (averaged brain activity), electrooculogram (eye movements) and nuchal muscles electromyogram. An AHI of ≥5 establishes the diagnosis of SDB/SA. OSA is defined as absence of airflow in the presence of chest wall and/or abdominal excursions. The severity of SA is based on the AHI, and classified as mild (AHI ≥5 to <15), moderate (AHI ≥15 to <30), and severe (AHI ≥30), according to the guidelines of the American Academy of Sleep Medicine Task Force [Report of American Academy of Sleep Medicine Task Force, 1999].

3.3 Clinical features

Obese patients with OSA have short and wide neck, large tongue, and excess pharyngeal soft tissues. Significant SA is present in 40% of obese individuals, and 70% of OSA patients are obese [Vgontzas AN, 1994; Resta O, 2001; Daltro C, 2007]. Not only excess weight but also fat distribution, i.e. intra-abdominal fat accumulation, plays a major role in the development of OSA [Shinohara, 1997; Schäfer, 2002; Vgontzas, 2003]. A recent study of Japanese patients with T2DM found that BMI and waist circumference (WC) were the strongest predictors of the severity of SDB [Kashine, 2011]. OSA is independently associated with insulin resistance, T2DM and hypertension [Idris, 2009]. Several reports found high incidence of SA in both Japanese [Katsumata, 1991] and Caucasian [Einhorn, 2007] diabetic patients.

3.4 Treatment

There are several options for treatment of SA [Rosenberg & Doghramji, 2009]. These include:

3.4.1 Lifestyle changes

Weight loss, especially visceral fat reduction through caloric diet and exercise, should be recommended for all overweight patients with SA. Avoidance of alcohol and sleeping pills is often beneficial.

3.4.2 Oral devices

Oral devices such as dental appliances have been used with some success to maintain an open airway during sleep [Ng, 2005].

3.4.3 Nasal Continuous Positive Airway Pressure (nCPAP)

Nasal continuous positive airway pressure (nCPAP) is the golden standard treatment of SA in which a mask is worn over the nose and/or mouth whilst sleeping. The mask is attached to a machine that delivers a continuous stream of compressed air. The positive pressure pneumatically maintains an open airway during sleep. Treatment of OSA is reported to improve daytime sleepiness and various other clinical features of Sa including insulin responsiveness [Hassaballa, 2005; Harsch, 2004].

3.4.4 Surgery

Surgery may be considered in some cases, particularly those with tonsillar and adenoidal hypertrophy, narrow nasal airways, or facial deformities such as small jaw, nasal polyp or deviated nasal septum [Sundaram, 2005; Lojander, 1996; Holty, 2010].

4. Type 2 diabetes and sleep apnea

SDB/SA is often observed in patients with T2DM, and known to be potentially associated with atherosclerosis, leading to ACVDs. The International Diabetes Federation (IDF) Taskforce on Epidemiology and Prevention [Shaw, 2008] stated that the pathophysiological consequences of hypoxemia and sleep fragmentation might be involved in the development of insulin resistance and pancreatic β-cell dysfunction through various biological mechanisms, such as direct effects of 1) intermittent hypoxia/desaturation and hypoxemia, 2) sympathetic nervous system activation (catecholamine) [Prabhakar & Kumar, 2010; Esler & Eikelis, 2006], 3) systemic inflammation (tumor necrosis factor-alpha [TNF-α], interluokin-6 [IL-6], high sensitivity C-reactive protein [hsCRP] and monocyte chemoattractant protein 1 [MCP-1]) [Drager, 2010; Sahlman, 2010; Romero-Corral, 2010], 4) hypothalamic-pituitary-adrenal dysfunction (cortisol) [Follenius, 1992; Henley, 2009; Vgontzas & Chrousos, 2002], 5) dysregulation of adipocytokines (plasminogen activator inhibitor-1 [PAI-1], adiponectin) [Lam, 2008], 6) sleep architecture [Wang & Teichtahl, 2007] and 7) other factors. Both SDB/SA and T2DM are strongly associated with ACVD [Bradley & Floras, 2009] (Figure 1).

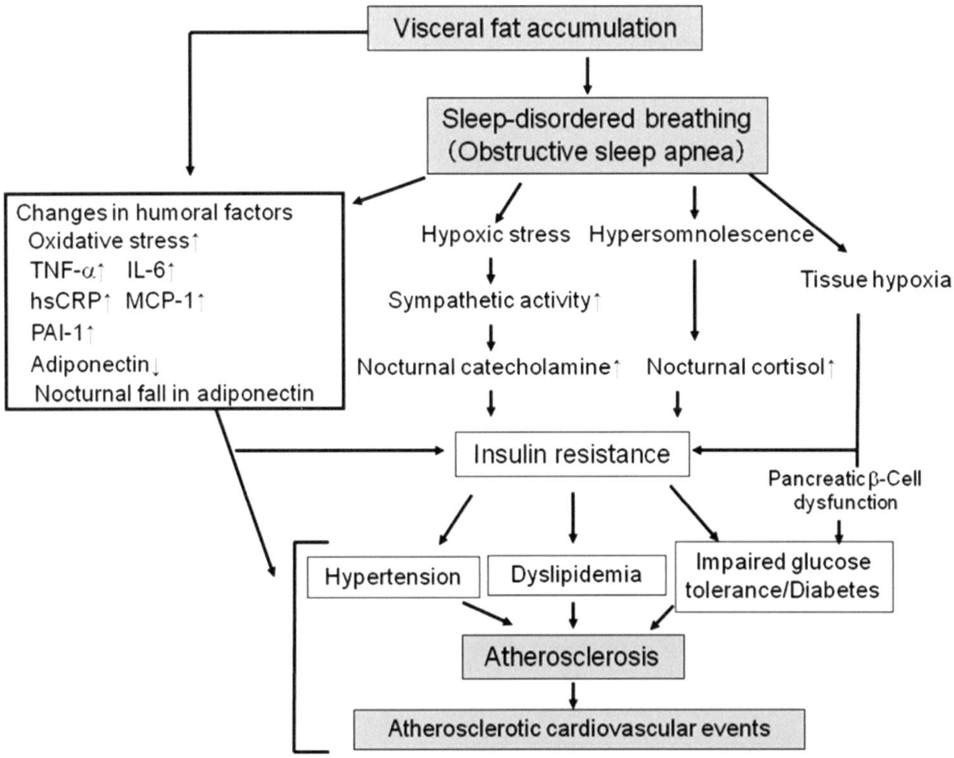

Fig. 1. Relationships among sleep-disordered breathing, visceral fat accumulation and atherosclerosis.

5. Type 2 diabetes mellitus and sleep-disordered breathing / sleep apnea: Role of adipocytokines

Both T2DM and SDB/SA have been linked to the metabolic syndrome based on visceral fat accumulation, with clustering of hyperglycemia, intra-abdominal fat accumulation, hypertension, hypertriglyceridemia, and hypo-high-density-lipoprotein-cholesterolemia [Rasche, 2010; Lui & Ip, 2010]. There is a broad overlap between the presumed mechanisms of that link T2DM and SDB/SA and features of the metabolic syndrome (Syndrome X) [Reaven, 1993], which is also known as "Syndrome Z" [Wilcox, 1998].

In addition to the localization and functional properties of visceral fat, experimental evidence links certain molecules in visceral fat to human disorders, especially insulin resistance and ACVD. An important question relates to the profile of molecules or genes expressed in subcutaneous and visceral fat. In order to answer this question, our group in collaboration with the human body map project team investigated the gene expression profile in human adipose tissue. This tissue had been traditionally regarded as a passive storage of excess energy in the form of triglycerides. Unexpectedly, we found that adipose tissues, especially visceral fat, abundantly express genes that encode secretory proteins including complement factors in the immune system, growth factors, and cytokines, most of which are important bioactive substances [Maeda, 1997; Matsuzawa, 2004]. We found PAI-1 [Shimomura, 1996] and HB-EGF [Matsumoto, 2002] in human visceral and subcutaneous fat cDNA library. Excess visceral fat overproduces and secretes PAI-1, which in turn increases the risk for thrombotic disorders [Shimomura, 1996]. Thus, it seems that visceral fat is directly linked to ACVD. Adipose tissue also produces a variety of the bioactive substances conceptualized as 'adipocytokines' [Funahashi, 1999; Matsuzawa, 2010]. Through systematic analysis of adipose tissue-expressed genes, we discovered a novel gene, designated adipose most abundant gene transcript 1 (apM1), for an adipocyte-derived secretory protein [Maeda, 1996], which was later named 'adiponectin'. At the same time, using different approaches, adiponectin was identified independently by three other groups, as adipocyte complement-related protein of 30 kDa (ACRP30) [Scherer, 1995], adipoQ [Hu, 1996], and gelatin binding protein of 28 kDa (GBP28) [Nakano, 1996]. Adiponectin is specifically expressed in the adipose tissue [Arita, 1999]. The molecule has two domains, namely a collagen-like fibrous domain and a C1q-like globular domain. The single molecules combine and form a high-ordered structure [Arita, 1999]. Adiponectin binds to collagens I, III, and V, which are present in the subendothelial intima [Okamoto, 2000]. In fact, adiponectin adheres to endothelium-injured arterial walls [Okamoto, 2000]. This is the reason why we named this protein 'adiponectin' [Arita, 1999]. Numerous experimental studies found that adiponectin has anti-atherosclerotic [Ouchi, 2003] and insulin sensitivity properties [Han, 2009].

The production and secretion of adipocytokines are dynamically regulated by nutritional status. Over-eating and physical inactivity result in visceral fat accumulation, which leads to visceral fat dysfunction and dysregulated production of adipocytokines (overproduction of offensive adipocytokines, such as PAI-1, TNF-α, HB-EGF and angiotensinogen, and underproduction of defensive adipocytokines, such as adiponectin), a state we call adipotoxicity. These changes are probably the major underlying mechanisms of lifestyle-related diseases [Kishida, 2011].

Daytime hypoadiponectinemia and nocturnal falls in circulating adiponectin concentrations in OSA patients with abdominal obesity, are in part, due to hypoxic stress [Nakagawa, 2008 & 2011]. A high frequency of SDB was identified in Japanese patients with poorly controlled T2DM, who also had intra-abdominal obesity with nocturnal dysregulated production of adiponectin [Kashine, 2010]. Obese East and South Asians including Japanese have a mild degree of adiposity, compared with European and American subjects [Wulan, 2010; Fujimoto, 1999; Tong, 2007; Kadowaki, 2006]. Unlike total body fat, body fat distribution, especially excess accumulation of visceral fat, correlates with various diabetogenic, atherogenic, prothrombotic and proinflammatory metabolic abnormalities in Japanese (referred to as the metabolic syndrome), that increase the risk of ACVD [Fujioka, 1987; Matsuzawa, 1994].

6. Conclusion

It is necessary to diagnose SDB from the standpoint of prevention of ACVD in diabetic patients. Weight reduction, particularly reduction of visceral fat, intensive glucose-lowering therapy, nCPAP therapy, or the combination of these therapies, have beneficial effects on the outcome of T2DM patients with SDB through improvement of dysregulated production of adipocytokines and SDB-related ACVD.

7. Acknowledgement

This work was supported in part by a Grant-in-Aid for Scientific Research No. (C) No. 21591177.

8. References

Trenell MI, et al. (2007) Sleep and metabolic control: waking to a problem? *Clinical and Experimental Pharmacology and Physiology*. Vol.34, No.1-2, (Jan-Feb 2007), pp.1-9

Boethel CD. (2002) Sleep and the endocrine system: new associations to old diseases. *Curr Opinion Pulmonary Medicine*. Vol.8, No.6, (Nov 2002), pp.502-505.

Knutson KL, Van Cauter E. (2008) Associations between sleep loss and increased risk of obesity and diabetes. *Annals of New York Academy of Sciences*. Vol.1129, pp.287-304.

Knutson KL, et al. (2007) The metabolic consequences of sleep deprivation. *Sleep Medicine Review*. Vol.11, No.3, (Jun 2007), pp.163-178.

Resnick HE, et al.; Sleep Heart Health Study. Diabetes and sleep disturbances: findings from the Sleep Heart Health Study. *Diabetes Care*. Vol.26, No.3, (Mar 2003), pp.702-709.

Kawakami N, et al. (2004) Sleep disturbance and onset of type 2 diabetes. *Diabetes Care*. Vol.27, No.1, (Jan 2004), pp.282-283.

Vgontzas AN, et al. (2000) Sleep apnea and daytime sleepiness and fatigue: relation to visceral obesity, insulin resistance, and hypercytokinemia. *Journal of Clinical Endocrinology and Metabolism*. Vol.85, No.3, (Mar 2000), pp.1151-1158.

Buxton OM, et al. (2010) Sleep restriction for 1 week reduces insulin sensitivity in healthy men. *Diabetes*. Vol.59, No.9, (Sep 2010), pp.2126-2133.

Van Cauter E, et al. (1997) Roles of circadian rhythmicity and sleep in human glucose regulation. *Endocrine Reviews*. Vol.18, No.5, (Oct 1997), pp.716-738.

Spiegel K, et al. (2005) Sleep loss: a novel risk factor for insulin resistance and Type 2 diabetes. *Journal of Applied Physiology*. Vol.99 No.5, (Nov 2005), pp.2008-2019.

Chasens ER. (2007) Obstructive sleep apnea, daytime sleepiness, and type 2 diabetes. *The Diabetes Educator*. Vol.33, No.3, (May-Jun 2007), pp.475-82.

Knutson KL, Van Cauter E. (2008) Associations between sleep loss and increased risk of obesity and diabetes. *Annals of the New York Academy of Sciences*. Vol.1129, (2008), pp.287-304.

Tishler PV, et al. (2003) Incidence of sleep-disordered breathing in an urban adult population: the relative importance of risk factors in the development of sleep-disordered breathing. *The Journal of American Medical Association*. Vol.289, No.17, (May 2003), pp.2230-2237.

Young T, et al. (1993) The occurrence of sleep-disordered breathing among middle-aged adults. *The New England Journal of Medicine*. Vol.328, No.17, (Apr 1993), pp.1230-1235.

Spiegel K, et al. (1999) Impact of sleep debt on metabolic and endocrine function. *Lancet*. Vol.354, No.9188, (Oct 1999), pp.1435-1439.

Sridhar GR, Madhu K. (1994) Prevalence of sleep disturbances in diabetes mellitus. *Diabetes Research and Clinical Practice*. Vol.23, No.3, (Apr 1994), pp.183-186.

Scheen AJ, et al. (1996) Relationships between sleep quality and glucose regulation in normal humans. *American of Journal Physiology*. Vol.271, No.2(Pt 1), (Aug 1996), pp.E261-270.

Ayas NT, et al. (2003) A prospective study of self-reported sleep duration and incident diabetes in women. *Diabetes Care*. Vol.26, No.2, (Feb 2003), pp.380-384.

Mallon L, et al. (2005) High incidence of diabetes in men with sleep complaints or short sleep duration: a 12-year follow-up study of a middle-aged population. *Diabetes Care*. Vol.28, No.11, (Nov 2005), pp.2762-2767.

Gottlieb DJ, et al. (2005) Association of sleep time with diabetes mellitus and impaired glucose tolerance. *Archives of Internal Medicine*. Vol.165, No.8, (Apr 2005), pp.863-867.

Mallon L, et al. (2005) High incidence of diabetes in men with sleep complaints or short sleep duration: a 12-year follow-up study of a middle-aged population. *Diabetes Care*. Vol.28, No.11, (Nov 2005), pp.2762-2767.

Yaggi HK, et al. (2006) Sleep duration as a risk factor for the development of type 2 diabetes. *Diabetes Care*. Vol.29, No.3, (Mar 2006), pp.657-661.

Chaput JP, et al. (2007) Association of sleep duration with type 2 diabetes and impaired glucose tolerance. *Diabetologia*. Vol.50, No.11, (Nov 2007), pp.2298-2304.

Nakajima H, et al. (2008) Association between sleep duration and hemoglobin A1c level. *Sleep Medicine*. Vol.9, No.7, (Oct 2008), pp.745-752.

Anonymous. (1999) Sleep-related breathing disorders in adults: recommendations for syndrome definition and measurement techniques in clinical research. The Report of an American Academy of Sleep Medicine Task Force. *Sleep*. Vol.22, No.5, (Aug 1999), pp.667-689.

Masood A, Phillips B. (2000) Sleep apnea. *Current Opinion in Pulmonary Medicine*. Vol.6, No.6, (Nov 2000), pp.479-484.

Bresnitz EA, et al. (1994) Epidemiology of obstructive sleep apnea. *Epidemiologic Reviews*. Vol.16, No.2, (1994), pp.210-227.

Gupta RK, et al. (2010) Obstructive sleep apnoea: a clinical review. *The Journal of Association of Physicians of India*. Vol.58, (Jul 2010), pp.438-441.

Wickwire EM, Collop NA. (2010) Insomnia and sleep-related breathing disorders. *Chest*. Vol.137, No.6, (Jun 2010), pp.1449-1463.

Jafari B, Mohsenin V. (2010) Polysomnography. *Clinics in Chest Medicine*. Vol.31, No.2, (Jun 2010), pp.287-297.

Collop NA, et al.; Portable Monitoring Task Force of the American Academy of Sleep Medicine. (2007) Clinical guidelines for the use of unattended portable monitors in the diagnosis of obstructive sleep apnea in adult patients. Portable Monitoring Task Force of the American Academy of Sleep Medicine. *Journal of Clinical Sleep Medicine*. Vol.3, No.7, (Dec 2007), pp.737-747.

Vgontzas AN, et al. (1994) Sleep apnea and sleep disruption in obese patients. *Archives of Internal Medicine*. Vo.154, No.15, (Aug 1994), pp1705-1711.

Resta O, et al. (2001) Sleep-related breathing disorders, loud snoring and excessive daytime sleepiness in obese subjects. *International Journal of Obesity Related Metabolic Disorders*. Vol.25, No.5, (May 2001), pp669-675.

Daltro C, et al. (2007) Prevalence and severity of sleep apnea in a group of morbidly obese patients. *Obesity Surgery*. Vol.17, No.6, (Jul 2007), pp.809-814.

Shinohara E, et al. (1997) Visceral fat accumulation as an important risk factor for obstructive sleep apnoea syndrome in obese subjects. *Journal of Internal Medicine*. Vol.241, No.1, (Jan 1997), pp.11-18.

Schäfer H, et al. (2002) Body fat distribution, serum leptin, and cardiovascular risk factors in men with obstructive sleep apnea. *Chest*. Vol.122, No.3, (Sep 2002), pp.829-839.

Vgontzas AN, et al. (2003) Metabolic disturbances in obesity versus sleep apnoea: the importance of visceral obesity and insulin resistance. *Journal of Internal Medicine*. Vol.254, No.1, (Jul 2003), pp.32-44.

Kashine S, et al. (2011) Effect of diabetes treatment on changes in sleep-disordered breathing and its related parameters in patients hospitalized with type 2 diabetes mellitus. *Journal of Atherosclerosis and Thrombosis*. in press.

Idris I, et al. (2009) Obstructive sleep apnoea in patients with type 2 diabetes: aetiology and implications for clinical care. *Diabetes,Obesity & Metabolism*. Vol.11, No.8, (Aug 2009), pp.733-741.

Katsumata K, et al. (1991) High incidence of sleep apnea syndrome in a male diabetic population. *Diabetes Research and Clinical Practice.* Vol.13, No.1-2, (Aug 1991), pp.45-51.

Einhorn D, et al. (2007) Prevalence of sleep apnea in a population of adults with type 2 diabetes mellitus. *Endocrine Practice*. Vol.13, No.4, (Jul-Aug 2007), pp.355-362.

Rosenberg R, Doghramji P. (2009) Optimal treatment of obstructive sleep apnea and excessive sleepiness. *Advances in Therapy*. Vol.26, No.3, (Mar 2009), pp295-312.

Ng A, et al. (2005) Oral appliance therapy for obstructive sleep apnea. *Treatment in Respiratory Medicine*. Vol.4, No.6, (2005), pp.409-422.

Hassaballa HA, et al. (2005) The effect of continuous positive airway pressure on glucose control in diabetic patients with severe obstructive sleep apnea. *Sleep & Breathing*. Vol.9, No.4, (Dec 2005), pp.176-180.

Harsch IA, et al. (2004) The effect of continuous positive airway pressure treatment on insulin sensitivity in patients with obstructive sleep apnoea syndrome and type 2 diabetes. *Respiration*. Vol.71, No.3, (May-Jun 2004), pp.252-259.

Sundaram S, et al. (2005) Surgery for obstructive sleep apnoea. *Cochrane Database of Systematic Reviews*. Vol.19, No.4, (Oct 2005), CD001004.

Lojander J, et al. (1996) Nasal-CPAP, surgery, and conservative management for treatment of obstructive sleep apnea syndrome. A randomized study. *Chest*. Vol.110, No.1, (Jul 1996), pp.114-119.

Holty JE, Guilleminault C. (2010) Surgical options for the treatment of obstructive sleep apnea. *The Medical Clinics of North America*. Vol.94, No.3, (May 2010), pp.479-515.

Shaw JE, et al.; International Diabetes Federation Taskforce on Epidemiology and Prevention. (2008) Sleep-disordered breathing and type 2 diabetes: a report from the International Diabetes Federation Taskforce on Epidemiology and Prevention. *Diabetes Res Clin Pract*. Vol.81, No.1, (Jul 2008), pp.2-12.

Prabhakar NR, Kumar GK. (2010) Mechanisms of sympathetic activation and blood pressure elevation by intermittent hypoxia. *Respiratory Physiology & Neurobiology*. Vol.174, No.1-2, (Nov 2010), pp.156-161.

Esler M, Eikelis N. (2006) Is obstructive sleep apnea the cause of sympathetic nervous activation in human obesity? *Journal of Applied Physiology*. Vol.100, No.1, (Jan 2006), pp.11-12.

Drager LF, et al. (2010) The impact of obstructive sleep apnea on metabolic and inflammatory markers in consecutive patients with metabolic syndrome. *PLoS One*. Vol.5, No,8, (Aug 2010), e12065.

Sahlman J, et al.; Kuopio Sleep Apnoea Group. (2010) The activation of the inflammatory cytokines in overweight patients with mild obstructive sleep apnoea. *J of Sleep Research*. Vol.19, No.2, (Jun 2010), pp.341-348.

Romero-Corral A, et al. (2010) Interactions between obesity and obstructive sleep apnea: implications for treatment. *Chest*. Vol.137, No.3, (Mar 2010), pp.711-719.

Follenius M, et al. (1992) Nocturnal cortisol release in relation to sleep structure. *Sleep*. Vol.15, No.1, (Feb 1992), pp.21-27.

Henley DE, et al. (2009) Hypothalamic-pituitary-adrenal axis activation in obstructive sleep apnea: the effect of continuous positive airway pressure therapy. *Journal of Clinical Endocrinology and Metabolism*. Vol.94, No.11, (Nov 2009), pp.4234-4242.

Vgontzas AN, Chrousos GP. (2002) Sleep, the hypothalamic-pituitary-adrenal axis, and cytokines: multiple interactions and disturbances in sleep disorders. *Endocrinology and Metabolism Clinics of North America*. Vol.31, No.1, (Mar 2002), pp.15-36.

Lam JC, et al. (2008) Hypoadiponectinemia is related to sympathetic activation and severity of obstructive sleep apnea. *Sleep*. Vol.31, No.12, (Dec 2008), pp.1721-1727.

Wang D, Teichtahl H. (2007) Opioids, sleep architecture and sleep-disordered breathing. *Sleep Medicine Reviews*. Vol.11, No.1, (Feb 2007), pp.35-46.

Bradley TD, Floras JS. (2009) Obstructive sleep apnoea and its cardiovascular consequences. *Lancet*. Vol.373, No.9657, (Jan 2009), pp.82-93.

Rasche K, et al. (2010) Obstructive sleep apnea and type 2 diabetes. *European Journal of Medical Research*. Vol.15, No. Suppl 2, (Nov 2010), pp152-1526.

Lui MM, Ip MS. (2010) Disorders of glucose metabolism in sleep-disordered breathing. *Clinics in Chest Medicine*. Vol.31, No.2, (Jun 2010), pp.271-285.

Reaven GM. (1993) Role of insulin resistance in human disease (syndrome X): an expanded definition. *Annual Review of Medicine*. Vol.44, (1993) pp.121-131.

Wilcox I, et al. (1998) 'Syndrome Z': The Interaction of Sleep Apnoea, Vascular Risk Factors and Heart Disease. *Thorax*. Vol.53, No.Supple3, (Oct 1998), pp.S25-28.

Maeda K, et al. (1997) Analysis of an expression profile of genes in the human adipose tissue. *Gene*. Vol.190, No.2, (May 1997), pp.227-235.

Matsuzawa Y, et al. (2004) Adiponectin and metabolic syndrome. *Arteriosclerosis, Thrombosis, and Vascular Biology*. Vol.24, No.1, (Jan 2004), pp.29-33.

Shimomura I, et al. (1996) Enhanced expression of PAI-1 in visceral fat: possible contributor to vascular disease in obesity. *Nat Med*. Vol.2, No.7, (Jul 1996), pp.800-803.

Matsumoto S, et al. (2002) Increased plasma HB-EGF associated with obesity and coronary artery disease. *Biochemical and Biophysical Research Communications*. Vol.292, No.3, (Apr 2002), pp.781-786.

Funahashi T, et al. (1999) Role of adipocytokines on the pathogenesis of atherosclerosis in visceral obesity. *Internal Medicine*. Vol.38, No.2, (Feb 1999), pp.202-206.

Matsuzawa Y. (2010) Establishment of a concept of visceral fat syndrome and discovery of adiponectin. *Proceedings of the Japan Academy. Series B, Physical and Biological Sciences*. Vol.86, No.2, (2010), pp.131-141.

Maeda K, et al. (1996) cDNA cloning and expression of a novel adipose specific collagen-like factor, apMa (Adipose Most Abundant gene transcript 1). *Biochemical and Biophysical Research Communications*. Vol.221, No.2, (Apr 1996), pp.286-289.

Scherer PE, et al. (1995) A novel serum protein similar to C1q, produced exclusively in adipocytes. *The Journal of Biological Chemistry*. Vol.270, No.45, (Nov 1995), pp.26746−26749.

Hu E, et al. (1996) AdipoQ is a novel adipose-specific gene dysregulated in obesity. *The Journal of Biological Chemistry*. Vol.271, No.18, (May 1996), pp.10697−10703.

Nakano Y, et al. (1996). Isolation and characterization of GBP28, a novel gelatin- binding protein purified from human plasma. *Journal of Biochemistry*. Vol.120, No.4 (Oct 1996), pp.803−812.

Arita Y, et al. (1999) Paradoxical decrease of an adipose-specific protein, adiponectin, in obesity. *Biochemical and Biophysical Research Communications*.Vol.257, No.1, (Apr 1999), pp.79-83.

Okamoto Y, et al. (2000) An adipocyte-derived plasma protein, adiponectin, adheres to injured vascular walls. *Hormone and Metabolic Research*. Vol.32, No.2, (Feb 2000), pp.47-50.
Ouchi N, et al. (2003) Obesity, adiponectin and vascular inflammatory disease. *Current Opinion in Lipidology*. Vol.14, No.6, (Dec 2003), pp.561-566.
Han SH, et al. (2009) Antiatherosclerotic and anti-insulin resistance effects of adiponectin: basic and clinical studies. *Progress in Cardiovascular Diseases*. Vol.52, No.2, (Sep-Oct 2009), pp.126-140.
Kishida K. et al. (2011) Visceral adiposity as a target for the management of the metabolic syndrome: A Japanese perspective. *Annals of Medicine*. in press.
Nakagawa Y, et al. (2008) Nocturnal reduction in circulating adiponectin concentrations related to hypoxic stress in severe obstructive sleep apnea-hypopnea syndrome. *American Journal of Physiology. Endocrinology and Metabolism*. Vol.294, No.4, (Apr 2008), pp.E778-784
Nakagawa Y, et al. (2011) Nocturnal falls of adiponectin levels in sleep apnea with abdominal obesity and impact of hypoxia-induced dysregulated adiponectin production in obese murine mesenteric adipose tissue. *Journal of Atherosclerosis and Thrombosis*. in press.
Kashine S, et al. (2010) Characteristics of sleep-disordered breathing in Japanese patients with type 2 diabetes mellitus. *Metabolism*. Vol.59, No.5, (May 2010), pp.690-696.
Wulan SN, et al. (2010) Ethnic differences in body composition and the associated metabolic profile: a comparative study between Asians and Caucasians. *Maturitas*. Vol.65, No.4, (Apr 2010), pp.315-319.
Fujimoto WY, et al. (1999) Visceral adiposity and incident coronary heart disease in Japanese-American men. The 10-year follow-up results of the Seattle Japanese-American Community Diabetes Study. *Diabetes Care*. Vo.22, No.11, (Nov 1999), pp.1808-1812.
Tong J, et al. (2007) Intra-abdominal fat accumulation predicts the development of the metabolic syndrome in non-diabetic Japanese-Americans. *Diabetologia*. Vol. 50, No.6, (Jun 2007), pp.1156-1160.
Kadowaki T, et al. (2006) Japanese men have larger areas of visceral adipose tissue than Caucasian men in the same levels of waist circumference in a population-based study. *International Journal of Obesity (London)*. Vol.30, No.7, (Jul 2006), pp.1163-1165.
Fujioka S, et al. (1987) Contribution of intra-abdominal fat accumulation to the impairment of glucose and lipid metabolism in human obesity. *Metabolism*. Vol.36, No.1, (Jan 1987), pp.54-59.
Matsuzawa Y, et al. (1994) Pathophysiology and pathogenesis of visceral fat obesity. *Diabetes Research and Clinical Practice*. Vol.24, No. Suppl, pp.S111-S116.

Part 5

Treatments and Therapy

15

Can Bariatric or Metabolic Surgery Cure Type 2 Diabetes?

Gustavo P. S. Miguel, Perseu Carvalho, João Luiz Azevedo,
Murilo Hosken Júnior, Évelyn Zambrana, Otávio Azevedo and Isaac Abreu
Federal University of Espírito Santo/ Cassiano Antônio Moraes University Hospital
Brazil

1. Introduction

Obesity is a multifactorial disease that affects millions of people worldwide. It is the main independent risk factor for developing type 2 diabetes mellitus (T2DM).[1,2] Most patients with T2DM and glucose intolerance (GI) are overweight, a condition known as diabesity.[2,3] In patients with the most severe form of obesity, i.e. morbid obesity, the likelihood of developing diseases associated with obesity is increased.[1,4]

We currently know that bariatric surgery provides sustained weight loss and well-documented remission of T2DM.[5,6] Patients who undergo bariatric surgery show long-term reduced mortality[7] from coronary artery disease, cancer and diabetes; 136 lives are saved per 10,000 surgical procedures performed.[8] Bariatric surgery is a relatively safe procedure that is becoming increasingly well-accepted; in 2007, approximately 170,000 bariatric procedures were performed in the USA.[6] Currently, bariatric surgery is the most effective choice of treatment of morbidly obese patients with diabetes.[9]

The surgical procedures that are currently performed to treat morbid obesity are divided into two main groups: gastric restrictive procedures and combination procedures; the latter combine gastric restriction and malabsorption.[10] The roux-en-Y gastric bypass (RYGB) is the combination procedure most frequently performed,[7,11] whereas sleeve gastrectomy (SG) is an emerging restrictive procedure.[12] SG can be performed as the first of a two-stage operation in patients at high risk of death,[13,14] or as a definitive surgical procedure.[15] It has shown good results with regard to weight loss[16] and glycemic control in various studies.[6,14,16,17] The potential advantages of SG include lower probability of vitamin and mineral deficiencies because this procedure has no malabsorptive component; access to the entire intestinal tract; no need for a subcutaneous access port or adjustments; absence of dumping syndrome and lower probability of intestinal obstruction. In addition, SG can be performed in patients who have inflammatory bowel disease or who have undergone bowel surgery, and it can be easily converted into RYGB.[12,15] Both SG and RYGB can be performed with or without the placement of a Silastic® ring.[18,19]

The metabolic control achieved with bariatric procedures has been demonstrated and reproduced in various medical centers worldwide.[6] Metabolic control can be achieved with gastric restrictive procedures such as vertical banded gastroplasty,[5] adjustable gastric banding[20] and, more recently, SG.[17] However, it has been shown that glucose homeostasis is affected by various intestinal mechanisms observed exclusively in procedures that include a malabsorptive element,[21] such as RYGB.[22-24]

A systematic review of 22,094 cases of morbidly obese patients submitted to bariatric surgery has shown that resolution of T2DM was achieved in 76.8% of the cases, improvement being achieved in 86% of cases.[25] Among the criteria used to diagnose metabolic syndrome, fasting glucose levels[26] are the first to return to normal in patients submitted to Silastic® ring gastric bypass (SRGB), a modification of the traditional RYGB which consists in adding a Silastic® ring to the gastric bypass operation. Normoglycemia after bariatric procedures, as well as diabesity itself, [27,28] is multifactorial.[6,29,30] Normoglycemia is observed as a result of dietary control,[20,21] decreased plasma levels of ghrelin,[32] weight loss and reduction of body fat[6], as well as of the release of gastrointestinal hormones that interfere with the function of pancreatic β cells (incretins).[23,24,33,34]

To compare the weight loss of morbidly obese patients submitted to either a Silastic® ring sleeve gastrectomy (SRSG) or an SRGB, as well as to compare the effects of both procedures on glucose homeostasis in morbidly obese patients, our research group developed a study that will be better described ahead.

2. Methods

2.1 Study protocol

This was a non-randomized, prospective, controlled clinical study. It was approved by the Research Ethics Committee of the University Hospital of the Federal University of Espírito Santo, Brazil (protocol no. 049/06) and registered in clinicaltrials.gov, identifier NCT00873405. In order to homogenize the sample, we adopted the following inclusion criteria: female patients aged 20-60 years, with BMI 40-45 (inclusive), who agreed on giving written informed consent. The exclusion criteria adopted were secondary obesity, alcohol or drug use, severe psychiatric disorder, binge-eating of sweets and previous stomach or bowel surgery.

2.2 Sample

Sixty-five female patients were included in the present study. The patients had a mean age of 36.03 years, mean BMI of 42.47 and mean waist circumference of 119.62 cm. Mean preoperative fasting glucose levels were 103.38 mg/dL (Table 1).

Variables	Mean, SD, minimum value, maximum value
Age (years)	36.03 ± 9.18 (20-59)
Body mass index (kg/m^2)	42.47 ± 1.64 (40-45)
Waist circumference (cm)	119.62 ± 8.06 (100-140)
Fasting glucose levels (mg/dL)	103.38 ± 36.5 (70-320)

Table 1. Anthropometric data and preoperative fasting glucose levels.

The diagnoses of diabetes and GI were based on the criteria adopted by the Brazilian Diabetes Society.[35] T2DM was found in 14 patients (21,5%) and GI, a transitional state to diabetes itself, was found in 12 patients (18,5%). Therefore, 40% of the morbidly obese patients analyzed in the present study presented with elevated fasting glucose levels (Table 2).

Fasting glucose levels	n	%
Normal	39	60%
Glucose intolerance	12	18,5%
Diabetes	14	21,5%

Table 2. Prevalence of preoperative type 2 diabetes mellitus and glucose intolerance.

Most of the diabetic patients used oral hypoglycemic agents (Table 3).

Therapy	n	%
Diet	6	9%
OHG	7	11%
OHG + Insulin	1	2%

OHG - oral hypoglycemic agent

Table 3. Preoperative antidiabetic therapy.

The 65 patients were divided into two groups; 33 patients (51%) were submitted to SRSG (SRSG group), whereas 32 (49%) patients were submitted to SRGB (SRGB group). Assessment was performed again 12 to 14 months after the surgery.

2.3 Surgical procedure

The surgical procedures were performed between December 08, 2006 and July 27, 2007 at *Hospital Universitário Cassiano Antonio Moraes from the Universidade Federal do Espírito Santo* (HUCAM/UFES, Cassiano Antonio Moraes University Hospital, Federal University of Espírito Santo). The procedures were performed by the same surgeon using a similar anesthetic technique (peridural anesthesia combined with general anesthesia).

The patients from the SRSG group were submitted to the following procedures: ligation of the vessels of the greater curvature of the body and fundus of stomach; resection of the fundus and part of the body of stomach using a linear stapler (80 mm, Tyco®) and a 32-Fr tube to calibrate the remaining stomach; placement of a 6.2 cm Silastic® ring around the stomach, 5.0 cm below the esophagogastric junction.

The patients of the SRGB group were submitted to the following procedures: creation of a small, proximal gastric pouch and exclusion of a large part of the stomach using a linear stapler (80 mm, Tyco®) and a 32-Fr tube to calibrate the gastric pouch; creation of an intestinal loop of 150 cm and a biliopancreatic loop of 40 cm; placement of a 6.2 cm Silastic® ring around the stomach, 5.0 cm below the esophagogastric junction.

In both groups, the stapled lines were sutured and a methylene blue test was performed to verify whether the staple line was secure. The patients were given a liquid diet on the first postoperative day and were to be discharged on the third postoperative day. They received dietary guidance and instructions regarding physical activities. In addition, patients from both groups were prescribed similar vitamin and mineral supplementation.

2.4 Assessment

Weight loss, BMI reduction and waist circumference reduction were assessed. The percentage of excess BMI loss was calculated as follows: preoperative BMI - current BMI ÷ preoperative BMI - 25 × 100.[36] Glucose homeostasis was assessed through the measurement of fasting glucose levels after the interruption of the pharmacological treatment.

2.5 Statistical analysis

Descriptive analysis was conducted and the results were expressed as means, standard deviations, medians, frequency (%), minimum values and maximum values. The Mann-Whitney test was applied to assess sample variation and homogeneity between groups. Fisher's exact test and chi-square test were employed to compare the results between the two groups. The ANOVA was used to assess glucose levels according to time and groups. Statistical significance was set at $p < 0.05$.

2.6 Results

In the preoperative period, no significant difference in age, BMI or waist circumference was found between patients from the SRSG group and patients from the SRGB group (Table 4).

Variable	Group	Mean, SD, minimum value, maximum value*
Age	SRSG	36.70 ± 9.4 (20-59)
	SRGB	35.34 ± 9.04 (21-58)
BMI	SRSG	42.33 ± 1.5 (40-45)
	SRGB	42.62 ± 1.78 (40.3-44.9)
Waist circumference (cm)	SRSG	118.70 ± 5.98 (107-131)
	SRGB	120.58 ± 9.76 (100-140)

BMI: body mass index. SRSG: Silastic® ring sleeve gastrectomy. SRGB: Silastic® ring gastric bypass. *No significant difference was observed between the groups.

Table 4. Comparison of age, preoperative body mass index and preoperative waist circumference between the groups.

Considering the entire sample, BMI decreased from 42.47 to 27.5 ± 2.67 ($p < 0.05$). Excess BMI loss was 86.18 ± 15% (46.6 - 114.6). In addition, we observed a reduction in waist circumference from 119.62 to 90.38 ± 7.9 cm (74 - 108) ($p < 0.05$). The results obtained with both surgical procedures were similar with regard to weight loss, BMI reduction, excess BMI loss and waist circumference reduction (Table 5).

Variables	SRSG	SRGB	p
Weight loss (%)	- 34.65 (6.43)	- 35.32 (6.20)	0.751
BMI loss (%)	- 35.11 (6.03)	- 35.35 (6.22)	0.893
Excess BMI loss	86.51 (14.20)	85.86 (15.97)	0.954
waist circumference reduction (%)	- 23.98 (5.42)	- 23.95 (7.86)	0.626

BMI = body mass index. SRSG: Silastic® ring sleeve gastrectomy. SRGB: Silastic® ring gastric bypass.

Table 5. Comparison of weight loss, BMI reduction, percentage of excess BMI reduction and waist circumference reduction between the groups.

Decreased fasting glucose levels were observed in the postoperative period ($p < 0.001$), as shown in Figure 1.

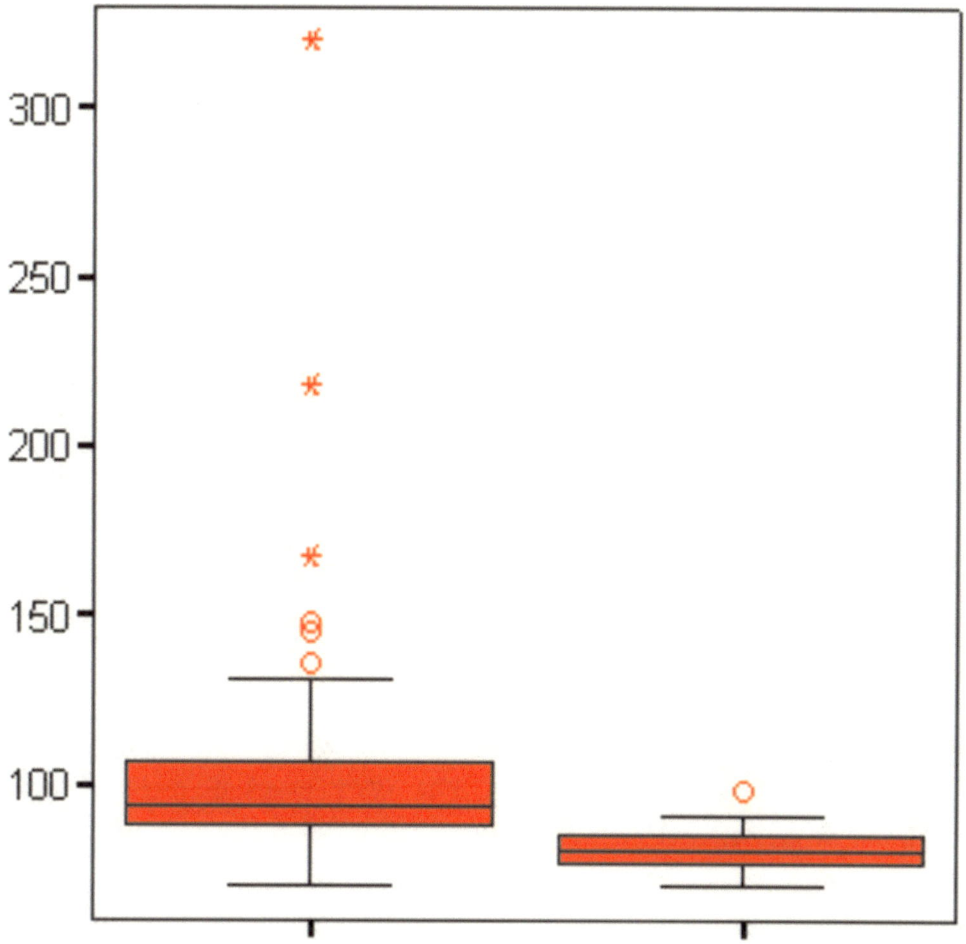

Fig. 1. Preoperative and postoperative fasting glucose levels mg/dl ($p < 0.001$).

This decrease was similar in both groups (Table 6).

Group*	Period**	Fasting glucose levels
SRSG	Preoperative	108.5 ± 43.76 (75-320)
	Postoperative	80.79 ± 6.47 (71-98)
SRGB	Preoperative	98.25 ± 27.18 (70-218)
	Postoperative	81.04 ± 5.22 (70-91)

SRSG: Silastic® ring sleeve gastrectomy. SRGB: Silastic® ring gastric bypass. *No significant difference was observed between groups. **$p < 0.001$.

Table 6. Preoperative and postoperative fasting glucose levels for both groups.

Both surgical procedures proved effective in promoting the resolution of T2DM and GI in the affected patients ($p < 0.001$), as shown in Table 7.

Preoperative T2DM and GI	Preoperative T2DM and GI		Total
	Absent	Present	
Absent	37	0	37
	60%	0%	60%
Present	25	0	25
	40%	0%	40%
Total	62	0	62

T2DM: type 2 diabetes mellitus. GI: glucose intolerance. Groups vs. time, $p < 0.001$.

Table 7. Remission of type 2 diabetes mellitus and glucose intolerance in the patients affected submitted to surgery.

All of the patients were able to discontinue the use of oral hypoglycemic agents or insulin, or both, during the follow-up period (Figure 2).

Glucose homeostasis box	Preoperative		Postoperative	
	n	%	n	%
Normal	39	60%	62	100%
Glucose intolerance	12	18%	0	0%
T2DM - diet	6	9%	0	0%
Oral hypoglycemic agents	7	11%	0	0%
Oral hypoglycemic agents + Insulin	1	2%	0	0%
Total	65	100%	62	100%

Fig. 2. Progress of glucose homeostasis and treatment of the patients submitted to surgery.

Although it was not the main focus of the present study, it was noteworthy that a fistula was developed at the staple line in two (6%) SRSG group patients ($p = 0.4936$). Both patients required reoperation. One of these patients died and the other was submitted to total gastrectomy, which led to the resolution of the fistula.

2.7 Discussion

The SG procedure has been increasingly used in bariatric surgery.[12-17] However, there are few prospective clinical studies in the literature that compare that emerging procedure with the gold standard.[12,17]

In the present study, SG was performed and a Silastic® ring was placed around the stomach. We obtained a small, functional stomach, like that obtained with traditional vertical gastroplasty, and removed the principal site of ghrelin production, which gave the SRSG the characteristics of both bariatric and endocrine surgery.[19] The removal of the principal site of ghrelin production led to a decrease in ghrelin levels, adding a hormonal element to SRSG, which other restrictive procedures such as adjustable gastric banding lack.[31] Some authors have reported the use of added restriction in SG in order to increase the intensity and duration of weight loss[19,37,38]. In addition, by placing a Silastic® ring around the stomach in all patients of our sample, both procedures became identical at the portion located above the ring.

Gastric bypass is the most used procedure in bariatric surgery and is considered by many the gold standard. Some researchers have reported that SG is less risky than RYGB.[12-14] However, in our sample, the most serious complications occurred in the SRSG group, which is, albeit not statistically significant, noteworthy.

Weight loss, BMI reduction, waist circumference reduction and excess BMI loss were expressive and similar in both groups. These findings are in accordance with those of some studies,[12,15,17] but in disagreement with those of other studies[13,14] that have regarded SG as the first stage of a definitive surgery. The good results of the present study are probably due to the judicious selection of the sample, which excluded BMI greater than 45 and patients with prior stomach or bowel surgery. In such cases, the results have been admittedly less effective. Other factors that might have contributed to the results of the present study include the calibration of the remaining stomach using a 32-Fr tube and the placement of a Silastic® ring. In other studies in which weight loss was less pronounced, tubes of greater caliber were used[39] and a Silastic® ring was not placed.[13,14]

Resolution of T2DM and decreased incidence of the disease have been well-documented in various types of bariatric surgery.[5] In two studies of patients submitted to SG, control of T2DM was achieved in 80% of the cases.[13,14] This remission rate was higher than that commonly reported for restrictive procedures such as vertical banded gastroplasty[5] and adjustable gastric banding;[20] it was, however, lower than that obtained with RYGB[9,26] and biliopancreatic diversion procedures.[21]

In the study described above, the rate of clinical remission of GI and T2DM was similar for both groups of patients (100%). The reduction in blood glucose levels was also similar for both groups, a surprising result that has been reported in another study.[17] Because SRSG is basically a restrictive procedure that theoretically does not affect incretin expression, it was expected that the results obtained with this procedure would be inferior to those obtained after procedures with duodenal switch with regard to glucose homeostasis.[23,24,29,30] In the present study, glucose levels might have decreased as a result of the expressive weight loss observed in both groups, which led to increased sensitivity to insulin and decreased production of leptin, followed by increased insulin secretion and remission of GI and T2DM[40]. Other hormones produced in the adipose tissue, such as resistin, might also have been involved in the glycemic control observed in the present study.[41,42]

We should also take into consideration that the patients submitted to surgery in the present study presented with mild GI or T2DM, the remission of which is more likely according to previous studies.[22,24]

The greatest limitation of our prospective, controlled study was the lack of randomization. This occurred because the Research Ethics Committee and the authors of this study considered that the often irreversible surgical procedures performed in the present study could not have been decided on without patient consent. A similar ethical issue was reported by the authors of the Swedish Obese Subjects study.[5] In order to overcome such limitations we selected patients with rather similar characteristics. Both groups comprised patients with similar age, BMI, waist circumference and fasting glucose levels in the preoperative period. This translated to a superiority of this study over other studies conducted previously, in which the groups investigated were not similar,[12] the sample was not homogeneous[15] and the patients included often presented with BMI < 40[12,15,17] and/or > 50.[12-17]

The surgical procedures performed in the present study, i.e. SRSG and SRGB, resulted in marked weight loss, BMI reduction, waist circumference reduction, excess BMI loss, improved glucose homeostasis and remission of GI and T2DM. These results were similar in both groups of morbidly obese patients. Further studies should be carried out adopting a longer follow-up period, as well as investigating other variables and possible hormonal changes, in order to consolidate SRSG.

With the satisfactory results obtained in the surgical treatment of T2DM through bariatric surgery in the last few years, has been evaluated the possibility of expanding the procedure indications for patients who are in a lesser degree of overweight. Such conduct has been accepted more liberally in patients with BMI between 30 and 35, but there are several clinical studies in subjects with BMI between 25 and 30. Recently, the IDF (International Diabetes Federation) classified as eligible for metabolic surgery, T2DM patients with BMI between 30 and 35.[43]

An Australian study, including patients with BMI between 30 and 40, comparing the intervention adjustable gastric band vs conventional therapy had remission of T2DM in 73% of the subjects against 13% in patients who underwent conventional therapy, with improvement in glucose levels, reduction of glycated hemoglobin and decrease of insulin plasma levels, demonstrating an improvement in insulinic sensitivity, measured by HOMA IR.[44]

Preliminary study report using the operation called laparoscopic mini-gastric bypass, performed in patients with BMI between 25 and 30, produced the resolution of hyperglycemia in 70% of operated patients.[45]

Double-blind randomized controlled trial including patients with BMI between 25 and 35 comparing the operations of gastric bypass vs sleeve gastrectomy showed remission of T2DM in both groups. However, the sleeve gastrectomy group remission occurred in 47% of patients and gastric bypass in group 93%. Demonstrating the superiority of gastric bypass in individuals with less overweight, probably due to the incretin action and the activity reduction of dipeptidyl peptidase-4.[46]

It should be noted in those patients with BMI between 25 and 35 the importance of a more detailed investigation in terms of T2DM pathogenesis, in order to reduce the possibility of submitting to surgery patients with complete failure of beta cells or autoimmune disease (DMT1ou LADA - Late autoimmune diabetes of adult). The preoperative evaluation of these patients should include: concentration of peptide C and tests for markers of pancreatic autoimmunity, as anti-glutamic acid dearboxylase (GAD) antibody and anti- Langerhans islet antibody.

3. Conclusion

The bariatric-metabolic surgery has unquestionable role in remission (cure?) of T2DM in subjects with BMI greater than 35. In this group of patients seems to be no difference in remission rates of T2DM between subjects undergoing gastric bypass or sleeve gastrectomy.

In subjects with less overweight, BMI between 30 and 35, nowadays eligible for metabolic surgery, gastric bypass seems to be more effective in producing remission of T2DM.

The metabolic surgery in patients with BMI between 25 and 30, still investigational, seems to show promising results in remission of T2DM, but further studies should be carried out to define its actual role.

4. References

[1] North American Association for the Study of Obesity (NAASO) and National Heart, Lung, and Blood Institute (NHLBI). The Practical Guide: Identification, Evaluation, and Treatment of Overweight and Obesity in Adults. NIH Publication #00-4084, Oct 2000.

[2] Must A, Spadano J, Coakley EH, Field AE, Colditz G, Dietz WH. The disease burden associated with overweight and obesity. JAMA. 1999;282:1523-1529.

[3] Gomes MB, Giannella Neto D, De Mendonça E, Tambascia MA, Fonseca RM, Réa RR, et al. Prevalência de sobrepeso e obesidade em pacientes com diabetes mellitus do tipo 2 no Brasil: Estudo multicêntrico nacional. Arq Bras Endocrinol Metab 2006;50:136-44.

[4] Venkat Narayan KM, Gregg EW, Fagot-Campagna A, Engelgau MM, Vinicor F. Diabetes: a common, growing, serious, costly, and potentially preventable public health problem. Diabetes Res Clin Pract. 2000;50:S77-84.

[5] Sjöström L, Narbro K, Sjöström D, Karason K, Larsson B, Wedel H, et al. Effects of bariatric surgery on mortality in swedish obese subjects. N Engl J Med. 2007;357:741-52.

[6] Bose M, Oliván B, Teixeira J, Pi-Sunyer FX, Laferrère B. Do incretins play a role in the remission of type 2 diabetes after gastric bypass surgery: what are the evidence? Obes Surg. 2009;19:217-29.

[7] Christou NV, Sampalis JS, Liberman M, Look D, Auger S, McLean APH, et al. Surgery decreases long-term mortality, morbidity, and health care use in morbidly obese patients. Ann Surg. 2004;240:416-424.

[8] Adams TD, Gress RE, Smith SC, Halverson RC, Simper SC, Rosamond WD, et al. Long-term mortality after gastric bypass surgery. N Engl J Med. 2007;357:753-61.

[9] Pories WJ, Swanson MS, MacDonald KG, Long SB, Morris PG, Brown BM, et al. Who would have thought it? An operation proves to be the most effective therapy for adult-onset diabetes mellitus. Ann Surg 1995;222:339-350.

[10] Buchwald H, Buchwald JN. Evolution of operative procedures for the management of morbid obesity 1950-2000. Obes Surg. 2002;12:705-17.

[11] Fobi MA. Why the operation I prefer is silastic ring banded gastric bypass. Obes Surg. 1991;1:423-6.

[12] Lee CM, Cirangle PT, Jossart GH. Vertical gastrectomy for morbid obesity in 216 patients: report of two-year results. Surg Endosc. 2007; 21:1810-6.
[13] Cottam D, Qureshi FG, Mattar SG, Sharma S, Holover S, Bonanomi G, et al. Laparoscopic sleeve gastrectomy as an initial weight-loss procedure for high-risk patients with morbid obesity. Surg Endosc 2006; 20:859-63.
[14] Silecchia G, Boru C, Pecchia A, Rizzelo M, Casella G, Leonetti F, et al. Effectiveness of laparoscopic sleeve gastrectomy (first stage of biliopancreatic diversion with duodenal switch) on co-morbidities in super-obese high-risk patients. Obes Surg 2006; 16:1138-44.
[15] Baltasar A, Serra C, Perez N, Bou R, Bengochea M, Ferri L. Laparoscopic sleeve gastrectomy: a multi-purpose bariatric operation. Obes Surg 2005; 15(8):1124-8.
[16] Moon Han S, Kim WW, Oh JH. Results of laparoscopic sleeve gastrectomy (LSG) at 1 year in morbidly obese Korean patients. Obes Surg 2005;15:1469-75.
[17] Vidal J, Ibarzabal A, Romero F, Delgado S, Momblán D, Flores L, et al. Type 2 diabetes mellitus and the metabolic syndrome following sleeve gastrecmomy in severely obese subjects. Obes Surg. 2008; 18:1077-82.
[18] Valezi AC, Brito EM, Souza JCL, Guariente ALM, Emori FT, Lopes VCH. A importância do anel de silicone na derivação gástrica em Y de Roux para o tratamento da obesidade. Rev Col Bras Cir. 2008; 35:18-22.
[19] Miguel GPS, Azevedo JLMC, Gicovate Neto C, Moreira CLCB, Viana EC, Carvalho PS. Glucose homeostasis and weight loss in morbidly obese patients undergoing banded sleeve gastrectomy: a prospective clinical study. Clinics 2009; 64: 1093-8.
[20] Dixon JB, O'Brien PE, Playfair J, Chapman L, Schachter LM, Skinner S, et al. Adjustable gastric banding and conventional therapy for the type 2 diabetes: a randomized controlled trial. JAMA. 2008;299:316-23.
[21] Scopinaro N, Adami GF, Marinari GM, Gianetta E, Traverso E, Friedman, et al. Biliopancreatic diversion. World J Surg. 1998;22:936-946.
[22] Schauer PR, Burguera B, Ikramuddin S, Cottam D, Gourash W, Hamad G, et al. Effect of laparoscopic Roux-en Y gastric bypass on type 2 diabetes mellitus. Ann Surg. 2003;238(4):467-485.
[23] Cummings DE, Overduin J, Foster-Schubert KE. Gastric bypass for obesity: mechanisms of weight loss and diabetes resolution. J Clin Endocrinol Metab. 2004;89:2608-2615.
[24] Rubino F, Forgione A, Cummings DE, Vix M, Gnuli D, Mingrone G, et al. The mechanism of diabetes control after gastrointestinal bypass surgery reveals a role of the proximal small intestine in the pathophysiology of type 2 diabetes. Ann Surg 2006;244:741-749.
[25] Buchwald H, Avidor Y, Braunwald E, Jensen MD, Pories W, Fahrbach K, et al. Bariatric surgery: a systematic review and meta-analysis. JAMA. 2004;292:1724-1737.
[26] Carvalho PS, Barelli MC, Moreira CLCB, Oliveira FH, Guzzo MF, Miguel GPS, et al. Can bariatric surgery cure metabolic syndrome? Arq Bras Endocrinol e Metab 2007;51(1):79-85.

[27] Cavaghan MK, Ehrmann DA, Polonsky KS. Interactions between insulin resistance and insulin secretion in the development of glucose intolerance. J Clin Invest. 2000;106(6):329-33.
[28] Wajchenberg BL. Beta-cell failure in diabetes and preservation by clinical treatment. Endocr Rev. 2007;28:187-218.
[29] Mason EE. The mechanism of surgical treatment of type 2 diabetes. Obes Surg. 2005;15:459-461.
[30] Martins MVD, Souza AAP. Mecanismos cirúrgicos de controle do diabetes mellitus tipo 2 após cirurgia bariátrica. Rev Col Bras Cir. 2007;34(5):343-346.
[31] Langer FB, Reza Hoda MA, Bohdjalian A, Felberbauer FX, Zacherl J, Wenzl E, et al. Sleeve gastrectomy and gastric banding: effects on plasma ghrelin levels. Obes Surg 2005; 15(7):1024-9.
[32] Nakazato M, Murakami N, Date Y, Kojima M, Matsuo H, Kangawa K, et al. A role for ghrelin in the central regulation of feeding. Nature. 2001;409:194-8.
[33] Pories WJ, Albrecht RJ. Etiology of type II diabetes mellitus: role of the foregut. World J Surg. 2001;25:527-531.
[34] Drucker DJ. Biological actions and therapeutic potential of the glucagon-like peptides. Gastroenterology. 2002;122:531-544.
[35] Sociedade Brasileira de Diabetes. Diretrizes: tratamento e acompanhamento do diabetes mellitus. 2007. Diagraphic editora.
[36] Deitel M, Gawdat K, Melissas J. Reporting weight loss 2007. Obes Surg. 2007; 17:565-568.
[37] Cai J, Zheng C, Xu L, Chen D, Li X, Wu J, et al. Therapeutic effects of sleeve gastrectomy plus gastric remnant banding on weigth reduction and gastric dilatation: na animal study. Obes Surg. 2008;18:1411-7.
[38] Greenstein AJ, Vine AJ, Jacob BP. When sleeve gastrectomy fails: adding a laparoscopic adjustable gastric band to increase restriction. Surg Endosc. 2009 Epub ahead of print.
[39] Braghetto I, Korn O, Valladares H, Gutiérrez L, Csendes A, Debandi A, et al. Laparoscopic sleeve gastrectomy: surgical technique, indications and clinical results. Obes Surg. 2007;17:1442-50.
[40] Meirelles K, Ahmed T, Culnan DM, Lynch CJ, Lang CH, Cooney R. Mechanisms of glucose homeostasis after Roux-en-Y gastric bypass surgery in the obese, insulin-resistant Zucker rat. Ann Surg. 2009;249:277-85.
[41] Diamond F. The endocrine function of adipose tissue. Growth: genetics & hormones 2002; 18:17-22.
[42] Steppan CM, Bailey ST, Bhat S, Brown EJ, Banerjee RR, Wrigt CM, et al. The hormone resistin links obesity to diabetes. Nature. 2001; 409:307-312.
[43] Available in:<http://www.idf.org/press-release/idf-announces-new-position-supporting-surgery-treat-type-2-diabetes> Accessed on May 2, 2011.
[44] Dixon JB, O'Brien PE, Playfair J, Chapman L, Schachter LM, Skinner S, Proietto J, Bailey M, Anderson M. Adjustable gastric banding and conventional therapy for type 2 diabetes: a randomized controlled trial. JAMA. 2008 Jan 23;299(3):316-323.

[45] Kim Z, Hur KY. Laparoscopic mini-gastric bypass for type 2 diabetes: the preliminary report. World J Surg. 2011 Mar;35(3):631-636.

[46] Lee WJ, Chong K, Ser KH, Lee YC, Chen SC, Chen JC, Tsai MH, Chuang LM. Gastric bypass vs sleeve gastrectomy for type 2 diabetes mellitus: a randomized controlled trial. Arch Surg. 2011 Feb;146(2):143-148.

16

Nuclear Imaging of Glucose Transport/Metabolism – An Interesting Tool to Screen Insulin Resistance, Refine Diagnosis of Type 2 Diabetes, Understand Disease Mechanisms, and/or Evaluate New Therapies

Perret P., Henri M., Slimani L., Fagret D. and Ghezzi C.
UJF-Grenoble 1/INSERM UMR 1039
France

1. Introduction

Over the past two decades, a striking increase in the number of people with type 2 diabetes has been observed. However, type 2 diabetes may remain undiagnosed for as long as 5 to 7 years before the appearance of clinical symptoms. Insulin resistance (IR) is the best prediction factor of type 2 diabetes (Reaven, 1988; Erikson et al., 1989; Taylor et al., 1994; Henry, 2003). Therefore, early IR detection is of major clinical interest (McLaughlin & Reaven, 2003). Resistance to insulin-mediated glucose uptake occurs in most insulin sensitive tissues: the skeletal muscle, myocardium and adipose tissue. Mechanisms underlying this defect are still not fully understood (for review Biddinger & Kahn, 2006; Muoio & Newgard, 2008; Samuel et al., 2010). Until now, there is no available technique in clinical routine that allows the non-invasive assessment of insulin sensitivity in specific tissues under physiologic or pathophysiologic conditions. This kind of approach is possible using appropriate radiolabelled tracers that can be detected non-invasively.
Indeed, a tracer is a compound that is chemically identical but separately detectable from the tracee, in this case glucose. Injected intravenously, the tracer is present in negligible quantities that do not themselves perturb metabolism, and its distribution in a given organ reflects the appearance or clearance rate of the tracee in this organ.
Radiolabelled glucose analogues have been used for many years (D-glucose, L-glucose, 2-deoxyglucose, 3-O-methyl-D-glucose) labelled with carbone 14 or tritium associated with hyperinsulinaemic euglycaemic clamp in animals, even in humans, to understand disease mechanisms and/or evaluate new therapies for type 2 diabetes. Modeling of washout curves of tracers allowed good estimation of glucose inward/outward transport and phosphorylation rates, but the use of these β- emitter radioisotopes is not always allowed in humans, moreover this technique does not permit to evaluate the regional location of metabolic events within tissues. In order to be less restrictive, the same approach has been developed in nuclear imaging, where radioactive tracers are injected to assess non-invasively biological processes *in vivo*. Thus, a couple of tracers have been evaluated in combination with hyperinsulinaemic euglycaemic clamp, such as ^{18}F-2-deoxy-D-glucose for

glucose metabolism (transport and phosphorylation), the most famous, or ^{11}C-3-*O*-methylglucose for glucose transport evaluation. Experimentally, with the recent development of nuclear imaging cameras with high resolution dedicated to small animals, and the increase of FDG disponibility, a couple of protocoles have been proposed to evaluate glucose uptake *in vivo* in rat and even in mice. But the necessity of the hyperinsulinaemic clamp conditions, which consist in a 3 hours perfusion of insulin and glucose, rendered this technique complicated and cumbersome for the patient and it cannot be used routinely. More recently, a new tracer, ^{123}I-6-iodo-6-deoxy-D-glucose has been proposed to evaluate insulin-stimulated glucose transport *in vivo* using a more simple and shorter protocole (Briat et al., 2007).

2. ^{18}F-2-deoxy-D-glucose (FDG)

The most widely used glucose analogue radiotracer in humans is ^{18}F-2-deoxy-D-glucose (FDG), developed for positron emission tomography (PET) imaging. FDG, a glucose analogue quite similar to 2-Deoxy-Glucose (2DG), is recognized and transported into the cells by glucose transporters, and phosphorylated by hexokinase to form ^{18}F-FDG-6-phosphate (Bessell et al., 1972, 1973; Gallagher et al., 1977,1978). It cannot act as a substrate for further glycolysis and so rapidly accumulates in cells that have increased activity of hexokinase and increased glucose transporter levels, such as tumour cells. That is the reason why FDG is extensively used for PET imaging in oncology and has been evaluated and established in clinical routine for initial staging and assessment of response to cancer therapy.

Since glucose transport defect in skeletal muscle is the main characteristic of insulin resistance, FDG and dynamic PET have also been developped to provide tissue-specific metabolic assessment of proximal steps of glucose metabolism in clinical investigations.

We often heard about round trips between bench and bedside, the development of FDG is a perfect example. First, animal studies to assess *in vivo* insulin resistance in tissues such as skeletal muscle were performed during hyperinsulinaemic clamp with an injection of ^{14}C-2DG, dissection of tissues, and extraction of 2DG-6-P to count carbon 14. *Ex vivo* or *in vitro*, this tracer was so usefull in so many fields (i.e. diabetology, oncology, neurology, cardiology...) that an analogue usable in humans was extensively searched for many years. When ^{18}FDG was obtained, PET imaging was not widely available. Nowadays with the increasing interest of this tracer in oncology, more and more medical centers are equiped with PET cameras and FDG is becoming more available and less expensive. Then PET cameras dedicated to small animals were developed and experimental studies can be performed.

To assess global insulin sensitivity, the hyperinsulinaemic euglycaemic clamp is the gold standard (DeFronzo et al., 1981). To evaluate insulin stimulated glucose uptake *in vivo* within individual tissues, the used of 2-[^{14}C]-DG injected as a bolus at the end of the insulin clamp, during steady state, has been developed first in concious rats by Kraegen and colleagues (Kraegen et al.,1983), and since then largely used, even in concious mice (Rossetti et al., 1997). Using this technique, tissue glucose metabolic rate or Rg′ can be assessed using plasma kinetic of 2DG over 45 minutes and tissue accumulation of 2-DG-6-P at that time. The main limitation of this technique is the labelling of 2DG with carbon 14, a low energy β- emitter, which involves the death of the animal, dissection of the tissue and a laborious preparation to count the radioactivity. This method involves also numerous blood samples which can represent another limitation especially in mice. FDG, labelled with a β+ emitter, can be detectable non invasively. This tracer is an analogue of 2DG, i.e. it enters the cell using the same transporter as glucose and once inside the cell FDG is phosphorylated. The kinetics of its uptake reflect both the transport and phosphorylation steps. In human, FDG was first used to evaluate glucose metabolism in brain using dynamic PET-imaging associated with compartimental modeling developped by Sokoloff and colleagues (Sokoloff et al., 1977). This method was afterwards adapted to heart and skeletal muscle, associated with hyperinsulinaemic euglycaemic clamp (Phelps et al., 1978; Nuutila et al., 1992). A tree-compartment model was applied to estimate inward transport, outward transport and phosphorylation rates. Nuutila and colleagues used this technique to demonstrate that the glucose-FFA cycle operates *in vivo* in both heart and skeletal muscles in humans (Nuutila et al., 1992). In the same manner, Selberg and colleagues showed that patients with liver cirrhosis presented significant insulin resistance, and kinetic constants using the three-compartment model indicated reduced glucose transport in skeletal muscle but unchanged phosphorylation of glucose (Selberg et al., 1993). Another interesting study concerned the evaluation of regional insulin resistance in lean, obese, and obese with type 2 diabetic patients (Kelley et al., 1996). Kelley and colleagues showed that during a hyperinsulinaemic clamp associated with FDG-PET-imaging of skeletal muscle, the rate constant for glucose phosphorylation was similar in obese and lean subjects but reduced in diabetic patients. These *in vivo* assessment, associated with an immunohistochemical study of GLUT 4 performed *ex vivo* in muscle biopsies of patients indicated that impaired glucose transport plays a key role in insulin resistance of diabetes and obesity, and that an additional impairment of glucose phosphorylation is evident in the insulin resistance of type 2 diabetes (Kelley et al., 1996) (Figure 1).

First experimental studies with FDG were performed in rabbits hindlimb that was secured between a single pair of coincidence gamma photon detectors positioned on the medial and lateral sides of the posterior thigh (Mossberg et al., 1989). The counting system consisted of two bismuth germanate oxide crystals interfaced to photomultiplier tubes. After signal amplification and filtering by discriminator units, the processed signals from each detector were sent to a coincidence logic unit. Animal has to be anesthetized, and FDG was injected as a bolus and then infused continuously through the experiment. Mossberg and colleagues used the method of graphical analysis of tissue and plasma radioactivity concentrations derived from Patlak and colleagues (Patlak & Blasberg, 1985) to quantitate the fractional rate of tracer phosphorylation. Briefly, the slope of the relationship between the integral of the plasma radioactivity concentration and the tissue radioactivity concentration during any given time interval yields the transfer constant, K, or the fractional rate of FDG phosphorylation. Multiplication of K by the plasma glucose concentration gives an index of the rate of glucose uptake (Rg'). During perturbation by electrical stimulation, an increased in the rate of tracer phosphorylation was observed, but no change of K was observed during hyperinsulinemia induced by a bolus of insulin. The next step was to introduced the hyperinsulinaemic clamp conditions in the method (Mossberg & Taegtmeyer, 1991, 1992). But the detection system was developed only by Mossberg and colleagues, and until the development of the first PET-cameras dedicated to small animals available on the market (2002 for Siemens Concorde R4), tissue insulin resistance was assessed with FDG mostly in humans.

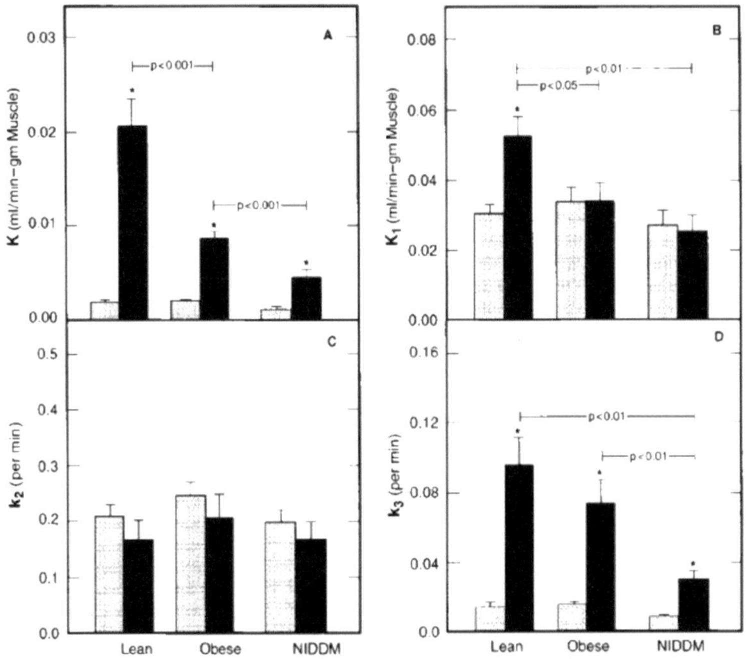

Fig. 1. Glucose transport and phosphorylation rates assessed with ^{18}FDG imaging and mathematical modeling in human skeletal muscle. In *A*, data from lean and obese nondiabetic and obese type 2 diabetic subjects during basal (*shaded bars*) and insulin stimulated (*solid bars*) conditions are shown for ^{18}FDG clearance (K) into midthigh muscle; in *B*, the rate constant for transport of ^{18}FDG (K_1) is shown; in *C*, the rate constant for outward transport (k_2) of ^{18}FDG is shown; and in *D*, the rate constant for ^{18}FDG phosphorylation (k_3) during basal and insulin-stimulated conditions is shown. *Significant within-group difference comparing basal and insulin-stimulated values ($P < 0.05$). [Figure from Kelley et al, 1996 with permission].

Paternostro and colleagues studied insulin resistance in patients with a history of myocardial infarction (Paternostro et al., 1996). Using PET imaging technique, they measured heart and skeletal muscle blood flow with $H_2{}^{15}O$ and glucose uptake with FDG during euglycaemic hyperinsulinaemic clamp. The authors showed that in these patients, insulin resistance affects both the myocardium and skeletal muscle and is independent of blood flow. Numerous studies have been then performed to measure regional insulin resistance, mainly in heart and skeletal muscle in various patients, type 1 or type 2 diabetic (vom Dahl et al., 1993; Voipio-Pulkki et al., 1993), with or without hypertension (Yokoyama et al., 1998), obese or non obese (Kelley et al., 1999), with or without hypertriglyceridemia (Kobayakawa et al., 1999). The technique was also usefull to evaluate the impact of new therapy. For example, Yokoyama and colleagues showed that troglitazone, one of the first available thiazolidinedione, could improve whole-body insulin resistance through the improvement of skeletal muscle glucose uptake but not through a decline in plasma free fatty acid concentration in patients with type 2 diabetes (Yokoyama et al., 2001).
In a way to simplify the technique, the activity in left ventricule or in aorta can be used as arterial input function (Iozzo et al., 2003 ; Keiding et al., 2000). Yokoyama and colleagues

proposed a even simpler method using static instead of dynamic imaging (Yokoyama et al., 2003).
The advent of small-animal PET technology allowed for the consecutive measurements of biochemical and physiological function in rodents. Sharp and colleagues provided an example of a cardiac imaging study using four radiotracers (^{15}O-water, 1-[^{11}C]-acetate, 1-[^{11}C]-palmitate and 1-[^{11}C]-glucose) injected into normal rats (Sharp et al., 2005), demonstrating that rats can be used for multiplc non invasive imaging studies with reproducible results over time with minimal or no change in hemodynamic or substrate levels. Using the same method, Welch and colleagues studied Zucker diabetic fatty (ZDF) rats showed that non invasive measurements of myocardial substrate metabolism were consistent with the expected early metabolic abnormalities that occur in this model of type 2 diabetes mellitus (Welch et al., 2006). To summarize, when compared with their lean controls, the ZDF rat showed (a) elevated insulin, glucose, and FFA levels; (b) elevated FFA utilization and oxidation; (c) preserved myocardial glucose utilization; and (d) a trend toward a lower MVO2. However, the micro-blood sampling technique is necessary to provide accurate blood input function measurements, and when multiple tracer studies are performed in the same animal, this technique is limited by the number of blood samples that can be withdrawn in small animals. Kim and colleagues proposed a factor analysis (FA) technique for extracting the blood input function and myocardial time-activity curve from dynamic small-animal PET images of the rodent heart (Kim et al., 2006). Indeed, CT scans were not available on PET cameras dedicated to small animals at that time rendering the design of ROI in left ventricule rather difficult. The FA method has been used to decompose dynamic images into component images and to determine their time-activity curves by analysis of the variance in the data (Barber, 1980). It has been reported that the FA method successfully extracts the input functions and myocardial time-activity curves from dynamic PET images of canines, humans, and monkeys (Wu et al., 1995 ; 1996). In rat and mice, the FA method enables reliable quantification of physiologic or biologic information generated in small-animal PET-FDG studies and does not require the drawing of ROIs on small structures, such as a rodent heart or other small organs of interest, or repeated blood sampling (Kim et al., 2006). Using small-animal PET, Shogi and colleagues confirmed alterations in myocardial glucose utilization and validated PET measurement of Muscle Glucose Uptake (MGU) against gene and protein expression of GLUTs in the heart of an animal model of type 2 diabetes (Shogi et al., 2008). A new method has been validated in mice, a hybrid image and blood sampling (HIBS) method to derive the input function for quantification of microPET mice data. The HIBS algorithm derives the peak of the input function from the image (on the heart), which is corrected for recovery, while the tail is derived from 5 to 6 optimally placed blood sampling points (Shogi et al., 2007). The method is now well established in rodents, and can be used for example to validate new animal model of type 2 diabetes induced by diet closer to the human disease than genetic animal model available (Ménard et al., 2010).
The compartmental model developed for FDG-PET imaging in skeletal muscle was initially used for PET data acquired in the central nervous system (CNS) and later modified. Bertoldo and colleagues proposed a muscle specific compartmental model, a modification that takes into account movement of FDG from plasma to interstitial space and from interstitial space into tissue via transmembrane glucose transport, as well as an irreversible compartment for formation of FDG-6-P (Bertoldo et al, 2001). Compared with the classic

model, the skeletal muscle-specific model reveals a more clearly defined effect of insulin on transmembrane glucose transport and an impairment of this response in obesity (Williams et al., 2003).

Resistance to insulin also occurs in adipose tissue. But methods available to study directly adipose tissue metabolism *in vivo* are limited in human beings and its investigation has been carried out mainly by indirect measurements in the whole body or in cannulated limbs. FDG-PET has been combined with microdialysis to investigate adipose tissue glucose metabolism in human during insulin stimulation. Using this method, Virtanen and colleagues confirmed that obese patients had insulin resistance in both adipose tissue and skeletal muscle (Virtanen et al., 2001).

More recently, Hirvonen and colleagues studied in humans the effects of insulin on brain glucose metabolism and cerebral blood flow in patients with impaired glucose tolerance and healthy subjects using FDG-PET associated to hyperinsulinemic clamp (Hirvonen et al., 2011). Their results suggest that insulin stimulation of brain glucose metabolism is maximal at fasting concentrations in healthy subjects but not in patients with impaired glucose tolerance. This study showed that it could be a very usefull technique to evaluate the role of insulin in the brain and the possible insulin resistance in some conditions of this organ which has been for a long time considered as a non insulin sensitive tissue.

3. 3-O-methyl-D-glucose (3-OMG)

Skeletal muscle glucose uptake requires delivery of glucose to the sarcolemma, transport across this membrane, and the irreversible phosphorylation of glucose by hexokinase inside the cell. Because these three processes are so tightly coupled, it is difficult to determine the role of each of these steps in controlling the rate of muscle glucose uptake *in vivo*. An alternative approach is the measurement of the steady-state distribution of a non metabolizable glucose analogue across the sarcolemma, which allows the calculation of the transsarcolemmal glucose gradient. Numerous *in vitro* and *in vivo* experiments have shown that 3-O-methyl-D-glucose (3-OMG) is an ideal glucose analogue to probe transmembrane transport, sharing the same transport system as glucose and with equivalent affinity for glucose transport proteins (Narahara & Ozand, 1963; Buschiazzo et al., 1970; Carruthers, 1990; O'Doherty et al., 1998).

Cobelli and colleagues have used the perfused forearm and euglycaemic hyperinsulinaemic clamp techniques in combination with a dual-tracer injection to measure basal and insulin-mediated glucose transport in normal subjects. L-[^{3}H]glucose, which is not transported, was used to trace extracellular glucose kinetics, and 3-O-[^{14}C]-methyl-D-glucose was used to monitor glucose transport across the cell membrane (Cobelli et al., 1989). A linear compartmental model was developed that accounts for blood flow heterogeneity. Using the same method, Bonadonna and colleagues have shown that transmembrane glucose transport was insulin resistant in the skeletal muscle of patients with type 2 diabetes and that this impairment was proportional to their degree of insulin resistance (Bonadonna et al., 1993). Halseth and colleagues adapted the technique for rat studies and showed that during exercice glucose phosphorylation becomes an important limitation to skeletal muscle (soleus) glucose uptake. During hyperinsulinaemia, both glucose delivery and glucose phosphorylation influence the rate of skeletal muscle glucose uptake more than under basal conditions (Halseth et al., 1998). The same group studied high fat diet rats showing a defect in skeletal muscle glucose transport under insulin conditions (Halseth et al., 2000), and the influence of muscle fiber types on the rate of insulin-stimulated muscle glucose uptake, with glucose delivery and transport being the primary limiting factors in type II muscle (Halseth et al., 2001; Petersen et al., 2003). Recently, *in vivo* rates of transmembrane glucose transport and intracellular glucose phosphorylation were determined by analyzing the dilution curves of D-mannitol, [^{14}C]3OMG, and D-[3-^{3}H]glucose, using a multicompartmental model of glucose kinetics in forearm tissues (Pendergrass et al., 2007). The authors concluded that *1*) obese non diabetic, lean type 2 diabetic, and offspring manifest moderate-to severe muscle insulin resistance and decreased insulin-stimulated glucose transport and glucose phosphorylation in forearm muscle; these defects in insulin action are not further reduced by the combination of obesity plus diabetes; and *2*) the increase in intracelullar glucose concentration under hyperinsulinaemic euglycaemic conditions in obese and type 2 diabetic groups suggests that the defect in glucose phosphorylation exceeds the defect in glucose transport (Pendergrass et al., 2007).

Concerning imaging studies, the fact that emission from ^{18}F can occur at either [^{18}F]FDG or [^{18}F]FDG-6-P, creates implicit uncertainty as to whether compartmental modeling achieves separate estimations of glucose transport and phosphorylation. Therefore dynamic PET imaging to isolate the step of transmembrane glucose transport in skeletal muscle based on chemical specificity of 3-OMG labeled with ^{11}C has been proposed (Bertoldo et al., 2005). High quality imaging can be obtained and a clear effect of insulin to modulate the amplitude and configuration of tissue tracer activity was observed. Initial application indicated a robust effect of insulin to stimulate glucose transport in skeletal muscle of lean, healthy, insulin-sensitive volunteers (Bertoldo et al., 2005). Using the same method, Pencek and colleagues showed that in healthy volunteers there was robust dose-responsive insulin stimulation of glucose transport in skeletal muscle (Pencek et al., 2006) (Figure 2).

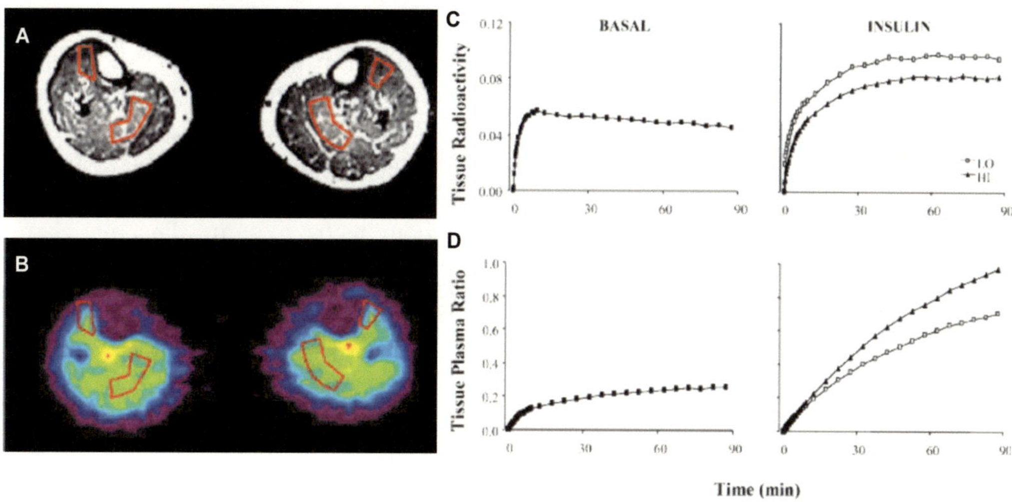

Fig. 2. Glucose transport assessment with ^{11}C-3-OMG in human skeletal muscle. MRI (**A**) and PET (**B**) images were carefully co-registered, and regions of interest (ROIs) were drawn within tibialis anterior and soleus muscle groups. ROIs were then applied to PET images to determine radioactivity accumulation within specific muscle groups. **C**: representative tissue activity curves during Basal (*left*), low-insulin (LO), and high-insulin (HI) conditions (*right*). **D**: representative tissue to plasma ratios (TPR) of ^{11}C-3-OMG radioactivity. [Figure adapted from Pencek et al, 2006 with permission].

There have been prior *in vivo* PET investigations in humans using [^{11}C]3-OMG to study glucose transport across the blood-brain barrier (Vyska et al., 1985; Feinendegen et al., 1986; Brooks et al., 1986a, 1986b). But the use of this tracer was limited by the fact that it is labelled with carbon 11, a short half-life radioisotope ($t_{1/2}$= 20 minutes) produced by cyclotron, which undoubtedly explains why very few studies have been devoted to this compound.

4. [^{123}I]-6-deoxy-6-iodo-D-glucose (6DIG)

Given the significant interest of a tracer to estimate alterations of glucose uptake *in vivo*, numerous researchers have tried for many years to develop glucose molecules labelled with a radioactive atom which is a pure γ-emitter, such as iodine 123, and which could be used routinely in Single Photon Emission Computed Tomography (SPECT), in all Nuclear Medicine centers (Kloster et al., 1983a, 1983b; Goodman et al., 1981a, 1981b; Lutz et al., 1991; Magata et al., 1992; Koumanov et al., 1997a, 1997b; Perret et al, 2004). [^{123}I]-6-deoxy-6-iodo-D-glucose (6DIG) was first synthetized by Wassenar and colleagues, but the biological evaluation was limited to tumor uptake and not evaluated further (Wassenaar et al., 1973). The synthesis of 6DIG has been performed again more recently, and its biological behavior was carrefully evaluated. It was similar to that of 3-OMG (Henry et al., 1997a). It is transported into the cell by glucose transporters, but is not phosphorylated or further metabolized and is then free to leave the cell using the same transporters. The cellular uptake of this tracer allows true transport rates to be measured. Moreover, an *in vitro* study on the adipocytes of diabetic rats and obese mice showed that 6DIG, like 3-OMG, could be used to determine alterations in glucose transport (Henry et al., 1997b). Our group then proposed to use 6DIG *in vivo* to assess insulin resistance by nuclear imaging. Studies in diabetic mice *db/db* and in insulin resistant fructose-fed rats showed that 6DIG was able to assess glucose transport defects *in vivo* (Slimani et al., 2002; Perret et al., 2003, 2007). In a preliminary study, we have shown in different rat models of insulin resistance that 6DIG could be used to assess non-invasively, using nuclear NaI probes, different degrees of cardiac insulin resistance without using hyperinsulinaemic clamp (Briat et al., 2007) (Figure 3). Based on these preliminary works, we further investigated the non-invasive assessment of cardiac and skeletal muscle insulin resistance using a gamma camera dedicated to small animals. We validated a simple protocol which is currently undergoing a clinical trial.

5. Conclusion

Nuclear imaging is routinely used to refine diagnosis in oncology and cardiology, but although his great potential not yet in diabetology. Probably because all the methods proposed until now were associated with complex protocoles. With the recent development of cameras for small animals, the development of new tracers is rendering easier and then can be proposed for new clinical insights, or experimentally for new drug testing or physiopathology studies. Considering the complexity of mechanisms involved in insulin resistance development, such tools, giving non invasivelly fonctionnal informations *in vivo* are of great interest.

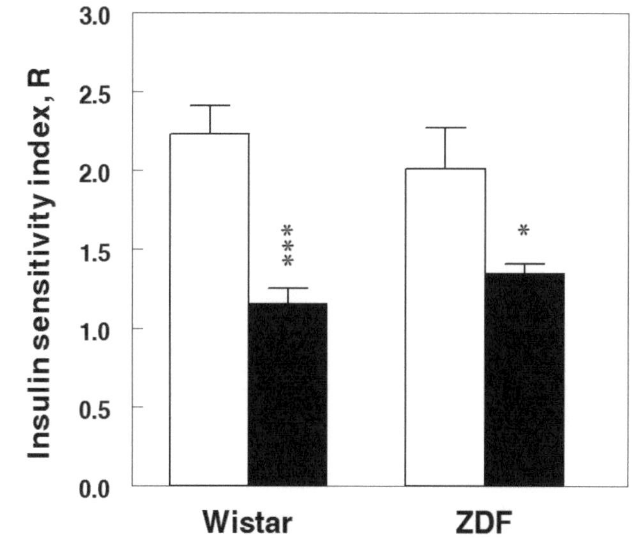

Fig. 3. Index of insulin sensitivity calculated as the ratio of 6DIG transport rate constant in insulin and basal conditions in rat myocardium (k_{in} insulin / k_{in} basal). White bars represent control animals (Wistar and lean ZDF rats) and solid bars insulin resistant animals (fructose-fed Wistar and Zucker Diabetic Fatty rats). *Comparison of insulin-resistant rats versus control rats, Mann-Whitney test: *$P < 0.05$, ***$P < 0.001$. [Unpublished figure from the Ghezzi laboratory].

6. References

Barber, D.C. (1980). *Physics in Medicine and Biology*. Vol.25, pp. 283–292.

Bertoldo, A.; Peltoniemi, P.; Oikonen, V.; Knuuti, J.; Nuutila, P. & Cobelli, C. (2001). *American Journal of Physiology*. Vol.281, pp. E524-E536.

Bertoldo, A.; Price, J.; Mathis, C.; Mason, S.; Holt, D.; Kelley, C.; Cobelli, C. & Kelley, D.E. (2005). *Journal of Clinical Endocrinology and Metabolism*. Vol.90, pp. 1752-1759.

Bessell, E.M.; Foster, A.B. & Westwood, J.H. (1972). *Biochemistry Journal*. Vol.128, No.2 (June), pp. 199-204.

Bessell, E.M. & Thomas, P. (1973). *Biochemistry Journal*. Vol.131, No.1(January), pp. 83-89.

Biddinger S.B. & Kahn, R.C. (2006) Annual Review of Physiology. Vol.68, pp. 123-158.

Bonadonna, R.-C.; Del Prato, S.; Saccomani, M.-P.; Bonora, E.; Gulli, G.; Ferrannini, E.; Bier, D.; Cobelli, C. & DeFronzo, R.A. (1993). *Journal of Clinical Investigation*. Vol.92, pp. 486-494.

Briat, A.; Slimani, L.; Perret, P.; Villemain, D.; Halimi, S.; Demongeot, J.; Fagret, D. & Ghezzi, C. (2007). *European Journal of Nuclear Medicine and Molecular Imaging*. Vol.34, No.11, pp. 1756-1764.

Brooks, D.; Beaney, R.; Lammertsma, A.; Herold, S.; Turton, D.; Luthra, S.; Frackowiak, R.; Thomas, D.; Marshall, J. & Jones, T. (1986a). *Journal of Cerebral Blood Flow and Metabolism*. Vol.6, pp. 230-239.

Brooks, D.; Gibbs, J.; Sharp, P.; Herold, S.; Turton, D.; Luthra, S.; Kohner, E.; Bloom, S. & Jones, T. (1986b) *Journal of Cerebral Blood Flow and Metabolism*. Vol.6, pp. 240-244.

Buschiazzo, P.; Terrell, E. & Regen, D. (1970). *American Journal of Physiology*. Vol.219, pp. 1505–1513.

Carruthers, A. (1990). *Physiological Reviews*. Vol.70, pp. 1135–1176.

Cobelli, C, Saccomani, MP, Ferrannini, E, Defronzo, RA, Gelfand, R, Bonadonna, R. (1989). *American Journal of Physiology, Endocrinology and Metabolism*. Vol.257, No.6 (December), pp. E943-E958.

DeFronzo, R.A.; Jacot, E.; Jequier, E.; Maeder, E.; Wahren, J. & Felber, J.P. (1981). *Diabetes*. Vol.30, pp. 1000-1007.

Eriksson, J.; Franssila-Kallunki, A.; Ekstrand, A.; Saloranta, C.; Widén, E.; Schalin, C. & Groop, L. (1989). *New England Journal of Medicine*. Vol.321, pp. 337-343.

Feinendegen, L.E.; Herzog, H.; Wieler, H.; Patton, D.D. & Schmid, A. (1986). *Journal of Nuclear Medicine*. Vol.27, No. 12 (December), pp. 1867-1877.

Gallagher BM, Ansari A, Atkins H, Casella V, Christman DR, Fowler JS, Ido T, MacGregor RR, Som P, Wan CN, Wolf AP, Kuhl DE, Reivich M. (1977). *Journal of Nuclear Medicine*. Vol.18, No.10 (October), pp. 990-996.

Gallagher BM, Fowler JS, Gutterson NI, MacGregor RR, Wan CN, Wolf AP. (1978). *Journal of Nuclear Medicine*. Vol.19, No.10 (October), pp. 1154-1161.

Goodman, M.M.; Kabalka, G.W.; Waterhouse, R.N. & Daniel, G.B. (1991a). *Journal of Labelled Compounds and Radiopharmaceuticals*. Vol.30, pp. 278-279.

Goodman, M.M.; Kabalka, G.W.; Meng, X. (1991b). *Journal of Labelled Compounds and Radiopharmaceuticals*. Vol.30, pp. 280-282.

Halseth, A.E.; Bracy, D.P. & Wasserman, D.H. (1998). *Journal of Applied Physiology*. Dec;Vol.85, No.6 (december), pp. 2305-2313.

Halseth, A.E.; Bracy, D.P. & Wasserman, D.H. (2000) *American Journal of Physiology, Endocrinology and Metabolism*. Vol.279, No.5 (November), pp. E1064-1071.

Halseth, A.E.; Bracy, D.P. & Wasserman, D.H. (2001). *American Journal of Physiology, Endocrinology and Metabolism*. Vol.280, No.6 (June), pp. E994-999.

Henry, C.; Koumanov, F.; Ghezzi, C.; Morin, C.; Mathieu, J.-P.; Vidal, M.; de Leiris, J. & Comet, M. (1997a). *Nuclear Medicine and Biology*. Vol.24, pp. 527-534.

Henry, C.; Tanti, J.F.; Grémeaux, T.; Morin, C.; Van Obberghen, E.; Comet, M. & Le Marchand-Brustel, Y. (1997b). *Nuclear Medicine and Biology*. Vol.24, No.1 (January), pp. 99-104.

Henry, R.R. (2003). *Clinical Therapeutics*. Vol.25, suppl.B, pp. B47-B63.

Hirvonen, J.; Virtanen, K.A.; Nummenmaa, L.; Hannukainen, J.C.; Honka, M.-J.; Bucci, M.; Nesterov, S.V.; Parkkola, R.; Rinne, J.; Iozzo, P. & Nuutila, P. (2011). *Diabetes*. Vol.60, pp. 443–447.

Iozzo, P.; Geisler, F.; Oikonen, V.; Maki, M.; Takala, T.; Solin, O.; Ferrannini, E.; Knuuti, J. & Nuutila, P. (2003). *Journal of Nuclear Medicine*. Vol.44, No.5 (May), pp. 682-689.

Israel, O; Weiler-Sagie, M; Rispler, S; Bar-Shalom, R; Frenkel, A; Keidar, Z; Bar-Shalev, A & Strauss, HW. (2007). *Journal of Nuclear Medicine*, Vol.48, pp. 234–239.

Kelley, D.E.; Mintun, M.A.; Watkins, S.C.; Simoneau, J.-A.; Jadali, F.; Fredrickson, A.; Beattie, J. & Thériault, R. (1996). *Journal of Clinical Investigation*. Vol.97, pp. 2705–2713.

Kelley, D.E.; Williams, K.V.; Price, J.C. & Goodpaster, B. (1999). *Journal of Nuclear Medicine*. Vol.40, No.11 (November), pp. 1798-1804.

Keiding, S.; Munk, O.L.; Schiøtt, K.M. & Hansen, S.B. (2000). *European Journal of Nuclear Medicine*. Vol.27, No.4 (April), pp. 407-412.

Kim, J.; Herrero, P.; Sharp, T.; Laforest, R.; Rowland, D.J.; Tai, Y.-C.; Lewis, J.S. & Welch, M.J. (2006). *Journal of Nuclear Medicine*. Vol.47, pp. 330–336.

Kloster, G.; Laufer, P.; Wutz, W.; & Stocklin, G. (1983a). *European Journal of Nuclear Medicine*. Vol.8, pp. 237-241.

Kloster, G.; Laufer, P. & Stocklin, G. (1983b). *Journal of Labelled Compounds and Radiopharmaceuticals*. Vol.20, pp. 391-415.

Kobayakawa, N.; Aoyagi, T.; Sugiura, S.; Ohtomo, K.; Sasaki, Y.; Omata, M. & Yazaki, Y. (1999). *Journal of Nuclear Medicine*. Vol.40, No.7 (July), pp. 1116-1121.

Koumanov, F.; Henry, C.; Ghezzi, C.; Bignan, G.; Morin, C.; Mathieu, J.-P.; Hamant, S.; Vidal, M.; de Leiris, J. & Comet, M. (1996). *Nuclear Medicine and Biology*. Vol.23, pp. 53-60.

Koumanov, F.; Henry, C.; Ghezzi, C.; Mathieu, J.-P.; Morin, C.; Vidal, M.; de Leiris, J. & Comet, M. (1997b). *Nuclear Medicine and Biology*. Vol.24, pp. 519-525.

Kraegen, E.W.; James, D.E.; Bennett, S.P. & Chisholm, D.J. (1983). *American Journal of Physiology*. Vol.245, No.1 (July), pp. E1-7.

Lutz, T.; Dougan, H.; Rihela, T.; Hudon, M.; Cohen, P.; Jamieson, W.R.E. & Lyster, D.M. (1991). *Journal of Labelled Compounds and Radiopharmaceuticals*. Vol.29, pp. 535-545.

Magata, Y.; Saji, H.; Ohmomo, Y.; Tanaka, C.; Konishi, J. & Yokoyama, A. (1992). *Journal of Labelled Compounds and Radiopharmaceuticals*. Vol.31, pp. 317-328.

McLaughlin, T.L. & Reaven, G.M. (2003). *American Journal of Medicine*. Vol.114, pp. 501-502.

Ménard, S.L.; Croteau, E.; Sarrhini, O.; Gélinas, R.; Brassard, P.; Ouellet, R.; Bentourkia, M.; van Lier, J.E.; Des Rosiers, C.; Lecomte, R. & Carpentier, A.C. (2010). *American Journal of Physiology: Endocrinology and Metabolism*. Vol.298, pp. E1049–E1057.

Mossberg, K.A. & Taegtmeyer, H. (1991) *Metabolism*. Vol.40, No.6 (June), pp. 594-599.

Mossberg, K.A. & Taegtmeyer, H. (1992). *Journal of Nuclear Medicine*. Vol.33, No.8 (August), pp. 1523-1529.

Mossberg, K. A., Rowe, R. W., Tewson, T. J. & Taegtmeyer, H. (1989). *Journal of Applied Physiology*. Vol.67, No.4, pp. 1569-1577.

Muoio, D.M. & Newgard, C.B. (2008). *Nature reviews: molecular cell biology*. Vol. 9 (March), pp. 193-205.

Narahara, H. & Ozand, P. (1963). *Journal of Biological Chemistry*. Vol.238, pp. 40–49.

Nuutila, P.; Koivisto, V.A.; Knuuti, J.; Ruotsalainen, U.; Teräs, M.; Haaparanta, M.; Bergman, J.; Solin, O.; Voipio-Pulkki LM, Wegelius, U. & Yki-Järvinen, H. (1992). *Journal of Clinical Investigation*. Vol.89, No.6 (June), pp. 1767-1774.

O'Doherty, R.; Halseth, A.; Granner, D.; Bracy, D. & Wasserman, D. (1998). *American Journal of Physiology*. Vol.274, pp. E287–E296.

Paternostro, G.; Camici, P.G.; Lammerstma, A.A.; Marinho, N.; Baliga, R.R.; Kooner, J.S.; Radda, G.K. & Ferrannini, E. (1996). *Journal of Clinical Investigation*. Vol.98, pp. 2094–2099.

Patlak, C.S. & Blasberg R.G. (1985). *Journal of Cerebral Blood Flow and Metabolism*. Vol.5, No.4 (December), pp. 584-590.

Pencek, R.R.; Bertoldo, A.; Price, J.; Kelley, C.; Cobelli, C. & Kelley, D.E. (2006). *American Journal of Physiology: Endocrinology and Metabolism* Vol.290, pp. E1124-E1130.

Pendergrass, M.; Bertoldo, A.; Bonadonna, R.; Nucci, G.; Mandarino, L.; Cobelli, C. & DeFronzo, R.A. (2007). *American Journal of Physiology: Endocrinology and Metabolism*. Vol.292, pp. E92–E100.

Perret, P.; Ghezzi, C.; Mathieu, J.P.; Morin, C. & Fagret, D. (2003). *Diabetes/Metabolism Research and Reviews*. Vol.19, pp. 306-312.

Perret, P.; Slimani, L.; Briat, A.; Ghezzi, C.; Villemain, D.; Halimi, S.; Demongeot, J. & Fagret, D. (2007). *European Journal of Nuclear Medicine and Molecular Imaging*. Vol.34, pp. 734-744.

Petersen, H.A.; Fueger, P.T.; Bracy, D.P.; Wasserman, D.H. & Halseth, A.E. (2003). *American Journal of Physiology: Endocrinology and Metabolism*. Vol.284, No. 3 (March), pp. E541-548.

Phelps, M.E.; Hoffman, E.J.; Selin, C.; Huang, S.C.; Robinson, G.; MacDonald, N.; Schelbert, H. & Kuhl, D.E. (1978). *Journal of Nuclear Medicine*. Vol.19, pp. 1311-1319.

Reaven, G.M. (1988). *Diabetes*. Vol. 37, pp. 1595-1607.

Rossetti, L.; Stenbit, A.E.; Chen, W.; Hu, M.; Barzilai, N.; Katz E.B. & Charron M.J. (1997). *Journal of Clinical Investigation*. Vol.100, pp. 1831-1839.

Samuel, V.T.; Petersen, K.F. & Shulman, G.I. (2010). *Lancet*. June Vol.26, Vol.375, No.9733 (June), pp. 2267–2277.

Selberg, O.; Burchert, W.; vd Hoff, J.; Meyer, G.J.; Hundeshagen, H.; Radoch, E.; Balks, H.J. & Müller, M.J. (1993). *Journal of Clinical Investigation*. Vol.91, No.5 (May), pp. 1897-1902.

Sharp, T.L.; Dence, C.S.; Engelbach, J.A.; Herrero, P.; Gropler, R.J. & Welch, M.J. (2005). *Nuclear Medicine and Biology*. Vol.32, pp. 875–884.

Shoghi, K.I.; Gropler, R.J.; Sharp, T.; Herrero, P.; Fettig, N.; Su, Y.; Mitra, M.S.; Kovacs, A.; Finck, B.N. & Welch, M.J. (2008). *Journal of Nuclear Medicine*. Vol.49, pp. 1320–1327.

Shoghi, K.I. & Welch, M.J. (2007). *Nuclear Medicine and Biology*. Vol.34, pp. 989–994.

Slimani, L.; Perret, P.; Briat, A.; Villemain, D.; Ghezzi, C.; Fagret, D. & Demongeot, J. (2002). *CR Biol*. Vol.325, No.4, pp. 529-546.

Slimani, L., Oikonen, V., Hällsten, K., Savisto, N., Knuuti, J., Nuutila, P. & Iozzo, P. (2006). *Journal of Clinical Endocrinology and Metabolism*. Vol.91, pp. 3394–3403.

Sokoloff, L.; Reivich, M.; Kennedy, C.; Des Rosiers, M.H.; Patlak, C.S.; Pettigrew, K.D.; Sakurada, O. & Shinohara, M. (1977). *Journal of Neurochemistry*. Vol.28, No.5 (May), pp. 897-916.

Taylor, S.I.; Accili, D. & Imai, Y. (1994). *Diabetes*. Vol. 43, pp. 735-740.

Virtanen, K.A.; Peltoniemi, P.; Marjamaki, P.; Asola, M.; Strindberg, L.; Parkkola, R.; Huupponen, R.; Knuuti, J.; Lonnroth, P. & Nuutila, P. (2001). *Diabetologia*. Vol.44, No.12 (December), pp. 2171-2179.

Voipio-Pulkki, L.-M.; Nuutila, P.; Knuuti, M.J.; Ruotsalainen, U.; Haaparanta, M.; Teras, M.; Wegelius, U. & Koivisto, V.A. (1993). *Journal of Nuclear Medicine*. Vol.34, 2064-2067.

Vom Dahl, J.; Herman, W.H.; Hicks, R.J.; Ortiz-Alonso, F.J.; Lee, K.S.; Allman, K.C.; Wolfe, E.R.Jr.; Kalff, V. & Schwaiger, M. 1993. *Circulation*. Vol.88, No.2 (August), pp. 395-404.

Vyska, K, Magloire, J, Freundlieb, C, Hock, A, Becker, V, Schmid, A, Feinendegen, L, Kloster, G, Stocklin, G, Schuier, F 1985 Eur J Nucl Med 11:97–106

Wassenaar, W & Tator, C.H. (1973). *Transactions of the American Neurological Association*. Vol.98, pp. 43-48.

Welch, M.J.; Lewis, J.S.; Kim, J.; Sharp, T.L.; Dence, C.S.; Gropler, R.J. & Herrero, P. (2006). *Journal of Nuclear Medicine*. Vol.47, pp. 689–697.

Williams, K.V.; Bertoldo, A.; Mattioni, B.; Price, J.C.; Cobelli, C. & Kelley, D.E. (2003). *Journal of Clinical Endocrinology and Metabolism*. Vol.88, No.3, pp. 1271–1279.

Yokoyama, I.; Ohtake, T.; Momomura, S.; Yonekura, K.; Yamada, N.; Nishikawa, J.; Sasaki, Y. & Omata. (1998). *Journal of Nuclear Medicine*. Vol.39, pp. 884-889.

Yokoyama, I.; Yonekura, K.; Moritan, T.; Tateno, M.; Momose, T.; Ohtomo, K.; Inoue, Y. & Nagai, R. (2001). *Journal of Nuclear Medicine*. Vol.42, No.7 (July), pp. 1005-1010.

Yokoyama, I.; Inoue, Y.; Moritan, T.; Ohtomo, K. & Nagai, R. (2003). *Journal of Nuclear Medicine* Vol.44, No.10 (October), pp. 1592-1598.

17

Targeting PKA Signaling to Prevent Metabolic Syndrome and Delay Aging

Enns, Linda C and Ladiges, Warren C
University of Washington, USA

1. Introduction

Protein kinase A (PKA) is a ubiquitous serine-threonine kinase that is activated by adenyl cyclase (AC)-mediated cAMP (Niswender et al., 1975). Canonically, the PKA signaling pathway is triggered when G-coupled receptors, a family of seven transmembrane domain proteins, are bound by extracellular hormones. The resultant dissociation of the Gs complex allows the stimulatory Gsα protein to bind to and activate membrane-bound adenylyl cyclases (ACs), which convert ATP to cAMP. The PKA holoenzyme has four subunits: 2 of which are catalytic (PKA C) and two of which are regulatory (PKA R). When associated, the heteroterameric enzyme is inactive. When cAMP binds to the regulatory subunits, the PKA C monomers are released, becoming catalytically active (Kirschner et al., 2009) (Fig. 1).

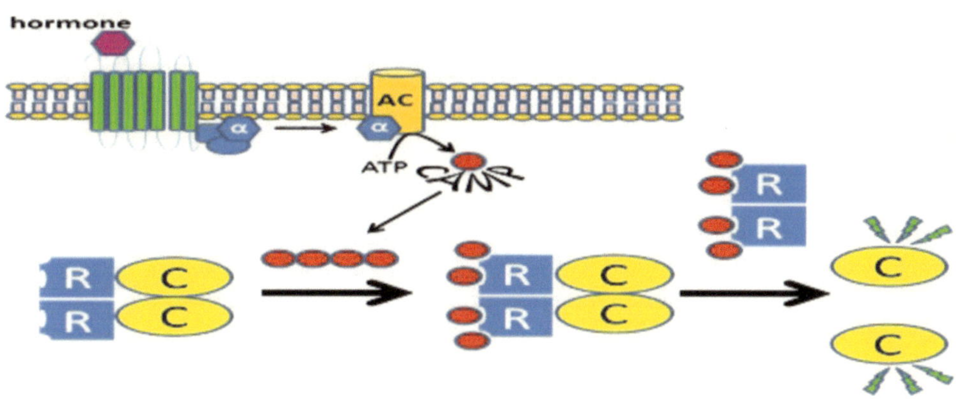

Fig. 1. cAMP activation of PKA.

PKA plays a role in numerous biological functions, with hundreds of PKA substrates identified in both the cytoplasm as well as the nucleus (Budovskaya et al., 2005; Huang et al., 2007; Neuberger et al., 2007; Gao et al., 2008). PKA signaling is known to influence cellular differentiation, ion channel activity, and plays a key role in the regulation of metabolism and triglyceride storage (Enns and Ladiges, 2010). This single enzyme is able to regulate such numerous and diverse processes by having isoforms and splice variants for both the catalytic and regulatory subunits, each of which has its own spatial and temporal patterns of expression, and each of which confers a different mutant phenotype when knocked out in mice (Table 1).

	Subunit	Expression	KO Phenotype
R	RIα	widespread	embryonic lethal (Amieux et al., 2002)
R	RIIα	widespread	no obvious phenotype (Burton et al., 1997)
R	RIβ	brain	deficits in neural plasticity (Brandon et al., 1995)
R	**RIIβ**	**brain, adipose**	**obesity resistant** (Cummings et al., 1996)
C	Cα	widespread	early postnatal lethality, growth retardation, sperm dysfunction (Skalhegg et al., 2002)
C	**Cβ**	**brain**	**obesity resistant** (Enns et al., 2009b)

Table 1. Different isoforms of regulatory and catalytic subunits of PKA.

The C and R subunits are encoded by three and four different isoforms, respectively: Cα, Cβ and Cγ for the catalytic subunit, and RIα, RIβ, RIIα and RIIβ for the regulatory subunit (Burton et al., 1997). Generally speaking, the α isoforms are constitutively expressed in most tissues, whereas the β isoforms are expressed at highest levels in the brain (Cadd and McKnight, 1989). Specific responses to different hormones and neurotransmitters is also believed to be achieved by the subcellular compartmentalization of PKA (Harper et al., 1985). RII subunits are thought to contribute to this type of regulation, by anchoring PKA in close proximity to its substrates through the binding of a family of A-kinase anchor proteins (AKAPs) (Lohmann et al., 1984; Rubin, 1994; Dell'Acqua et al., 1997). AKAPs anchor PKA by interacting with specific R subunits, and thus determine the subcellular localization of the PKA holoenzyme by what type of R subunit is present. The type-I PKA holoenzyme contains RI subunits (RIα and RIβ) and is primarily cytoplasmic, while the type II holenzyme contains RII subunits (RIIα and RIIβ) and is associated with particulate subcellular fractions (McConnachie et al., 2006).

Different and specific roles for the various subunits of PKA have been verified using conventional gene knockout mouse models. Deletion of the Cα subunit causes perinatal lethality, or, in the case of survivors, severe growth retardation (Skalhegg et al., 2002), while up until recently, it was believed that knockout (KO) mice for Cβ are phenotypically indistinguishable from their WT littermates (Qi et al., 1996). Complete loss of function of the R1α subunit leads to embryonic death early during gestation caused by abnormal mesodermal development (Amieux et al., 2002), while mice heterozygous for the knockout allele are predisposed to develop the myoxymas and endocrine tumors associated with Carney Complex (CNC) in humans (Kirschner et al., 2005). RIβ KO mice have deficiencies in synaptic plasticity (Brandon et al., 1995).

Yet loss of function of various elements of the PKA signaling pathway have also been shown to have health and lifespan benefits. Some of these beneficial PKA functions have been conserved evolutionarily from yeast to mammals, as evidenced by lifespan studies in yeast, worms, flies and mice. In yeast, loss of function of CYR1, an adenylyl cyclase, increases lifespan (Longo, 2003) as do mutations in the GTP-GDP exchange factors CDC35 and CDC25. Reduced function of TPK1, 2 and 3, functionally redundant yeast PKA catalytic subunits which are homologous to those in both mouse and human, also promotes longevity (Lin et al., 2000). PKA activity also mediates age-related decline in flies (Yamazaki et al., 2007; Laviada et al., 1997), and recent studies in mice have described delayed cardiac aging and extended lifespan by deletion of the adenylyl cyclase, AC5 (Yan et al., 2007) and obesity resistance, increased lifespan and healthy aging by disruption of specific PKA subunit genes (Cummings et al., 1996; Enns et al., 2009a, 2009b). This chapter will focus on recent studies describing the health benefits of disruption of two different PKA subunits, the regulatory isoform RIIβ, and the catalytic subunit Cβ. The proposed mechanisms behind these effects will be discussed as well as future work required to further investigate the potential of these subunits as pharmaceutical targets for the treatment of aging and age-related disease in humans.

2. Disruption of subunits of PKA leads to obesity resistance and leptin sensitivity

Most mammals maintain their body composition within a narrow range of fat mass. For example, following caloric restriction and a subsequent weight loss, rats increase food intake and decrease energy expenditure until they return to their original body weight (Mitchel and Keesey, 1977). Likewise, obese rats which have been induced to overeat by electrical stimulation of the lateral hypothalamus, return to original body weights and blood glucose levels when the stimulus is removed (Steffens, 1975). In order to accomplish energy homeostasis, an animal must be able to sense the amount of energy available in adipose tissue as well as sense and integrate opposing signals; it also must be able to regulate both energy intake and expenditure in response to this information. The main tissues responsible for both the sensing of as well as the response to nutrient status are the hypothalamus, which controls body weight and appetite, brown adipose tissue (BAT), which controls thermogenesis and energy expenditure, and white adipose tissue (WAT), which is involved in energy storage (Cypess & Kahn, 2010). The AC/cAMP/PKA pathway plays a major role in the genetic regulation of obesity and energy balance, as evidenced by mouse studies showing that disruption of specific PKA subunits leads to a more lean phenotype under 'normal' conditions, as well as to obesity resistance when challenged with either a high fat/high carbohydrate diet or with age-induced obesity.

2.1.1 PKA and obesity resistance

Disruption of the regulatory RIIβ subunit of PKA causes obesity resistance (Cummings et al., 1996). RIIβ is known to play a role in energy homeostasis. The RIIβ regulatory isoform of PKA is abundant in brown and white adipose tissue and the brain, with limited expression elsewhere. As mentioned earlier, these three tissues are the key players in the coordination of adiposity through regulation of energy storage, energy expenditure, and feeding behaviour. Disrupting the RIIβ gene in these tissues does not cause any overt abnormalities, but RIIβ null mutants are remarkably lean, with fat pad weights about half that of their wild-type littermates. Body composition differences are only a result of a reduction in fat; these mutants do not suffer from decreases in muscle mass. In addition, disrupting the RIIβ gene protects the obesity-susceptible C57/BL6 strain of mice from high fat/high carbohydrate (HF/HC) diet-induced both obesity and fatty livers (Cummings et al., 1996). Obesity resistance caused by deletion of the RIIβ subunit has also been observed in aging C57/BL6 mice, the WT which we have found to gain body weight post-maturity due to the accumulation of fat (Enns et al., 2009a). At the peak of obesity, aging male WT mice, maintained on a regular diet, had 25% body fat, while RIIβ null mice only had about 15% body fat; aging WT females and RIIβ null mice showed average maximum body fat percentages of about 30% and 15%, respectively. This same study also found that WT mice, with age, developed livers up to twice their original size due to an accumulation of fat, and that disruption of RIIβ prevented this from occurring. RIIβ thus represents a potential pharmacological target for the treatment of diet and age-induced obesity and fatty liver.

Our studies have indicated that the Cβ catalytic subunit of PKA also plays a role in maintaining a set point of adiposity (Enns et al., 2009b). Young Cβ null mice appear overtly normal when maintained on a regular chow diet, but when challenged with a HF/HC diet, show resistance to the obesity and fatty liver disease suffered by their WT littermates. This obesity resistance is not due to reduced food intake, which is similar between genotypes, nor to increased locomoter activity, which also shows no differences between genotypes. In addition, knocking out Cβ protects aging mice on a regular diet from developing age-related obesity and fatty livers (Enns, In Press).

2.1.2 PKA and thermogenesis

The leanness of RIIβ null mutants had been thought in the past to be due to changes in PKA activity in brown adipose tissue (BAT). BAT is a major contributor to non-shivering, diet-induced thermogenesis, or heat production (Rothwell and Stock, 1979). Thermogenesis is caused by the uncoupling of oxidative phosphorylation from ATP production in the mitochondria by uncoupling protein-1 (UCP1), which results in the energy from the proton motive force being dissipated as heat. Increases in thermogenesis occur in response to marked increases in energy intake, such as those that occur in HF/HC diet-challenged mice. Non-shivering thermogenesis is in part regulated by the sympathetic nervous system, and can be stimulated by hormones such as norephinephrine and leptin. It is known that PKA plays a mediating role in this process, phosphorylating perilipin, the main regulator of lipolysis, in response to these hormones (Souza et al., 2007). Loss of the RIIβ subunit in BAT is associated with a compensatory increase in the RIα isoform, which has a higher affinity for binding cAMP. The resultant increase in basal PKA activity in the BAT of RIIβ null mutants leads to an increase in UCP, an elevated metabolic rate and an increase in body temperature, suggesting that mutants are metabolically inefficient and waste food calories as heat (Cummings et al., 1996). The hypothesis that metabolic inefficiency is the cause of the RIIβ null lean phenotype is, however, confounded by data showing that disrupting UCP1 in RIIβ null mice reduces basal oxygen consumption but does not prevent the lean phenotype (Nolan et al., 2004). Regardless, the brain is believed to regulate adiposity in part through modulating sympathetic stimulation of PKA in BAT, resulting in changes in UCP expression and facultative energy expenditure (Himms-Hagen, 1990), and chronic activation of PKA in adipose tissue through β-adrenergic stimulation is being investigated for its potential in obesity therapy. While UCP1 induction does not appear to be required for the maintenance of the lean phenotype in RIIβ null mice, it is still essential to sustain their increased basal oxygen consumption, a process important to the regulation of energy expenditure and metabolic setpoint. Understanding the role that RIIβ may play in this process is important for determining pharmaceutical targets that may also be useful for the development of anti-obesity drugs.

Altered thermogenesis does not appear to play a role in the PKA Cβ null obesity-resistant phenotype. We did not find body temperature differences between Cβ null mice and their WT littermates, nor did we observe differences in UCP1 levels in the BAT between genotypes maintained on either a regular chow or a HF/HC diet. Taken together, the RIIβ and Cβ mutant data indicates that while RIIβ is involved in regulating energy expenditure through induction of thermogenesis, upregulation of this process in particular is not essential in either of these mutants for obesity resistance to occur.

2.1.3 PKA and WAT signaling

In white adipose tissue (WAT), PKA is known to integrate a number of hormonal signals in order to regulate the lipolysis, or the catabolism of stored triglycerides into fatty acids and glycerol by hormone-sensitive lipase (HSL) (Planas et al., 1999). Lipolysis is in part increased by β-adrenergic agonists, which stimulate PKA to both activate HSL (Stralfors et al.,1984; Anthonsen et al., 1998) as well as promote its translocation to lipid droplets (Egan et al., 1992; Hirsch & Rosen, 1984). PKA also inhibits the expression of a number of lipogenic genes. In RIIβ mutant WAT, there is an elevated basal rate of lipolysis when measured *in vitro*, and a blunted lipolytic response to β-AR stimulation that is observed both *in vitro* and *in vivo*. It is unknown if these changes in WAT metabolism could play a role in the lean phenotype and obesity resistance observed in the RIIβ null mutants. We have not yet characterized the WAT metabolism of Cβ null mutants.

2.1.4 PKA and leptin sensitivity

Studies on RIIβ using the leptin-deficient, obese *ob/ob* mouse (*ob*) indicate an important role for this particular PKA subunit in the leptin-dependent regulation of energy homeostasis (Newhall et al., 2005). Leptin is a well-known peptide hormone that is produced by adipose tissue. It plays a key role in the regulation of energy intake and energy expenditure, including appetite and metabolic rate. The level of circulating leptin is directly proportional to the amount of fat stored in the body, and acts on receptors in the hypothalamus of the brain where it regulates the activity or synthesis of many neuropeptides that are important in appetite and metabolic control. The region of hypothalamus which serves to integrate signals controlling feeding and energy expenditure is called the arcuate nucleus region (ARC). Two distinct populations of leptin-responsive neurons exist here: one that expresses the anabolic neuropeptides, NPY and agouti-related protein (AgRP) and one that expresses a precursor protein for the catabolic neuropeptide α-MSH, called proopiomelanocortin (POMC) (Cone 2005; Morton et al., 2006). Both sets of neurons project into the paraventricular hypothalamus (PVH) where the Gs-coupled melanocortin receptor MC4R is activated by α-MSH; this activation is antagonized by AgRP. Activation of the MC4R receptor is believed to decrease food intake and increase energy expenditure. PKA is a downstream mediator for many of these neuropeptides, (Schwartz et al., 2000; Flier, 2004). Generally speaking, catabolic and anabolic neuropeptides signal through pathways that increase and decrease PKA activity, respectively. Leptin inhibits NPY and AgRP release from the paraventricular nucleus, which normally leads to the activation of anabolic pathways through a decrease in PKA activity. Conversely, leptin stimulates the release of α-MSH, leading to an increase in PKA activity and the activation of catabolic pathways (Fig. 2).

Studies on RIIβ null mice indicate that this mutation may confer leptin sensitivity. Even when fed only standard rodent chow, leptin serum levels in mutants were found to be threefold lower than for WT mice (Schreyer et al., 2001). When maintained on the HF/HC diet, serum leptin levels increased differently between genotypes. Both genotypes experienced elevations in serum leptin levels, but these increases were delayed in the mutants compared to WT, consistent with their delayed weight gain. In spite of lower leptin levels, when standardized to body weight, food intake was actually slightly higher in the mutants, indicative of leptin sensitivity.

This hypothesis was verified by knocking out the RIIβ subunit in other mouse mutants known to have problems with leptin signaling. The *ob* mouse is hyperphagic, hypoactive, hypothermic and hyperinsulinemic (Bray & York, 1979), due to decreased expression of β-adrenergic receptors (β-ARs) and UCP in BAT (Reichling et al., 1988; Collins et al., 1994). The obese phenotype can be rescued by administration of leptin, which decreases their food intake and increases their metabolic rate in addition to restoring normal expression levels of adipose β-AR and UCP1 (Weigel et al., 1995; Mistry et al., 1997; Phelleymounter et al., 1995; Halaas et al., 1995; Campfield et al., 1995; Breslow & Berkowitz, 1997; Commins et al., 1999). The phenotype of the *ob* mouse can also be rescued by knocking out RIIβ. The double mutant shows decreased body weight, increased energy expenditure, and activation of BAT resulting in increased thermogenesis (Newhall et al., 2004). RIIβ is expressed in high levels in the hypothalamus (Planas et al., 1999). An increase in basal PKA activity here, due to the disruption of the RIIβ subunit could lead to increased stimulation of leptin sensitive catabolic pathways.

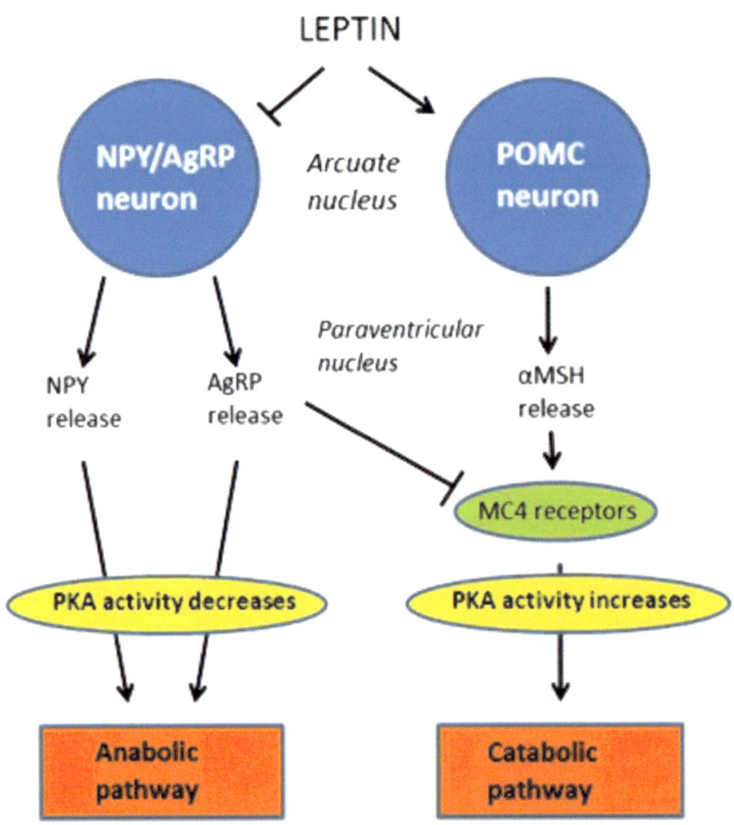

Fig. 2. Leptin signaling pathway as mediated by PKA.

Disruption of RIIβ also reverses the obesity syndrome found in agouti lethal yellow mice (A^y), which express agouti-related protein (AgRP) ectopically due to a genetic rearrangement at the agouti locus (Czyzyk et al., 2007). Constitutive expression of AgRP, such as occurs in A^y mice, leads to hypoactivity, hyperphagy, hyperglycemia and hyperinsulinemia (Yen et al., 1994; Manne et al., 1995). Disruption of RIIβ reduces both food intake and adiposity in these mice, indicating that the signaling pathway downstream of the agouti antagonism has been modified. It has been suggested that the known compensatory increase in the more cAMP-affinitive type I PKA, observed in RIIβ KO tissues, results in an overall increase in the basal activity of PKA that is downstream and thus independent of AgRP antagonism in hypothalamic neurons.

We have also found that Cβ null mice are leptin sensitive in addition to being obesity resistant (In Press). After several weeks of being maintained on a high fat diet, WT mice had elevated leptin serum levels that were 2.5-fold higher than Cβ null mutants. In spite of lower serum leptin, mutants were found to be hypophagic and hypermetabolic, indicative of leptin sensitivity. Although mutants maintained on a regular diet showed metabolic rates similar to WT, as determined using indirect calorimetry to measure the rate of O_2 consumption (VO_2), we did observe a higher metabolic rate in the Cβ null mutants compared to WT when both genotypes were maintained on a HF/HC diet (Enns, In Press). To directly test leptin sensitivity in the mutants, at the end of the HF/HC dietary challenge, both WT and mutants were injected with 4.0 ug leptin/g mouse, twice daily, for a period of a week. Mutants, but not WT mice, showed significant weight loss, indicating that the WT mice had become leptin resistant on the HF/HC diet, while the Cβ null mice had not. Leptin sensitivity in the Cβ null mice was verified by injecting young both mutants and WT mice, maintained on a regular diet, with leptin twice daily. While weight loss and food intake were not affected differently between genotypes, by the end of the week-long injections, Cβ null mice were showing significantly higher rates of oxygen consumption compared to WT mice. Thus it is possible that Cβ, like RIIβ, acts downstream of leptin signaling in the hypothalamus. The Cβ gene encodes three isoforms: Cβ1 is expressed in most tissues, while Cβ2 and Cβ3 are neural-specific (Guthrie et al., 1997). Measurements of brain PKA activity in the PKA Cβ null mutant have shown that knocking out all Cβ isoforms does not result in changes in total PKA activity, at least in the amygdala and hippocampus, as Cα protein levels are upregulated in order to compensate. It does, however, result in a 26% decrease in basal activity (without added cAMP) that may affect kinase activity at low cAMP concentrations (Howe et al., 2002). This data would appear to be at odds with that showing that increased PKA activity is responsible for leptin sensitivity and obesity resistance in the RIIβ null mutant. It is unknown how PKA activity is affected in the hypothalamus of Cβ null mice, but there are a number of possibilities. It may be affected differently than in other regions of the brain (ie. it may increase). Conversely, Cα1 and Cβ1 have diverged by about 10% in amino acid sequence in the mouse, but these sequence differences are strictly maintained with almost perfect fidelity across mammalian species (Uhler et al., 1986), suggesting that each has an important and unique function. If Cα plays a specific role in the leptin signaling pathway compared to Cβ, it may be that the compensatory increase in Cα activity in the Cβ null mutant is what is increasing signaling downstream of the MC4R receptor. Regardless, this leptin sensitivity is likely the cause of the obesity resistant phenotype observed in both age and HF/HC diet-challenged Cβ null mutants.

3. Disruption of subunits of PKA protects against diet-induced insulin resistance and dyslipidemia

In addition to inducing obesity, the HF/HC diet used in our studies is known to induce diabetes in C57/BL6 mice (Surwit et al., 1988; Surwit et al., 1991). It is also common for mice fed this diet to develop hyperlipidemia, or an elevation of lipids in the blood, reflected by serum increases in low density and very low density lipoproteins (LDL and VLDL) (Kirk et al., 1995; Srivastava et al., 1991; Ishida et al., 1991; LeBoeuf et al., 1993). Studies on HF/HC diet-fed PKA mutants have clearly illustrated an important role for PKA in the mediation of diet-induced insulin resistance and lipid disorder.

3.1.1 PKA and insulin sensitivity

RIIβ null mutants are resistant to HF/HC diet-induced insulin resistance. Knocking out the RIIβ subunit of PKA resulted in mice with 26% lower serum insulin levels than WT when maintained on a regular diet. When maintained on a HF/HC diet for 15 weeks, both genotypes developed hyperinsulinemia, however insulin levels were much higher for WT mice (Schreyer et al., 2001). Blood glucose levels increased similarly for both genotypes when challenged with the HF/HC diet, but the observation that RIIβ null mice achieve similar glucose levels with less insulin indicates improved insulin sensitivity. In keeping with this, loss of the RIIβ subunit resulted in improved glucose disposal in mice maintained on a regular chow diet, with lower blood glucose levels in the mutants compared to WT at all time points following a glucose injection. Also, while there were no differences in blood glucose between genotypes raised on a regular chow diet, RIIβ null mice were resistant to the marked reduction suffered by WT mice in the percentage of blood glucose cleared following an insulin injection after 15 weeks on the HF/HC diet.

It is believed that since RIIβ expression is absent from pancreatic islets, these effects are not directly due to changes in insulin secretion in response to circulating glucose. It was proposed by Shreyer et al. that RIIβ null mice are at least in part protected from diet-induced insulin resistance due to their resistance to obesity under a HF/HC dietary challenge. They were unable to test the null hypothesis due to a lack of sufficient number of RIIβ null mice that had white adipose tissue weights similar to those of their WT littermates; however, when insulin-mediated glucose disposal was corrected for differences in body weight, it was found that the HF/HC diet-fed RIIβ null mice cleared glucose in response to insulin at a similar rate to regular chow-fed mutants, while WT mice on the HF/HC diet showed decreased glucose disposal per gram mouse weight when compared with those on the regular diet. This suggests that loss of RIIβ improves insulin sensitivity at least in part via a mechanism independent of adiposity. One proposed mechanism is a reduction in PKA's known ability to antagonize insulin's activation of the mitogen-activated protein kinase (MAPK) cascade in adipose tissue (Sevetson et al., 1993). Although it is known that in this particular tissue, the compensation for RIIβ by the more cAMP-affinitive RIα causes a four- to fivefold increase in basal PKA activity, is is possible that inhibition of this particular cascade, probably at the level of ras or raf, is dependent on an RIIβ-containing PKA holoenzyme.

Similarly, we have found that PKA Cβ also plays a role in insulin sensitivity. As with RIIβ null mice, Cβ null mice are significantly protected against HF/HC diet-induced insulin resistance, showing improved glucose dispersal in response to insulin, compared to WT (Enns et al., 2009). Interestingly, we have found that Cβ null mice are extremely sensitive to insulin compared to their WT littermates, even when maintained on a regular chow and without major differences in adiposity levels. In fact, on a regular diet, at least for females, young Cβ null mice show insulin sensitivity in spite of having slightly higher body fat percentages than WT. In other words, insulin sensitivity of the Cβ null mutant is independent of adiposity, and the loss of the Cβ null mutant has direct effects on insulin sensitivity. Given the similarity between the Cβ and the RIIβ null phenotypes, it would be logical to propose that these two mutations are acting on insulin sensitivity via a similar mechanism. This would support the hypothesis of Shreyer et al. that PKA directly affects insulin sensitivity of adipose tissue, and that this particular mechanism is dependent on a specific subunit composition of PKA, specifically one containing either RIIβ or Cβ.

3.1.2 PKA and dyslipidemia

Dyslipidemia, another problem often observed in conjunction with obesity and diabetes, was found to be reduced in both RIIβ and Cβ null mutants when challenged with a HF/HC diet. Plasma both total cholesterol as well as very low density and low density lipoproteins (VLDL and LDL) were significantly lower in RIIβ null mice compared to WT (Schreyer, 2001). Cβ null mutants, at least for males, when challenged with the HF/HC diet were resistant to the increases in LDL and VLDL and partially resistant to the increases in high density lipoprotein (HDL) observed in the serum of WT mice (Enns et al., 2009b). Because insulin inhibits the assembly and release of VLDLs from the liver (Koo & Montminy, 2006), it is possible that the reduced serum VLDL levels seen in both types of mutants is an indirect effect of their insulin sensitivity. Whether the marked loss of lipoproteins from the VLDL/LDL fraction of the diet-challenged RIIβ null mice and of lipoproteins from both the HDL and VLDL/LDL fraction of the diet-challenged Cβ null mice is due to direct effects of the mutations on lipoprotein production or clearance, or is a result of indirect influences due to their insulin sensitivity or obesity resistance, is unknown.

4. Disruption of PKA protects against cardiac hypertrophy and dysfunction

Cardiac hypertrophy is an increase in the mass of the heart in response to and to compensate for an increased workload. Prolonged stress leads to impaired diastolic and eventually systolic properties of the left ventricle, leading to heart failure (Shapiro & Sugden, 1996). Altered PKA signaling has been implicated in cardiomyopathy by many previous studies (Enns et al., 2010; Lohse & Engelhardt, 2001). For example, it is believed that the muscle-specific A-kinase Anchoring Protein (mAKAP) targets PKA to the perinuclear region of the cell where it can modulate cardiomyocyte size. Inhibiting mAKAP expression suppresses the ability of leukemia inhibitory factor (LIF), which acts by increasing ERK5 activity, to induce cardiac hypertrophy (McConnachie et al., 2006). Deficiencies in PKA signaling have been linked to human cardiomyopathy due to reduced phosphorylation of downstream targets such as cardiac troponin I (Zakhary et al., 1999) and to preservation of cardiac function against pressure overload in mice (Okumura et al., 2003a; Okumura et al., 2003b). We have found that the Cβ subunit of PKA plays an important role in the development of cardiac hypertrophy and dysfunction in response to both angiotensin II-induced as well as age-induced hypertension.

Cβ null mice are resistant to angiotensin II- and age-induced cardiac hypertrophy and dysfunction (Enns et al., 2010; Enns et al., In Press). Angiotensin (ang) II is the effector of the renin-angiotensin system (RAS) and increases blood pressure by causing potent vasoconstriction through stimulation of angiotensin receptors in the vascular system (Ito et al., 1995). When ang II was administered to Cβ null mice and their WT littermates at a continuous rate and over a period of 4 weeks, both genotypes experienced similar and significant increases in both systolic and diastolic blood pressure. In spite of experiencing similar hypertension, the hearts of the Cβ null mice were smaller and showed improved cardiac function in 4 of 5 echocardiographical parameters measured including left ventricular mass index (a measure of the thickness of the ventricular wall), fractional shortening (a measure of contractility of the left ventricle), ratio of early to late diastolic filling (a measure of compensation by the left atrium for left ventricle failure), and ratio of aortic to left atrial diameter (a measure of left atrial enlargement due to overcompensation for left ventricular failure). We have also recently shown that as C57/BL6J mice age, they have a natural tendency to develop hypertension (Enns et al, In Press). As with angiotensin II-challenged mice, aged (24 month-old) WT mice of this strain also experience significant cardiac hypertrophy, some showing hearts twice the size of those found in young (4 month-old) mice. In addition to enlarged hearts, aged WT mice, like those challenged with ang II, show thickened ventricular walls, reduced fractional shortening of the left ventricle, reduced early to late diastolic filling ratios, and enlarged left atria. An additional parameter of global left ventricular function, myocardial performance index (MPI) was also found to worsen in aging WT mice. Disruption of the Cβ subunit did not protect aging C57/BL6 mice from hypertension, but did make mice resistant to both the cardiac hypertrophy experienced by the aging WT mice, as well as to their decline in cardiac performance in all parameters measured. Effects of disruption of RIIβ on age and ang II-induced cardiac decline have not yet been assessed.

PKA Cβ thus appears to play an important role in the mediation of hypertension and its myopathological effects. The β-adrenergic (β-AR)/adenylyl cyclase/PKA pathway, central to stimulating cardiac function, is known to be dysfunctional in heart failure (Bristow et al., 1982). Blockade of β-AR receptors improves survival in heart failure patients (Bristow, 2000) and transgenic mouse studies have shown that chronic activation of the cAMP-PKA pathway by cardiac-specific overexpression of β-AR, Gsα, and the α-catalytic subunit of PKA result in cardiomyopathy (Lohse & Engelhardt, 2001; Antos et al., 2001). PKA is known to cause cardiac hypertrophy in response to elevation of cAMP by β-adrenergic agonists (Rockman et al., 2002). There are, however, conflicting data in the literature to support the idea that activation of the β-AR/cAMP/PKA pathway may play a protective role in response to hemodynamic overload. In humans, phosphorylation of troponin I (TnI) by PKA is reduced in dilated cardiomyopathy (Zakhary et al., 1999), and in mice, overexpression of two types of cardiac adenylyl cyclases results in improved cardiac function (Lipskaia et al., 2000; Gao et al., 1999). The RIIβ mutant is thought to be sensitive to β-AR activation (McKnight et al., 1998; Montovani et al., 2009), an idea supported by their exaggerated response to amphetamine (Brandon et al., 1998). Given the other phenotypic similarities between the RIIβ and Cβ mutants, it is possible that the Cβ null mouse has a similar sensitivity, and that an overactive β-AR pathway is protecting their hearts against pressure overload.

PKA plays many other roles in cardiac signaling, and any of these may play a role in cardiac hypertrophy and dysfunction. For example, activation of cAMP/PKA signaling in the heart has been shown to inhibit smooth muscle proliferation (Indolfi et al., 1997). Calcium signaling pathways also play a role in cardiac hypertrophy (Passier et al., 2000; Minamisawa et al., 1999), supported by the finding that in the presence of hypertension, its development can be prevented by L-type calcium channel blockers (Zou et al., 2002). PKA has multiple downstream targets involved in calcium signaling in the heart, including the L-type Ca^{2+} channel in the sarcolemma, the ryanodine receptor (RyR2), and phospholamban in the sarcoplasmic reticulum (Antos et al., 2001). The Cβ subunit of PKA may play a specific role in the activation of one or more of these substrates.

5. PKA and longevity

Given that disruption of either the RIIβ or Cβ subunit of PKA in mice confers resistance to a number of health problems associated with aging, including obesity, leptin and insulin resistance, and cardiac hypertrophy and dysfunction, it was of interest to determine whether or not knocking out either of these genes would also lengthen the murine lifespan. Lifespan studies revealed an increase in both the median and maximum lifespans for RIIβ null males with an increase in median lifespan from 884 days to 1005 days, and an increase in the 80% lifespan (80% deaths of the cohort) from 941 to 1073 days. There was no difference in either median or 80% lifespan between genotypes in females (Enns et al., 2009a). Lifespan cohorts for Cβ null mice showed no effect on either the median or maximium lifespan for females, and a reduced lifespan for Cβ null males.

Whether or not the attenuation of an age-related health problem translates to an increase in lifespan for a particular strain of mouse depends on its contribution to that strain's probable cause of death. We have determined that adiposity plays a significant role in the lifespan of the male, but not the female C57BL/6J WT mouse (Enns et al., 2009a). As mentioned earlier, this strain of mouse is susceptible to age-related obesity, and individuals continue to put on body weight in the form of body fat for many months post-maturity. This gain in adiposity was found to be variable between individuals, however, and when the lifespan of individual WT mice was plotted against their maximal body weight, a strong correlation was found for males (R^2=0.4795), but not for females (R^2=0.0369). Age-related obesity is thus a strong risk factor for mortality in male C57BL/6J mice, and it is not surprising that disruption of a gene such as RIIβ, that removes this risk factor would also lengthen their lifespan .

Lifespan analyses can be an indicator for whether or not disrupting a gene also confers detrimental effects. For example, the shortened lifespan of the Cβ null male mouse implies that this PKA subunit plays a role in other necessary functions. When mice heterozygous for the Cβ null mutation are bred , male homozygous nulls are born at a lower than expected frequency, indicating that the Cβ subunit of PKA may be important to males during their embryonic development. That disruption of either RIIβ or Cβ does not lengthen the female lifespan is not necessarily surprising, given that we found no correlation between adiposity and lifespan for C57BL/6J females. However, it can also be said for females that there appear to be no detrimental effects, at least those which would impact lifespan, of disrupting either of these PKA subunits. This is important for validating either of these subunits as a potential pharmaceutical target for the treatment of age-related disease in humans.

6. Conclusions

The Cβ and RIIβ subunits of PKA represent promising pharmaceutical targets for the treatment of metabolic syndrome, a name for a group of risk factors that together increase the risk of coronary disease, stroke, and type II diabetes and a problem which is rapidly becoming the predominant cause of poor health and reduced lifespan in industrialized nations. Mouse mutants lacking either of these subunits display a number of health benefits, including resistance to age and diet-induced obesity, protection against age and diet-induced leptin and insulin sensitivity, and resistance to cardiac hypertrophy and dysfunction.

The potential of a protein or protein subunit as a pharmaceutical target depends on whether or not its disruption also causes negative effects. Lifespan analyses show that in C57BL/6J mice, there appear to be no major detrimental health effects either on males and females from disrupting the RIIβ subunit, or on females from disrupting the Cβ subunit. Disrupting the Cβ subunit in males appears to carry some detriment, possibly during embryonic development, that affects the overall lifespan of the mouse, but pharmaceutical treatment of obesity and aging in humans would presumably occur beyond the age of maturity. Conditional mouse mutants need to be constructed to determine if knocking out the gene later in life removes the detrimental effects on the male PKA Cβ null lifespan.

Future work needs to address the many unanswered questions that have arisen from these studies. Are the phenotypes we are observing the result of the loss of the RIIβ and Cβ subunits, or of the known compensation by other PKA isoforms? Do these subunits affect the nature of the downstream targets of PKA, and if so, what are those targets, and what is their potential for pharaceutical targeting? Is leptin sensitivity the sole cause of the obesity resistance in the RIIβ and Cβ null mutants, or are there other mechanisms? By what direct mechanism is RIIβ and Cβ influencing insulin sensitivity, and what is its specific contribution to healthy aging and lifespan? What are the mechanisms behind the resistance to cardiac hypertrophy and dysfunction? Finally, how can we discover or develop pharaceuticals that will specifically target these PKA isoforms? Answering these questions will both validate the potential of these subunits as pharmaceutical targets, as well as identify new potential targets for the treatment of age-related metabolic syndrome in humans.

7. References

Ahima, R.S. (2009). Connecting obesity, aging and diabetes. *Nat. Med.,* Vol. 15, pp.996-997

Amieux, P.S.; Howe, D.G.; Knickerbocker, H.; Lee, D.C.; Su, T.; Laszlo, G.S.; Idzerda, R.L. & McKnight, G.S. (1997). Compensatory regulation of RIα protein levels in protein kinase A mutant mice. *J. Biol. Chem.* Vol. 272, pp. 3993-3998

Anthonsen, M.W.; Ronnstrand, L.; Wernstedt, C.; Degerman, E. & Holm, C. (1998). Identification of novel phosphorylation sites in hormone-sensitive lipase that are phosphorylated in response to isoproterenol and govern activation properties in vitro. *J. Biol. Chem.,* Vol. 273, pp.215-221

Antos, C.L.; Frey, H.; Marx, S.O.; Reiken, S.; Gaburjakova, M.; Richardson, J.A.; Marks, A.R. & Olson, E.N. (2001). Dilated cardiomyopathy and sudden death resulting from constitutive activation of protein kinase A. *Circ. Res.* Vol. 89, pp.997-1004

Brandon, E.P.; Zhuo, M.; Huang, Y.Y.; Qi, M; Gerhold, K.A.; Burton K.A.; Kandel, E.R.; McKnight, G.S. & Idzerda, R.L. (1995). Hippocampal long-term depression and depotentiation are defective in mice carrying a targeted disruption of the gene encoding the RI beta subunit of cAMP-dependent protein kinase. *PNAS*, Vol. 92, pp. 8851-8855

Brandon, E.P.; Logue, S.F.; Adams, M.R.; Qi, M.; Sullivan, S.P.; Matsumoto, A.M., Dorsa, D.M., Wehner, J.M., McKnight, G.S. & Idzerda, R.L. (1998). Defective motor behaviour and neural gene expression in RIIβ-protein kinase A mutant mice. *J. Neurosci.*, Vol. 18, pp. 3639-3649

Bray, G.A. & York, D.A. (1979). Hypothalamic and genetic obesity in experimental animals: an autonomic and endocrine hypothesis. *Physiol. Rev.* Vol. 59, pp. 719-809

Breslow, M.J.; An, Y. & Berkowitz, D.E. (1997). β-3 adrenoceptor (β-3AR) expression in leptin treated OB/OB mice. *Life Sci.*, Vol. 61, pp. 59-64

Bristow, M.R.; Ginsburg, R.; Minobe, W.; Cubicciotti, R.S.; Sageman, W.S.; Lurie, K.; Billingham, M.E.; Harrison, D.C. & Stinson, E.B. (1982). Decreased catecholamine sensitivity and β-adrenergic-receptor density in failing human hearts. *N. Engl. J. Med.* Vol. 307, pp.205-211

Bristow, M.R. (2000). β-Adrenergic receptor blockade in chronic heart failure. *Circ.* Vol. 101, pp. 558-569

Burton, K.A.; Johnson, B.D.; Hausken, Z.E.; Westenbroek, R.E.; Idzerda, R.L.; Scheuer, T.; Scott, J.D.; Catterall, W.A. & McKnight, G.S. (1997). Type II regulatory subunits are not required for the anchoring-dependent modulation of Ca^{2+} channel activity by cAMP-dependent protein kinase. *Proc. Natl. Acad. Sci. USA*, Vol. 94, pp. 11067-11072

Budovskaya, Y.V.; Stephan, J.S.; Deminoff, S.J. & Herman, P.K. (2005). An evolutionary proteomics approach identifies substrates of the cAMP-dependent protein kinase. *PNAS*, Vol. 102, pp. 13933-13938

Cadd, G. & Mcknight, G.S. (1989). Distinct patterns of cAMP-dependent protein kinase gene expression in mouse brain. *Neuron*, Vol. 3, pp. 71-79

Campfield, L.A.; Smith, F.J.; Guisez, Y.,; Devos, R. & Burn, P. (1995). Recombinant mouse OB protein: evidence for a peripheral signal linking adiposity and central neural networks. *Science*, Vol. 269, pp.546-549

Collins, S.; Daniel, K.W.; Rohlfs, E.M.; Ramkumar, V.; Taylor, I.L. & Gettys, T.W. (1994). Impaired expression and functional activity of the β3- and β1-adrenergic receptors in adipose tissue of congenitally obese (C57BL/6J ob/ob) mice. *Mol. Endocrinol.*, Vol. 8, pp. 518-527

Commins, S.P.; Watson, P.M.; Padgett, M.A.; Dudley, A.; Argyropoulos, G. & Gettys, T.W. (1999). Induction of uncoupling protein expression in brown and white adipose tissue by leptin. *Endocrinol.*, Vol. 140, pp.292-300

Cummings, D.E.; Brandon, E.P.; Planas, J.V.; Motamed, K; Idzerda, R.L. & McKnight, G.S. (1996). Genetically lean mice result from targeted disruption of the RIIβ subunit of protein kinase A. *Nature*, Vol. 382, pp. 622-626

Cone, R.D. (2005). Anatomy and regulation of the central melanocortin system. *Nat. Neurosci.*, Vol. 8, pp.571-578

Cypess, A.M. & Kahn, C.R. (2010). The role and importance of brown adipose tissue in energy homeostasis. *Curr. Opin. Pediatr.*, Vol. 22, pp.478-484

Czyzyk, T.A.; Sikorski, M.A.; Yang, L. & McKnight, G.S. (2007). Disruption of the RIIβ subunit of PKA reverses the obesity syndrome of agouti lethal yellow mice. *PNAS,* Vol. 105, pp.276-281

Dell'Acqua, M.L. & Scott, J.D. (1997). Protein kinase A anchoring. *J. Biol. Chem.,* Vol. 272, pp. 12881-12884

Egan, J.J.; Greenberg, A.S.; Chang, M.K.; Wek, S.A.; Moos, M.C. Jr. & Londos, C. (1992). Mechanism of hormone-stimulated lipolysis in adipocytes: translocation of hormone-sensitive lipase to the lipid storage droplet. PNAS, Vol. 89, pp.8537-8541

Enns, L.C.; Morton, J.F.; Emond, M.J.; Wolf, N.S.; McKnight, Rabinovitch, P.S. & Ladiges, W.C. (2009a). Disruption of protein kinase A in mice enhances healthy aging. *PLoS ONE,* Vol. 4, e5963

Enns, L.C.; Morton, J.F.; Mangalindan, R.S.; McKnight, G.S.; Schwartz, M.W.; Kaeberlein, M.R.; Kennedy, B.K.; Rabinovitch, P.S. & Ladiges, W.C. (2009b). Attenuation of age-related metabolic dysfunction in mice with a targeted disruption of the Cβ subunit of protein kinase A. *J. of Gerontol.,* Vol. 64, pp.1221-1231

Enns, L.C. & Ladiges, W. (2010). Protein kinase A signaling as an anti-aging target. *Ageing. Res. Rev.,* Vol. 9, pp. 269-272

Enns, L.C.; Pettan-Brewer, C. & Ladiges, W.C. (2010). Protein kinase A is a target for aging and the aging heart. *Aging,* Vol. 2, pp.238-243

Enns, L.C.; Bible, K.L. & Ladiges, W.C. (2010). Mice lacking the Cβ subunit of PKA are resistant to angiotensin II-induced cardiac hypertrophy and dysfunction. *BMC Res. Notes,* Vol. 3, pp.307

Gao, M.H.; Lai, N.C.; Roth, D.M.; Zhou, J.Y.; Zhu, J.; Dalton, N.; Anzai, T. & Hammond, K. (1999). Adenylyl cyclase increases responsiveness to catecholamine stimulation in transgenic mice. *Circ.,* Vol. 99, pp.1618-1622

Gao, X.; Jin, C.; Ren, J.; Yao, X. & Xue, Y. (2008). Proteome-wide prediction of PKA phosphorylation sites in eukaryotic kingdom. *Genomics,* Vol. 92, pp. 457-463

Guthrie, C.R.; Skalhegg, B.S. & McKnight, G.S. (1997). Two novel brain-specific splice variants of the murine Cβ gene of cAMP-dependent protein kinase. *J. Biol. Chem.,* Vol. 272, pp.29560-29565

Hirsch, A.H. & Rosen, O.M. (1984). Mechanism of hormone-stimulated lipolysis in adipocytes: translocation of hormone-sensitive lipase to the lipid storage droplet. *J. Lipid Res.* Vol. 25, pp.665-677

Halaas, J.L.; Gajiwala, K.S.; Maffei, M.; Cohen, S.L.; Chait, B.T.; Rabinowitz, D.; Lallone, R.L.; Burley, S.K. & Friedman, J.M. (1995). Weight-reducing effects of the plasma protein encoded by the obese gene. *Science,* Vol. 269, pp. 543-546

Harper, J.F.; Haddox, M.K.; Johanson, R.A.; Hanley, R.M. & Steiner, A.L. (1985). Compartmentation of second messenger action: immunocytochemical and biochemical evidence. *Vitam. Horm.,* Vol. 42, pp. 197-252

Himms-Hagen, J. (1990). Brown adipose tissue thermogenesis: interdisciplinary studies. *FASEB J.* Vol. 4, pp.2890-2898

Howe, D.G.; Wiley, J.C. & McKnight, G.S. (2002). Molecular and behavioural effects of a null mutation in all PKA Cβ isoforms. *Mol. Cell. Neurosci.,* Vol. 20, pp.515-524

Huang, S.Y.; Tsai, M.L.; Chen, G.Y.; Wu, C.J. & Chen, S.H. (2007). A systematic MS-based approach for identifying in vitro substrates of PKA and PKG in rat uteri. *J. Proteome. Res.,* Vol 6, pp. 2674-2684

Indolfi, C.; Awedimento, E.V.; Di Lorenzo, E.; Esposito, G.; Rapacciulo, A.; Giuliano, P.; Grieco, D.; Cavuto, L.; Stingone, A.M.; Ciullo, I.; Condorelli, G.; Chiariello, M. (1997). Activation of cAMP-PKA signaling in vivo inhibits smooth muscle cell proliferation induced by vascular injury. *Nature Med.* Vol. 3, pp. 775-779

Ishida, B.Y.; Blanche, P.J.; Nicols, A.V.; Yashar, M. & Paigen, B. (1991). Effects of atherogenic diet consumption on lipoproteins in mouse strains C57BL/6 and C3H. *J. Lipid Res.* Vol. 32, pp.559-568

Ito, M.; Oliverio, M.I.; Mannon, P.J.; Best, C.F.; Maeda, N.; Smithies, O. & Coffman, T.M. (1995). Regulation of blood pressure by the type 1A angiotensin II receptor gene. *PNAS,* Vol.92, pp.3521-3525

Kirk, E.A.; Moe, G.L.; Caldwell, M.T.; Lernmark, J.A.; Wilson, D.L. & LeBoeuf, R.C. (1995). Hyper- and hypo-responsiveness to dietary fat and cholesterol among inbred mice: searching for level and variability genes. *J. Lipid Res.,* Vol. 36, pp.1522-1532

Kirschner, L.S.; Kusewitt, D.F.; Matyakhina, L.; Towns, W.H. II; Carney, J.A.; Westphal, H. & Stratakis, C.A. (2005). A mouse model for the Carney complex tumor syndrome develops neoplasia in cyclic AMP-responsive tissues. *Cancer Res.,* Vol. 65, pp.4506-4514

Kirschner, L.S.; Yin, Z.; Jones, G.N. & Mahoney, E. (2009). Mouse models of altered protein kinase A signaling. *Endocrine-Related Cancer,* Vol 16, pp. 773-793

Koo, S.-H. & Montminy, M. (2006). Fatty acids and insulin resistance: A perfect storm. *Mol. Cell.,* Vol. 21, pp.449-450

Laviada, I.D.; Galve-Roperh, I.; Malpartida, J.M. & Haro, A. (1997). cAMP signalling mechanisms with aging in the *Ceratitis capitata* brain. *Mechanisms of Aging and Development,* Vol 97, pp. 45-53

LeBoeuf, R.C.; Tsao, W.; Kirk E. & Childs, M.T. (1993). Cholesterol feeding induced cholesterol-rich VLDL in atherosclerosis-susceptible mice regardless of dietary fat content. *Nutrition Res.,* Vol. 13, pp.549-561

Lin, S.-J.; Defossez, P.A. & Guarente, L. (2000). Requirement of NAD and SIR2 for lifespan extension by calorie restriction in *Saccharomyces cerevisiae. Science,* Vol. 289, pp.2126-2128

Lipskaia, L.; Defer, N.; Esposito, G.; Hajar, I.; Garel, M.C.; Rockman, H.A. & Hanoune, J. (2000). Enhanced cardiac function in transgenic mice expressing a Ca^{2+}-stimulated adenylyl cyclase. *Cir. Res.,* Vol. 86, pp.795-801

Lohmann, S.M.; DeCamilli, P., Einig, I. & Walter, U. (1984). High-affinity binding of the regulatory subunit (RII) of cAMP-dependent protein kinase to microtubule-associated and other cellular proteins. *PNAS,* Vol. 81, pp. 6723-6727

Lohse, M.J. & Engelhardt, S. (2001). Protein kinase A transgenes: the many faces of cAMP. *Circ. Res.* Vol. 89, pp. 938-940

Longo, V.D. (2003). The Ras and Sch9 pathways regulate stress resistance and longevity. *Exp. Gerontol.,* Vol. 38, pp.807-811

Manne, J.; Argeson, A.C. & Siracusa, L.D. (1995). Mechanisms for the pleiotropic effects of the agouti gene. *PNAS,* Vol. 92, pp.4721-4724

McConnachie, G.; Langeberg, L.K. & Scott, J.D. (2006). AKAP signaling complexes: getting to the heart of the matter. Trends Mol. Med., Vol. 12, pp. 317-323

McKnight, G.S.; Cummings, D.E.; Motamed, K.; Brandon, E.P.; Wailes, L.A.; Le, K. & Idzerda, R.L. (1998). Cyclic AMP, PKA , and the physiological regulation of adiposity. *Recent Prog. Hormone Res.*, Vol. 53, pp.139-161

Minamisawa, S.; Hoshijima, M.; Chu, G.; Ward, C.A.; Frank, K.; Gu, Y.; Martone, M.E.; Wang, Y.; Ross, J. Jr.; Kranias E.G.; Giles, W.R., & Chien, K.R. (1999). Chronic phospholamban-sarcoplasmic reticulum calcium ATPase interaction is the critical calcium cycling defect in dilated cardiomyopathy. *Cell*, Vol. 99, pp.313-322

Mistry, A.M.; Swick, A.G.; Romsos, D.R. (1997). Leptin rapidly lowers food intake and elevates metabolic rates in lean and ob/ob mice. *J. Nutr.*, Vol. 127, pp.2065-2072

Mitchel, J.S., & Keesey, R.E. (1977). Defense of a lowered weight maintenance level by lateral hypothalamically lesioned rats: evidence from a restriction-refeeding regimen. *Physiol. Behav.*, Vol. 18, pp.1121-1125

Montovani, G.; Bondioni, S.; Alberti, L.; Gilardini, L.; Invitti, C.; Corbetta, S.; Zappa, M.A.; Ferrero, S.; Lania, A.G.; Bosari, S.; Beck-Peccoz, P. & Spada, A. (2009). Decreased R2B expression and activity in adipocytes from obese subjects. *Diabetes*, Vol. 58, pp. 620-626

Morton, G.J.; Cummings, D.E.; Baskin, D.G.; Barsh, G.S. & Schwartz, M.W. (2006). Central nervous system control of food intake and body weight. *Nature*, Vol. 443, pp. 289-295

Newhall, K.J.; Cummings, D.E.; Nolan, M.A. & McKnight, G.S. (2005). Deletion of the RIIβ-subunit of protein kinase A decreases body weight and increases energy expenditure in the obese, leptin-deficient ob/ob mouse. *Mol. Endocrinol.*, Vol. 19, pp. 982-991

Neuberger, G.; Schneider, G. & Eisenhaber, F. (2007). pkaPS: prediction of protein kinase A phosphorylation sites with the simplified kinase-substrate binding model. *Biol. Dir.*, Vol 2, pp. 1

Niswender, C.M.; Ishihara, R.W.; Judge, L.M.; Zhang, C.; Shokat, K.M. & McKnight, G.S. (1975). Protein engineering of protein kinase A catalytic subunits results in the acquisition of novel inhibitor sensitivity. *J. Biol. Chem.*, Vol. 277, pp. 28916-28922

Nolan, M.A.; Sikorski, M.A. & McKnight, G.S. (2004). The role of uncoupling protein 1 in the metabolism and adiposity of RIIβ-protein kinase A-deficient mice. *Mol. Endocrinol.*, Vol., 18, pp. 2302-2311

Okumura, S.; Takagi, G.; Kawabe, J.; Yang, G.; Lee, M.C.; HOng, C.; Liu, J.; Vatner, D.E.; Sadoshima, J.; Vatner, S.F. & Ishikawa, Y. (2003a). Disruption of type 5 adenylyl cyclase gene preserves cardiac function against pressure overload. *PNAS*, Vol. 100, pp. 9986-9990

Okumura, S., Kawabe, J.; Yatani, A.; Takagi, G.; Lee, M.C.; Hong, C.; Liu, J.; Takagi, I.; Sadoshima, J.; Vatner, D.E.; Vantner, S.F.; Ishikawa, Y. (2003). Type 5 adenylyl cyclase disruption alters not only sympathetic but also parasympathetic and calcium-mediated cardiac regulation. *Circ. Res.*, Vol. 93, pp. 364-374

Passier, P.; Zeng, H.; Frey, N.; Naya, F.J.; Nicol, R.L.; McKinsey, T.A.; Overbeek, P.; Richardson, J.A.; Grant, S.R. & Olson, E.N. (2000). CaM kinase signaling induces cardiac hypertrophy and activates the MEF2 transcription factor in vivo. *J. Clin. Invest.*, Vol. 105, pp.1395-1406

Pelleymounter, M.A.; Cullen, M.J.; Baker M.B.; Hecht, R.; Winters, D.; Boone, T. & Collins, F. (1995). Effects of the obese gene product on body weight regulation in ob/ob mice. *Science*, Vol. 269, pp.540-543

Planas, J.V.; Cummings, D.E.; Idzerda, R.L. & McKnight, G.S. (1999). Mutation of the RIIβ subunit of protein kinase A differentially affects lipolysis but not gene induction in white adipose tissue. *J. Biol. Chem.* Vol. 274, pp.36281-36287

Qi, M.; Zhuo, M., Skalhegg, B.S.; Brandon, E.P.; Kandel, E.R.; McKnight, G.S. & Idzerda, R.L. (1996). Impaired hippocampal plasticity in mice lacking the Cβ1 catalytic subunit of cAMP-dependent protein kinase. *PNAS*, Vol. 93, pp. 1571-1576

Reichling, S.; Patel, H.V.; Freeman, K.B.; Kates, A.L.; Himms-Hagen, J. (1988). Attenuated cold-induced increase in mRNA for uncoupling protein in brown adipose tissue of obese (ob/ob) mice. *Biochem. Cell. Biol.*, Vol. 66, pp. 193-198

Rothwell, N.J. & Stock, M.J. (1979). A role for brown adipose tissue in diet-induced thermogenesis. *Nature*, Vol. 281, pp.31-35

Rubin, C.S. (1994). A kinase achor proteins and the intracellular targeting of signals carried by cyclic AMP. *Biochim. Biophys. Acta*, Vol. 1224, pp. 467-479

Rockman, H.A.; Koch, W.J. & Lefkowitz, R.J. (2002). Seven-transmembrane-spanning receptors and heart function. *Nature* Vol. 415, pp. 206-212

Schreyer, S.A.; Cummings, D.E.; McKnight, G.S. & LeBoeuf, R.C. (2001). Mutation of the RIIβ subunit of protein kinase A prevents diet-induced insulin resistance and dyslipidemia in mice. *Diabetes*, Vol. 50, pp.2555-2562

Sevetson, B.R.; Kong, X. & Lawrence, J.C. Jr. (1993). Increasing cAMP attenuates activation of mitogen activated protein kinase. *PNAS*, Vol. 90, pp.10305-10309

Shapiro, L.M. & Sugden, P.H. (1996). Left ventricular hypertrophy, In: *Diseases of the Heart*. 2 edition. Edited by: Julian, D.G.; Damm, A.J.; Fox, K.M.; Hall, R.T.C.; Poole-Wilson, P.A. London: Saunders

Skalhegg, B.S.; Huang, Y., Su, T., Idzerda, R.L., McKnight, G.S. & Burton, K.A. (2002). Mutation of the Cα subunit of PKA leads to growth retardation and sperm dysfunction. *Mol. Endocrinol.* Vol. 16, pp. 630-639

Souza, S.C.; Christoffolete, M.A.; Ribeiro, M.O.; Miyoshi, H.; Strissel, K.J.; Stancheva, Z.S.; Rogers, N.H.; D'Eon, T.M.; Perfield, J.W. 2nd; Imachi, H.; Obin, M.S.; Bianco, A.C. & Greenberg, A.S. (2007). Perilipin regulates the thermogenic actions of norepinephrine in brown adipose tissue. J. Lipid Res. Vol. 6, pp.1273-1279

Srivastava, R.A.; Jiao, S.; Tang, J.J.; Pfleger, B.A.; Kitchens, R.T. & Schonfeld, G. (1991). In vivo regulation of low-density lipoprotein receptor and apolipoprotein B gene expressions by dietary fat and cholesterol in inbred strains of mice. *Biochim. Biophys. Acta*, Vol. 1086, pp.29-43

Steffens, A.B. (1975). Influence of reversible obesity on eating behaviour, blood glucose, and insulin in the rat. *Am. J. Physiol.*, Vol. 288, pp.1738-1744

Stralfors, P.; Bjorgell, P. & Belfrage, P. (1984). Hormonal regulation of hormone-sensitive lipase in intact adipocytes: identification of phosphorylated sites and effects on the phosphorylation by lipolytic hormones and insulin. *PNAS*, Vol. 81, pp. 3317-3321

Surwit, R.S.; Kuhn, C.M.; Cochrane, C.; McCubbin, J.A. & Feinglos, M.N. (1988). Diet induced type II diabetes in C57BL/6J mice. *Diabetes,* Vol. 37, pp.1163-1170

Surwit, R.S.; Seldin, M.F.; Kuhn, C.M.; Cochrane, C. & Feinglos, M.N. (1991). Control of expression of insulin resistance and hyperglycemia by different genetic factors in diabetic C57BL/6J mice. *Diabetes,* Vol. 40, pp. 82-87

Weigle, D.S.; Bukowski, T.R.; Foster, D.C.; Holderman, S.; Kramer, J.M.; Lasser, G.; Lofton-Day, C.E.; Prunkard, D.E.; Raymond, C. & Kuijper, J.L. (1995). Recombinant ob protein reduces feeding and body weight in the ob/ob mouse. *J. Clin. Invest.*, Vol. 96, pp.2065-2070

Uhler, M.D.; Carmichael, D.F.; Lee, D.C.; Chrivia, J.C.; Krebs, E.G. & McKnight, G.S. (1986). Isolation of cDNA clones coding for the catalytic subunit of mouse cAMP-dependent protein kinase. *PNAS,* Vol. 83, pp.1300-1304

Yamazaki, D.; Horiuchi, J.; Nakagami, Y.; Nagano, S.; Tamura, T. & Saitoe, M. (2007). The *Drosophila DCO* mutation supresses age-related memory impairment without affecting lifespan. *Nature Neurosci.,* Vol. 10, pp. 478-484

Yan, L.; Vatner, D.E.; O'Connor, J.P.; Ivessa, A.; Ge, H.; Chen, W.; Hirotani, S.; Ishikawa, Y.; Sadoshima, J. & Vatner, S.F. (2007). Type 5 adenylyl cyclase disruption increases longevity and protects against stress. *Cell,* Vol. 130, pp.247-258

Zakhary, D.R.; Moravec, C.S.; Stewart, R.W. & Bond, M. (1999). Protein Kinase A (PKA)-dependent Troponin-I phosphorylation and PKA regulatory subunits are decreased in human dilated cardiomyopathy. *Circ.,* Vol. 99, pp. 505-510

Zho, Y.; Yamazaki, T.; Nakagawa, K; Yamada, H.; Iriguchi, N.; Toko, H.; Takano, H.; Akazawa, H., Nagai, R., Komuro, I. (2002). Continuous blockade of L-type Ca^{2+} channels suppresses activation of calcineurin and development of cardiac hypertrophy in spontaneously hypersensitive rats. *Hypertens. Res.* Vol. 25, pp. 117-124

18

Targeting AMPK for Therapeutic Intervention in Type 2 Diabetes

Mohamed Kodiha and Ursula Stochaj
McGill University
Canada

1. Introduction

This chapter begins with general information on the role of 5'-AMP activated kinase (AMPK) in human physiology and the molecular mechanisms that control this kinase. We discuss the functions of AMPK in different tissues and their relationship to type 2 diabetes. AMPK substrates in different subcellular organelles and compartments are described, and we speculate how the localized action of AMPK could help to control type 2 diabetes. Our review concludes with future directions that are based on the compartment-specific action of AMPK to develop new therapeutic strategies for patients with type 2 diabetes.

1.1 AMPK activity is critical to cell physiology in different tissues and organs

AMPK functions as a ser/thr kinase which provides an evolutionary conserved cellular energy sensor. This kinase is a focal point for metabolic control in all eukaryotes, where it regulates many aspects of physiology (Hardie, 2008a; Kim et al., 2009a; Li & McCullough, 2010; Lopaschuk, 2008; Ronnett et al., 2009; Steinberg & Kemp, 2009; Zhang, et al., 2009). It is well-established that AMPK and its yeast ortholog Snf1 control a large number of diverse processes; they include the response to nutrient limitation or other environmental changes, transcription, transport across the nuclear envelope, cell growth, cell cycle progression, mitosis, cell polarity, development, auto- and mitophagy (Amato et al., 2011; Bungard et al., 2010; Egan et al., 2010; Lee et al., 2007; Li & McCullough, 2010; Mirouse et al., 2007; Nagata & Hirata, 2009; Narbonne & Roy, 2009; Quan et al., 2007; Steinberg & Kemp, 2009; Viollet et al., 2009a; Wang et al., 2010; Witczak et al., 2008). As a result of these contributions, AMPK is vital to the function of several organs and tissues in metazoans (Fig. 1).

Owing to its pivotal role in the control of glucose homeostasis, carbohydrate, lipid and protein metabolism AMPK is a key player in many human diseases and disorders (Fogarty & Hardie, 2010; Lage et al., 2008; Towler & Hardie, 2007; Viollet et al., 2009b). In particular, the low activation state of AMPK could contribute to the increase in type 2 diabetes and obesity (Hardie et al., 2006). Moreover, as essential regulator of glucose homeostasis and lipid metabolism, AMPK has become an important therapeutic target in type 2 diabetes and obesity. This is exemplified by metformin and thiazolidinedione derivatives (TZDs); these drugs are used for therapeutic intervention in type 2 diabetes and lead to the activation of AMPK.

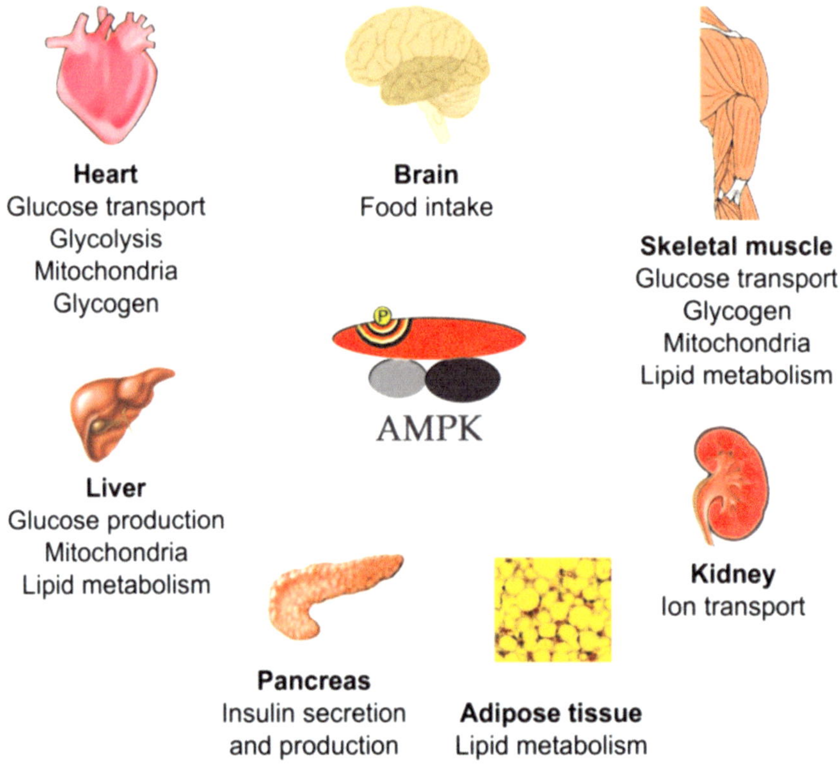

Fig. 1. The role of AMPK in different organs and tissues. AMPK controls the physiology of multiple organs which are critical to type 2 diabetes, obesity and other metabolic diseases. As such, AMPK regulates both anabolic and catabolic pathways as well as the function and biogenesis of organelles. See text for details.

2. Organization and activation of AMPK

AMPK senses a drop in cellular energy as it is induced by a reduction in glucose availability or other metabolic stresses. The overall consequence of AMPK activation is a change in metabolism; thus, when the AMP/ATP ratio increases AMPK becomes activated in order to rescue the energy balance. As a result of AMPK activation, the cellular metabolism switches from anabolic to catabolic processes. This metabolic shift is accomplished by the AMPK-dependent phosphorylation of multiple targets which are located in different cellular organelles and compartments (see below).

The heterotrimeric enzyme AMPK (Fig. 2; αβγ) contains one catalytic α subunit that is encoded by two genes (α1 and α2). The regulatory β and γ subunits are encoded by two and three genes, respectively (Hardie et al., 2006). The two β subunits (β1, β2) can be myristoylated and phosphorylated, and these modifications may impact the activation and intracellular localization of AMPK (Oakhill et al., 2010; Warden et al., 2001; see below). The γ subunits (γ1, γ2, γ3) bind AMP and ATP in a mutually exclusive fashion, this AMP binding is important to the activation of the enzyme. The subunit composition of AMPK heterotrimers varies in different tissues and can affect the activation of the kinase (Canto & Auwerx, 2010; Cheung et al., 2000; Steinberg & Kemp, 2009; Viollet et al., 2010).

2.1 Control of AMPK activity by phosphorylation and changes in AMPK concentration

The importance of AMPK as a key regulator in cellular metabolism requires a tight control of the enzyme. The rapid regulation of AMPK activity is based on at least three mechanisms that contribute to AMPK activation (Oakhill et al., 2010; Sanders et al., 2007; Shackelford & Shaw, 2009; Steinberg & Kemp, 2009). (a) The most important step for AMPK activation is the phosphorylation of Thr172 of the α subunit which can be modified by the upstream kinases LKB1, CaMKKβ and TAK1 (Fig. 2). Thr172 is phosphorylated when the energy state of the cell is low, i.e. when the AMP/ATP ratio rises. Under these conditions, AMP binding to the regulatory γ subunit promotes the subsequent Thr172 phosphorylation. LKB1 is the major upstream kinase for this event in tissues like skeletal muscle. The effect of AMP binding depends on the type of γ subunit (Cheung et al., 2000). Specifically, AMP-binding to γ2 subunits leads to the largest increase in AMPK activity. By contrast, a relative small change is observed for the γ3 subunit which is mostly synthesized in glycolytic skeletal muscle. Recent data suggest that the β subunits also play a crucial role in AMPK activation. It was proposed that β subunit myristoylation provides a switch that is a prerequisite for Thr172 phosphorylation (Oakhill et al., 2010). (b) Aside from changes in the AMP/ATP ratio, a rise in intracellular Ca^{2+} concentrations triggers Thr172 phosphorylation. This modification is mediated by CaMKKβ and particularly important in tissues where LKB1 is not the predominant kinase for Thr172. At present, the role of TAK1 in AMPK activation is not fully understood. (c) AMPK activation can be prolonged by preventing the dephosphorylation of Thr172, a process catalyzed by phosphatases PP2A and PP2C (Kim et al., 2009a; Nagata & Hirata, 2010).

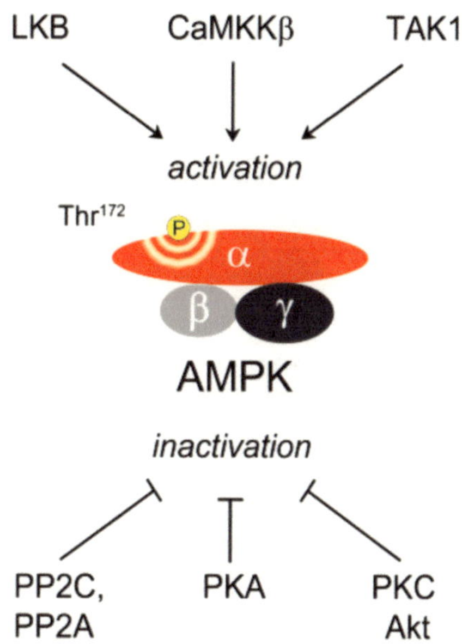

Fig. 2. Organization of AMPK and regulation of kinase activity by phosphorylation. AMPK is a heterotrimeric enzyme that is activated by phosphorylation on Thr172 of the α subunit. Several upstream kinases can modify Thr172; they include LKB, CaMKKβ and TAK1. The activity of AMPK can be reduced by different mechanisms. For example, PP2A and PP2C mediate the dephosphorylation of phospho-Thr172. In addition, PKC and Akt phosphorylate Ser485/491 of the α chain which decreases AMPK activity. Furthermore, PKA-dependent modification of Ser173 diminishes AMPK activity.

Aside from the dephosphorylation of phospho-Thr172, a negative regulation of AMPK involves the phosphorylation of Ser485/491 by PKC and possibly Akt, whereas the decline in activity by Ser173 phosphorylation was ascribed to PKA (Djouder et al., 2010). Such modification on Ser173 may help to fine tune lipid metabolism in adipose tissue.

The tissue-specific regulation of AMPK activity is likely achieved by the combined effects of upstream activating kinases, inactivating phosphatases as well as the synthesis and degradation of AMPK subunits. For example, LKB1 is particularly important to activate AMPK in skeletal muscle, whereas CaMKKβ is crucial in the brain (Ronnett et al., 2009). On the other hand, TNFα alters AMPK activation by modulating the synthesis of PP2C (Lu et al., 2010; Steinberg et al., 2006). Aside from the rapid control of AMPK activation by phosphorylation, changes in the expression of subunit genes or the turnover of AMPK subunits can help to fine tune AMPK activity in some tissues (Barry et al., 2010; Fukuyama et al., 2007; Hallows et al., 2006; Qi et al., 2008; Niesler et al., 2007; Steinberg et al., 2003).

2.2 Pharmacological compounds and other factors that alter AMPK activity

Previous work established the essential role of AMPK in the regulation of carbohydrate, protein and lipid metabolism; this made AMPK a key target for the treatment of type 2 diabetes, obesity and metabolic syndrome (Gruzman, Babai & Sasson, 2009; Hardie, 2008b; Steinberg & Kemp, 2009; Viollet et al., 2010; Viollet et al., 2009b). Indeed, in a clinical setting AMPK activity is altered with the anti-diabetic drug metformin and other biguanides. The drug-induced activation of AMPK has important consequences for the patient; among these is the improvement of insulin resistance.

Pharmacological drugs have also been critical to define how AMPK mediates metabolic control (see Table 1). These compounds employ a variety of molecular mechanisms that culminate in AMPK activation (Gruzman et al., 2009; Hawley et al., 2010; Mantovani & Roy, 2011). For example, the kinase can be activated by a rise in the AMP/ATP ratio, generation of an AMP mimetic or increase in intracellular Ca^{2+} concentrations (Hawley et al., 2010). Metformin impacts several biological processes that ultimately activate AMPK. These include changes in the respiratory chain, increased synthesis of the protein deacetylase SIRT1 (which activates LKB1) and activation of TAK1 (Caton et al., 2010; Hawley et al., 2002; Hawley et al., 2010; Xie et al., 2006). Phenphormin promotes the LKB1-dependent activation of AMPK by inhibiting mitochondrial complex I (Hawley et al., 2010). Resveratrol prevents the acetylation and concomitant inactivation of the upstream kinase LKB1, this compound also inhibits mitochondrial ATP synthase and may increase the concentration of adiponectin (Hawley et al., 2010; Wang et al., 2011). AICAR generates the AMP mimetic 5-amino-4-imidazolecarboxamide ribotide (ZMP) and causes a drop in cellular ATP and ADP, which leads to AMPK activation (Hawley et al., 2010). Aside from drugs that activate AMPK, compound C serves as an ATP-competitive inhibitor of AMPK that has been used widely. All of the compounds discussed here are established pharmacological tools that alter AMPK activation or enzymatic activity; they have been useful for the analysis of AMPK *in vitro*, in growing cells and in whole animals. The following table summarizes how AMPK activity can be affected *in vitro*, growing cells, organs or whole organisms.

Compounds, physiological processes and stress	Mode of action and effect on AMPK
(A) Drugs and other compounds	
AICAR (5-aminoimidazole-4-carboxamide-1-b-D-ribo-furanoside)	Generation of ZMP, which functions as an analog of AMP; activation
Metformin (Biguanide)	Reduces mitochondrial ATP production; activation
Phenformin	Inhibition of respiratory chain, activation
Resveratrol	Change in ATP synthase activity; prevents acetylation of LKB1 via modulation of SIRT1; upregulation of adiponectin synthesis and multimerization; activation
Thiazolidinedione derivatives (TZDs, troglitazone; rosiglitazone, pioglitazone)	Stimulate the expression and secretion of adiponectin; increase in AMP concentration; activation of PPARγ; AMPK activation
Antimycin A	Inhibition of respiratory chain; activation
Sodium azide	Inhibition of respiratory chain; activation
NO	Inhibition of respiratory chain; activation
Oligomycin	Inhibition of ATP synthase; activation
Dinitrophenol	Uncoupler of electron transfer/ATP synthesis; activation
2-Deoxyglucose	Inhibition of glycolysis; activation
Arsenite	Inhibition of TCA cycle; activation
β-guanadinopropionic acid	Creatine analog; increases AMP/ATP ratio; activation
A23187	Activation by increase in cytosolic calcium ions
A769662	Direct AMPK activator
Compound C (dorsomorphin)	Reversible, ATP-competitive inhibitor
(B) Hormones, cytokines, physiological processes and environmental stressors	
Insulin	Inhibition of AMPK activation; mediated by Akt kinase
Ghrelin	Tissue-specific effects; activation in heart and hypothalamus; reduced activity in liver and adipose tissue
Adiponectin	Activation by increase in AMP concentration
Resistin	Tissue-specific effects; reduction of AMPK activity in skeletal muscle
Leptin	Tissue-specific effects; activates α2 heterotrimers; activation in muscle and fat tissue; reduces activity in hypothalamus
TNFα	Acute and chronic effects; acute: activation; chronic: reduction in activity; increase in PP2C

Compounds, physiological processes and stress	Mode of action and effect on AMPK
IL-6	Increase in AMP/ATP ratio; activation (note that IL-6 can have different effects on insulin sensitivity)
CNTF (Ciliary neurotrophic factor)	Tissue-specific effects; activation in muscle; activity reduced in hypothalamus
UCP1, UCP3	Uncoupling proteins in mitochondria, change in energy status; activation
Reduction in glucose availability	Change in energy status; activation
Rise in Ca^{2+} concentration, osmotic stress	CaMKKβ activation
Exercise	Skeletal muscle contraction; activation
Heat shock, oxidative stress	Environmental stressors; transient activation
Ischemia/hypoxia, reactive oxygen species	Metabolism/oxidative stress; activation

Table 1. Modulators of AMPK activity.

The data in Table 1 are compiled from several publications that describe the molecular mechanisms and tissue-specific effects on AMPK activity in detail (Caton et al., 2010; Dzamko & Steinberg, 2009; Hawley et al., 2010; Maeda et al., 2001; Nagata & Hirata, 2010; Steinberg et al., 2009; Viollet et al., 2010). It should be noted that although in most cases a correlation between treatment and changes in AMPK activity has been demonstrated, the molecular mechanisms are not always fully understood. For example, hormone or cytokine-dependent changes in AMP/ATP ratios may be secondary to other signaling events, such as changes in cAMP concentrations. For some of the treatments, it has yet to be established whether AMPK is *essential* for the downstream physiological effect. More recent experiments with knockout cells and animal models will help to fill these gaps (Viollet et al., 2009a).

3. AMPK functions in different tissues and organs

Although AMPK is present in different tissues and organs, the subunit composition varies, and changes in cell physiology can also alter the profile of expressed subunits (Mahlapuu et al., 2004; Pulinilkunnil et al., 2011; Putman et al., 2007; Quentin et al., 2011; Stapleton et al., 1996; Turnley et al., 1999). Of particular importance at the cellular, organ and organismal level is the ability of AMPK to switch from anabolic to catabolic processes when energy supplies are low. AMPK regulates metabolism and other aspects of cell physiology both under normal and disease conditions; studies with different cells or tissues emphasize the significance of AMPK for cellular metabolism and the response to various forms of stress. Thus, AMPK controls several metabolic pathways that are directly relevant to diabetes and other metabolic diseases or syndromes (Steinberg & Kemp, 2009; Viollet et al., 2010; Zhang et al., 2009). However, AMPK not only provides a sensor for nutrient availability, the kinase is also activated by hormonal signals in peripheral tissues and the hypothalamus (Jorda et al., 2010; Ronnett et al., 2009). Notably, this signaling in the central nervous system contributes to the regulation of food uptake. Research with hepatic, skeletal muscle, adipose, pancreatic and kidney cells is particularly important to our understanding of type 2 diabetes as these cell types are crucial to the etiology or pathophysiology of the disease (Fig. 1). In general, the consequences of AMPK activation can be divided into acute and long-term effects (Mantovani & Roy, 2011; Viollet et al., 2010). Whereas the phosphorylation of key enzymes produces a fast downregulation of ATP-consuming metabolic pathways, long-term effects involve changes in the expression of target genes that control metabolism. Since several recently published excellent reviews covered these topics extensively, Table 2 only summarizes the impact of AMPK activation on tissues that are critical to type 2 diabetes.

Tissue or cell type	Physiological process	Enzyme or process affected by AMPK
Liver	activation of fatty acid oxidation, inhibition of lipogenesis	inhibition of acetyl-CoA carboxylase ACC (Acc1, Acc2)
	reduced cholesterol synthesis	HMG-CoA reductase
	stimulation of fatty acid uptake	CD36 (a fatty acid translocase) moves to the plasma membrane
	changes in lipogenesis and glycolysis due to reduced concentration of transcriptional regulators SREBP1 (sterol response element binding protein-1) and ChREBP (carbohydrate response-element binding protein)	inhibits ChREBP by phosphorylation, reduces the transcription of genes encoding SREBP1 and ChREBP
	increase in mitochondrial biogenesis	increased expression of PGC1α and other genes required for mitochondrial biogenesis
	glycogen synthesis reduced	inhibition of glycogen synthase
	inhibition of gluconeogenesis and hepatic glucose production	changes in the activity, concentration or localization of key enzymes or transcriptional regulators; (phosphoenol pyruvate carboxy kinase, HNF4; TORC2, p300)
Skeletal muscle	stimulation of glucose uptake; fusion of GLUT4 (glucose transporter) containing vesicles with plasma membrane	phosphorylation of AS160 may promote trafficking of vesicles; increased transcription of GLUT4 gene by phosphorylation of HDAC5
	increase in mitochondrial biogenesis	increased expression of PGC1α and other genes required for mitochondrial biogenesis
	increased fatty acid uptake and oxidation	inhibition of ACC
	reduction in protein synthesis	inhibition of mTOR pathway via modification of mTOR, TSC2 and eEF2 kinase
	control of glycogen metabolism	inactivation of glycogen synthase

Tissue or cell type	Physiological process	Enzyme or process affected by AMPK
Adipose tissue	increase in fatty acid oxidation	inactivation of ACC
	inhibition of lipolysis	phosphorylation of HSL, reduced association of HSL with lipid droplets
Pancreas	inhibition of glucose-induced insulin secretion in β cells	reduced trafficking of vesicles containing insulin
	inhibition of transcription of the preproinsulin gene in β cells; stimulation of glucagon secretion in α cells	molecular mechanisms not fully understood
Heart	stimulation of glucose uptake by translocation of GLUT4 to the plasma membrane	fusion of GLUT4 containing vesicles with the plasma membrane
	stimulation of glycolysis	activation of 6-phosphofructo-2-kinase → enhances production of fructose 2,6-bisphosphate → stimulates 6-phosphofructo-1-kinase
	increase in fatty acid oxidation	inactivation of ACC
	control of glycogen metabolism	contributions of AMPK activity not completely understood at the molecular level
Kidney	ameliorates changes linked to diabetic nephropathy	inhibition of mTOR, inhibition of CFTR and other ion channels
Brain	food intake; multiple pathways affected in the hypothalamus; adiponectin, leptin, insulin and ghrelin control AMPK	control of neuropeptide synthesis

Table 2. AMPK-dependent modulation of cell physiology.
Some of the tissue-specific reactions regulated by AMPK and relevant to type 2 diabetes are listed. A comprehensive description of these processes can be found in several recent reviews (Hardie, 2008a; Ix & Sharma, 2010; Lieberthal & Levine, 2009; Steinberg & Kemp, 2009; Viollet et al., 2009a; Viollet et al., 2010) and original publications (da Silva Xavier et al., 2003; Leclerc et al., 2011; Takiar et al., 2011; van Oort et al., 2009).

4. AMPK modulates targets in different subcellular organelles and compartments

4.1 Subcellular distribution of AMPK substrates

The combination and integration of different subcellular events regulated by AMPK enables cells, tissues and organs to coordinate different metabolic pathways in order to achieve and maintain the proper energy balance of the whole organism. Fig. 3 depicts established AMPK substrates according to their presence in different subcellular compartments. Table 3 expands this information and specifies how the AMPK-dependent phosphorylation of individual substrates alters their functions.

It is obvious from Fig. 3 that AMPK phosphorylates a large number of proteins that are associated with distinct organelles or subcellular compartments. Cytoplasmic and mitochondrial substrates of the kinase include enzymes that are involved in fat, protein, glucose and glycogen metabolism. Kinase targets in the plasma membrane consist of ion channels, carriers and receptors, whereas other substrates are linked to the function or trafficking of intracellular membranes. This includes the transport of vesicles containing the glucose transporter GLUT4, because GLUT4 translocation to the plasma membrane is a pre-requisite for efficient glucose uptake in skeletal muscle and other tissues. AS160 and TBC1D1 likely play a role in these processes (Table 3). In the nucleus, the AMPK-mediated modification of transcription factors, transcriptional regulators and a subunit of RNA-polymerase I control the expression of genes that are implicated in specific anabolic and catabolic reactions. The phosphorylation of several of these targets is also critical to the biogenesis of mitochondria and the assembly of ribosomes.

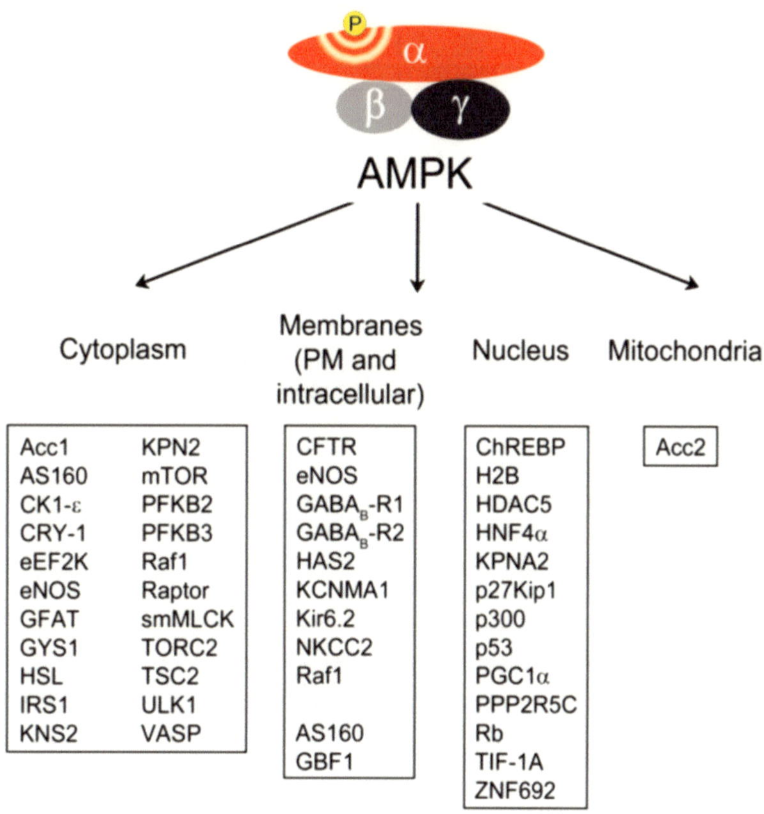

Fig. 3. AMPK affects functions in various cellular compartments and organelles. Examples are shown for the proteins that AMPK modifies in distinct sub-cellular locations. Some of the substrates are present in multiple compartments. PM, plasma membrane. See text and Table 3 for details.

Given the diverse types of AMPK substrates and their presence in different cellular locations, it is helpful to recapitulate their functions (Table 3). This knowledge is a prerequisite to understand how the dynamic association and action of AMPK in different compartments will impact downstream events.
Substrates that have been established for AMPK heterotrimers that contain the α1 or α2 subunit are shown. For different AMPK substrates the function, effect of AMPK-dependent phosphorylation and the major subcellular localization are depicted. For some substrates, there are cell-type specific differences, and the effect of AMPK-dependent phosphorylation may not be fully understood or controversial. The list of AMPK substrates was compiled from PhosphoSitePlus (phosphosite.org).

Substrates for AMPKα1	**Function**	**Effect of phosphorylation**	**Primary intracellular localization**	**References**
Acc1; Subunit of acetyl-CoA carboxylase, ACC	Carboxylates acetyl-CoA, thereby generating malonyl-CoA; this step is rate-limiting for FA biosynthesis.	inhibition	cytoplasm	Sun et al., 2006
Acc2; Subunit of acetyl-CoA carboxylase, ACC	Carboxylates acetyl-CoA, thereby generating malonyl-CoA; this step is rate-limiting for FA biosynthesis.	inhibition	mitochondria (outer mitochondrial membrane)	Reihill et al., 2007
AMPKα1	Catalytic subunit of AMPK	potential autoregulation	cytoplasm, nucleus	Stein et al., 2000
AMPKβ1	Regulatory subunit of AMPK	enzymatic activity, localization	cytoplasm, nucleus	Warden et al., 2001
CFTR	Cystic fibrosis transmembrane conductance regulator, chloride channel	inhibits PKA-dependent stimulation of CFTR	plasma membrane, ER, cytoplasmic vesicle; early endosome	King et al., 2009; Kongsuphol et al., 2009; Takiar et al., 2011
ChREBP	Transcription factor; repressor	inactivation of DNA binding	nucleus, cytoplasm	Kawaguchi et al., 2002
CK1-ε (CK1 epsilon)	Ser/thr kinase; member of the casein kinase 1 (CK1) family; phosphorylates mPer2	increase of CK1-ε activity; control of circadian clock	cytoplasm, nucleus, cell junction, centrosome	Um et al., 2007
CRY1 (cryptochrome)	DNA photolyase, regulates circadian rhythm	phosphorylation leads to destabilization	nucleus, mitochondria, cytoplasm	Lamia et al., 2009

Substrates for AMPKα1	Function	Effect of phosphorylation	Primary intracellular localization	References
CRTC-1	CREB-regulated transcriptional coactivator	phosphorylation causes cytoplasmic retention	nucleus, cytoplasm	Mair et al., 2011
eEF2K (eEF2 kinase)	Protein kinase; eEF2K modifies and thereby inactivates eEF2	activation of kinase activity	cytoplasm	Brown et al., 2004
eNOS	Endothelial nitric oxide synthase (constitutive), EC 1.14.13.39; regulation of cytoskeletal reorganization	activation, promotes deacetylation by SIRT1	plasma membrane, Golgi	Chen et al., 2010; Sun et al., 2006
$GABA_B$-R1	$GABA_B$ receptor subunit; G-protein coupled receptor	increase in receptor function, promotes functional coupling to K^+ channels	plasma membrane, ER, dendrite, axon, postsynaptic membrane	Kuramoto et al., 2007
$GABA_B$-R2	$GABA_B$ receptor subunit; G-protein coupled receptor	increase in receptor function, promotes functional coupling to K^+ channels	plasma membrane, ER, dendrite, axon, postsynaptic membrane	Kuramoto et al., 2007
GBF1; Golgi-specific brefeldin A resistance factor	Guanine nucleotide exchanger for ARF5; mediates ARF5 activation; Golgi to ER trafficking	triggers disassembly of Golgi apparatus	Golgi membrane	Miyamoto et al., 2008
GFAT	glutamine-fructose-6-phosphate transaminase 1; EC 2.6.1.16; regulates glucoseflux to hexosamine pathway	1.4 fold increase in enzymatic activity	cytoplasm	Li et al., 2007
GYS1	Glycogen synthase; EC 2.4.1.11	inhibits enzymatic activity	cytoplasm	Skurat, et al., 2000
H2B	Histone H2B	activates stress-induced transcription	nucleus	Bungard et al., 2010

Substrates for AMPKα1	Function	Effect of phosphorylation	Primary intracellular localization	References
HDAC5	Histone deacetylase 5; EC3.5.1.98; transcriptional regulator, cell cycle progression, development	reduced binding to GLUT4 promoter → enhanced GLUT4 expression	nucleus (cytoplasm)	McGee et al., 2008
HNF4 alpha	Hepatocyte nuclear factor 4 alpha; transcription factor, control of gene expression in hepatocytes	reduced DNA-binding	nucleus	Hong et al., 2003
HSL	Hormone sensitive lipase; EC 3.1.1.79; involved in triglyceride lipolysis	inhibition; change in the association with lipid droplets	cytoplasm, lipid droplets	Garton et al. 1989; ; Watt et al., 2006
IRS1; adaptor protein	Insulin receptor substrate 1, adaptor protein	modulation of PI3 kinase signaling	cytoplasm	Jakobsen et al., 2001; Tzatsos & Tsichlis, 2007
KCNMA1 iso4; α subunit of BK_{Ca} channel	Potassium channel, activated in response to membrane depolarization, oxygen sensing in carotid body	inhibition of potassium currents	integral membrane protein, plasma membrane, axon	Ross et al., 2011
Kir6.2 (KCNJ11)	Potassium channel, voltage dependent, inward rectifying	might play a role in insulin secretion	plasma membrane	Chang et al., 2009
KNS2	Kinesin 2; kinesin light chain 1, motor protein	biological role of modification not known	cytoplasm, microtubules	McDonald et al., 2009, 2010
KPNA2, importin-α1	Adaptor for classical nuclear import	interferes with nuclear import of HuR	cytoplasm, nucleus, nuclear envelope	Wang et al., 2004
mTOR	Ser/thr kinase; EC 2.7.11.1; catalytic subunit of mTORC1 and mTORC2	links nutrient supply to translation	cytoplasm	Cheng et al., 2004
NKCC2 (SLC12A1)	Electroneutral transporter; reabsorption of Na^+ and Cl^-; controls cell volume	regulation of transporter activity	plasma membrane	Fraser et al., 2007

Substrates for AMPKα1	**Function**	**Effect of phosphorylation**	**Primary intracellular localization**	**References**
p27Kip1 (CDKN4)	Cyclin-dependent kinase inhibitor 1B, controls cell cycle progression at G1	stabilization of p27; linked to autophagy	nucleus	Liang et al., 2007
p300	Protein (histone) acetyltransferase; EC2.3.1.48; transcriptional co-activator	inhibits interaction with nuclear receptors, such as PPARγ	nucleus	Yang et al., 2001
p53	Tumor suppressor, transcription factor, cell cycle arrest, DNA repair, apoptosis	stabilization of p300-p53 interaction; controls cell cycle progression	nucleus	Dornan & Hupp, 2001
PFKFB2	6-Phosphofructo-2-kinase/ fructose-2,6-bisphosphatase 2; EC 2.7.1.105 or EC 3.1.3.46; glycolysis	activation; stimulation of glycolysis	cytoplasm	Marsin et al., 2000
PFKFB3; iPFK2	similar to PFKFB2; inducible in monocytes	activation	cytoplasm	Marsin et al., 2002
PPP1R3C (R5/PTG)	Regulatory subunit of protein phosphatase PP1; controls PP1 activity; targets PP1 to glycogen; stimulation of glycogen synthase	promotes ubiquitination and thereby degradation	glycogen granules	Vernia et al., 2009
PPP2R5C (B56 γ)	Regulatory subunit of protein phosphatase PP2A; possible role in the regulation and targeting of PP2A	increases PP2A activity	nucleus, chromosomes	Kim et al., 2009b
Raf1	Ser/thr kinase; EC 2.7.11.1; component of Ras→Raf→MEK1/2→ERK 1/2 signaling pathway		cytoplasm, plasma membrane	Sprenkle et al., 1997
Raptor	Regulation of mTORC1 (mammalian target of rapamycin complex 1); functions as scaffold	inhibition of mTORC1; cell cycle arrest	cytoplasm	Gwinn et al., 2008
Rb	Retinoblastoma protein; regulates cell cycle progression at G1; functions as transcriptional co-regulator; tumor suppressor	control of brain development	nucleus	Dasgupta & Milbrandt, 2009

Substrates for AMPKα1	Function	Effect of phosphorylation	Primary intracellular localization	References
smMLCK	Smooth muscle myosin light chain kinase; ser/thr protein kinase; EC2.7.11.18	reduces activity of smMLCK	cytoplasm	Horman et al., 2008
TBC1D1	GTPase activating protein Rab family members; regulates glucose transport	induces binding to 14-3-3 proteins	ER	Chen et al., 2008
TIF-IA	Transcription initiation factor for RNA-pol I	reduced rDNA transcription	nucleolus	Hoppe et al., 2009
TORC2 (CRTC2)	Transducer of regulated CREB protein 2; transcriptional regulator	phosphorylation causes cytoplasmic retention	nucleus, cytoplasm	Koo et al., 2005
TSC2 (tuberin)	Generates heterodimer with hamartin (TSC1); TSC1/TSC2 functions as GTPase activator of Rheb	enhances TSC2 activity → inhibition of mTOR	cytoplasm	Inoki, et al., 2003
ULK1	Ser/thr kinase; EC 2.7.11.1; binds to mTORC1 via raptor, binding controlled by nutrient supply	control of autophagy	cytoplasm	Egan et al., 2011
VASP	Vasodilator-stimulated phosphoprotein; actin regulator	impairs endothelial actin assembly	cytoplasm, cytoskeleton	Blume et al., 2007
ZNF692 (AREBP)	Transcriptional regulator, contains zinc finger	reduction in DNA binding	nucleus	Inoue & Yamauchi, 2006

Substrates for AMPKα2	Function	Effect of phosphorylation	Primary intracellular localization	References
ACC1	See above description of AMPKα1 targets		cytoplasm	
AS160 (TBC1D4; Akt substrate of 160k)	GTPase activating protein for Rab; implicated in GLUT4 exocytosis in skeletal muscle	not fully understood; may regulate glucose uptake	cytoplasm	Eguez et al., 2005; Treebak et al., 2010
HAS2	Hyaluronic acid synthase 2; EC 2.4.1.212; integral membrane protein	inhibition of enzymatic activity	plasma membrane	Vigetti et al., 2011

HDAC5	See above description of AMPKα1 targets		nucleus	
p53	See above description of AMPKα1 targets		nucleus	
PGC1α	PPAR γ coactivator-1; transcriptional co-activator; association with PPARγ; binds to CREB and nuclear respiratory factors; controls mitochondrial biogenesis	phosphorylation alters activity as transcriptional regulator	nucleus	Jager et al., 2007
PLD1	Phospholipase D1 phophatidylcholine specific; EC 3.1.4.4; linked to Ras signaling; involved in membrane trafficking	activation of enzymatic activity	Golgi, ER	Kim et al., 2010

Table 3. Substrates of AMPK heterotrimers containing the α1 or α2 subunit

4.2 Subcellular distribution and trafficking of AMPK

AMPK is associated with different organelles and subcellular compartments; however, little is known about the dynamic nature of this distribution. Analyses of other signaling pathways have demonstrated that the subcellular localization of kinases is critical for the proper response to extra- and intracellular stimuli, and it is likely that the same scenario applies to AMPK. We will therefore briefly review what is currently known about the subcellular localization and trafficking of AMPK.

AMPK is found in the nucleus and cytoplasm which reflects functions for the enzyme in both locations (Kodiha et al., 2007; Witczak et al., 2008). Although the kinase is associated with multiple compartments, α1 and α2 subunits differ in their nucleocytoplasmic distribution. Under normal growth conditions, α1 is predominantly in the cytoplasm, whereas α2 locates to both the nucleus and cytoplasm (Salt et al., 1998). It was further shown that the nuclear localization sequence (NLS) present in the α2 subunit is required for AMPK nuclear translocation (Suzuki et al., 2007), suggesting that the catalytic α subunit is essential for the proper intracellular localization of the holoenzyme. Our current model of AMPK trafficking proposes that the kinase shuttles between the nucleus and the cytoplasm. Data from our group and others support this idea, as they demonstrated that the nuclear carrier Crm1 is essential for AMPK export from the nucleus to the cytoplasm (Kazgan et al., 2010; Kodiha et al., 2007).

How the β subunit impacts the proper targeting of the holoenzyme is at present not entirely clear. The β1 subunit can be modified posttranslationally, both by phosphorylation and myristoylation, and these modifications were linked to the subcellular targeting of the β1 subunit (Suzuki et al., 2007; Warden et al., 2001). It was proposed that AMPK concentrates in the cytoplasm when the heterotrimeric enzyme contains the β1 subunit (Suzuki et al., 2007). However, this model is difficult to reconcile with the fact that both β1 and β2 subunits can be detected in the nucleus (Kodiha et al., 2007). Furthermore, recent studies suggest that the myristoylation of β1 and β2 subunit is particularly important for AMPK activation, as AMP-dependent myristoylation provides a switch that triggers Thr172 phosphorylation (Oakhill et al., 2010). Although the contribution of β subunits to nuclear and membrane targeting of the holoenzyme is not completely understood at this point, the importance of the β subunit for glycogen binding is well established (Polekhina et al., 2003).

In contrast to the α and β subunits, little is known about the trafficking of AMPK γ subunits. In *Drosophila*, the single γ subunit migrates into the nucleus of the fat body with the onset of autophagy during normal development, and a potential NLS was detected in this subunit (Lippai et al., 2008). It was speculated that this nuclear accumulation contributes to the expression of genes that are necessary for autophagy.

Several studies support the model that the intracellular distribution of AMPK in human and other cells is dynamic. This is particularly important in the context of disease, because the distribution of AMPK can be modulated by physiological and environmental stimuli. For example, the α2 subunit translocates to the cell nucleus upon exercise or environmental stress (Kodiha et al., 2007; McGee et al., 2003), indicating that the adaptation of skeletal muscle during exercise or metabolic stress is at least in part mediated by the subcellular relocation of AMPK. Examples of the relocation of AMPK α subunits in human cells exposed to oxidative stress or depleted for energy are shown in Fig. 4 (Kodiha et al., 2007).

The relocation of AMPK subunits in response to physiological changes is not restricted to the α subunits; our previous experiments demonstrated that AMPK β subunits accumulate in the nucleus as well when cells are exposed to oxidative and other forms of stress (Kodiha et al., 2007). Moreover, AMPK localization could be regulated by the circadian rhythm. Specifically, changes in the expression of AMPK subunits may depend on the circadian rhythm; this change in expression will then alter the intracellular distribution of AMPK (Lamia et al., 2009). Since these studies were carried out with mice, it has yet to be shown whether the same applies to humans.

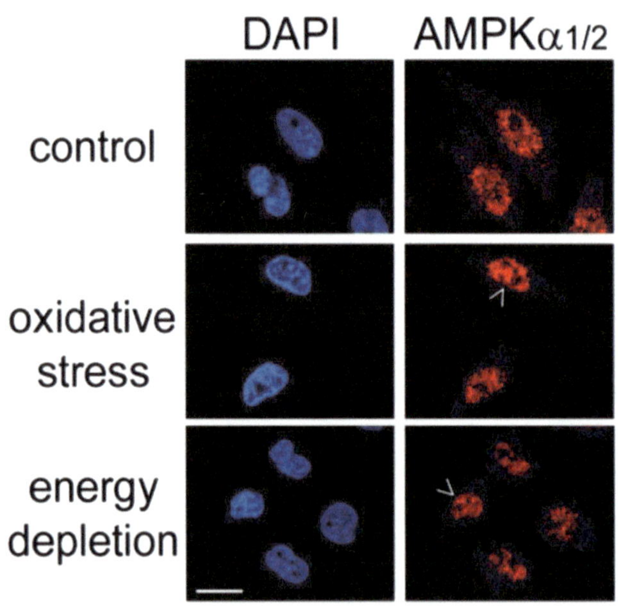

Fig. 4. AMPKα concentrates in nuclei when cells are exposed to oxidative stress or depleted for energy. HeLa cells were treated with diethyl maleate to induce oxidative stress or with a combination of sodium azide and 2-deoxyglucose for energy depletion. The distribution of AMPKα1 and α2 subunits was examined by indirect immunofluorescence; DNA was stained with DAPI (Kodiha et al., 2007). Note that the α-subunits are more concentrated in nuclei of stressed cells. Several nuclei are marked with arrowheads. Size bar is 20 μm.

Studies from several laboratories, including our group, defined the signals and mechanisms that determine the trafficking and intracellular distribution of AMPK. Our work also suggested crosstalk between other signaling cascades and the localized action of AMPK (Kodiha et al., 2007 and unpublished). Ultimately, such crosstalk will add to the complexity of downstream events that are modulated by AMPK. Taken together, previous research suggests that AMPK subunits move between different subcellular locations, and it can be expected that the compartment-specific actions of the kinase are linked to the physiological response of cells and tissues.

4.3 How does the compartment-specific action of AMPK impact cellular functions that are relevant to type 2 diabetes?

Type 2 diabetes is associated with the increased risk of a growing number of diseases and pathologies. This is exemplified by renal nephropathy, myocardial disease, stroke, Alzheimer's and Parkinson's disease (Almdal et al., 2004; Biessels et al., 2006; Burdo et al., 2009; Hallows et al., 2010; Hu et al., 2007; Maher & Schubert, 2009; Schernhammer et al., 2011). Several drugs are currently used in the clinical setting to activate AMPK in patients suffering from type 2 diabetes or obesity. However, it should be kept in mind that AMPK activation can be beneficial as well as harmful in the ischemic heart, and AMPK activation may be linked to neurodegeneration (Lopaschuk, 2008; Spasic, Callaerts & Norga, 2009; Thornton et al., 2011; Vingtdeux et al., 2011). Thus, activation of AMPK throughout the whole organism or the entire cell of a particular tissue may not always be advantageous. As an alternative approach, we put forward the concept of a compartment-specific modulation of AMPK action. Since AMPK activation can be damaging in the context of some of the complications associated with type 2 diabetes, our approach applies both to the localized activation as well as inhibition of the kinase. We believe that the confined action of AMPK will provide a better therapeutic approach in the future that could reduce the side-effects of AMPK modulators. The simplified model in Fig. 5 summarizes the possible changes of cellular functions that will be induced by targeting AMPK in different subcellular compartments.

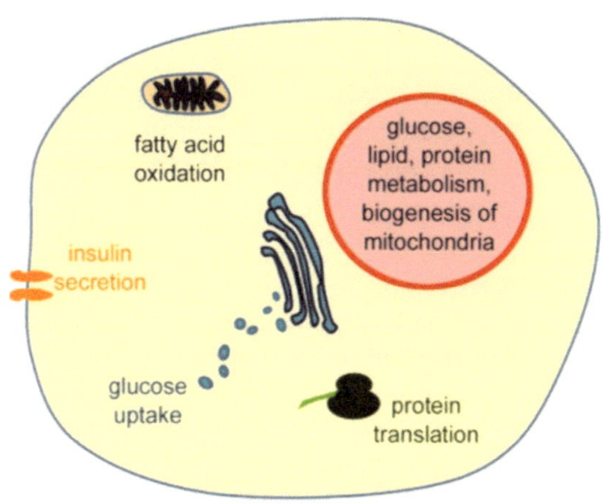

Fig. 5. Localized modulations of AMPK activity. The possible changes induced by the compartment-specific alteration of AMPK activity are depicted. Note that there are cell-type dependent differences for the processes regulated by AMPK.

In the past few years, significant progress has been made with the identification of AMPK substrates and their links to human disease. As shown in Fig. 3 and Table 3, AMPK modifies targets in different subcellular compartments or organelles. We propose that the modification of these substrates relies on (a) the amount of active AMPK and (b) the intracellular distribution of AMPK. The combination of AMPK activation and subcellular localization will then determine the level of phosphorylation of its substrates and the subsequent changes in cell physiology. Such changes will affect both the rapid response to specific stimuli as well as the long-term modification of metabolism and other processes. In the following, we focus on some of the processes that are controlled by AMPK and linked to type 2 diabetes or the complications associated with the disease.

4.3.1 AMPK targets the protein synthesis apparatus in the cytoplasm

Several of the cytoplasmic substrates of AMPK are essential to promote a fast cellular response to changes in nutrient supply. For example, AMPK phosphorylates cytoplasmic targets, such as eEF2 kinase and mTOR, which regulate protein translation. AMPK-dependent modification of these substrates results in downregulation of protein synthesis. Under some conditions, it could be desirable to preferentially modulate these processes that are associated with cytoplasmic AMPK targets. A possible example of such a scenario is the diabetic kidney (Cammisotto et al., 2008; Hallows et al., 2010; Lee et al., 2007; McMahon et al., 2009). Diabetes-induced renal hypertrophy correlates with diminished AMPK activity and, at the same time, with increased protein synthesis under high glucose conditions (Hallows et al., 2010). AICAR and metformin reduce protein synthesis triggered by high glucose (Lee et al., 2007), but these compounds also produce effects that are unrelated to AMPK activation (Mantovani & Roy, 2011). Thus, stimulating AMPK in the cytoplasm could provide a more focused approach to reduce damage in the diabetic kidney.

4.3.2 AMPK targets associated with the plasma membrane and vesicular trafficking

Several channels and transporters in the plasma membrane are phosphorylated by AMPK and control the secretion of insulin, hyperpolarization of β-cells under low glucose concentration and the response to hypoxia (Beall et al., 2010; Chang et al., 2009; Düfer et al., 2010; Evans et al., 2009; Hallows, 2005; Zheng et al., 2008). Although details of the molecular mechanisms are not always clear and in part controversial, altering the AMPK activity at the plasma membrane has the potential to modify β-cell function. The same principle could also apply to the heart and kidney, where several integral proteins of the plasma membrane are modified by AMPK.

4.3.3 AMPK substrates in the nucleus

In the nucleus, AMPK directly regulates the transcription of genes that control metabolism as well as the biogenesis of mitochondria and ribosomes. As such, AMPK modifies HNF4α, HDAC5, p300, histone H2B, the tumor suppressor p53, PGC1α, and TIF-1A (see Fig. 3 and Table 3). AMPK-dependent phosphorylation of these targets is critical to alter the transcriptional profile, which in turn is necessary to adjust metabolic activities in skeletal muscle, heart, liver and adipose tissues in response to changes in glucose availability. It is reasonable to assume that the modification of transcription factors and transcriptional regulators will rely to a large extent on AMPK in the nucleus. This model is supported by a recent study that shows AMPK to move along genes together with the transcriptional machinery (Bungard et al., 2010). Activation of AMPK in the nucleus could enhance the effects of AMPK on the transcription of several target genes. One of the possible benefits of the activation of nuclear AMPK will be the increase in mitochondrial biogenesis. In the long-term, this could help to stimulate the oxidation of fatty acids and limit the lipotoxicity that is linked to type 2 diabetes (Schrauwen & Hesselink, 2004).

4.3.4 AMPK targets associated with mitochondria

Acc2 is associated with mitochondria and important for the synthesis of malonyl-CoA, an intermediate of fatty acid biosynthesis. AMPK phosphorylates and thereby inactivates Acc, which leads to a reduction in malonyl-CoA concentration. As a consequence, *de novo* fatty acid synthesis is reduced and fatty acid oxidation is upregulated. It is conceivable that the localized Acc2 inhibition by AMPK could stimulate CPT-1 (carnitine palmitoyltransferase-1) dependent transport of fatty acids into mitochondria for subsequent degradation. This in turn could reduce the load of peroxidation products of fatty acids in the cytoplasm and the subsequent damage to mitochondria (Schrauwen & Hesselink, 2004).

5. Development of drugs that alter the compartment-specific activity of AMPK

In order to modulate AMPK activity in a fashion that is more localized as compared to the currently used drugs, a number of questions will have to be addressed. This includes the ability to regulate AMPK (a) in different organs or tissues and (b) in specific subcellular locations. Oral administration of metformin is believed to preferentially alter liver metabolism, whereas TZDs and their derivatives affect adipose tissue, skeletal muscle and probably β-cells (Gruzman et al., 2009). One possibility to enhance the tissue-specific action of AMPK will rely on the development of drugs that *directly* bind to AMPK; indeed such compounds have been described (Hawley et al., 2010). Since tissue-specific differences in AMPK subunits have been established, developing compounds that preferentially interact with individual subunits or specific subunit combinations of heterotrimers could provide a means to increase the specificity of AMPK action. For example, the γ3 subunit is predominantly synthesized in glycolytic skeletal muscle and could therefore serve as a target to alter AMPK in this tissue.

Taking into account differences in AMPK subunits could further be exploited to regulate the kinase in different subcellular locations (see section 4.2). Thus, it is believed that the α2 subunit is more concentrated in the nucleus as compared to the α1 subunit; this difference could help to activate mainly nuclear or cytoplasmic pools of the kinase. This line of reasoning could be expanded to the posttranslational modifications of the β subunit, as phosphorylation and myristoylation of the β subunits are implicated in the subcellular distribution of the kinase.

In addition to taking advantage of the differences in AMPK heterotrimers, developing AMPK modulators that accumulate in distinct subcellular compartments will be useful. This strategy could be based on the generation of combimolecules with multiple properties (Rachid et al., 2007). Combimolecules that combine DNA-binding with AMPK activation could enhance the modification of nuclear substrates and thereby alter the gene expression profile. On the other hand, such combimolecules could exploit the differences in lipid composition of intracellular membranes to control the AMPK-dependent phosphorylation of mitochondrial Acc2 or channels residing in the plasma membrane.

6. Conclusions

AMPK and its substrates are critical to the etiology and pathology of type 2 diabetes and other metabolic diseases. Several of the current therapeutic regimens for type 2 diabetes alter AMPK activity, either by affecting the cellular energy status or the concentration of AMPK modulators. More recent studies led to the identification of compounds that directly bind AMPK and change its enzyme activity. We propose that the future design of drugs that takes into account the dynamic subcellular distribution of the kinase and its substrates will help to regulate AMPK not only in different tissues and organs, but also at the subcellular level. In the long term this approach will help to fine-tune AMPK action and the downstream events that rely on the phosphorylation of its targets.

7. References

Almdal, T., Scharling, H., Jensen, J. S. & Vestergaard, H. (2004). The Independent Effect of Type 2 Diabetes Mellitus on Ischemic Heart Disease, Stroke, and Death: A Population-Based Study of 13 000 Men and Women With 20 Years of Follow-up. *Arch Intern Med* 164, 1422-1426.

Amato, S., Liu, X., Zheng, B., Cantley, L., Rakic, P. & Man, H. Y. (2011). AMP-Activated Protein Kinase Regulates Neuronal Polarization by Interfering with PI 3-Kinase Localization. *Science* 332, 247-251.

Barry, S. P., Lawrence, K. M., McCormick, J. et al. (2010). New targets of urocortin-mediated cardioprotection. *J Mol Endocrinol* 45, 69-85.

Beall, C., Piipari, K., Al-Qassab, H., Smith, M. A., Parker, N., Carling, D., Viollet, B., Withers, D. J. & Ashford, M. L. J. (2010). Loss of AMP-activated protein kinase alpha2-subunit in mouse beta-cells impairs glucose-stimulated insulin secretion and inhibits their sensitivity to hypoglycaemia. *Biochem J* 429, 323-333.

Biessels, G. J., Staekenborg, S., Brunner, E., Brayne, C. & Scheltens, P. (2006). Risk of dementia in diabetes mellitus: a systematic review. *Lancet Neurol* 5, 64-74.

Blume, C., Benz, P. M., Walter, U., Ha, J., Kemp, B. E. & Renne, T. (2007). AMP-activated Protein Kinase Impairs Endothelial Actin Cytoskeleton Assembly by Phosphorylating Vasodilator-stimulated Phosphoprotein. *J Biol Chem* 282, 4601-4612.

Browne G. J., Finn, S. G. & Proud, C. G. (2004) Stimulation of the AMP-activated Protein Kinase Leads to Activation of Eukaryotic Elongation Factor 2 Kinase and to Its Phosphorylation at a Novel Site, Serine 398. *J Biol Chem* 279, 12220-12231.

Bungard, D., Fuerth, B. J., Zeng, P. Y., Faubert, B., Maas, N. L., Viollet, B., Carling, D., Thompson, C. B., Jones, R. G. & Berger, S. L. (2010). Signaling kinase AMPK activates stress-promoted transcription via histone H2B phosphorylation. *Science* 329, 1201-1205.

Burdo, J. R., Chen, Q., Calcutt, N. A. & Schubert, D. (2009). The pathological interaction between diabetes and presymptomatic Alzheimer's disease. *Neurobiol Aging* 30, 1910-1917.

Cammisotto, P. G., Bendayan, M., Cammisotto, P. G. & Bendayan, M. (2008). Adiponectin stimulates phosphorylation of AMP-activated protein kinase alpha in renal glomeruli. *J Mol Histol* 39, 579-584.

Canto, C. & Auwerx, J. (2010). AMP-activated protein kinase and its downstream transcriptional pathways. *CMLS* 67, 3407-3423.

Caton, P. W., Nayuni, N. K., Kieswich, J., Khan, N. Q., Yaqoob, M. M. & Corder, R. (2010). Metformin suppresses hepatic gluconeogenesis through induction of SIRT1 and GCN5. *J Endocrinol* 205, 97-106.

Chang, T. J., Chen, W. P., Yang, C., Lu, P. H., Liang, Y. C., Su, M. J., Lee, S. C. & Chuang, L. M. (2009). Serine-385 phosphorylation of inwardly rectifying K^+ channel subunit (Kir6.2) by AMP-dependent protein kinase plays a key role in rosiglitazone-induced closure of the K(ATP) channel and insulin secretion in rats. *Diabetologia* 52, 1112-1121.

Chen, S., Murphy, J., Toth, R., Campbell, D. G., Morrice, N. A. & Mackintosh, C. (2008). Complementary regulation of TBC1D1 and AS160 by growth factors, insulin and AMPK activators. *Biochem J* 409, 449-459.

Chen, Z., Peng, I. C., Cui, X., Li, Y. S., Chien, S. & Shyy, J. Y. (2010). Shear stress, SIRT1, and vascular homeostasis. *Proc Natl Acad Sci USA* 107, 10268-10273.

Cheng, S. W. Y., Fryer, L. G. D., Carling, D. & Shepherd, P. R. (2004). Thr2446 Is a Novel Mammalian Target of Rapamycin (mTOR) Phosphorylation Site Regulated by Nutrient Status. *J Biol Chem* 279, 15719-15722.

Cheung, P. C., Salt, I. P., Davies, S. P., Hardie, D. G. & Carling, D. (2000). Characterization of AMP-activated protein kinase gamma-subunit isoforms and their role in AMP binding. *Biochem J* 346, 659-669.

Da Silva Xavier, G., Leclerc, I., Varadi, A., Tsuboi, T., Moule, S. K. & Rutter, G. A. (2003). Role for AMP-activated protein kinase in glucose-stimulated insulin secretion and preproinsulin gene expression. *Biochem J* 371, 761-774.

Dasgupta, B. & Milbrandt, J. (2009). AMP-Activated Protein Kinase Phosphorylates Retinoblastoma Protein to Control Mammalian Brain Development. *Developm Cell* 16, 256-270.

Djouder, N., Tuerk, R. D., Suter, M., Salvioni, P., Thali, R. F., Scholz, R., Vaahtomeri, K., Auchli, Y., Rechsteiner, H., Brunisholz, R. A., Viollet, B., Makela, T. P., Wallimann, T., Neumann, D. & Krek, W. (2010). PKA phosphorylates and inactivates AMPKα to promote efficient lipolysis. *EMBO J* 29, 469-481.

Dornan, D. & Hupp, T. R. (2001). Inhibition of p53-dependent transcription by BOX-I phospho-peptide mimetics that bind to p300. *EMBO Rep*, 139–144.

Düfer, M., Noack, K., Krippeit-Drews, P. & Drews, G. (2010). Activation of the AMP-activated protein kinase enhances glucose-stimulated insulin secretion in mouse beta-cells. *Islets* 2, 156-163.

Dzamko, N. L. & Steinberg, G. R. (2009). AMPK-dependent hormonal regulation of whole-body energy metabolism. *Acta Physiologica* 196, 115-127.

Egan, D. F., Shackelford, D. B., Mihaylova, M. M. et al. (2011). Phosphorylation of ULK1 (hATG1) by AMP-activated protein kinase connects energy sensing to mitophagy. *Science* 331, 456-461.

Eguez, L., Lee, A., Chavez, J. A., Miinea, C. P., Kane, S., Lienhard, G. E. & McGraw, T. E. (2005). Full intracellular retention of GLUT4 requires AS160 Rab GTPase activating protein. *Cell Metabolism* 2, 263-272.

Evans, A. M., Hardie, D. G., Peers, C. , et al. (2009). Ion Channel Regulation by AMPK. *Annals New York Acad Sci* 1177, 89-100.

Fogarty, S. & Hardie, D. G. (2010). Development of protein kinase activators: AMPK as a target in metabolic disorders and cancer. *Biochim Biophys Acta* 1804, 581-591.

Fraser, S. A., Gimenez, I., Cook, N., Jennings, I., Katerelos, M., Katsis, F., Levidiotis, V., Kemp, B. E. & Power, D. A. (2007). Regulation of the renal-specific Na^{+}-K^{+}-$2Cl^{-}$ co-transporter NKCC2 by AMP-activated protein kinase (AMPK). *Biochem J* 405, 85-93.

Fukuyama, Y., Ohta, K., Okoshi, R., Suehara, M., Kizaki, H. & Nakagawa, K. (2007). Hypoxia Induces Expression and Activation of AMPK in Rat Dental Pulp Cells. *J Dental Res* 86, 903-907.

Garton, A. J., Campbell, D.G., Carling, D., Hardie, D. G., Colbran, R.J. & Yeaman, S. J. (1989). Phosphorylation of bovine hormone-sensitive lipase by the AMP-activated protein kinase. *Eur J Biochem* 179, 249-254.

Gruzman, A., Babai, G. & Sasson, S. (2009). Adenosine Monophosphate-Activated Protein Kinase (AMPK) as a New Target for Antidiabetic Drugs: A Review on Metabolic, Pharmacological and Chemical Considerations. *Rev Diabetic Studies* 6, 13-36.

Gwinn, D. M., Shackelford, D. B., Egan, D. F., Mihaylova, M. M., Mery, A., Vasquez, D. S., Turk, B. E. & Shaw, R. J. (2008). AMPK Phosphorylation of Raptor Mediates a Metabolic Checkpoint. *Mol Cell* 30, 214-226.

Hallows, K. R. (2005). Emerging role of AMP-activated protein kinase in coupling membrane transport to cellular metabolism. *Current Opinion Nephrol Hypertens* 14, 464-471.

Hallows, K. R., Fitch, A. C., Richardson, C. A., Reynolds, P. R., Clancy, J. P., Dagher, P. C., Witters, L. A., Kolls, J. K. & Pilewski, J. M. (2006). Up-regulation of AMP-activated Kinase by Dysfunctional Cystic Fibrosis Transmembrane Conductance Regulator in Cystic Fibrosis Airway Epithelial Cells Mitigates Excessive Inflammation. *J Biol Chem* 281, 4231-4241.

Hallows, K. R., Mount, P. F., Pastor-Soler, N. M. & Power, D. A. (2010). Role of the energy sensor AMP-activated protein kinase in renal physiology and disease. *American Journal of Physiology-Renal Physiology* 298, F1067-F1077.

Hardie, D. G. (2008a). AMPK: a key regulator of energy balance in the single cell and the whole organism. *Int J Obesity* 32 S4, S7-12.

Hardie, D. G. (2008b). Role of AMP-activated protein kinase in the metabolic syndrome and in heart disease. *FEBS Lett* 582, 81-89.

Hardie, D. G., Hawley, S. A. & Scott, J. W. (2006). AMP-activated protein kinase - development of the energy sensor concept. *J Physiol* 574, 7-15.

Hawley, S. A., Gadalla, A. E., Olsen, G. S. & Hardie, D. G. (2002). The Antidiabetic Drug Metformin Activates the AMP-Activated Protein Kinase Cascade via an Adenine Nucleotide-Independent Mechanism. *Diabetes* 51, 2420-2425.

Hawley, S. A., Ross, F. A., Chevtzoff, C. et al. (2010). Use of cells expressing gamma subunit variants to identify diverse mechanisms of AMPK activation. *Cell Metabolism* 11, 554-565.

Hong, Y. H., Varanasi, U. S., Yang, W. & Leff, T. (2003). AMP-activated Protein Kinase Regulates HNF4α Transcriptional Activity by Inhibiting Dimer Formation and Decreasing Protein Stability. *J Biol Chem* 278, 27495-27501.

Hoppe, S., Bierhoff, H., Cado, I., Weber, A., Tiebe, M., Grummt, I. & Voit, R. (2009). AMP-activated protein kinase adapts rRNA synthesis to cellular energy supply. *Proc Natl Acad Sci USA* 106, 17781-17786.

Horman, S., Morel, N., Vertommen, D. et al. (2008). AMP-activated Protein Kinase Phosphorylates and Desensitizes Smooth Muscle Myosin Light Chain Kinase. *J Biol Chem* 283, 18505-18512.

Hu, G., Jousilahti, P., Bidel, S., Antikainen, R. & Tuomilehto, J. (2007). Type 2 Diabetes and the Risk of Parkinson's Disease. *Diabetes Care* 30, 842-847.

Inoki, K., Zhu, T. & Guan, K. L. (2003). TSC2 Mediates Cellular Energy Response to Control Cell Growth and Survival. *Cell* 115, 577-590.

Inoue, E. & Yamauchi, J. (2006). AMP-activated protein kinase regulates PEPCK gene expression by direct phosphorylation of a novel zinc finger transcription factor. *BBRC*351, 793-799.

Ix, J. H. & Sharma, K. (2010). Mechanisms Linking Obesity, Chronic Kidney Disease, and Fatty Liver Disease: The Roles of Fetuin-A, Adiponectin, and AMPK. *J Am Soc Nephrol* 21, 406-412.

Jager, S., Handschin, C., St.-Pierre, J. & Spiegelman, B. M. (2007). AMP-activated protein kinase (AMPK) action in skeletal muscle via direct phosphorylation of PGC-1alpha. *Proc Natl Acad Sci USA* 104, 12017-12022.

Jakobsen, S. N., Hardie, D. G., Morrice, N. & Tornqvist, H. E. (2001). 5'-AMP-activated Protein Kinase Phosphorylates IRS-1 on Ser-789 in Mouse C2C12 Myotubes in Response to 5-Aminoimidazole-4-carboxamide Riboside. *J Biol Chem* 276, 46912-46916.

Jordan, S. D., Konner, A. C. & Bruning, J. C. (2010). Sensing the fuels: glucose and lipid signaling in the CNS controlling energy homeostasis. *CMLS* 67, 3255-3273.

Kawaguchi, T., Osatomi, K., Yamashita, H., Kabashima, T. & Uyeda, K. (2002). Mechanism for Fatty Acid "Sparing" Effect on Glucose-induced Transcription. *J Biol Chem* 277, 3829-3835.

Kazgan, N., Williams, T., Forsberg, L. J. & Brenman, J. E. (2010). Identification of a Nuclear Export Signal in the Catalytic Subunit of AMP-activated Protein Kinase. *Mol Biol Cell* 21, 3433-3442.

Kim, A. S., Miller, E. J. & Young, L. H. (2009a). AMP-activated protein kinase: a core signalling pathway in the heart. *Acta Physiologica* 196, 37-53.

Kim, K., Baek, A., Hwang, J.-E., Choi, Y. A., Jeong, J., Lee, M.-S., Cho, D. H., Lim, J.-S., Kim, K. I. & Yang, Y. (2009b). Adiponectin-Activated AMPK Stimulates Dephosphorylation of AKT through Protein Phosphatase 2A Activation. *Cancer Res* 69, 4018-4026.

Kim, J. H., Park, J.-M., Yea, K., Kim, H. W., Suh, P.-G. & Ryu, S. H. (2010). Phospholipase D1 Mediates AMP-Activated Protein Kinase Signaling for Glucose Uptake. *PLoS ONE* 5, e9600.

King, J. D., Jr., Fitch, A. C., Lee, J. K., McCane, J. E., Mak, D. O., Foskett, J. K. & Hallows, K. R. (2009). AMP-activated protein kinase phosphorylation of the R domain inhibits PKA stimulation of CFTR. *Am J Physiol-Cell Physiol* 297, C94-101.

Kodiha, M., Rassi, J. G., Brown, C. M. & Stochaj, U. (2007). Localization of AMP kinase is regulated by stress, cell density, and signaling through the MEK-->ERK1/2 pathway. *Am J Physiol-Cell Physiol* 293, C1427-1436.

Kongsuphol, P., Cassidy, D., Hieke, B., Treharne, K. J., Schreiber, R., Mehta, A. & Kunzelmann, K. (2009). Mechanistic insight into control of CFTR by AMPK. *J Biol Chem* 284, 5645-5653.

Koo, S.-H., Flechner, L., Qi, L. et al. (2005). The CREB coactivator TORC2 is a key regulator of fasting glucose metabolism. *Nature* 437, 1109-1111.

Kuramoto, N., Wilkins, M. E., Fairfax, B. P. et al. (2007). Phospho-Dependent Functional Modulation of GABA(B) Receptors by the Metabolic Sensor AMP-Dependent Protein Kinase. *Neuron* 53, 233-247.

Lage, R., Diéguez, C., Vidal-Puig, A. & López, M. (2008). AMPK: a metabolic gauge regulating whole-body energy homeostasis. *Trends Mol Med* 14, 539-549.

Lamia, K. A., Sachdeva, U. M., DiTacchio, L. et al. (2009). AMPK Regulates the Circadian Clock by Cryptochrome Phosphorylation and Degradation. *Science* 326, 437-440.

Leclerc, I., Sun, G., Morris, C., Fernandez-Millan, E., Nyirenda, M. & Rutter, G. (2011). AMP-activated protein kinase regulates glucagon secretion from mouse pancreatic alpha cells. *Diabetologia* 54, 125-134.

Lee, M.-J., Feliers, D., Mariappan, M. M., Sataranatarajan, K. et al. (2007). A role for AMP-activated protein kinase in diabetes-induced renal hypertrophy. *Am J Physiol – Renal Physiol* 292, F617-F627.

Li, J. & McCullough, L. D. (2010). Effects of AMP-activated protein kinase in cerebral ischemia. *J Cereb Blood Flow Metab* 30, 480-492.

Li, Y., Roux, C. l., Lazereg, S., LeCaer, J.-P., Lapravote, O., Badet, B. & Badet-Denisot, M.-A. (2007). Identification of a Novel Serine Phosphorylation Site in Human Glutamine:Fructose-6-phosphate Amidotransferase Isoform 1 *Biochem* 46, 13163-13169.

Liang, J., Shao, S. H., Xu, Z.-X., Hennessy, B., Ding, Z., Larrea, M., Kondo, S., Dumont, D. J., Gutterman, J. U., Walker, C. L., Slingerland, J. M. & Mills, G. B. (2007). The energy sensing LKB1-AMPK pathway regulates p27kip1 phosphorylation mediating the decision to enter autophagy or apoptosis. *Nat Cell Biol* 9, 218-224.

Lieberthal, W. & Levine, J. S. (2009). The Role of the Mammalian Target Of Rapamycin (mTOR) in Renal Disease. *J Am Soc Nephrol* 20, 2493-2502.

Lippai, M., Csikos, G., Maroy, P., Lukacsovich, T., Juhasz, G. & Sass, M. (2008). SNF4Agamma, the Drosophila AMPK gamma subunit is required for regulation of developmental and stress-induced autophagy. *Autophagy* 4, 476-486.

Lopaschuk, G. D. (2008). AMP-activated protein kinase control of energy metabolism in the ischemic heart. *Int J Obesity* 32, S29-S35.

Lu, J., Wu, D. M., Zheng, Y. L., Hu, B., Zhang, Z. F., Shan, Q., Zheng, Z. H., Liu, C. M. & Wang, Y. J. (2010). Quercetin activates AMP-activated protein kinase by reducing PP2C expression protecting old mouse brain against high cholesterol-induced neurotoxicity. *J Pathology* 222, 199-212.

Maeda, N., Takahashi, M., Funahashi, T. et al. (2001). PPARγ Ligands Increase Expression and Plasma Concentrations of Adiponectin, an Adipose-Derived Protein. *Diabetes* 50, 2094-2099.

Maher, P. A. & Schubert, D. R. (2009). Metabolic links between diabetes and Alzheimer's disease. *Expert Rev Neurotherapeutics* 9, 617-630.

Mahlapuu, M., Johansson, C., Lindgren, K. et al. (2004). Expression profiling of the gamma-subunit isoforms of AMP-activated protein kinase suggests a major role for gamma3 in white skeletal muscle. *Am J Physiol - Endocrinol Metabol* 286, E194-E200.

Mair, W., Morantte, I., Rodrigues, A. P. C., Manning, G., Montminy, M., Shaw, R. J. & Dillin, A. (2011). Lifespan extension induced by AMPK and calcineurin is mediated by CRTC-1 and CREB. *Nature* 470, 404-408.

Mantovani, J. & Roy, R. (2011). Re-evaluating the general(ized) roles of AMPK in cellular metabolism. *FEBS Letters* 585, 967-972.

Marsin, A.-S., Bouzin, C., Bertrand, L. & Hue, L. (2002). The Stimulation of Glycolysis by Hypoxia in Activated Monocytes Is Mediated by AMP-activated Protein Kinase and Inducible 6-Phosphofructo-2-kinase. *J Biol Chem* 277, 30778-30783.

Marsin, A. S., Bertrand, L., Rider, M. H. et al. (2000). Phosphorylation and activation of heart PFK-2 by AMPK has a role in the stimulation of glycolysis during ischaemia. *Curr Biol* 10, 1247-1255.

McDonald, A., Fogarty, S., Leclerc, I., Hill, E. V., Hardie, D. G. & Rutter, G. A. (2009). Control of insulin granule dynamics by AMPK dependent KLC1 phosphorylation. *Islets* 1, 198-209.

McDonald, A., Fogarty, S., Leclerc, I., Hill, E. V., Hardie, D. G. & Rutter, G. A. (2010). Cell-wide analysis of secretory granule dynamics in three dimensions in living pancreatic beta-cells: evidence against a role for AMPK-dependent phosphorylation of KLC1 at Ser517/Ser520 in glucose-stimulated insulin granule movement. *Biochem Soc Transactions* 38, 205-208.

McGee, S. L., Howlett, K. F., Starkie, R. L., Cameron-Smith, D., Kemp, B. E. & Hargreaves, M. (2003). Exercise Increases Nuclear AMPK alpha2 in Human Skeletal Muscle. *Diabetes* 52, 926-928.

McGee, S. L., van Denderen, B. J. W., Howlett, K. F., Mollica, J., Schertzer, J. D., Kemp, B. E. & Hargreaves, M. (2008). AMP-Activated Protein Kinase Regulates GLUT4 Transcription by Phosphorylating Histone Deacetylase 5. *Diabetes* 57, 860-867.

McMahon, K. W., Zanescu, D. I., Sood, V. & Prabhakar, S. S. (2009). The Role of 5'-AMP-Activated Protein Kinase (AMPK) in Diabetic Nephropathy: A New Direction? *Curr Enzyme Inhibition* 5, 44-50.

Mirouse, V., Swick, L. L., Kazgan, N., St Johnston, D. & Brenman, J. E. (2007). LKB1 and AMPK maintain epithelial cell polarity under energetic stress. *J Cell Biol* 177, 387-392.

Miyamoto, T., Oshiro, N., Yoshino, K., Nakashima, A., Eguchi, S., Takahashi, M., Ono, Y., Kikkawa, U. & Yonezawa, K. (2008). AMP-activated protein kinase phosphorylates Golgi-specific brefeldin A resistance factor 1 at Thr1337 to induce disassembly of Golgi apparatus. *J Biol Chem* 283, 4430-4438.

Nagata, D. & Hirata, Y. (2010). The role of AMP-activated protein kinase in the cardio-vascular system. *Hypertens Res* 33, 22-28.

Narbonne, P. & Roy, R. (2009). Caenorhabditis elegans dauers need LKB1/AMPK to ration lipid reserves and ensure long-term survival. *Nature* 457, 210-214.

Niesler, C. U., Myburgh, K. H. & Moore, F. (2007). The changing AMPK expression profile in differentiating mouse skeletal muscle myoblast cells helps confer increasing resistance to apoptosis. *Experim Physiol* 92, 207-217.

Oakhill, J. S., Chen, Z. P., Scott, J. W., Steel, R., Castelli, L. A., Ling, N., Macaulay, S. L. & Kemp, B. E. (2010). beta-Subunit myristoylation is the gatekeeper for initiating metabolic stress sensing by AMP-activated protein kinase (AMPK). *Proc Natl Acad Sci USA* 107, 19237-19241.

Polekhina, G., Gupta, A., Michell, B. J. et al. (2003). AMPK β Subunit Targets Metabolic Stress Sensing to Glycogen. *Curr Biol* 13, 867-871.

Pulinilkunnil, T., He, H., Kong, D., Asakura, K., Peroni, O. D., Lee, A. & Kahn, B. B. (2011). Adrenergic Regulation of AMP-activated Protein Kinase in Brown Adipose Tissue in Vivo. *J Biol Chem* 286, 8798-8809.

Putman, C. T., Martins, K. J. B., Gallo, M. E., Lopaschuk, G. D., Pearcey, J. A., MacLean, I. M., Saranchuk, R. J. & Pette, D. (2007). alpha-Catalytic subunits of 5'AMP-activated protein kinase display fiber-specific expression and are upregulated by chronic low-frequency stimulation in rat muscle. *Am J Physiology-Regul Integr Comp Physiol* 293, R1325-R1334.

Qi, J., Gong, J., Zhao, T., Zhao, J., Lam, P., Ye, J., Li, J. Z., Wu, J., Zhou, H.-M. & Li, P. (2008). Downregulation of AMP-activated protein kinase by Cidea-mediated ubiquitination and degradation in brown adipose tissue. *EMBO J* 27, 1537-1548.

Quan, X., Yu, J., Bussey, H. & Stochaj, U. (2007). The localization of nuclear exporters of the importin-beta family is regulated by Snf1 kinase, nutrient supply and stress. *Biochim Biophys Acta-Mol Cell Res* 1773, 1052-1061.

Quentin, T., Kitz, J., Steinmetz, M., Poppe, A., Bär, K. & Krätzner, R. (2011). Different expression of the catalytic alpha subunits of the AMP activated protein kinase - an immunohistochemical study in human tissue. *Histol Histopathol* 26, 589-596.

Rachid, Z., Katsoulas, A., Williams, C., Larroque, A.-L., McNamee, J. & Jean-Claude, B. J. (2007). Optimization of novel combi-molecules: Identification of balanced and mixed bcr-abl/DNA targeting properties. *Bioorg Med Chem Lett* 17, 4248-4253.

Reihill, J. A., Ewart, M. A., Hardie, D. G. & Salt, I. P. (2007). AMP-activated protein kinase mediates VEGF-stimulated endothelial NO production. *BBRC* 354, 1084-1088.

Ronnett, G. V., Ramamurthy, S., Kleman, A. M., Landree, L. E. & Aja, S. (2009). AMPK in the brain: its roles in energy balance and neuroprotection. *J Neurochem* 109, 17-23.

Ross, F. A., Rafferty, J. N., Dallas, M. L. et al. (2011). Selective Expression in Carotid Body Type I Cells of a Single Splice Variant of the Large Conductance Calcium- and Voltage-activated Potassium Channel Confers Regulation by AMP-activated Protein Kinase. *J Biol Chem* 286, 11929-11936.

Salt, I., Celler, J. W., Hawley, S. A., Prescott, A., Woods, A., Carling, D. & Hardie, D. G. (1998). AMP-activated protein kinase: greater AMP dependence, and preferential nuclear localization, of complexes containing the alpha2 isoform. *Biochem J* 334, 177-187.

Sanders, M. J., Grondin, P. O., Hegarty, B. D., Snowden, M. A. & Carling, D. (2007). Investigating the mechanism for AMP activation of the AMP-activated protein kinase cascade. *Biochem J* 403, 139-148.

Schernhammer, E., Hansen, J., Rugbjerg, K., Wermuth, L. & Ritz, B. (2011). Diabetes and the Risk of Developing Parkinson's Disease in Denmark. *Diabetes Care*, in press.

Schrauwen, P. & Hesselink, M. K. C. (2004). Oxidative Capacity, Lipotoxicity, and Mitochondrial Damage in Type 2 Diabetes. *Diabetes* 53, 1412-1417.

Shackelford, D. B. & Shaw, R. J. (2009). The LKB1-AMPK pathway: metabolism and growth control in tumour suppression. *Nat Rev Cancer* 9, 563-575.

Skurat, A. V., Dietrich, A. D. & Roach, P. J. (2000). Glycogen synthase sensitivity to insulin and glucose-6-phosphate is mediated by both NH2- and COOH-terminal phosphorylation sites. *Diabetes* 49, 1096-1100.

Spasic, M., Callaerts, P. & Norga, K. K. (2009). AMP-Activated Protein Kinase (AMPK) Molecular Crossroad for Metabolic Control and Survival of Neurons. *Neuroscientist* 15, 309-316.

Sprenkle, A. B., Davies, S. P., Carling, D., Hardie, D. G. & Sturgill, T. W. (1997). Identification of Raf-1 Ser621 kinase activity from NIH3T3 cells as AMP-activated protein kinase. *FEBS Letters* 403, 254-258.

Stapleton, D., Mitchelhill, K. I., Gao, G. et al. (1996). Mammalian AMP-activated Protein Kinase Subfamily. *J Biol Chem* 271, 611-614.

Stein, S. C., Woods, A., Jones, N. A., Davison, M. D. & Carling, D. (2000). The regulation of AMP-activated protein kinase by phosphorylation. *Biochem. J.* 345, 437-443.

Steinberg, G. R. & Kemp, B. E. (2009). AMPK in Health and Disease. *Physiol Rev* 89, 1025-1078.

Steinberg, G. R., Michell, B. J., van Denderen, B. J. W. et al. (2006). Tumor necrosis factor alpha-induced skeletal muscle insulin resistance involves suppression of AMP-kinase signaling. *Cell Metabolism* 4, 465-474.

Steinberg, G. R., Rush, J. W. E. & Dyck, D. J. (2003). AMPK expression and phosphorylation are increased in rodent muscle after chronic leptin treatment. *Am J Physiol-Endocrin Metabol* 284, E648-E654.

Steinberg, G. R., Watt, M. J. & Febbraio, M. A. (2009). Cytokine regulation of AMPK signalling. *Front Biosci* 14, 1902-1916.

Sun, W., Lee, T.-S., Zhu, M., Gu, C., Wang, Y., Zhu, Y. & Shyy, J. Y.-J. (2006). Statins Activate AMP-Activated Protein Kinase In Vitro and In Vivo. *Circulation* 114, 2655-2662.

Suzuki, A., Okamoto, S., Lee, S., Saito, K., Shiuchi, T. & Minokoshi, Y. (2007). Leptin Stimulates Fatty Acid Oxidation and Peroxisome Proliferator-Activated Receptor α Gene Expression in Mouse C2C12 Myoblasts by Changing the Subcellular Localization of the α2 Form of AMP-Activated Protein Kinase. *Mol Cell Biol* 27, 4317-4327.

Takiar, V., Nishio, S., Seo-Mayer, P., King, J. D., Li, H., Zhang, L., Karihaloo, A., Hallows, K. R., Somlo, S. & Caplan, M. J. (2011). Activating AMP-activated protein kinase (AMPK) slows renal cystogenesis. *Proc Natl Acad Sci USA* 108, 2462-2467.

Thornton, C., Bright, N. J., Sastre, M., Muckett, P. J. & Carling, D. (2011). AMP-activated protein kinase (AMPK) is a tau kinase, activated in response to amyloid beta-peptide exposure. *Biochem J* 434, 503-512.

Towler, M. C. & Hardie, D. G. (2007). AMP-activated protein kinase in metabolic control and insulin signaling. *Circulation Res* 100, 328-41.

Treebak, J. T., Taylor, E. B., Witczak, C. A., An, D., Toyoda, T., Koh, H.-J., Xie, J., Feener, E. P., Wojtaszewski, J. r. F. P., Hirshman, M. F. & Goodyear, L. J. (2010). Identification of a novel phosphorylation site on TBC1D4 regulated by AMP-activated protein kinase in skeletal muscle. *Am J Physiol-Cell Physiol* 298, C377-385.

Turnley, A. M., Stapleton, D., Mann, R. J., Witters, L. A., Kemp, B. E. & Bartlett, P. F. (1999). Cellular Distribution and Developmental Expression of AMP-Activated Protein Kinase Isoforms in Mouse Central Nervous System. *J Neurochem* 72, 1707-1716.

Tzatsos, A. & Tsichlis, P. N. (2007). Energy Depletion Inhibits Phosphatidylinositol 3-Kinase/Akt Signaling and Induces Apoptosis via AMP-activated Protein Kinase-dependent Phosphorylation of IRS-1 at Ser-794. *J Biol Chem* 282, 18069-18082.

Um, J. H., Yang, S., Yamazaki, S., Kang, H., Viollet, B., Foretz, M. & Chung, J. H. (2007). Activation of 5'-AMP-activated Kinase with Diabetes Drug Metformin Induces Casein Kinase 1ε (CKIε)-dependent Degradation of Clock Protein mPer2. *J Biol Chem* 282, 20794-20798.

van Oort, M. M., van Doorn, J. M., Hasnaoui, M. E., Glatz, J. F., Bonen, A., van der Horst, D. J., Rodenburg, K. W. & JJ, P. L. (2009). Effects of AMPK activators on the sub-cellular distribution of fatty acid transporters CD36 and FABPpm. *Arch Physiol Biochem* 115, 137-146.

Vernia, S., Solaz-Fuster, M. C., Gimeno-Alcaniz, J. V. et al. (2009). AMP-activated Protein Kinase Phosphorylates R5/PTG, the Glycogen Targeting Subunit of the R5/PTG-Protein Phosphatase 1 Holoenzyme, and Accelerates Its Down-regulation by the Laforin-Malin Complex. *J Biol Chem* 284, 8247-8255.

Vigetti, D., Clerici, M., Deleonibus, S., Karousou, E., Viola, M., Moretto, P., Heldin, P., Hascall, V. C., De Luca, G. & Passi, A. (2011). Hyaluronan Synthesis Is Inhibited by

Adenosine Monophosphate-activated Protein Kinase through the Regulation of HAS2 Activity in Human Aortic Smooth Muscle Cells. *J Biol Chem* 286, 7917-7924.

Vingtdeux, V., Davies, P., Dickson, D. & Marambaud, P. (2011). AMPK is abnormally activated in tangle- and pre-tangle-bearing neurons in Alzheimer's disease and other tauopathies. *Acta Neuropathol* 121, 337-349.

Viollet, B., Athea, Y., Mounier, R., Guigas, B., Zarrinpashneh, E., Horman, S., Lantier, L., Hebrard, S., Devin-Leclerc, J., Beauloye, C., Foretz, M., Andreelli, F., Ventura-Clapier, R. & Bertrand, L. (2009a). AMPK: Lessons from transgenic and knockout animals. *Front Biosc* 14, 19-44.

Viollet, B., Lantier, L., Devin-Leclerc, J., Hebrard, S., Amouyal, C., Mounier, R., Foretz, M. & Andreelli, F. (2009b). Targeting the AMPK pathway for the treatment of Type 2 diabetes. *Front Biosci* 14, 3380-3400.

Viollet, B., Horman, S., Leclerc, J., Lantier, L., Foretz, M., Billaud, M., Giri, S. & Andreelli, F. (2010). AMPK inhibition in health and disease. *Crit Rev Biochem Mol Biol* 45, 276-295.

Wang, A., Liu, M., Liu, X., Dong, L. Q., Glickman, R. D., Slaga, T. J., Zhou, Z. & Liu, F. (2011). Up-regulation of adiponectin by resveratrol: The essential roles of the Akt/FOXO1 and AMPK signaling pathways and DsbA-L. *J Biol Chem* 286, 60-66.

Wang, T., Yu, Q., Chen, J., Deng, B., Qian, L. & Le, Y. (2010). PP2A Mediated AMPK Inhibition Promotes HSP70 Expression in Heat Shock Response. *PLoS ONE* 5, e13096.

Wang, W., Yang, X., Kawai, T., de Silanes, I. L. p., Mazan-Mamczarz, K., Chen, P., Chook, Y. M., Quensel, C., KÃ¶hler, M. & Gorospe, M. (2004). AMP-activated Protein Kinase-regulated Phosphorylation and Acetylation of Importin α1. *J Biol Chem* 279, 48376-48388.

Warden, S. M., Richardson, C., O'Donnell, J., Stapleton, D., Kemp, B. E. & Witters, L. A. (2001). Post-translational modifications of the beta-1 subunit of AMP-activated protein kinase affect enzyme activity and cellular localization. *Biochem J* 354, 275-283.

Watt, M. J., Holmes, A. G., Pinnamaneni, S. K., Garnham, A. P., Steinberg, G. R., Kemp, B. E. & Febbraio, M. A. (2006). Regulation of HSL serine phosphorylation in skeletal muscle and adipose tissue. *Am J Physiol-Endocrin Metabol* 290, E500-E508.

Witczak, C., Sharoff, C. & Goodyear, L. (2008). AMP-activated protein kinase in skeletal muscle: From structure and localization to its role as a master regulator of cellular metabolism. *CMLS* 65, 3737-3755.

Xie, M., Zhang, D., Dyck, J. R. B. et al. (2006). A pivotal role for endogenous TGF-beta-activated kinase-1 in the LKB1/AMP-activated protein kinase energy-sensor pathway. *Proc Natl Acad Sci USA* 103, 17378-17383.

Yang, W., Hong, Y. H., Shen, X.-Q., Frankowski, C., Camp, H. S. & Leff, T. (2001). Regulation of Transcription by AMP-activated Protein Kinase. *J Biol Chem* 276, 38341-38344.

Zhang, B. B., Zhou, G. & Li, C. (2009). AMPK: An Emerging Drug Target for Diabetes and the Metabolic Syndrome. *Cell Metabolism* 9, 407-416.

Zheng, D., Perianayagam, A., Lee, D. H., Brannan, M. D., Yang, L. E., Tellalian, D., Chen, P., Lemieux, K., Marette, A., Youn, J. H. & McDonough, A. A. (2008). AMPK activation with AICAR provokes an acute fall in plasma [K+]. *Am J Physiol-Cell Physiol* 294, C126-C135.

19

Design and Evaluation of a Complex Phytoceutical Formulation for Circulatory Diseases

Olalde J, Antoshechkin A, del Castillo O, Guzmán R and Améndola, F
Centro Medico Docente Adaptogenos
Venezuela

1. Introduction

Although herbal/natural remedies have been, and are still being used, in the treatment of chronic degenerative diseases, little is known about basic principles –or theory- to combine these components and attain synergistic, gene modulating, as well as clinical health improving effects. This chapter is divided into six sections. Section 2 reviews the background which gives origin and establishes the Systemic Theory and Systemic Medicine. The section also provides the general precepts to structure Circulat -a complex herbal formulation- for the treatment of circulatory chronic degenerative diseases. Section 3 is an outline of an investigation into the aforementioned formulation's role and capability to modulate various gene expression levels -in cultured human fibroblasts- including those associated with diabetes. On the other hand, Section 4 presents a review of Circulat´s clinical properties through a Diabetic Foot management Study. An abbreviated limited Phase 2 GSPECT evaluated Chronic Ischemic Disease –another circulatory chronic disease- study is presented in Section 5. Finally, Section 6 provides some conclusions concerning the use of a complex herbal formulation as well as some reflections on the future design of such compositions.

2. The origin of Systemic theory and Systemic medicine: Relevance to complementary and alternative medicine

Past and Present Phytomedicine and natural practitioners: Tomorrow's Systemics? Recent past -and even present- successful phytomedicine practitioners and naturalists share a long and honorable tradition of knowledge and pride in the cure of illnesses, which goes back to written history and beyond. These qualities have been substantiated by the successes of the Chinese (Chen *et al.*, 2004; Wago & Deng, 2004), Kampo (Teresawa, 2004; Yamada, 2004), Ayurvedic (Naik *et al.*, 2003), Chumash (Adams and Garcia, 2005) or Mayan (Peña, 2002) traditional medicines among many others. These traditional medicines 'demonstrated that every culture is capable of understanding and "inventing" the meaning of disease and its cure, even when it is different from our modern medical views' (Peña, 2002). The variability and extent of cultures to provide answers -or traditional medicines- to pathologies are embedded in the curiosity and observational capabilities of the human race. There are also collective factors such as 'a background of extensive family in traditional medicine' (Vandenbroek *et al.*, 2004) which play an important role in the communication and survival of medicinal plant knowledge among ethnic groups. A potential issue, though, is the possible curtailment of the wisdom -and therapies- of traditional medicines within geographical and ethnic boundaries. In any case, the amount of plants, potential formulations or properties are a massive concern for any given individual caregiver or group to understand, store and transmit. Some exceptional individuals seem to have come by this ability. One of these gifted health care practitioners was Maurice Messegue, whom Mistinguet and Konrad Adenaur -among his famous patients- swore that only he could treat their illnesses. More recently, both, Dr. Rusudan Lomidze, using the Georgian Kohlkian traditional medicine, and Lonrig Dangar, a Tibetan physician who applied the rich Tibetan traditional medicine have also obtained significant success. These gifted individuals have shown that traditional medicine is a successful medicine. But a question still hangs in the air. Might a theory be devised by which regular practitioners, health care specialists devoid of the naturalists' extensive background, formulate natural organic therapeutic protocols? Furthermore, is it possible to set up a system -or periodic table- where plants and other natural remedies could, according to superior therapeutic properties, be arranged to produce specific formulae that provide well-being for a given pathology? The treatment of circulatory pathologies with substances which act only on function and structure might be an incomplete approach. Whether the investigations in circulatory chronic disease studies –and their results- can be generalized in confirmation of a systemic approach is something that should be pursued as this may pave the way for a new integral vision of therapeutics in general and/or in circulatory chronic diseases such as Diabetes in particular.

2.1 Prior developments of a natural therapeutic protocol: Systemic Theory

Aggressors or stressors were identified by Professor Hans Selye, and described and classified in over 1500 articles and 32 books. He formulated the General Adaptation Syndrome (Selye, 1976), which classified effects on animals and humans affected by threats (exhaustion, disease, fear, extreme cold …) as: alarm (body's recognition of danger and its preparation to deal with threats); resistance (or adaptation, in which the body adapts to resist stress); and exhaustion (condition in which the body's energy supply is depleted). The next step was taken by Soviet scientists led by Lazarev and Brekhman, who investigated properties of substances, with the ability to increase adaptability and resistance to stress. They named these 'adaptogens'. By 1960 more than 1000 studies had been published by Soviet scientists concerning the use of adaptogens. In 1962, *Eleutherococcus senticosus*, *Rhaponticum carthamoides* and *Rhodiola rosea*, all adaptogens, were included in the Soviet Union's Pharmacopoeia. Since then many other plants and sources have been found to have similar properties (Brekman and Ivanov, 1969; Khasina *et al.*, 1983; Bhattacharya and Muruganandam, 2003; Dhuley, 2000) and increasing resistance to stressors as depicted by Selye, enhancing energy, and regulating immune, neuroendocrine and cellular function. Although the adaptogen definition in science is questioned by some researchers, most concur on their health enhancing properties (Davydov and Krikorian, 2000). Figure 1 (Olalde, 2005a) is an interpretation of Energy drop (E↓) in relation to Selye's description of biochemical collapse (I↓) and organic dysfunction (O↓). This paved the way to the E, I and O triangle.

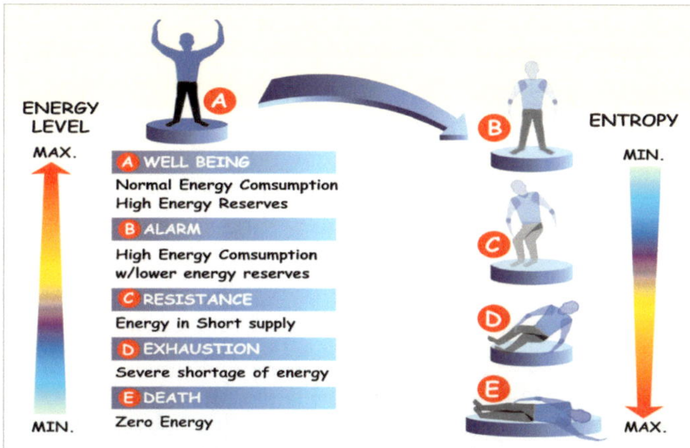

Fig. 1. Functional energy reserve ladder. Energy drop affects the human organism, going from a state of well being with high Energy reserves and low entropy - low disorder- through various stages and finally to that of death, or state of zero energy and maximun disorder

2.1.1 Life and negentropy: Rationalization for the use of phytomedicines

The second law of thermodynamics states that a system logically tends to go from a state of higher energy and order to one of lower energy and disorder. This is more so in living systems where internal entropy tends to increase in its journey through life, going from health, energy and physiological order towards sickness, asthenia (the loss or lack of bodily strength; weakness) and physiological disorder. Illness, however, can be countered based on quantum physicist's Erwin Schrödinger's notion that the general change of entropy in an open system, such as a living (biological) system, consists of (i) internal entropy variations and (ii) entropy exchange of the system with the environment; i.e. $\triangle S = \triangle S$ internal + $\triangle S$ exchange. Internal entropy in a biological organism, by definition, tends to be greater than zero due to inner irreversible processes. Therefore, the increase in entropy of an open biological system, and thus illness, may be reduced (von Stockar and Liu, 1999) by providing negative entropy -or negentropy- from the environment. This is pivotal as nature provides a source of negative entropy. '… The decrease of entropy in living systems is provided by free energy, released when nutrients consumed from the outside dissociate, i.e. at the expense of the sun's energy. Thus, the flow of negative entropy is essential to compensate for inner destructive processes as well as for the decrease of available free energy dissipated by spontaneous metabolic reactions. This last, is the key point, circulation and transformation of free energy, which drives the functions of living systems …' (Korotkov *et al.*, 2004).

2.2 ↑ Health ↔ entropy ↓

How does life defy entropy? In physics, entropy is defined as the measure of disorder in a system. Disorder, in turn, can be mathematically expressed by the probability of random occurrence. All pathologies, by definition, result from a higher than normal organic entropy; thus, to induce health, entropy must first be reduced; this is bi-conditional. Contemporary thermodynamics defines entropy (or chaos) in an intelligent system as a deficiency in energy and/or information. Therefore, entropy is inversely related to information and energy availability. According to Shannon -father of the Information Theory- and Weaver 'information is always a measure of the decrease of uncertainty at a receiver or molecular machine' (Shanon and Weaver, 1999). Thus was born the concept of informational entropy, which they concluded was equivalent to a shortage of information content in a message. About the same time, Weiner (Weiner, 1954) established the possibility of interpreting information carried by a message as '... essentially the negative entropy, and the negative logarithm of its probability' since 'the relationship between information (J) and thermodynamic entropy (S) is constant (S + J = const)' (Korotkov, 1988). Thus, the work of such eminent minds as: Boltzmann (Lindley, 2001), Gibbs (Deltete, 1995), Szilard (Leff & Rex, 1990), Von Neumann (Heims *et al.*, 1980), Schrödinger (1992), Prigogine (1984), Shannon and Weaver (1999) and Weiner (Heims *et al.*, 1980; Weiner, 1954), brought about the dawn of new emergent fields, including: informational thermodynamics, information theory, biological information theory and cybernetics all dealing with energy, information and entropy in mechanical and living systems. A basic common premise in the new thinking proposes that information and energy had an inverse, i.e. opposite, correlation with entropy. In other words, evidence suggests that no suitable organization can be attained in living systems that possess reduced levels of information or energy. Disease, therefore, may be defined as a state of disorganization, i.e. higher organic entropy, corresponding with a low energo-informational status of the system. In consequence, if a reduction in illness is to be achieved, entropy must be reduced. A comprehensive way of accomplishing this, is administering negative entropy, or order, through matter which stimulates the production of energy and provides survival information to the immune, neuroendorine and cellular systems. To recap, the tendency to reach order depends on the energy and information available within the system, which determines the possible level of stable organization possible. The quantity of true information (conceptual data, not noise) transferred to the system's modulating intelligence allows for chaos and/or confusion management and, enhances the system's ability to attain a higher organization level. Moreover by definition, only an intelligent system can process information and energy to reduce entropy. This unequivocal fact demonstrates the existence of a regulating biological intelligence within the human body. Intelligence is the way in which life affronts entropy.

2.2.1 The E, I and O health triangle

All living systems are functional units that seek maximum survival. The cell is the simplest form of a living system that functions as a basic building block of the living universe, just as an atom does in matter. Conversely, a virus is the simplest living unit, which in some situations acts as destroyer of living systems. **I** (or Intelligence) is the backbone of every living system in equilibrium. **I** controls, regulates, adapts and develops the living system. Chaos occurs in its absence. The proof of this is that no living system can exist without intelligence. The intelligence of the system, **I,** creates and utilizes **E** (or Energy) with the primary role of achieving **O** (Organization) and evolving into a higher system (Owens and Van de Castle, 2004). **I** also creates/builds **O** with the primary end of producing **E**. There can be a corollary: as a consequence, **I** cannot act optimally when subjected to a severe deficiency of **E**. Finally, **I** is the most important side of the health triangle since it concurrently generates both energy (**E**) and organization (**O**). One phytoceutical that can increase all sides is *Panax ginseng* (Figure 2).

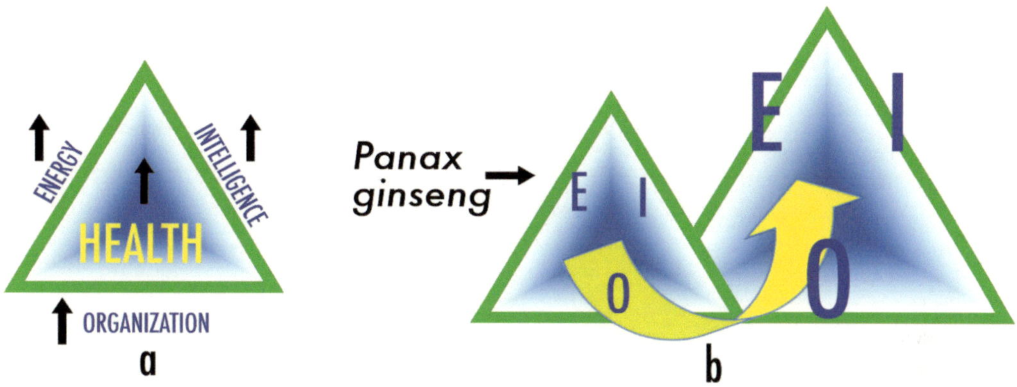

Fig. 2. (a) Example of a living system's health triangle. (b) Evolution from a given health situation and initial E, I, O triangle (left) to an improved E, I, O triangle (right). All sides are boosted due to negative entropy provided by *Panax ginseng*.

2.2.2 Example of I, E and O increase by providing *Panax ginseng*

Panax ginseng active principles are bonded to beta-adrenoceptors in the cellular membrane, triggering a secondary transmitting message system (cyclic AMP) which travels through a transducer pathway to the mitochondria to increase MDH, SDH and CTS activity, enzymes of the glycolisis or tricarboxylic acid cycle. ATP generation is thus increased, raising energy levels using glucose as fuel (Figure 3a). Thus, either the ATP/ADP ratio increase or the binding of ginsenosides to cell membrane receptors results in the KATP channel closure and insulin secretion (Rotsheyn & Zito, 2004) (Figure 3b). Thus with the increase of energy a larger health triangle is obtained and the system's intelligence has acquired more capacity to organize. *Panax ginseng* provides an example of a remarkable phytomedicine which is capable of enhancing **I**, **E** and **O** simultaneously in the living system.

2.3 Significance of the intelligence (I) within the systemic triangle. What is intelligence?

The importance (and significance) of a system's intelligence is pivotal. How can this controversial and subjective concept be defined accurately? Olalde (2005a) confronted this dilemma by examining its definition in different fields. Table 1 lists different concepts of the term intelligence.

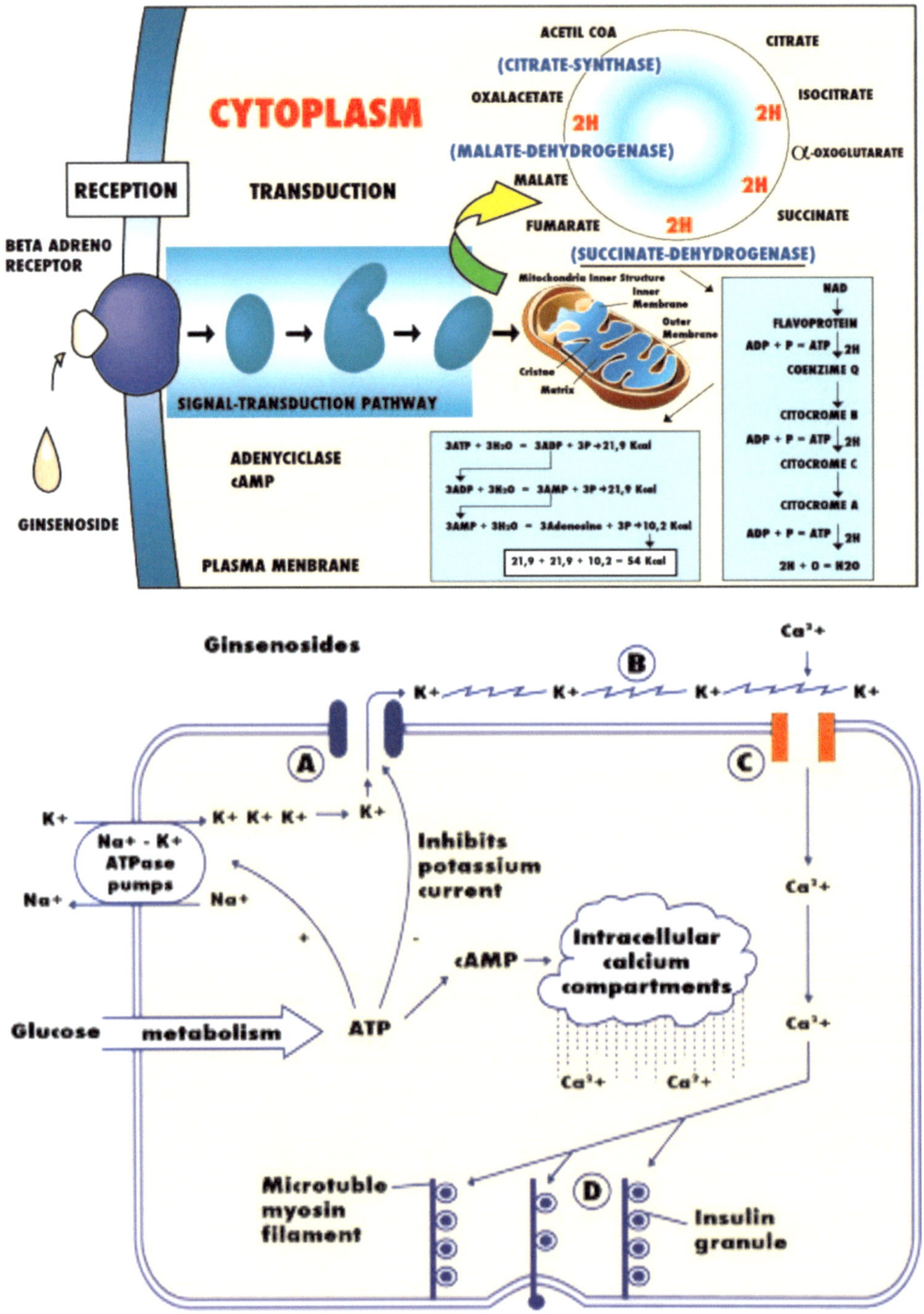

Fig. 3. a: (top) *Panax* intracellular action mechanism results in ATP synthesis stimulation, whose hydrolysis produces energy; b: (bottom) shows the Sodium–potassium ATP pump, illustrating ATP generation by administering ginsenosides in *Panax ginseng* to the Living System.

Domain	Reference	Definition of intelligence
Cybernetics	Wiener, 1954	That whose core concepts are communication, control and learning, by means of feedback mechanisms.
Physics		Refers to regulation processes.
Biophysics		Living system's endogenous regulation processes effectively constitute intelligence.
Encyclopedic Neufeldt V, Guralnik D (Eds)	Webster's New World Dictionary(1988)	(a) Ability to learn or understand from experience. (b) Ability to acquire and retain knowledge. (c) Ability to respond quickly and successfully to a new situation. (d) Use of the faculty of reason in resolving problems, directing conduct, etc. effectively. (e) An intelligent spirit or being. (f) Having knowledge, understanding or awareness.
Multivarious	World Wide Web	a) Ability of a system to process general information to react appropriately to specific events; b)The product of communication, resulting from the collection, processing, integration, analysis, evaluation and interpretation of available information; c)Ability to acquire, store, retrieve, process and generate information; d) Ability to learn or understand or to deal with new or challenging situations; e) Accumulation of experiences together with the understanding of how these experiences are connected; f)Capacity to act purposefully, to think rationally, to communicate and to deal effectively with his or her environment. (g) Entity. (h) Emergent.

Table 1. Definitions of Intelligence

2.3.1 Intelligence = Informational entity

By analyzing common traits within the definitions given in Table 1, intelligence may be defined as that emergent informational entity, capable of learning, exerting control, emitting and receiving communication, handling energy flows, establishing feedback mechanisms and creating organization for survival. Emergent implies a higher level of intelligence of the whole, stemming from the intelligence of its parts. According to Laszlo, living systems are special third-stage systems, self-creating and self-replicating, that engender order out of chaos (Lazlo, 1987). However, Wiener states 'It is my thesis that the physical functioning of the living individual and the operation of some of the newer communications machines are precisely parallel in their analogous attempts to control entropy through feedback' (Wiener, 1954). The notion of intelligence that Olalde (2005) adopts is that of an informational entity, i.e. one which is emergent, can generate, process and exchange informational flows in order to control entropy. The concept of intelligence becomes more objective, and functional, when treated as an informational entity, one dependent on information exchange, which as we know has a thermodynamic interpretation. A change of entropy ($\triangle S$) will produce a change or variation in information availability, and therefore a change in intelligence and order in the biological system. Any entity that can exchange informational flows can also generate changes of entropy. Thus, informational flow ↔ change in entropy ↔ change in intelligence. According to Stonier's proposed theory 'Pure energy can perform no 'useful' work (entropy reducing) without a concomitant input of information (Stonier, 1996). Conversely, all expenditures of energy lead to a reorganization of the universe, hence a change in its information status. Energy and information are inter-convertible'. This theory could provide additional support for the indispensable existence of an intelligent entity to handle information, since information without intelligence is without value. A possible corollary is: intelligence is that entity which can causatively alter entropy; and vice versa, entropy changes will also affect intelligence. Figure 4 shows an intelligent cell, an example of an informational entity capable of modifying entropy.

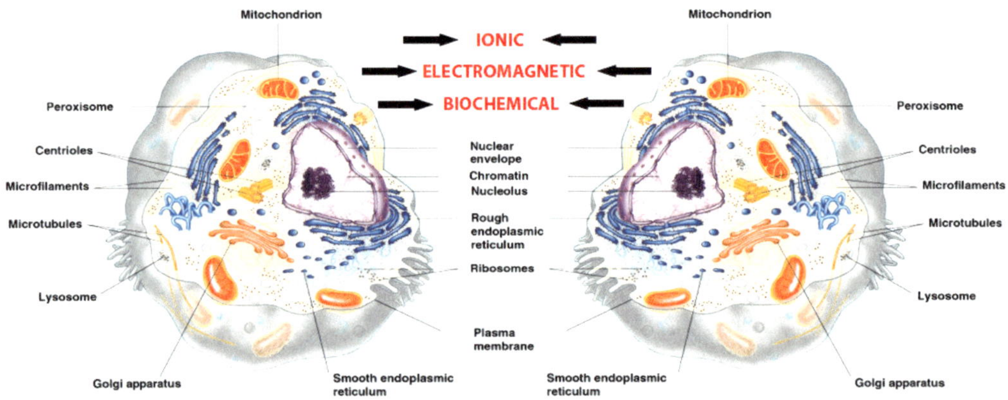

Fig. 4. A living system possesses intelligence and is capable, as human cells demonstrate, of an informational flow and exchange with other cells, organs and living systems. This communicational flow may have various 'vehicles' and 'avenues'.

2.4 Synergy and informational systems

Synergy is a quality of informational systems. It may be understood as emergent, i.e. the informational participation of each fractal member of the system in order to achieve a higher plateau of self-organization and survival (Haken, 2005). It can also be understood as the resulting effect that is greater than the algebraic sum of the parts. Synergy is an important characteristic of third-stage systems. The increase of energy availability within a third-stage, living, system also decreases its entropy, potentially generating an endogenous tendency for informational flow and a heightened intelligence; this in turn generates organization. By analogy, an increase of information will, on its own, raise intelligence which will positively influence energy and organization. In synergic terms, each of the three elements shown above has the capacity to affect (increase or decrease) the other two. Thus we derive the following synergic bi-conditionals, inherent to any third-stage system: survival potential = health = $\uparrow I \leftrightarrow \uparrow E \leftrightarrow \uparrow O \leftrightarrow S \downarrow$ and also demise = sickness = $\downarrow I \leftrightarrow \downarrow E \leftrightarrow \downarrow O \leftrightarrow S \uparrow$.

2.4.1 Informational substantiation of biological intelligence

If there is communication, intelligence exists. Communication is a manifestation of intelligence. The existence of biochemical and bio-photonic communication in cells has been corroborated: biochemical communication, for example, between the neurological and immune systems, has been examined, among others, by Blalock (1989), Cavagnaro and Lewis (1989) and more recently Takeda and Okomura (2004) and Cooper (2004). The biophotonic communication concept was discovered by Alexander Gurwitsch in 1923, as an 'ultraweak' photon emission from living systems (Gurwitsch, 1991). About the same time, Frolich, father of the 'coherent' notion of living systems, discovered that nucleated cells are capable of picking up, storing and broadcasting information about the environment. The term biophotons '...denotes a permanent spontaneous photon emission from all living systems...' and explains '... biological phenomena like intracellular and intercellular communication, cell growth and differentiation, interactions among biological systems and microbial infections...' (Popp, 2003). Different scientific groups have confirmed the existence of (and suggested some uses for) this subtle photon emission in: Australia (Tilbary & Quickenden, 1988; Trushin 2003), Japan (Kobayashi *et al., 1996*; Takeda *et al.*, 1998), Poland (Slawinska & Slawinski, 1987) and Germany (Popp, 2003). Other prominent scientists in the study of biophotons are Professor Voeikov (Voikov, 2003) and Dr. Albrecht-Buehler. This last sustains the thesis that cells are intelligent: 'capable of deriving abstract data and emitting near infrared signals' (Albrecht-Buehler, 1998, 1985).

2.4.2 Biological Intelligence (BI)

Intelligence is best measured by its manifestations. In structural terms, the BI is 'omnipresent' in the organism due to the intelligent nature of all cells (Gurwitsch, 1991); however, in functional terms, the BI's common denominator is comprised of the immune intelligence (II), cellular intelligence (CI) and biochemical (or neuroendocrine) intelligence (BI) (Blalock, 1989; Cavagnaro and Lewis, 1989; Cooper, 2004; Takeda and Okomura, 2004). The BI functions as an emergent informational entity, oriented towards survival, capable of auto-regulation, bidirectional communication, generating, processing and manipulating energy flows within the body. It is in charge of establishing, maintaining and restituting the organization. Figure 5 shows the interaction between neuroendocrine, immune and cellular intelligence. CI is the most important of BI's constituents since it regulates genetics and metabolism of each and every organic cell and gives birth to the autonomous II and BI. These three elements also constitute a synergistic trio, since none of them can exist in the absence of another, due to essential feedback and information exchange amongst them (Blalock, 1989; Cavagnaro and Lewis, 1989; Cooper, 2004; Takeda and Okomura, 2004). BI could also be represented schematically as a triangle, since alterations to one side of a triangle always affect the other two. Its healing potential may be defined as the mathematical product of its immune, cellular and neuroendocrine state, i.e. BI (Healing Potential) = $I^I \times C^I \times B^I$. In consequence, it is possible to enhance BI by increasing any of its three essential components, for example with immune modulators (Bocharova *et al.*, 2003; Geng *et al.*, 2005; Kidd, 2000; Kohguchi *et al.*, 2004; Kormosh *et al.*, 2004). The opposite also holds true, a collapse of any component will affect the other two.

2.5 From Systemic theory to Systemic medicine

At the beginning of this section a question was posed. Was it possible to set up a system -or periodic table- where plants and other natural remedies could, according to their superior medicinal properties, be arranged to produce specific formulae that provide well-being for a given pathology? The Systemic Theory was set forth to provide an answer to this crucial question. Systemic Theory postulates that Health (H) is directly proportional to the integrity of a living system's Energy (E), Bio-Intelligence (I) and Organization (O). Systemic Theory also established a common denominator to all sickness and ascertains the cause of all diseases to be an entropy increase: 'disorder augmenting within the biologically open system, stemming from energo-informational and organizational impacts, either of external or internal nature' (Olalde, 2005c). Systemic Therapeutics -or Medicine- should then include a negentropy supply to enhance the system's: energy-work capacity or E (i.e. physiological mechanisms associated with ATP synthesis, such as oxidative phosphorolysis, Krebbs cycle, β-oxidation etc.), its informational potential intelligence or I (i.e. the entity responsible for regulating neuroendocrine, biochemical, immune and cellular processes) and finally structure and functional organization or O. Systemic Medicine's (SM) treatment strategy is based on identifying and prescribing superior herbs—tonic or adaptogenic—or any nutraceuticals or medicine with potential to strengthen E, I, O by providing energo, informational and organizational aid to the overall network of intelligent cells and cell systems that constitute the body. The main premise proposes that when all three factors are brought back to ideal levels patients' conditions begin recovery to normal health. Table 2 provides a list of some E, I and O ceuticals -or superior medicines- whose capacity to enhance E, I and O have been studied and referenced.

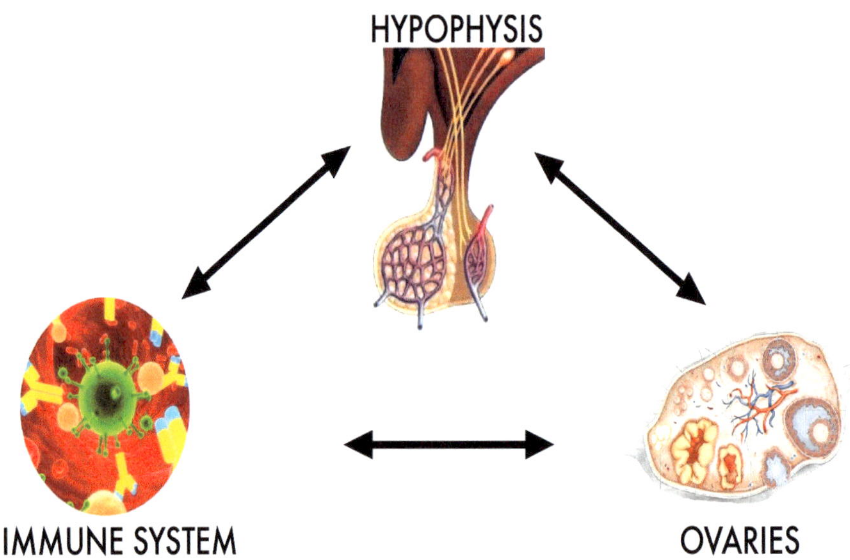

Fig. 5. An example of known cross-talk communication, bidirectional and bi-conditional, between the I^I (immune intelligence), C^I (cellular intelligence) and B^I (biochemical or neuroendocrine intelligence) in a human living system.

E-Energoceuticals that enhance mitochondrial ATP synthesis and resynthesis		**I- Infoceuticals that enhance biointelligence on cellular, neuroendocrine and immune levels**		**O-Organoceuticals that specifically enhance organ function and structure**	
Names	References	Names	References	Names	References
Acantopanacis senticosus	Wu *et al.* Gaffney *et al.*	*Uncaria tomentosa*	Sheng *et al* ; Akesson *et al.*	*Glycyrrhiza glabra*	Acharya *et al.*
Cornu Cervi pantotrichum	Kim KS *et al.* Zhang *et al.*	*Aloe vera*	Kim HS *et al.*	*Curcuma Longa*	Chainani-Wu
Ilex paraguariensis	Gorgen *et al.*	*Andrographis paniculata*	Matsuda *et al* ; Puri *et al.*	*Ulmus fulva*	Brown *et al.*
Lepidium meyenii	Lopez-Fando *et al.*	*Astragalus membranaceus*	Wang *et al* ; Shao *et al.*	*Angelica sinensis*	Mei *et al*; Yin
Ocimum sanctum	Agrawal *et al.*	*Croton lechleri*	Risco *et al.*	*Chondroitin/ glucosamine*	Houpt *et al.*
Panax ginseng	Yang *et al.*	*Echinacea purpurea and E. angustifolia*	Randolph *et al.*, Cundell	*Chitin fiber*	Jing *et al.*
Panax quinquefolius	Wang *et al.*	*Ganoderma lucidum*	Kohguchi *et al* ; Jiang *et al.*	*Crataegus oxyacantha*	Rigelsky and Sweet ; Lacaille-Dubois *et al.*
Pfaffia paniculata	Kotsiuruba *et al*; Tashmukhamedova *et al.*	*Grifola frondosa*	Odama *et al* ; Lin *et al.*	*Dioscorea villosa*	Shealy; Ladriere *et al.*
Ptychopetalum olacoides	Siqueira *et al.*	*Hydrastis canadensis*	Rehman *et al.*	*Plants enzymes*	Popiela *et al.*
Rhaponticum carthamoides	Kutuzova *et al.*	*Morinda citrifolia*	Su *et al.*	*Equisetum arvense*	Blumenthal *et al*; Fleming
Rhodiola rosea	Maslova *et al* ; Spasov *et al.*	*Petiveria alliacea*	Ruffa *et al*; Malpezzi *et al.*	*Ginkgo bilova*	Kubota *et al* ; Pepe *et al.*
Schizandra chinensis	Antoshechkin	*Sutherlandia frutescens*	Bence and Crooks; Jang *et al.*	*Gotu kola*	Incandela *et al.*
l-arginine	Gupta *et al.*	*Tabebuia avellaneda*	Planchon *et al*; Li *et al.*	*Sargassum fusiforme*	Ji *et al.*
Ubiquinone (Coenzyme Q10)	Baggio *et al.*	*Valeriana officinalis*	Dietz *et al.*	*Harpagophytum procumbens*	Chrubasik *et al.*
		Vitex agnus castus	Kobayakawa and Sato-Nishimori; Ohyama *et al.*	*Vitamins*	Carrero *et al.*
		Lentinus edodes	Borchers *et al*; Wasser and Weis	*Minerals*	Hercberg *et al.*
		Coriolus versicolor	Sun and Zhu, Sun *et al.*	*Ptycopetalum olacoides*	Bucci; Siqueira *et al.*

E-Energoceuticals that enhance mitochondrial ATP synthesis and resynthesis	I- Infoceuticals that enhance biointelligence on cellular, neuroendocrine and immune levels		O-Organoceuticals that specifically enhance organ function and structure	
	Cordyceps sinensis	Leu *et al.*	*Pygeum africanum*	Freeman and Solomon, Santa Maria Margalef *et al.*
			Rhamnus purshiana	Ma et al.
			Ruscus aculeatus	Redman, Bouaziz *et al.*
			Salix alba	Chrubasik *et al.*
			Sena alejandrina	Franz
			Serenoa repens	Goldmann *et al* ; Iguchi
			Silibum marianum	Halim *et al*; Chrungoo *et al.*
			Smilax china	Lee *et al.*
			Tribulus terrestris	Hong *et al.*
			Vaccinium myrthillus	Zaragoza *et al*; Savickiene *et al.*
			Viburnum spp.	Calle *et al.*
			Zingiber officinalis	Young *et al.*

Table 2. Examples of ceuticals -or superior medicines- whose capacity to enhance E, I and O has been studied and referenced

2.5.1 The case for a systemic complex herbal formulation: Circulat

Thus a composition was formulated taking into account the precepts established in both the Systemic Theory and Medicine. Circulat is a systemic standardized HPLC fingerprinted plant extract combination which consists of: 1) Energy plants (**E**) associated with ATP synthesis (such as tricarboxylic acid cycle, oxidative phosphorylation, etc) which boost the system's energy-work capacity: *Eleutherococcus senticosus, Leuzea carthamoides, Panax ginseng, Panax quinquefolius, Pfaffia paniculata,* and *Rhodiola rosea*; 2) Bio-Intelligence plants (**I**) which modulate the neuroendocrine and immunological systems and cellular processes enhancing the system's informational potential intelligence (specifically in this formulation they increase insulin production, insulin receptor sensitivity, improve intracellular glucose uptake, contribute anti-microbial properties, improve inflammation as well as humoral and unspecific cellular immunity): *Echinacea angustifolia, Echinacea purpurea, Ganoderma lucidum, Grifola frondosa, Hydrastis canadensis, Petiveria alliacea, Sutherlandia frutescens,* and *Uncaria tomentosa;* and finally 3) Organizational plants (**O**) which enhance the structure and functional organization of specific organs supporting overall health (in Circulat's case, among others, promoting vasodilatation, tissular perfusion improvement, regeneration and skin scarring): *Angelica sinensis, Crataegus oxyacantha, Croton lechleri, Ginkgo biloba, Hydrocotyle asiatica, Ruscus aculeatus, Vaccinium myrthillus,* and *Tabebuia avellanedae.* Although some of these plants act predominantly over one of the factors that influence individual's overall health (E, I, and O), some act over more than one factor (i.e. *Panax* and *Ganoderma*). Please, see Table 3.

Energy plants	
Panax ginseng and *Panax quinquefolius*	Increases ATP synthesis by stimulating activities of enzymes related to tricarboxylic acid cycle and oxidative-phosphorylation, such as succinate dehydrogenase, malate dehydrogenase, citrate synthetase, cytochrome oxidase, and phosphorylase (Wang *et al;*, 2003).
Eleutherococcus senticosus	Increases ATP synthesis by stimulating activities of enzymes related to tricarboxylic acid cycle, such as succinate dehydrogenase and malate dehydrogenase (Sugimura *et al.*, 1989).
Leuzea carthamoides and *Pfaffia paniculata*	Increase ATP synthesis, stimulates activities of enzymes related to tricarboxylic acid cycle, such as succinate dehydrogenase. Also, normalize NADH dehydrogenase activity, enzyme related to the oxidative phosphorylation processes, contributing to buildup the electrochemical potential used to produce ATP (Tashmukhamedova *et al.*, 1986).
Rhodiola rosea	Activates ATP synthesis/resynthesis in mitochondria, stimulates reparative energy processes (Abidov *et al.*; 2003).
Anti-inflamatory-Inmunostimulant plants (Immune Intelligence)	
Tabebuia avellanedae	Inhibits NO, iNOS, COX-2 and PGE(2) release. Attenuates expression of mRNA and pro-inflammatory cytokines proteins, such as interleukin (IL)-1beta, IL-6 and tumor necrosis factor (TNF)-alpha. Suppresses NF-kappaB activation by blocking IkappaBalpha degradation and downregulating ERK, p38 mitogen-activated protein kinase (MAPK) and Akt pathway (Moon *et al.*, 2007).
Echinacea angustifolia and *Echinacea purpurea*	Due to: a) reduction of IL-2 production (Sasagawa *et al.*, 2006); and b) down-regulation of COX-2 expression (Groom *et al*, 2007). Immune-stimulant due to: a) macrophage phagocytosis stimulation (Raso *et al.*, 2002); b) cellular immunity and neutrophils' phagocytosis stimulation. Increases number of leucocytes and lymphocytes, especially T lymphocytes (Jurkstiene *et al.*, 2004); c) Significant enhancement of IgM specific antibody forming cell response (Freier *et al.*, 2003); d) complement properdin increases (Kim *et al.*, 2002).
Ganoderma lucidum	Promotes phagocytosis and cytotoxicity of macrophages (Zhu *et al.*, 2007).
Grifola frondosa	Antiinflamatory: because it inhibits cyclooxygenase (COX) enzyme (Zhang *et al.*, 2002). Inmunoestimulant because it: Increases IL-10, NO and IFN-gamma. Enhances both the innate and adaptive arms of the immune response (Kodama *et al.*, 2004).
Hydrastis canadensis	Antiinflamatory due to a prostaglandin E2 production reduction as a result of AP-1 binding inhibition (Kuo *et al.*, 2004).
Sutherlandia frutescens	Antiinflamatory, inhibits COX-2 and through activation of activator protein-1 (AP-1) (Kundu *et al.*, 2005).
Uncaria tomentosa	Antiinflamatory achieved by a TNFalpha and PGE2 production inhibition (Piscoya *et al.*, 2001). Inmunostimulant because it stimulates macrophage phagocytosis (Groom *et al.*, 2007).
Panax ginseng and *Panax quinquefolius*	Antiinflamatory: It inhibit iNOS and COX-2 protein expression, and activates the transcription factor, NF-kappaB (Park *et al.*, 2004). Inmunomodulator: Increases neutrophiles and macrophages phagocytosis, stimulates humoral and cell immune factors and induces important regulating cytokins—interferone gamma and tumor necrosis factor (Smolina *et al.*, 2001).

Eleutherococcus senticosus	Inmunoestimulant: Activates B cells and macrophages (Han *et al.*, 2003).
Pfaffia paniculata	Increases macrophage activity (Pinello *et al.*, 2006)
Angelica sinensis	Immunomodulatory activity by regulating expression of Th1 and Th2 related cytokines (Yang *et al.*, 2006).
Hypoglycemic plants (Biochemical Intelligence)	
Panax ginseng	Reduces blood glucose levels (Reay *et al.*, 2005). Inhibits glycated hemoglobin formation (Bae and Lee, 2004).
Panax quinquefolius	Decreases postprandial glicemia (Vuksan *et al.*, 2000)
Eleutherococcus senticosus	Lowers circulating glucose and lipids, and enhances insulin action (Park *et al.*, 2006). Improves insulin sensitivity (Liu *et al.*, 2005).
Ganoderma lucidum	Stimulates glucose uptake, stimulating the activity of phosphatidylinositol 3-kinase, Protein kinase B, AMP-activated protein kinase which are regulatory molecules in the glucose uptake pathway (Jung *et al.*, 2006). Lowers glucose levels through insulin-releasing activity due to facilitation of Ca2+ inflow to pancreatic beta cells (Zhang and Lin, 200 4).
Grifola frondosa	Decreases fasting plasma glucose levels and increases insulin sensitivity (Hong *et al.*, 2007).
Hydrastis canadensis	Stimulates glucose uptake via: increasing GLUT1 activity and adenosine monophosphate-activated protein kinase and acetyl-coenzyme A carboxylase phosphorylation (Zhou *et al.*, 2007); and through AMP-AMPK-p38 MAPK pathway (Cheng *et al.*, 2006). Inhibitor of aldose reductase (Feng *et al.*, 2005).
Petiveria alliacea	Decreases: a) blood glucose levels (Lores and Cires Puyol, 1990); and b) fasting glucose, post-prandial glucose levels, and hemoglobin A1c in type 2 diabetic patients, by acting downstream in the insulin signaling pathway (Kim *et al.*, 2007).
Sutherlandia frutescens	Normalizes insulin levels and increases glucose uptake (Chadwick *et al.*, 2007). Decreases fasting glucose, post-prandial glucose levels, and hemoglobin A1c in type 2 diabetic patients, by acting downstream in the insulin signaling pathway (Kim *et al.*, 2007).
Antimicrobial and Skin Scarring plants (Organization)	
Tabebuia avellanedae	Antibacterial activity against methicillin-resistant S. aureus, S. epidermidis and S. haemolyticus strains, being the two last ones hetero-resistant to vancomycin (Pereira *et al.*, 2006).
Petiveria alliacea	Broad spectrum of antimicrobial activity (Kim *et al.*, 2006).
Hydrastis canadensis	Broad spectrum of antimicrobial activity (Scazzocchio *et al.*, 2001).
Sutherlandia frutescens	Antibacterial against against S. aureus, E. faecalis and E. coli (Katerere and Elfo, 2005).
Uncaria tomentosa	Antimicrobial activity on Enterobacteriaceae, S. mutans and Staphylococcus spp. (Ccahuana-Vasquez *et al.*, 2007).
Croton lechleri	Potent anti-bacterial activity (Chen *et al.*, 1994). Cicatrizant effect because it increases the migration of skin fibroblasts (Vaisberg *et al.*, 1989).
Hydrocotyle asiatica	Promotes fibroblast proliferation and extracullar matrix synthesis in wound healing because it upregulates 54 genes with known functions for cell proliferation, cell-cycle progression and synthesis of the extracellular matrix (Lu *et al.*, 2004).

Table 3. Circulat´s E, I and O –referenced- components and action mechanisms.

3. Assessment of Circulat´s capability to modulate diabetes related gene expression levels in cultured human fibroblasts

Circulat had provided an auspicious early clinical proof of its effectiveness (Olalde *et al.*, 2005) in the treatment of Diabetic Foot –a circulatory disease. However, a pending assignment was to confirm its molecular activity. One way to test this characteristic was to identify the modulating and/or synergistic roles that such formulation could have in diseases such as Diabetes Mellitus (I and II). The study called 'Analysis of the Effects of the Herbal preparation Circulat on Gene Expression Levels in Cultured Human Fibroblasts' was carried out in cooperation with the Pennsylvania State University, Department of Genetics (Antoshechkin *et al.*, 2007).

3.1 Materials and methods

Circulat whole composition -a lyophilized ethanol/water extract of 22 known medical plants in different ratios- and its three E, I and O fractions (or components 1, 2 and 3) identical and in the same proportion as in the formula were tested using microarray analysis using the Affymetrix GeneChip Human Genome U133 Plus 2.0 arrays that provide full genomic coverage and contain probes for more than 47 000 unique transcripts corresponding to more than 38 500 human genes. This allowed monitoring simultaneously the expression levels of practically all annotated genes of the human genome in an unbiased manner. Following hybridization and scanning, raw data in the form of image files were converted to gene expression files using the Affimetrix GeneChip Operating Software (GCOS) which utilizes MAS 5.0 algorithm for data normalization, background subtraction, and the estimation of nonspecific binding, calculation of detection p-values and generation of presence calls. Two-tailed Taylor Student's t-test assuming unequal sample variance was used to identify genes that displayed significant changes in the mean expression levels between control and each of the treated samples with the t-test-p value less than 0.05 and the mean fold change of at least 2. By comparing up and down regulated genes in each individual fraction and whole Circulat, additional genes were identified that were regulated between 1.5 and 2 fold in the whole preparation and followed the same trend as in individual fractions, where they were up -or down-regulated by at least 2 fold.

3.1.1 Results

The Affymetrix GeneChip represents state of the art in microarray design and features both perfectly matched and off-by-one probes that together with sophisticated processing algorithm allow distinguishing precisely between specific and non-specific hybridization signals. It has been proven to produce highly reliable data, which in combination with the high quality of starting RNA and sufficient number of replicates virtually eliminates false-positives. Significant changes in the mean expression levels between control and treated samples resulted in a list of 87, 96, 24 and 187 genes (probes) that were significantly up - or down- regulated upon treatment with components 1, 2, 3 and whole Circulat, respectively. The genes regulated by the individual components and the whole Circulat formula showed a significant overlap, as expected. More than 80% of the genes affected by the individual fractions were also affected by the whole preparation. Analysis of the data for each of the three components also identifies a sizable number of genes (23) that did not show up in the whole Circulat analysis. On the other hand, 55 genes the expression of which changed significantly after Circulat treatment were not observed in any of the three fractions. The regulation of these 32 genes by Circulat is more likely due to the interaction between active ingredients of the three components that produce a synergistic effect on gene regulation. Taken together the data demonstrates that: 1) Treatment of human fibroblast cells with either Circulat or its components result in marked changes in gene expression patterns; 2) Significant interactions between the active ingredients of Circulat exist resulting in a more complex pattern of gene expression in the complete preparation when compared with those of the isolated components which can be understood to be synergistic. Figure 6.

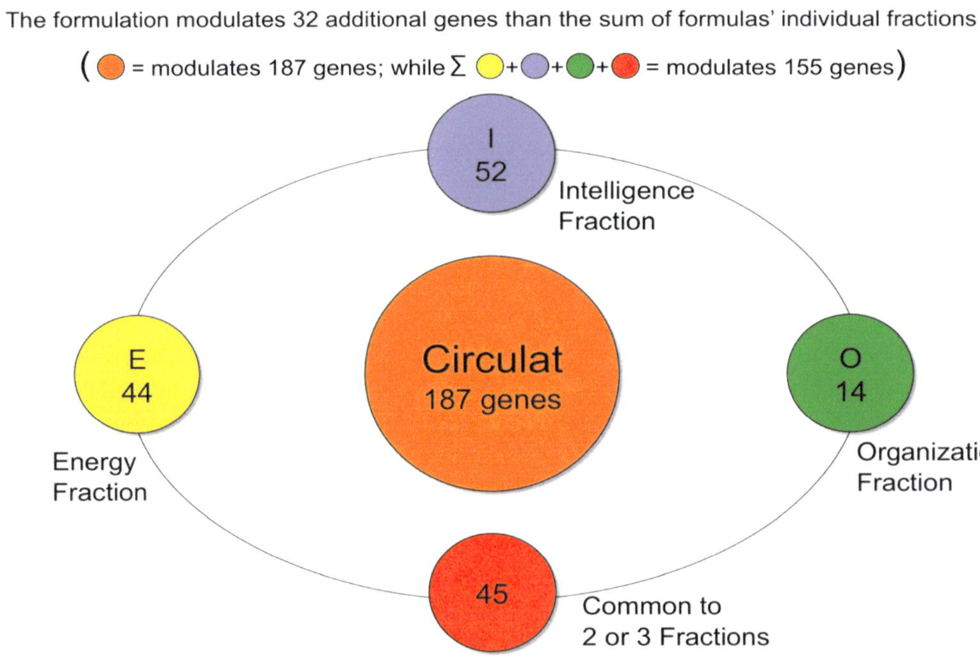

Fig. 6. Circulat -as a whole- modulates 187 genes, 32 genes more than the sum of the E, I and O fractions that make it up.

3.1.2 Analysis of processes and pathway affected by circulat

Examination of the biological process subset of Gene Ontology (GO) terms (Ashburner *et al.*, 2000) associated with each gene and their distribution revealed that genes affected by Circulat are involved in a variety of cellular processes including protein, nucleic acid, lipid and carbohydrate metabolism, regulation of transcription, response to endogenous and external stimuli and stress, signal transduction and cell communication, cell growth and proliferation, development, protein modification and biosynthesis, generation of precursor metabolites and energy, etc. The broad spectrum of processes potentially regulated by Circulat (Figure 7) is consistent with the established ability of Circulat to prevent the development of severe manifestations of type 2 diabetes, which is a complex syndrome involving many intracellular signaling cascades and pathways as well as cell-cell interactions.

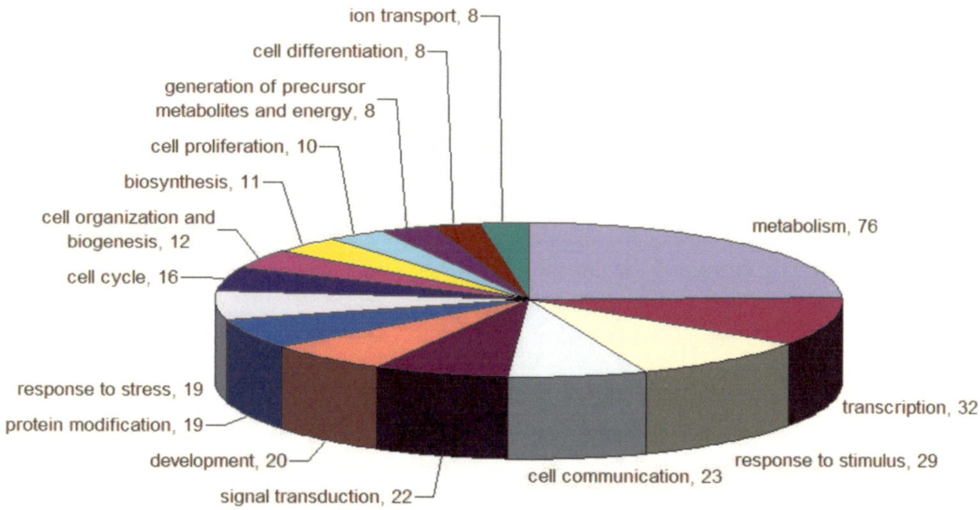

Fig. 7. Number of genes involved in a particular process that were affected by treatment is indicated. Numbers correspond to the number of probes that are annotated within a particular process.

Many of those pathways are involved in energy generation and are regulated on both transcriptional and post-transcriptional levels in response to endogenous or exogenous stimuli. A high proportion of genes identified in the experiments are implicated in the regulation of transcription (e.g.ATF3, Kruppel-like factor 4 Zinc finger protein 117, SATB2), energy production and glucose metabolism (thioredoxin domain containing 11, ATP5F1, PGK1) and signal transduction corroborating the hypothesis that Circulat is capable of normalizing molecular processes perturbed in the course of type 2 diabetes. Specially, Circulat proves to be effective in the treatment of diabetic gangrene, which is often resistant to common treatments. Previous studies have suggested that impaired fibroblast function such as proliferation, cell migration, growth factor production and collagen synthesis may be part of the mechanism of diabetic necrotic damage. Fibroblasts are central to the processes of extracellular matrix deposition and remodeling that take place during tissue repair process. It functions both as a synthetic cell, depositing a collagen-rich matrix, and a signaling cell, secreting the growth factors important for cell-cell communication during the tissue repair process. Many Circulat-regulated genes play roles in signal transduction and cell communication (ADAM32, TRIO, RAB7), response to endogenous and exogenous stimuli, an essential component in wound healing (FANCB, SLC19A2, C4A), growth factor-mediated signaling and cell motility (IL6, CXCL2, VIM), cell proliferation and biosynthesis (PBEF1, ABP1, PTGS2) corroborating Circulat's effectiveness in tissue repair. Furthermore, tissue remodeling involves both the generation of new cell types as well as regulated cell death, and several genes important for cell differentiation and apoptosis were identified in the experiment (KLF4, RTN1,

PDCD5). It was also observed that significantly down-regulated genes are enriched for members of signaling cascades known to regulate transcription and progression through the mitotic cycle such as FOSB, SNF1-like kinase and PRKAR1A (cAMP-dependent protein kinase regulatory subunit), cyclin L2. Up-regulated genes also contain a high number of genes involved in progression through the cell cycle as well as in DNA damage response, including cyclin M. GTSE1, FANCB and BR1P1 (BRCA1 interacting protein C-terminal helicase 1), cyclin-dependent kinase inhibitor C2 (CDKN2C). A number of transcription factors and members of protein degradation machinery (ubiquitin-conjugating enzyme E2E 3, Ring finger and WD repeat domain 2) are also present among those genes. Data suggest that one of the reasons for Circulat's therapeutic effects is derived from its ability to stimulate cellular activities that respond to internal and external stress by slowing or arresting the cell cycle to allow repair of cellular components that could be damaged in the course of the disease, such as DNA and proteins, to be carried out by repair enzymes.

3.2 Discussion

It was shown that four genes, IL6, HMGA1, SLC19A2 and C4A that are known to be involved in the development and progression of diabetes are strongly regulated by Circulat. This not only validated the experimental approach, but also allowed for the first time to suggest an explanation for the clinical effectiveness of Circulat at the molecular level. The role of interleukin-6 (1L6) in diabetes type 1 and 2 is thoroughly documented (for a review see Kristiansen and Mandrup-Poulsen, 2005). Low-grade inflammation has been proposed to be involved in the pathogenic processes causing type 2 diabetes and inflammatory mechanisms are known to play a key role in the pathogenesis of type 1 diabetes. As a mediator of inflammation, IL6 is thought to be involved in events causing both types of the disease when present at elevated levels. In addition, IL6 can also regulate glucose homeostasis and metabolism directly and indirectly by both increasing the destruction of insulin producing β-cells by promoting apoptosis and playing a role in mounting insulin resistance in skeletal muscle, adipocytes and other tissues. Since elevated levels of IL6 are the known predisposition factors for development of diabetes, reduction of IL6 concentration should have the opposite therapeutic effect. The results demonstrate that Circulat treatment reduces IL6 expression more than two fold. (0.42, $p = 0.002$) providing a solid link between the molecular events and the clinical manifestations taking place upon Circulat treatment. HMGA1 expression levels were elevated by more than two fold (2.07, $p = 0.02$) in samples treated with Circulat. Mutations in this small nuclear protein that acts as an architectural transcription factor have been detected in individuals suffering from type 2 diabetes (Foti *et al.,* 2005). This correlated with the insulin receptor's expression reduction and consequent development of insulin resistance. Deletion of HMGA1 gene in mice resulted in almost a complete loss of insulin receptor expression, development of insulin resistance and type 2 diabetes-like symptoms. HMGA1 thus plays a crucial role in glucose homeostasis and its increased expression promoted by Circulat may counteract deleterious effects caused by the loss of insulin receptor observed in type 2 diabetic patients. Two other genes, SLC19A2 and C4A, that are affected by Circulat (0.43, $p = 0.03$ and 0.48, $p = 0.02$, respectively) have also been unequivocally linked to diabetes. SLC19A2 encodes a thiamine transporter protein and causes thiamine-responsive megaloblastic anemia (TRMA) also known as Rogers syndrome, when mutated (Labay *et al.*, 1999). Diabetes (both type 1 and 2) is the primary disease that defines the syndrome. C4A encodes the acidic form of complement factor 4, part of the classical activation pathway. Deficiency of this protein is associated with systemic lupus erythematosus and type 1 diabetes mellitus (Palsdottir *et al.*, 1983). While no direct link between C4A and diabetes type 2 has been found thus far, it has been suggested that the two types of the disease share many of the underlying processes thus making C4A involvement in type 2 diabetes a real possibility. Precise molecular mechanisms of SLC19A2 and C4A involvement in the disease development are not established as well as for IL6 and HMGA1. Nevertheless, their link to diabetes is indisputable and the ability of Circulat to influence their expression suggests additional possible Circulat action mechanisms. Analysis of genes affected by Circulat also reveals that 26 of them have been implicated in many human diseases other than diabetes. It is possible that some of those diseases and syndromes could be caused by misregulation of the same (or similar) genetic pathways that are perturbed in type 2 diabetes, which could be one of the explanations for this observation. On the other hand, it raises an exciting possibility that Circulat could be effective for treatment of conditions other than type 2 diabetes. Finally, analysis of genes regulated by the total Circulat and its individual components demonstrated the existence of significant interactions between the active ingredients of Circulat suggesting that the full therapeutic effects can only be achieved by administration of the complete preparation.

3.3 Significance of gene expression analyses

The application of full-genome expression analyses to phytopharmacology opens new horizons for carrying out scientific studies of herbal remedies and integration of herbal-based treatments into mainstream medicine. Using this approach, the physiologically active fractions of effective herbal extracts can be isolated and their specific activities can be determined. Such separation of different activities of a particular extract may enable researchers to selectively regulate the expression of specific genes (or gene groups) by varying the composition of the herbal preparation. It is likely therefore, that expression-profiling-based approaches to studies of herbal medicines will become standard in phytopharmacology in the near future. This section, explained Circulat´s molecular modulating capabilities. Section 4 will examine its clinical effectiveness through a diabetic foot study synthesis.

4. Circulat´s therapeutic properties in diabetic foot: Synthesis

The World Health Organization estimated that more than 220 million people worldwide have diabetes (WHO, 2011). This number was likely to more than double by 2030. Diabetic foot ulcers are one of the most frequent complications of this disease. The prevalence of diabetic foot ulcers has been estimated, at the time of the study, between 2.2 and 15%. Differences being attributed to risk factor diversity: ethnicity, age, sex, education level, health service quality, and others (Table 4). Diabetic foot ulcers represent a large emotional and economic burden on patients and caregivers, as well (Gulam-Abbas *et al*, 2002). Foot complications are caused by diabetic neuropathy or peripheral ischemic vessel disease or a combination of both (Ratzmann *et al*, 1994) and are the most frequent reason for hospitalization in patients with diabetes.

Diabetic foot ulcers prevalence	Country	References
2.2 %	UK	Abbott *et al*, 2002
3-8%	Sweden	Apelqvist and Larsson, 2000
4.6%	Kenya	Nyamu *et al*, 2003
5.3-5.6%	Finland	Lehto *et al*, 1996
5.4 - 7.3%	USA	Moss *et al*, 1996
10.2%	Sri Lanka	Fernando, 1996
15%	Tanzania	Gulam-Abbas *et al*, 2002

Table 4. Examples of diabetic foot ulcer prevalence by country and references

Diabetic foot complications are the most common cause of non-traumatic lower extremity amputations in the industrialized world. The risk of lower extremity amputation is 15 to 46 times higher in diabetics than in persons who do not have diabetes mellitus (Armstrong, 1997). Approximately 40-60% of all lower extremity amputations are performed in patients with diabetes. More than 85% of these amputations are precipitated by a foot ulcer deteriorating to deep infection or gangrene (Apelqvist and Larsson, 2000). In people with healed diabetic foot ulcers, the 5 year cumulative rate of ulcer recurrence is 66% and of amputation is 12% (Apelqvist *et al.*, 1993). The high amputation incidence and healing failure after lower extremity amputation for the treatment of diabetic foot ulcer (Malay *et al.*, 2006) is a distinct signal that the efficiency of conventional medical treatments used is less than optimal. This substantiates the need to search for effective therapeutic alternatives and diminish the suffering and high economic and social costs caused by this common diabetic patient complication. Various medicinal plants have been used traditionally for the treatment of circulatory obstructive diseases. In the last couple of decades many of their active principles and action mechanisms have been discovered. Also, traditional healing know-how has been proven to be effective in many cases. This raised the possibility of using herbal therapeutic protocols to complement conventional treatments for complications in diabetes. Specially, since there was mounting evidence which demonstrated that medicinal plants contained synergistic and/or side-effect neutralizing combinations (Thyagarajan *et al.*, 2007; Gilani and Rahman, 2005). In contrast to synthetic pharmaceuticals based upon single chemicals, phytomedicines exert their beneficial effects through the additive or synergistic action of their multitude of constituents acting at single or multiple target sites (Dalby-Brown *et al.*, 2005); because of their primary and secondary metabolite roles (Greenspan *et al.*, 1994) and the adjuvant substances which enhance the activity of components actually responsible for the effect (Gilbert *et al.*, 2003). In order to take the maximum advantage of the therapeutic properties as well as benefits of the synergistic action of the active principles in medicinal plants, it is necessary to use herbal combinations. Herbal formulations have been used for hundreds of years, however, little was known about the methodology to combine plants and obtain effective compositions. The Systemic Theory provided fundamentals which allowed the formulation of an effective herbal composition for treating diabetic foot (Olalde, 2005; Olalde *et al.*, 2005). The previous section revealed that Circulat's active principles exerted therapeutic effects through a synergistic action, as well as its potential for genetic normalization in diabetic patients (Antoshechkin *et al.*, 2007).

4.1 Objective, research design and methods

The aim was to appraise the clinical efficacy of Circulat in healing diabetic foot, measure the amputation rate and determine patient's tolerance to the treatment. Thus, a retrospective, cohort, study of patients with type 2 diabetes and foot ulcerations from 50 medical centers, from 2004 to 2007. Patients were classified in accordance with The University of Texas Health Science Center Diabetic Wound Classification System (Lavery *et al.*, 1997). Patients were being administered ten Circulat 800 mg capsules twice per day, on an outpatient basis, during a period of two to four months. Each case was followed-up during a period of six months, after the end of the treatment. A patient was considered to attain clinical improvement if the lesion visibly decreased in size and depth, or closure or scarring of the wound was attained. All patients received conventional treatment for metabolism correction, local topic cures and systemic antibiotics. The Inclusion criteria of the study were: Patients of any age and gender diagnosed with Diabetes mellitus type 2, grades D1, D2 and D3 (University of Texas Diabetic Wound classification).

4.1.1 Results and discussion

The total number of patients which completed the treatment in accordance with the study's inclusion criteria was 174. The mean was 61.3 years of age. The gender classification was: 101 male (58.1%) and 73 female (41.9%). Clinical results are reflected in Table 5. Amputations were prevented in 88.55% ($p < 0.00001$, 99.9999%) of all 174 patients in the D1-D3 categorization. The treatment was well tolerated; only 4 patients (2.3%) had minor gastrointestinal unrest which did not warrant treatment suspension. Conventional diabetic foot treatments, based on: risk factors control, affected area's functional relaxation, metabolism correction, topical cures, antibiotics, rheology improving agents, prostanoid vasoactive therapy, platelet aggregation inhibitors, thrombolytic agents, tricyclic antidepressants or benzodiacepines for neuropathies and invasive treatments, such as endovascular, endarterectomy, by-pass or sympathectomy surgeries, do not manage to prevent small and large amputations which occur in 1.86 to 5.9 per every 1.000 diabetics per year (Bilenko et al, 2006; Winell et al, 2006; Rayman et al, 2004; Lavery et al, 2003; Trautner *et al*, 2001). Circulat- in combination with conventional therapy- prevented more amputations than various conventional treatments reported (Figure 8).

University of Texas Diabetic Wound classification Grade	N	Total scarring	Improvement	Total scarring + Improvement	Amputation
D1: Infected ischemic superficial wounds, no tendon, capsule, or bone.	88	52 (59.09%)	36 (40.9%)	88/88 (100%)	-
D2: Infected ischemic wounds, penetrating to tendon or capsule.	80	32 (40%)	30 (37.5%)	62/80 (77.5%)	18/80 (22.5%)
D3: Infected ischemic wounds, penetrating to bone or joint.	6	4 (66.6%)	-	4/6 (66.6%)	2/6 (33.3%)
Total	174	88 (50.57%)	66 (37.9%)	154/174 (88.5%)	20/174 (11.5%)

Table 5. Results of Circulat treatment in Diabetic foot

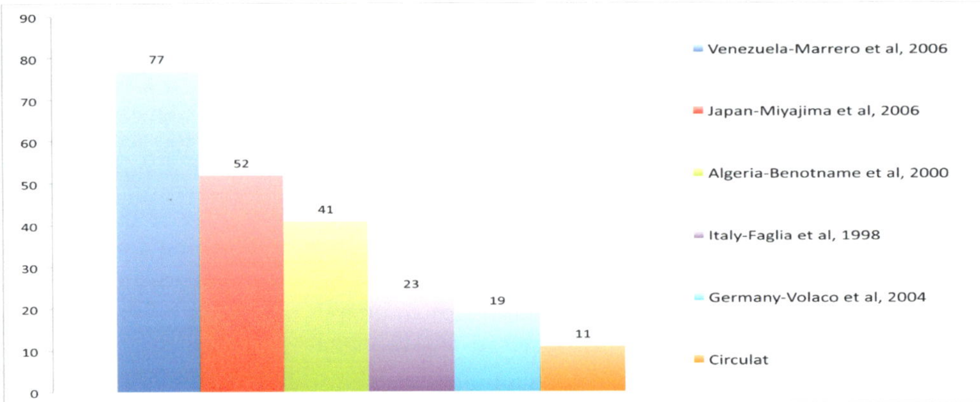

Fig. 8. Examples of Diabetic Foot Amputation rates (%) in various countries

5. Formulation´s potential in chronic ischemic heart disease treatment

Context: The previous clinical study (Olalde *et al.*, 2008) demonstrated a significant improvement in 174 diabetic foot patients. These encouraging outcomes and further evidence that other complex herbal formulations could help reduce atherosclerotic endothelium intima thickness (Tripathi *et al.*, 2005) prompted us to evaluate the formulation by measuring the arterial intima-media thickness, a structural marker of early atherosclerosis that relates to the severity and extent of artery disease (Järvisalo *et al.*, 2001), using high-resolution ultrasound (Celermajer *et al.*, 1992). The study (unpublished) showed that treatment with this herbal combination significantly reduced the arterial intima-media thickness. These results further encouraged the formulation of a new hypothesis: could similar results be obtained in the treatment of IHD? If so, is there a potential for CAM complex herbal formulations' intervention in the treatment of Ischemic Heart Disease? Objective: Assess the hypothesis that myocardial perfusion, in chronic ischemic heart disease patients, might safely improve with Circulat. This was evaluated with Gated Single Photon Emission Computerized Tomography (GSPECT) imaging.

5.1 Introduction

Ischemic heart disease (IHD) is the leading cause of death -in both genders- worldwide and a major public health problem in the world. WHO (2009) has estimated this to be 7.2 million deaths per year. IHD is the generic designation for a group of pathophysiologically related syndromes resulting from myocardial ischemia (an imbalance between supply -perfusion- and demand for oxygenated blood by the heart). IHD is caused by the atherosclerotic narrowing of one or more coronary arteries and endothelial dysfunction (Thadani, 2004, 2003, 1999). IHD brings oxygen insufficiency and reduces the availability of nutrients as well as the removal of metabolites. For this reason, IHD is generally less well tolerated by the heart than pure hypoxia, such as may be seen in severe anemia, cyanotic heart disease or advanced lung disease. Today much attention is being paid to Chronic Ischemic Heart Disease. This last is increasingly recognized as a dynamic condition. In addition to over acute myocardial infarction, which can precipitate at any time in patients with stable angina pectoris, clinical and sub-clinical ischemic events may accumulate and in the long term generate diverse states of chronic cardiac dysfunction. Repetitive episodes of ischemia, whether stress induced or spontaneous, symptomatic or silent, may progressively impair myocardial contractile performance through myocardial stunning or hibernation, and eventually lead to left ventricular remodeling and heart failure. Evidence is accumulating that genetic variability and altered gene and protein expressions contribute to clinical outcomes in ischemic heart disease. Severe ischemic heart disease remains a clinical challenge; many patients have undergone myocardial revascularization procedures due to the extension and diffuseness of the disease. Also, viable options are becoming available for the 'no option' patients with chronic IHD. Instead of revascularization of the highly diseased epicardial coronary arteries, scientists and clinicians are looking -among other- at providing symptomatic relief in these patients via a biological bypass such as a 'master' cardiac stem cell for intra-coronary and intra-myocardial injections (Bu *et al.*, 2009). Current treatments include pharmacological agents such as nitrates, aspirin, beta-adrenoceptor antagonists and calcium channel blockers as well as invasive therapies aimed at restoring blood flow, e.g. coronary artery bypass graft (CABG) and improved percutaneous coronary intervention - PCI (Tin-Hay *et al.*, 2010). On the other hand, various medicinal plants are being used - and researched- for the treatment of coronary heart disease and angina pectoris in China and East Asia, and are referenced in *Chinese Materia Medica* (Tam *et al.*, 2009; Ling *et al.*, 2008; Duan *et al.*, 2008; Zhao *et al.*, 2007). This last does not preclude quite the contrary it demands, additional pharmacotherapy analysis and herbal medicines drug interaction research (Izzo *et al.*, 2005). Nevertheless, the study and development for synthetic (Yamaguchi *et al.*, 2009; Hirata *et al.*, 2009) and medicinal plant in cardiac treatments continues (Chen *et al.*, 2010; *Luo et al.*, 2009).

5.1.1 Study materials and methods

Inclusion Criteria: Patients diagnosed with Chronic Ischemic Cardiopathy. Exclusion Criteria: Acute Coronary Syndrome, severe aortic valve stenosis, arrhythmia with hemodynamic repercussion, acute pericarditis, acute myocarditis, decompensated cardiac insufficiency, acute aortic syndrome, severe anemia, pulmonary embolism, severe arterial hypertension, severe pulmonary arterial hypertension, chronic debilitating diseases, second or third degree atrioventricular block, hypertrophic obstructive cardiomyopathy and valvular cardiomyopathy with hemodynamic compromise. Patients: 20 patients diagnosed with Chronic Ischemic Heart Disease were evaluated. Prior to treatment, tests had determined that 4 of these patients had cardiac ischemia, assessed with cardiac angiography and non invasive methods, and the other 9 patients tested positive for cardiac ischemia with the exercise treadmill testing protocol (Bruce). Initial cardiac ischemia diagnosis was also corroborated by GSPECT control imaging prior to treatment. Patients were receiving treatment with aspirin, ß-blockers, statins, nitrates, clopidogrel and anti-hypertensive medication (diuretics, ACE inhibitors, angiotensin II receptor antagonists, calcium channel blockers). Patients were given a complete physical examination at screening, each month and at the end of the treatment (sixth month). The patients' baseline factors, relevant cardiac conditions and ongoing treatments were established in Table 6. The most pervasive baseline condition risk, evidenced from patients' clinical history (Table 6) was Hypercholesterolemia (14/20; 70%). On the other hand, the most common treatment was aspirin (17/20; 85%).

Description	Patient Number																			
	1	2	3	4	5	6	7	8	9	10	11	12	13	14	15	16	17	18	19	20
Gender	M	F	M	M	M	M	M	F	M	F	F	F	M	M	F	M	F	M	M	M
Age	68	78	69	64	67	41	61	57	59	73	75	53	58	48	66	80	67	57	59	68
Myocardial infarction	N	Y	N	Y	N	N	N	N	Y	Y	N	N	N	N	Y	Y	Y	Y	Y	Y
CABG	N	N	N	N	N	N	N	N	N	N	N	N	N	N	N	Y	N	N	N	N
PCI	N	N	N	N	N	N	Y	N	N	N	N	N	N	N	N	N	N	N	N	N
Diabetes	N	N	N	N	N	Y	N	N	N	N	N	N	N	N	N	Y	N	N	N	Y
Former smoker ≥ 30d	N	N	N	N	N	N	N	N	Y	N	N	N	Y	N	Y	N	N	N	Y	Y
Hypertension	N	Y	Y	Y	N	N	Y	N	Y	Y	N	N	N	N	Y	Y	Y	N	N	Y
Hypercholesterolemia	Y	Y	N	N	Y	Y	N	Y	N	Y	N	N	Y	Y	Y	Y	Y	Y	Y	Y
BAA	N	N	N	N	Y	Y	N	Y	Y	N	Y	N	N	N	Y	N	Y	N	N	Y
Statins	N	N	Y	Y	N	N	Y	N	N	Y	N	N	N	Y	Y	Y	Y	Y	Y	Y
Aspirin	Y	N	Y	N	Y	N	Y	Y	Y	Y	Y	Y	Y	Y	Y	Y	Y	Y	Y	Y
Oral Anti-diabetics	N	N	N	N	N	Y	N	N	N	N	N	N	N	N	N	Y	N	N	N	Y
ACEI or ARB	N	N	Y	N	N	Y	N	N	Y	N	Y	N	N	N	Y	Y	Y	N	N	Y
Ca^{2+}-channel antagonist	N	N	N	N	N	N	N	N	N	N	N	N	N	N	N	N	N	N	N	N
Diuretics	N	N	N	N	N	Y	N	N	Y	N	Y	N	N	N	Y	Y	Y	N	N	Y

Legends. ACEI: Angiotensin Converting Enzyme Inhibitor; **ARB:** Angiotensin -type I-Receptor Blocker; **BAA:** Beta Adrenoceptor Antagonists; **CABG:** Coronary Artery Bypass Graft; **d:** days, **Female:** F; **Male:** M; **N:** No; **PCI:** Percutaneous Coronary Intervention.
Y: Yes. All data determined from patients' clinical histories.

Table 6. Patients' Baseline Characteristics

Patients were instructed to receive ten 800 mg capsules b.i.d., of the herbal composition. Assessment of cardiac functions: The Bruce test, named after Dr. Robert A. Bruce, involves walking on a slanted treadmill while patient's time resistance is measured and the heart is monitored by an electrocardiograph. Patients' Pre -and Post- treatment, treadmill resistance time (Functional Capacity Time or FCT) were determined and reflected in Figure 9.

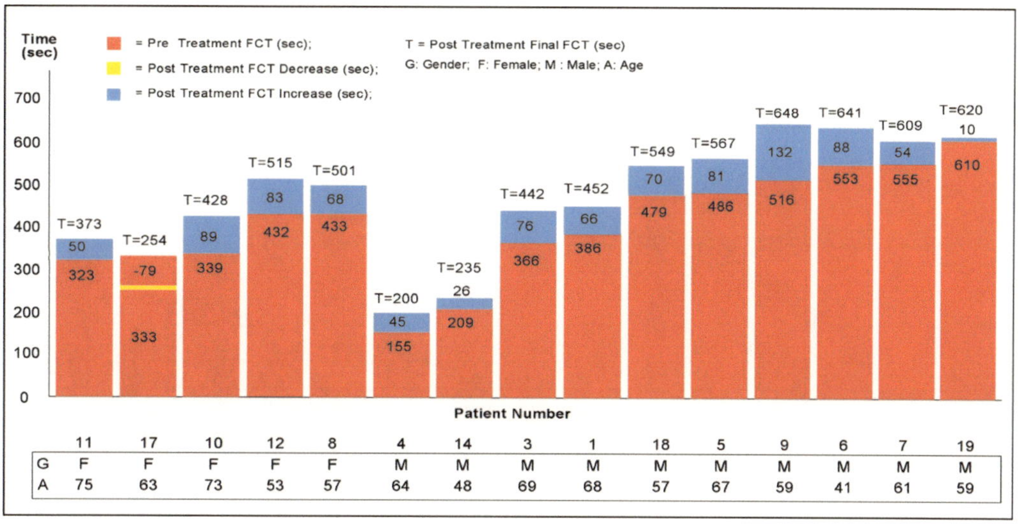

Note: Patients 2, 13, 15, 16 and 20 were unable to carry out the test due to physical limitations.

Fig. 9. Pre and Post (After) Treatment Functional Capacity Time per patient

5.2 Assessment of regional myocardial perfusion defect

Patient's -before and after Circulat treatment- post-effort -left ventricle- myocardial perfusion defect percentages were assessed by GSPECT imaging with technetium 99m-tetrofosmin injection. This technique uses imaging procedures for detection with the help of gamma rays. In the procedure, the radioisotope is used on the patient and the gamma ray emitted by the technetium 99 that is in the radioisotope is captured on a special gamma camera. The total scanning time for the heart of a patient takes around twenty minutes which is enough time given the half life span of technetium 99. This isotope has a short half life -about six hours- and this small longevity is very useful for medical purposes. Recollection of data [imaging] is quick and the amount of radiation which a patient undergoes through is very low in intensity. GSPECT myocardial perfusion imaging is a widely used nuclear imaging procedure for diagnosis and management of coronary artery disease -which is the most common cause of heart failure. It is extensively available with superb standardization and reproducibility (Chen *et al.*, 2008). For this study, the Phillips Forte (2007 model) AZ Spect Dual Headed Camera with an AUTOQUANT -quantitative algorithm- program for image processing was used. A 20 segment analysis was performed. Results of Perfusion Defect evolution are reflected in Figure 10.

5.2.1 Results

Clinical: Patients' Pre and Post Treatment Functional Capacity Time (treadmill evaluation) comparison (Figure 9) revealed that all patients who were physically capable to carry test out -except patient 17- improved their timed resistance [Female Improvement Median = 42.2 sec; Male Improvement Median = 64.8 sec]. Finally, patients' Post-Effort Left Ventricle Perfusion Defect imaging percentage values (Figure 10) were compared before and after six months treatment. Of the study group, 15 patients [75%] improved their perfusion defect. Statistics: The significance of the results was determined with the Wilcoxon Matched-Pairs Signed-Ranks Test ($p \leq 6.104$ e-05; %=99.9999). All statistical data was determined using

SPSS 17.0 for Windows. Adverse events: No patients suffered any adverse events during the treatment.

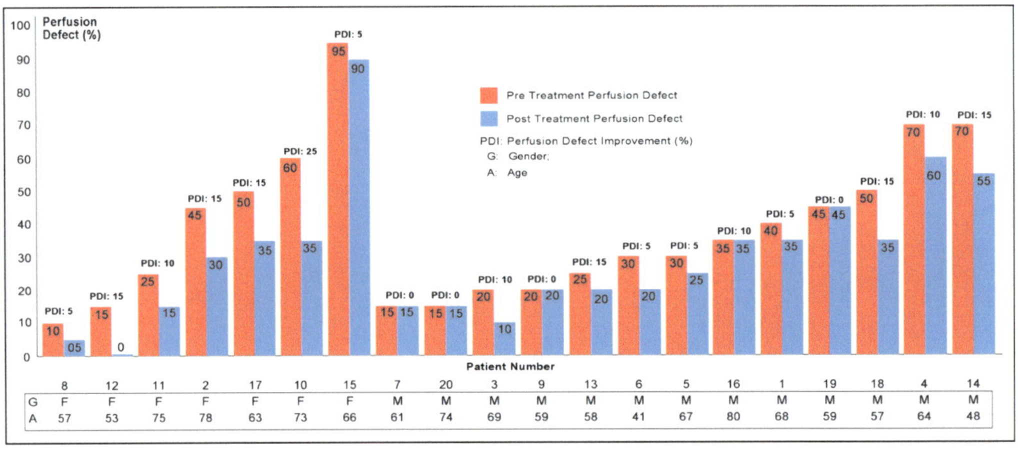

Fig. 10. Patient Cardiac Perfusion Defect Evolution (Ranked by age and gender)

5.3 Discussion on ischemic heart treatment

The results answered the formulated [raised] hypothesis. Indeed, CAM -and Circulat- can have a role in the treatment of Ischemic Chronic Heart Disease. This is supported by the number of patients (15 out of 20) which quantitatively improved their left ventricular perfusion capacity. Effects of this treatment are thought to be caused, among others, by vascular endothelium structure and function improvement, angiogenesis and tissue perfusion enhancement. Also to be noticed is patients' disease evolution according to initial perfusion defect -reflected in Figure 10. There seems to be a correlation suggesting that initial stages of ischemia development -corresponding to lower Pre-Treatment perfusion defect- are more precociously responsive to a short (6 month) treatment, thus advocating use of the formulation as a preventive remedy against chronic ischemic heart disease. **However, to measure the treatment's potential effectiveness, in patients with acute perfusion defect, a longer lasting treatment -of at least one year is necessary. Just as pathologies -with critical conditions- warrant longer management periods.**

6. Conclusions on chapter

A theory is as good as the praxis that backs it up. On one hand the gene expression study (Antoscheckin *et al*, 2007) established that a complex herbal formulation, designed in accordance with Systemic Theory precepts, had synergistic properties as well as the capacity to modulate genes implicated in diabetes development, energy metabolism, protein synthesis, glucose metabolism and signaling pathways. It also demonstarted that four genes (IL6, HMGA1, SLC19A2 and C4A) involved in the development and progression of diabetes are strongly regulated by Circulat. These bio-molecular results were confirmed with the further evaluation of diabetic foot management (Olalde *et al.*, 2008) which provided clinical substantiation that a complex herbal formulation could be successful in providing therapeutic response to such a circulatory chronic disease. However, the result obtained in the reduction of perfusion defect in Chronic Ischemic patients was unexpected. It also requires further validation. The authors are prolonging the length of the treatment -and the study- to one year. From this distance a better image of its potential therapeutic use can be assessed. However, there is room for cautious optimism. Evidence is accumulating that genetic variability and altered gene and protein expressions contribute to clinical outcomes in ischemic heart disease. It is likely therefore, that expression-profiling-based approaches to chronic degenerative diseases such as diabetes and ischemic heart disease with herbal medicines will become standard in phytopharmacology in the very near future. Resuming: a)The confirmation of Circulat's synergistic synergistic gene modulating capabilities (in 32 genes, among which are four significant genes related to diabetes; b) The clinical outcomes of diabetic foot management which prevented the amputation of 88.5% of the study's total population ; and c) The good response to therapy in 75% of the patients ($p \leq 6.104e\text{-}05$; % = 99.9999) by the composition in a GSPECT evaluated limited Phase II Chronic Ischemic Heart Disease suggest that treatment of circulatory pathologies with substances which act only on function and structure might be an incomplete approach. Whether the findings in circulatory chronic disease studies -and their results- can be generalized in confirming the systemic approach (E, I and O) is something that should be continued in medicinal science. Since this may pave the way for a new integral vision of therapeutics in general having started to proove its validity in circulatory chronic diseases in particular.

7. Acknowledgement

The authors wish to thank Dr. Edwin L. Cooper for his trust and invaluable guidance. Few can vouch such a supportive professor. Also, our appreciation to En Jose Olalde whose vision prompted a new therapeutic approach to chronic degenerative diseases recognizing that '...the essence of science...' is to have the valour to '...ask an impertinent question...' and get us on the road '...to a pertinent answer...' (Jacob Bronowski). Last but not least to Daniel Tucci, who although does not appear as an author provided figures and graphs, the art, that rounds up the science we all are so passionate about.

8. References

Abbott, CA.; Carrington, AL. & Ashe, H. (2002). The North-West Diabetes Foot Care Study: incidence of, and risk factors for new diabetic foot ulceration in a community-based patient cohort. *Diabet Med* Vol.19,No.5(2002),pp.377-84,ISSN 1464-5491

Abidov, M.; Crendal, F.; Grachev, S.; Seifulla, R. & Ziegenfuss, T. (2003). Effect of extracts from *Rhodiola rosea* and *Rhodiola crenulata* (*Crassulaceae*) roots on ATP content in mitochondria of skeletal muscles. *Bull Exp Biol Med* Vol.136, No.6 (2003) PP. 585-7, ISSN 1573-8221

Acharya, SK.; Dasarathy, S.; Tandon, A.; Joshi, YK. & Tandon BN.(1993). A preliminary open trial on interferon stimulator (SNMC) derived from *Glycyrrhiza glabra* in the treatment of subacute hepatic failure. *Indian J Med Res* Vol. 98,(1993), pp.69–74, ISSN: 0019-5359

Adams, JD. & Garcia C. (2005). The adavantages of traditional Chumash healing. *Evid Based Complement Alternat Med*; Vol.2, No.1 (June 2005), pp.19–23, ISSN 1741-427X

Agrawal, P.; Rai, V. & Singh, RB.(1996). Randomized placebo-controlled, single blind trial of holy basil leaves in patients with noninsulin-dependent diabetes mellitus. *Int J Clin Pharmacol Ther* Vol.34,No.9 (1996); pp.406–9,ISSN 0174-4879

Akesson, C.; Lindgren, H. & Pero, RW. (2003) An extract of *Uncaria tomentosa* inhibiting cell division and NF-kappa B activity without inducing cell death. *Int Immunopharmacol* Vol.3,No.13-14 (Dec 2003), pp.1889–900, ISSN 0074-0276

Albrecht-Buehler G. 1998. Altered drug resistance of microtubules in cells exposed to infrared light pulses: are microtubules the 'nerves' of cells? *Cell Motil Cytoskel* Vol.40, No.2 *(Dec* 1998), pp.183–92. ISSN (electronic): 1097-0169.

Albrecht Buehler, G. (1985) Is cytoplasm intelligent too?, In:*Cell Muscle Motility,* J.W. Shay, (Ed.), 1–21, Plenum Press, ISBN 90 6450 5020, New York-London

Antoshechkin, A. (2001). The Primary Adaptogens. Ceptoma Publishing Co., Clearwater, USA

Antoshechkin, A.; Olalde, J.; Magarici, M.; Muhammad, A.; Salom, A.; Suarez, J. & Amendola, F. (2007). Analysis of effects of the herbal preparation Circulat on gene expression levels in cultured human fibroblasts. *Phytotherapy Research* Vol.21,No.6,(August, 2007), pp. 777-789,ISSN 1099-1573

Apelqvist, J.; Larsson, J. & Agardh, CD. (1993). Long-term prognosis for diabetic patients with foot ulcers. *J Intern Med* Vol. 233, No.6,(1993) pp.485–491,ISSN 1939-1676

Apelqvist, J. & Larsson, J. (2000). What is the most effective way to reduce incidence of amputation in the diabetic foot? *Diabetes Metab Res Rev* Vol.16,Suppl 1,(Oct 2000),pp.S75-83, ISSN 1520-7560.

Armstrong, DG.; Lavery, LA.; Quebedeaux, TL. & Walker, SC. (1997). Surgical morbidity and the risk of amputation due to infected puncture wounds in diabetic versus nondiabetic adults. *South Med J* 90:384-9, ISSN 1541-8243

Ashburner, M., Ball, CA.; Blake, JA.; Botstein, D.; Butler, H.; Cherry, JM. & Davis, AP. (2000). The Gene Ontology Consortium. Gene Ontology tool for the unification of Biology. *Nature Genet* Vol.25 (2000),pp.25-29, ISSN 1061-4036

Bae, JW. & Lee, MH. (2004). Effect and putative mechanism of action of *ginseng* on the formation of glycated hemoglobin in vitro. *J Ethnopharmacol* Vol.91,No.1,(Mar 2004),pp.137-40, ISSN 1539-3704

Baggio, E.; Gandini, R.; Plancher, AC.; Passeri, M. & Carmosino, G. (1994) Italian multicenter study on the safety and efficacy of coenzyme Q10 as adjunctive therapy in heart failure. CoQ10 Drug Surveillance Investigators. *Mol Aspects Med* Vol.15,Suppl.1(1994),pp.S287–94,ISSN 1872-9452

Bence, AK. & Crooks, PA. (2003).The mechanism of l-canavanine cytotoxicity: arginy 1tRNA synthetase as a novel target for anticancer drug discovery. *J Enzyme Inhib Med Chem* Vol.18,No.5,(2003),pp.383–94,ISSN 1475-6374

Benotmane, A.; Mohammedi, F. & Ayad, F. (2000). Diabetic foot lesions: etiologic and prognostic factors. *Diabetes Metab* Vol. 26,No. 2,(April 2000),pp.113-7,ISSN 1520-7560

Bhattacharya, SK. & Muruganandam, AV. (2003). Adaptogenic activity of *Withania somnifera*: an experimental study using a rat model of chronic stress. *Pharmacol Biochem Behav* Vol. 75,No.3,(Jun 2003),pp.547–55,ISSN 0091-3057

Bilenko, V.; Bilenko, N.; Harman-Boehm, I.; Atar, D.; Rosen, S. & Weitzman, S. (2006). [Trends and characteristics of diabetes-related lower limb amputations in the Negev, 1996-1999] Harefuah Vol.145,No.10,pp.709-12

Blalock, JE. (1989). A molecular basis for bidirectional communication between the immune and neuroendocrine systems. *Physiol Rev* Vol.69,No.1,(Jan 1989),pp.1-32,ISSN 1522-1210.

Blumenthal, M.; Busse, WR.; Goldberg,A. & Gruenwald, J. (ed(s)). (1998). The Complete German Commission E Monographs., 1998,ISBN 0-96555-550-X,American Botanical Council, Austin, USA

Bocharova, OA.; Lyzhenkova, MA.; Mezentseva, MV.; Semernina, VV. & Knyazhev, VA. (2003). Phytoadaptogen for preventive oncology: immune biological criteria of composition. *Bull Exp Biol Med* Vol.136,No. 6,(Dec 2003),pp.591-4,ISSN 1573-8221

Borchers, AT.; Stern, JS.; Hackman, RM.; Keen, CL. & Gershwin, ME. (1999). Mushrooms, tumors, and immunity. *Proc Soc Exp Biol Med* Vol.221,No.4,(Sept 1999),pp.281-93, ISSN 0037-9727

Bouaziz, N.; Michiels, C. & Janssens, D. (1999). Effects of *Ruscus* extract and hesperidin methylchalcone on hypoxia-induced activation of endothelial cells. *Int Angiol* Vol.18,No.4,(Dec 1999),pp. 306-12, ISSN 0392-9590

Brekhman, II. & Dardymov, IV. (1969). New Substances of plant origin which increase non-specific resistance. *Annu Rev Pharmacol* Vol.9,(1969),pp.419-30, ISSN 0362-1642

Brown, AC.; Hairfield, M.; Richards, DG.; McMillin, DL.; Mein, EA. & Nelson, CD. (2009). Medical nutrition therapy as a potential complementary treatment for psoriasis-five case reports. *Altern Med Rev* Vol.9,No.3,(Sep 2004),pp. 297-307, ISSN 1089-5159

Bu, L.; Jiang, X.; Martin-Puig, S.; Caron, L.; Zhu, S.; Shao, Y.; Roberts, DJ.; Huang, PL.; Domian, IJ. & Chien, KR.(2009). Human ISL1 heart progenitors generate diverse multipotent cardiovascular cell lineages. *Nature* Vol. 460, No.7251, (July 2009), pp.113-117, ISSN 1476-4687

Bucci, LR. (2000). Selected herbals and human exercise performance. *Am J ClinNutr* Vol.72, S.2,(Aug 2000), pp.624S-36,ISSN 1938-3207

Calle, J.; Toscano, M.; Pinzon, R.; Baquero, J. & Bautista, E. (1999) Antinociceptive and uterine relaxant activities of *Viburnum toronis* alive (Caprifoliaceae). *J Ethnopharmacol* Vol.66,No.1,(July 1999),pp.71-3, ISSN 1539-3704

Carrero, JJ.; Lopez-Huertas, E.; Salmeron, LM.; Baro, L. & Ros, E. (2005). Daily supplementation with (n-3) PUFAs, oleic acid, folic acid, and vitamins B-6 and E increases pain-free walking distance and improves risk factors in men with peripheral vascular disease. *J Nutr* Vol.135,No. 6,(June 2005),pp.1393-9, ISSN 1541-6100.

Cavagnaro, J. & Lewis, RM. (1989). Bidirectional regulatory circuit between the immune and neuroendocrine systems. *Year Immunol* Vol.4,(1989),pp.241-52,ISSN 0256-2308

Ccahuana-Vasquez, RA.; Santos, SS.; Koga-Ito, CY. & Jorge, AO. (2007). Antimicrobial activity of *Uncaria tomentosa* against oral human pathogens. *Pesqui Odontol Bras* Vol.21,No.1,(Jan-Mar 2007), pp.46-50, ISSN 1517-7491

Celermajer, DS.; Sorensen, KE.; Gooch, VM.; Spiegelhalter, DJ.; Miller, OI.; Sullivan, ID.; Lloyd, JK. Deanfield, JE. (1992) Non-invasive detection of endothelial dysfunction in children and adults at risk of atherosclerosis. *Lancet* Vol.340, No.8828,(Nov 1992),pp.1111-1115, ISSN ONLI-2296

Chadwick, WA.; Roux, S.; van de Venter, M.; Louw, J. & Oelofsen, W. (2007). Anti-diabetic effects of *Sutherlandia frutescens* in Wistar rats fed a diabetogenic diet. *J Ethnopharmacol* Vol.109,No.1,(July 2006),pp.121-7, ISSN 1539-3704

Chainani-Wu N. (2003) Safety and anti-inflammatory activity of curcumin: a component of tumeric (*Curcuma longa*). *J Altern Complement Med* Vol.9,No.1,(Feb 2003), pp.161–8,ISSN 1557-7708

Chen, H.; Peng, P.; Cheng, L.; Lin, X.; Chung, S. & Li, M. (2010). Reconstitution of coronary vasculature in ischemic hearts by plant-derived angiogenic compounds. *Int J Cardiol* (Epub Dec 2010) ISSN: 0167-5273

Chen, J.; Bax, J.; Henneman, M.; Boogers, MJ. & Garcia, EV. (2008). Is nuclear imaging a viable technique to assess dyssynchrony? *Eurospace* Vol.10, S.iii,(Nov 2008), pp.101-105, ISSN 1532-2092

Chen, ZP.; Cai, Y & Phillipson, JD. (1994). Studies on the anti-tumour, anti-bacterial and wound-healing properties of dragon's blood. *Planta Med* Vol.60,No.6(1994),pp.541-5,ISSN 1439-0221

Chen, C.; Shum, Y.; & Yang, S. (2004). The modernization of traditional Chinese medicine in Taiwan -past, present and future. In: *Complementary and Alternative Approaches to Biomedicine*, E. L. Cooper,N. Yamaguchi, (Ed(s)), 167–79, Kluwer Academic/Plenum Publishers, ISBN 978-030-6482-88-5, New York, USA

Cheng, Z.; Pang, T.; Gu, M.; Gao, AH.; Xie, CM.; Li, JY.; Nan, FJ. & Li, J. (2006). Berberine-stimulated glucose uptake in L6 myotubes involves both AMPK and p38 MAPK. *Biochim Biophys Acta* Vol. 1760, No.11 (Nov 2006), pp.1682-9, ISSN 0006-3002

Chrubasik, S.; Kunzel, O.; Model, A.; Conradt, C. & Black, A. (2001). Treatment of low back pain with a herbal or synthetic anti-rheumatic: a randomized controlled study. Willow bark extract for low back pain. *Rheumatology* (Oxford) Vol. 40,No.12,(Dec 2001), pp.1388–93, ISSN 1462-0332

Chrubasik, S.; Model, A.; Black, A. & Pollack, S. (2003). A randomized double blind pilot study comparing Doloteffin and Vioxx in the treatment of lower back pain. *Rheumatology* (Oxford) Vol.42, No. 1, (Jan 2003), pp.141–8, ISSN 1462-0332

Chrungoo, VJ.; Singh, K. & Singh, J. (1997). Silymarin mediated differential modulation of toxicity induced by carbontetrachloride, paracetamol and d-galactosamine in freshly isolated rat hepatocytes. *Indian J ExpBiol* Vol.35 No.6, (Jun 1997), pp.611–7, ISSN 0975-1009

Cooper, EL. (2004). Commentary on CAM and NK cells by Kazuyoshi Takeda and Ko Okumura. *Evid Based Complement Alternat Med* Vol.1,No.1,(Jun 2004), pp. 29–34, ISSN 1741-4288

Cundell, DR.; Matrone, MA.; Ratajczak, P. & Pierce, JDJr. (2003). The effect of aerial parts of *Echinacea* on the circulating white cell levels and selected immune functions of the aging male Sprague-Dawley rat. *Int Immunopharmacol* Vol.3, No.7, (Jul 2003), pp.1041–8, ISSN 0074-0276

Dalby-Brown, L.; Barsett, H.; Landbo, AK.; Meyer, AS. & Mølgaard, P. (2005). Synergistic antioxidative effects ofalkamides, caffeic acid derivatives, and polysaccharide fractions from *Echinacea purpurea* on in vitro oxidation of human low-density lipoproteins. *Agric Food Chem* Vol.53, No.24 (Nov 2005), pp. 9413-23, ISSN 1684–5315

Davydov, M. & Krikorian, AD. (2000). *Eleutherococcus senticosus* (Rupr. & Maxim.) Maxim. (Araliaceae) as an adaptogen: a closer look. *J Ethnopharmacol* Vol.72, No.3, (Oct 2000), pp.345–93, ISSN 1539-3704

Dhuley, JN. (2000). Adaptogenic and cardioprotective action of ashwagandha in rats and frogs. *J Ethnopharmacol* Vol.70, No.1 (April 2000), pp.57–63, ISSN: 1539-3704

Dietz, BM.; Mahady, GB,.; Pauli, GF. & Farnsworth, NR. (2005). Valerian extracts and valerenic acid are partial agonists of the 5-HT5a receptor in vitro. *Brain Res Mol Brain Res* Vol.138, No.2,(August 2005), pp.191–7, ISSN 0169-328X

Duan, X.; Zhou L, Wu.; T, Liu, G.; Qiao, J.; Wei, J.; Ni, J.; Zheng, J.; Chen, X & Wang, Q. (2008). Chinese herbal medicine suxiao jiuxin wan for angina pectoris. *Cochrane Database Syst Rev* (Jan 2008) CD004473, ISSN 1469-493X

Faglia, E.; Favales, F.; Aldeghi, A.; Calia, P.; Quarantiello, A.; Barbano, P.; Puttini, M.; Palmieri, B.; Brambilla, G.; Rampoldi, A.; Mazzola, E.; Valenti, L.; Fattori, G.; Rega, V.; Cristalli, A.; Oriani, G.; Michael, M. & Morabito, A. (1998). Change in major amputation rate in a center dedicated to diabetic foot care during the 1980s: prognostic determinants for major amputation. J Diabetes Complications Vol. 12, No.2,(March-April 1998), pp.96-102, ISSN 1935-5548

Farnsworth, NR.; Kinghorn, AD.; Soejarto, DD. Waller, DP. (1985). Siberian ginseng (*Eleutherococcus senticosus*): current status as an adaptogen. In: Economic and Medicinal Plant Research, Vol.1, H. Wagner, H. Hikino, NR. Farnsworth, (Ed(s)), 217-284, Academic Press, London, UK,

Feng, CG.; Zhang, LX. & Liu, X. (2005). [Progress in research of aldose reductase inhibitors in traditional medicinal herbs]. *Zhongguo Zhong Yao Za Zhi* Vol.30, No.19, (Oct 2005), pp.1496-500, ISSN: 1001-5302

Fernando, DJ. (1996). The prevalence of neuropathic foot ulceration in Sri Lankan diabetic patients. *Ceylon Med J* Vol.41, No.3, (Sept 1996), pp.96-8, ISSN 0009-0875

Foti, D.; Chiefari, E.; Fedele, M.; Iuliano, R.; Brunetti, L.; Paonessa, F.; Manfioletti, G.; Barbetti, F.; Brunetti, A.; Croce, CM.; Fusco, A. & Brunetti, A. (2005). Lack of Architectural factor HMGA1 causes insulin resistance and diabetes in humans and mice. *Nat Med* Vol.11, No.7,(May 2005),pp.765-773, ISSN 1078-8956

Franz, G. (1993). The senna drug and its chemistry. *Pharmacology* Vol.47, S.1, (Oct 1993), pp. S2-6, ISSN 0031-7012

Freeman, MR. & Solomon, KR. (2004). Cholesterol and prostate cancer. *J Cell Biochem* Vol.91, No.1, pp.54–69,ISSN 1460-2105

Freier, DO.; Wright, K.; Klein, K. & Voll, D. (2003). Enhancement of the humoral immune response by*Echinacea purpurea* in female Swiss mice. *Immunopharmacol Immunotoxicol* Vol.25, No.4,(Nov 2003), pp.551-60, ISSN 1532-2513

Gaffney, BT.; Hugel, HM. & Rich, PA. (2001). *Panax ginseng* and *Eleutherococcus senticosus* may exaggerate an already existing biphasic response to stress via inhibition of enzymes which limit the binding of stress hormones to their receptors. *Med Hypotheses* Vol.56,No.5,(May 2001), pp.567–72, ISSN 0306-9877

Geng, XX.; Yang, Q.; Xie, RJ.; Luo, XH.; Han, B.; Ma, L.; Li, CX & Cheng, ML.(2005). *In vivo* effects of Chinese herbal recipe, Danshaohuaxian, on apoptosis and proliferation of hepatic stellate cells in hepatic fibrotic rats. *World J Gastroenterol* Vol.11,No.4,(Jan 2005),pp.561–6,ISSN 1007-9327

Gilani, AH. & Rahman, AU. (2005). Trends in ethnopharmocology. *J Ethnopharmacol* Vol.100,No. 1-2,(Jan 2005), pp.43-49, ISSN 1539-3704

Gilbert, B. & Alves, LF. (2003). Synergy in plant medicines. *Curr Med Chem* Vol.10, No.1, (Jan 2003), pp.13-20, ISSN 1568-0266

Goldmann, WH.; Sharma, AL.;Currier, SJ.; Johnston, PD.; Rana, A. & Sharma, CP.(2001). *Saw palmetto* berry extract inhibits cell growth and Cox-2 expression in prostatic cancer cells. *Cell Biol Int* Vol.25,No.11,(2001),pp.1117–24,ISSN 1423–0313

Gorgen, M.; Turatti, K. & Medeiros, AR. (2005). Aqueous extract of *Ilex paraguariensis* decreases nucleotide hydrolysis in rat blood serum. *J Ethnopharmacol* Vol.97, No.1, (Feb 2005), pp.73–7, ISSN: 1539-3704

Greenspan, HC.; Aruoma, OI. & Arouma, O. (1994). Could oxidative stress initiate programmed cell death in HIV infection? A role for plant derived metabolites having synergistic antioxidant activity. *Chem BiolInteract* Vol.91, No.2-3, (Jun 1994), pp. 187-97, ISSN 1421–9794

Groom, ST.; Johns, T. & Oldfield, PR. (2007). The potency of immunomodulatory herbs may be primarily dependent upon macrophage activation. *J Med Food* Vol.10, No.1, (Mar 2007), pp.73-9. ISSN: 1096-620X

Ghulam-Abbas, Z.; Lutale, JK.; Morbach, S. & Archibald, LK. (2002). Clinical outcome of diabetes patients hospitalized with foot ulcers, Dar el Salaam, Tanzania. *Diabet Med* Vol.19, No.7 (Jul 2002), pp.575-9, ISSN: 1464-5491

Gupta, V.; Gupta, A.; Saggu, S.; Divekar, HM.; Grover, SK. & Kumar, R. (2005). Anti-stress and adaptogenic activity of l-arginine supplementation. *Evid Based Complement Alternat Med* Vol.2, No.1, (Dec 2004), pp.93–7, ISSN 1741-4288

Gurwitsch, AG. (1991). *Principles of Analytical Biology and of the Theory of Cellular Fields*. Nauka, ISBN 90-806902-1-X, Moscow

Haken, H. (2000). Information and Self-Organization. A Macroscopic Approach to Complex Systems. Springer-Verlag, ISBN 0-521-62436-3, New York, USA

Halim, AB.; el-Ahmady, O.; Hassab-Allah, S.;Abdel-Galil, F.; Hafez, Y. & Darwish, D. (1997).Biochemical effect of anti-oxidants on lipids and liver function in experimentally-induced liver damage. *Ann Clin Biochem* Vol.34, Part 6, (Nov 1997), pp.656–63, ISSN 1758-1001

Han, SB.; Yoon, YD.; Ahn, HJ.; Lee, HS.; Lee, CW.; Yoon, WK.; Park, SK. & Kim, HM. (2003). Toll-like receptor-mediated activation of B cells and macrophages bypolysaccharide isolated from cell culture of *Acanthopanax senticosus*. *Int Immunopharmacol* Vol.3, No.9, (Sep 2003), pp.1301-12, ISSN 1567-5769

Heims SJ, von Neumann J, Wiener N. (1980). From Mathematics to the Technologies of Life and Death. MIT Press, ISBN 0262081059, Cambridge, USA

Hercberg, S.; Galan, P.; Preziosi, P.; Bertrais, S.; Mennen, L.; Malvy, D.; Roussel, AM.; Favier, A. & Briançon, S. (2004). The SU.VI.MAX Study: a rando-mized, placebo-controlled trial of the health effects of antioxidant vitamins and minerals. *Arch Intern Med* Vol.164,No.21,(Nov 2004), pp.2335–42. ISNN 0003-9926

Hirata, Y.; Soeki, T.; Aikake, M.; Sakai, Y.; Igarashi, T. & Sata, M. (2009). Synthetic prostacycline agonist, ONO-131, ameliorates left ventricular dysfunction and cardiac fibrosis in cardiomyopathic hamsters. *Biomed Pharmacother* Vol.63, No.19, (Sept 2009), pp 781-6, ISSN 1950-6007

Hong, CH.; Hur, SK.; Oh, OJ.; Kim, SS.; Nam, KA. & Lee, SK. (2002). Evaluation of natural products on inhibition of inducible cyclooxigenase (COX-2) and nitric oxide synthase (iNOS) in cultured mouse macrophage cells. *J Ethnopharmacol* Vol.83, No.1-2, (Nov 2002), pp.153–9. ISSN 0378-8741

Hong, L.; Xun, M. & Wutong, W. (2007). Anti-diabetic effect of an alpha-glucan from fruit body of maitake (*Grifola frondosa*) on KK-Ay mice. *J Pharm Pharmacol.* Vol.59, No.4, (Apr 2007), pp.575-82. ISSN 0022-3573

Houpt, JB.; Mc Millan, R.; Wein, C. & Paget-Dellio, SD. (1999). Effect of Glucosamine Hydrochloride in the treatment of pain of osteoarthritis of the knee. *J Rheumatol* Vol.26,No.11,(Nov 1999), pp.2423-30, 0315-162X

Huang, W.; Ye, X.; Li, X.; Zhao, Z.; Lan, P.; Wang, L.; Liu, M.; Gao, Y.; Zhu J.; Li, P.& Feng, P. (2010). [The inhibition activity of chemical constituents in hawthorn fruit and their synergistic action to HMG-CoA reductase]. *Zhongguo Zhong Yao Za Zhi* Vol.35,No.18,(Sept 2010),pp.2428-31, ISSN 1001-5302

Iguchi, K.; Okumura, N.; Usui, S.; Sajiki, H.; Hirota, K. & Hirano, K. (2001). Myristoleic acid, a cytotoxic component in theextract from *Serenoa repens*, induces apoptosis and necrosis in human prostatic LNCaP cells. *Prostate* Vol.47, No.1, (Apr 2001), pp.59-65, ISSN 0270-4137

Incandela, L.; Cesarone, MR. & Cacchio, M. (2001). Total triterpenic fraction of *Centella asiatica* in chronic venous insufficiency and in high-perfusion microangiopathy. *Angiology* Vol.52, Suppl.2,(Oct 2001),pp.S9-13, ISSN 0003-3197

Izzo, AA.; Di Carlo, G.; Borrelli, F. & Ernst, E. (2005). Cardiovascular pharmacotherapy and herbal medicines: the risk of drug interaction. *Int J Cardiol* Vol.98, No. (Jun 2006), pp.1-14. ISSN: 0167-5273

Jang, MH.; Jun DO.; Rue, SW.; Han, K.; Park, W. & Kim, YH. (2001). Arginine antimetabolite l-canavanine induces apoptotic cell death in human Jurkat T cells via caspase-3 activation regulated by Bcl-2 or Bcl-xL. *Biochem Biophys Res Commun* Vol.295, No.2,(Jul 2002),pp.283-8, 0006-291X

Järvisalo, MJ.; Jartti, L.; Nänto-Salonen, K.; Irjala, K.; Rönnemaa, T.; Hartiala, JJ.; Celermajer, DS.& Raitakari, OT. (2001). Increased aortic intima-media thickness: a marker of preclinical atherosclerosis in high-risk children. *Circulation* Vol.104, No.24,(Dec 2001), pp.2943-2947, ISSN 1524-4539

Ji, YB.; Gao, SY. & Zhang, XJ. (2004). [Influence of *Sargassum fusiforme* polysaccharide on apoptosis of tumor cells]. *Zhongguo Zhong Yao Za Zhi* Vol.29,No.3, (Mar 2004),pp.245-7, ISSN 1001-5302

Jiang, J.; Slivova, V.; Valachovicova, T.; Harvey, K. & Sliva, D. (2004). *Ganoderma lucidum* inhibits proliferation and induces apoptosis in human prostate cancer cells PC-3. *Int J Oncol* Vol.24, No.5, (May 2004),pp.1093-9, ISSN 1019-6439

Jing, SB.; Li, L.; Ji, D.; Takiguchi, Y. & Yamaguchi, T. (1997). Effect of chitosan on renal function in patients with chronic renal failure. *J Pharm Pharmacol* Vol.49,No.7,(Jul 1997),pp.721-3, ISSN 0022-3573

Jung, KH.; Ha, E.; Kim, MJ.; Uhm, YK.; Kim, HK.; Hong, SJ.; Chung, JH. & Yim, SV. (2006). *Ganoderma lucidum* extract stimulates glucose uptake in L6 rat skeletalmuscle cells. *Acta Biochim Pol* Vol.53,No.3,(Sep 2006),pp.597-601, 0001-527X

Jurkstiene, V.; Kondrotas, AJ. & Kevelaitis, E. (2004). [Compensatory reactions of immune system and action of Purple Coneflower (*Echinacea purpurea* L.) (Moench) preparations]. *Medicina (Kaunas)* Vol.40,No.7,(2004),pp.657-62,ISSN 1648-9144

Katerere, DR. & Eloff, JN. (2005). Antibacterial and antioxidant activity of *Sutherlandia frutescens* (Fabaceae), a reputed anti-HIV/AIDS phytomedicine. *Phytother Res* Vol.19,No.9, (Sept 2005), pp.779-81. ISSN 0951-418X

Khasina, EI.; Dardymov, IV. & Brekhman, II. (1983). [Effects of *Eleutherococcus* extract on the re-adaptation processes after 7 hour hypokinesia in rats]. *Kosm Biol Aviakosm Med* Vol.17, No.5, (Sept-Oct 1983),pp.55–8, ISSN 0321-5040

Kidd, PM. The use of mushrooms glucans and proteoglycans in cancer treatment. *Altern Med Rev* 2000 Vol.5, No. 1, (Feb 2000),pp.4–27, ISSN 1089-5159

Kim, HS.; Kacew, S. & Lee, BM. (1999). In vitro chemopreventive effects of plant polysaccharides (*Aloe barbadensis* miller, *Lentinus edodes, Ganoderma lucidum* and *Coriolus versicolor*. *Carcinogenesis* Vol.20,No.8,(Aug 1999),pp.1637–40, ISSN 0143-3334

Kim, KS.; Choi, YH.; Kim, KH.; Lee, YC.; Kim, CH.; Moon, SH.; Kang, SG. & Park, YG. (2004). Protective and anti-arthritic effects of deer antler aqua-acupunture (DAA), inhibiting dihydroorotate dehydrogenase, on phosphate ionsmediated chondrocyte apoptosis and rat collagen-induced arthritis. *Int Immunopharmacol* Vol.4,No.7,(Jul 2004), pp.963–73, ISSN 1567-5769

Kim, LS.; Waters, RF.& Burkholder, PM. (2002). Immunological activity of larch arabinogalactan and *Echinacea*: a preliminary, randomized, double-blind, placebo-controlled trial. *Altern Med Rev* Vol.7,No.2, (Apr 2002),pp.138-49, ISSN 1089-5159

Kim, MJ.; Yoo, KH.; Kim, JH.; Seo, YT.; Ha, BW.; Kho, JH.; Shin, YG. & Chung, CH.(2007).Effect of pinitol on glucose metabolism and adipocytokines in uncontrolledtype 2 diabetes. *Diabetes Res Clin Pract* Suppl.1,(Apr 2007), pp.S247-51, ISSN: 0168 8227

Kim, S.; Kubec, R. & Musah, RA. (2005). Antibacterial and antifungal activity of sulfur-containing compoundsfrom *Petiveria alliacea L. J Ethnopharmacol* Vol.104,No.1-2,(Mar 2006),pp.188-92, ISSN 0378-8741

Kobayakawa, J. & Sato-Nishimori, F. (2004). G2-M arrest and antimitotic activity mediated by casticin, a flavonoid isolated from *Viticis Fructus* (*Vitex rotundifolia* Linne fil.). *Cancer Lett* Vol.208, No.1,(May 2004),pp.59–64, ISSN 0304-3835

Kobayashi, M.; Devaraj, B.; Usa, M.; Tanno, Y.; Takeda, M. & Inaba, H (1996). Development and applications of new technology for two-dimensional space-time characterization and correlation analysis of ultraweak biophoton information. *Front Med Biol Eng* Vol.7,No.4,(1996),pp.299–309, 0921-3775

Kodama, N.; Murata, Y. & Nanba, H. (2004). Administration of a polysaccharide from *Grifola frondosa* stimulates immune function of normal mice. *J Med Food* Vol.7,No.2,(2004),pp.141-5, ISSN 1096-620X

Kohguchi, M.; Kunikata, T.; Watanabe, H.; Kudo, N.; Shibuya, T.; Ishihara, T.; Iwaki, K.; Ikeda, M.; Fukuda, S. & Kurimoto, M. (2004).Immuno-potentiating effects of the antler shaped fruiting body of *Ganoderma lucidum*. *Biosci Biotechnol Biochem* Vol.68,No.4,(Apr 2004),pp.881–7, ISSN 0916-8451

Kormosh, N.; Laktionov, K. & Antoshechkina, M. (2006). Effect of a combination of extract from several plants on cell-mediated and humoral immunity of patients with advanced ovarian cancer. *Phytother Res* Vol.20,No.5,(May 2006),pp.424-5,ISSN 0951-418X

Korotkov, K.; Williams, B. & Wisneski, LA. (2004).Assessing biophysical energy transfer mechanisms in living systems: the basis of life processes. *J Altern Complement Med* Vol.10,No.1,(Feb 2004),pp.49–57, ISSN 1075-5535

Korotkov, K. (1988). Light after Life. Backbone Publishing Co., ISBN 0-9644311-5-7 Fair Lawn, USA

Kotsiuruba, AV.; Bukhanevych, OM.; Tarakanov, SS. & Kholodova, IuD. (1993). [Modulation of intracellular pools of cyclic purine nucleotides by biologically active oxysterol-ecdysterone and vitamin D3]. *Ukr Biokhim Zh* Vol.65,No.5,(Sep-Oct 1993),pp.76–83, ISSN 0201-8470

Kristiansen, OP.; Mandrup-Poulsen T. (2005). Interleukin-6 and diabetes: the good, the bad, or the indifferent? Disbetes Vol.2 Suppl.1(2005),pp.S114-124, ISSN

Kubota, Y.; Tanaka, N.; Umegaki, K.; Takenaka, H.; Mizuno, H.; Nakamura, K.; Shinozuka, K.& Kunitomo, M. (2001). *Gingko biloba* extract induced relaxation of rat aorta is associated with increase in endothelial intracellular calcium level. *Life Sci* Vol.69,No.20,(Oct 2001),pp.2327–36, ISSN 0024-3205

Kundu, JK.; Mossanda, KS.; Na, HK. & Surh, YJ. (2005). Inhibitory effects of the extracts of *Sutherlandia frutescens* (L.) R. Br. and *Harpagophytum procumbens* DC. on phorbol ester-induced COX-2 expression in mou-se skin: AP-1 and CREB as potential upstream targets. *Cancer Lett* Vol.218,No.1,(Jan 2005),pp.21-31,ISSN 0304-3835

Kuo, CL.; Chi, CW. & Liu, TY.(2004).The anti-inflammatory potential of berberine in vitro and in vivo. *CancerLett* Vol.203,No.2,(Jan 2004),pp.127-37,ISSN 0304-3835

Kutuzova, NM.; Filippovich, IuB.; Kholodova, IuD. & Miladera, K. (1991). [Ecdysterone induces the activity of multiple forms of acid phosphatase and malate dehydrogenase]. *Ukr Biokhim Zh* Vol.63,No.3,(May-Jun 1991),pp.41–5,ISSN 0201-8470

Labay, V.; Raz, T.; Baron, D.; Mandel, H.; Williams, H.; Barrett, T.; Szargel, R.; McDonald, L.; Shalata, A.; Nosaka, K.; Gregory, S. & Cohen, N.(1999). Mutations in SlC19A2 cause thiamine-responsive megaloblastic anaemia associated with diabetes mellitus and deafness. *Nat Genet* Vol.22, No.3,(Jul 1999),pp.300-304, ISSN 1061-4036

Lacaille-Dubois, MA.; Franck, U. & Wagner, H. (2001). Search for potential angiotensin converting enzyme (ACE)-inhibitors from plants. *Phytomedicine* Vol.8,No.1,(Jan 2001),pp.47-52,ISSN 0944-7113

Ladriere, L.; Laghmich, A.; Malaisse-Lagae, F. & Malaisse, WJ. (1997). Effect of dehydroepiandrosterone in hereditarily diabetic rats. *Cell Biochem Funct* Vol.15,No.4,(Dec 1997),pp.287–92,ISSN 0263-6484

Laszlo, E. (1987). Evolution, The Grand Synthesis. Shambhala Publications Inc., ISBN 2-88124-491-2,Boston,USA

Lavery, LA.; Armstrong, DG. & Harkless, LB. (1997). Classification of diabetic foot wounds. *Ostomy Wound Manage* Vol.43,No.2, (Mar 1997),pp.44-8, 50, 52-3, ISSN 0889-5899

Lavery, La.; Armstrong, DG.; Wunderlich. RP.; Tredwell, J. & Boulton, AJ. (2003). Diabetic Foot Syndrome: Evaluating the prevalence and incidence of foot pathology in Mexican American and non-Hispanic whites from a diabetes management cohort. *Diabetes Care* Vol.26, No.5,(May 2003),pp.1435-1438, ISSN 0149-5992

Lee, SE.; Ju, EM. & Kim, JH. (2001). Free radical scavenging and antioxidant enzyme fortifying activities of extracts from *Smilax china* root. *Exp Mol Med* Vol.33,No.4(Dec 2001),pp.263–8,ISSN 1226-3613

Lee, SY. & Rhee, HM.(1990).Cardiovascular effects of mycelium extract of *Ganoderma lucidum*: inhibition of sympathetic outflow as a mechanism of its hypotensive action. *Chem Pharm Bull (Tokyo)* Vol.38,No.5,(May 1990),pp.1359-64,ISSN 0009-2363

Leff, HS. & Rex, AF. (eds). (1990). Maxwell's Demon: Entropy, Information, Computing. Princeton University Press, ISBN 0-7503-0759-5,Princeton, USA

Lehto, S.; Ronnemaa, T.; Pyorala, K. & Laakso, M.(1996). Risk factors predicting lower extremity amputations in patients with NIDDM. *Diabetes Care* Vol.19,No.6,(Jun 1996),pp.607–612, ISSN: 0149-5992

Leu, SF.; Chien, CH.; Tseng, CY.; Kuo, YM. & Huang, BM. (2005). The in vivo effect of *Cordyceps sinensis* mycelium on plasma corticosterone level in male mouse. *Biol Pharm Bull* Vol.28,No.9,(Sep 2005),pp.1722–5, ISSN 0918-6158

Li, CJ.; Wang, C. & Pardee, AB.(1995). Induction of apoptosis by b-lapachone in human prostate cancer cells. *Cancer Res* Vol.55,No.17,(Sep 1995),pp.3712–5,ISSN 0008-5472

Lin, H.; She, YH.; Cassileth, BR.; Sirotnak, F.& Cunningham Rundles, S. (2004).Maitake beta-glucan MD-fraction enhances bone marrow colony formation and reduces doxorubicin toxicity in vitro. *Int Immunopharmacol* Vol.4,No.1, (2004),pp.91–9, ISSN 1567-5769

Lindley, D. (2001).Boltzmann's Atom: The Great Debate that Launched a Revolution in Physics. Free Press, ISBN 0-684-85186-5, New York, USA

Ling, S.; Nheu, L.; Dai, A.; Guob, Z. & Komaseroff, P.(2008). Effects of four medicinal herbs on human vascular endothelial cells in culture. *Int J Cardiol* Vol.128,No.3,(Aug 2008), pp.350-58, ISSN: 1874-1754

Lishmanov, IuB.; Naumova, AV.; Afanas'ev, SA. & Maslov LN.(1997).[Contribution of the opioid system to realization ofinotropic effects of *Rhodiola rosea* extracts in ischemic and reperfusion heart damage in vitro]. *Eksp Klin Farmakol* Vol.60,No.3,(May-Jun 1997),pp.34-6,ISSN 0869-2092

Liu, JC.; Chan, P.; Chen, YJ.; Tomlinson, B.; Hong, SH. & Cheng, JT.(1999). The antihypertensive effect of the berberine derivative 6-protoberberine in spontaneously hypertensive rats. *Pharmacology* Vol.59,No.6,(Dec 1999),pp.283-9,ISSN 0031-7012

Liu,TP.; Lee, CS.; Liou, SS. & Cheng, JT.(2005). Improvement of insulin resistance by *Acanthopanax senticosus* root infructose-rich chow-fed rats. *Clin Exp Pharmacol Physiol* Vol.32,No.8,(Aug 2005),pp.649-54, ISSN 0305-1870

Lopez-Fando, A.; Gomez-Serranillos, MP.; Iglesias, I.; Lock, O.; Upamayta, UP. & Carretero, ME. (2004). *Lepidium peruvianum chacon* restores homeostasis impaired by restraint stress. *Phytother Res* Vol.18,No.6,(2004),pp.471–4,ISSN 0951-418X

Lores, RI. & Cires Pujol, M.(1990). *Petiveria alleaceae L.*(anamu). Study of the hypoglycemic effect. *Med Interne Vol.*28, No.4,(Oct-Dec 1990),pp.347-52, ISSN 0377-1202

Lu, L.; Ying, K.; Wei, S.; Fang, Y.; Liu, Y.; Lin, H.; Ma, L. & Mao, Y.(2004). Asiaticoside induction for cell-cycle progression, proliferation and collagen synthesis in human dermal fibroblasts. *Int J Dermatol* Vol.43,No.11,(Nov 2004),pp.801-7, ISSN 0011-9059

Luo, XY.; Zhang, FR. & He, RM. (2009) [Efficacy of shenfu injection as adjuvant therapy in treating patients of ischemic cardiomyopathy with Heart insufficiency] *Zhuongguo Zhong Xi Yi Jie He Za Zhi* Vol.29,No.8,(Aug 2009),pp.685-7,ISSN 1003-5370

Ma, T.; Qi, QH.; Xu, J.; Dong, ZL. & Yang, WX. (2004). Signal pathways involved in emodin-induced contraction of smooth muscle cells from rat colon. *World J Gastroenterol* Vol.10,No.10,(May 2004),pp.1476–9, ISSN 1007-9327

Malay, DS.; Margolis, DJ.; Hoffstad, OJ. & Bellamy, S.(2006). The incidence and risks of failure to heal after lower extre- mity amputation for the treatment of diabetic neuropathic foot ulcer. *J Foot Ankle Surg* Vol.45,No.6,(Nov-Dec 2006),pp.366-74,ISSN 1542-2224

Malpezzi, EL.; Davino, SC.; Costa, LV.; Freitas, JC.; Giesbrecht, AM. & Roque, NF. (1994). Antimitotic action of extracts of *Petiveria alliacea* on sea urchin egg development. *Braz J Med Biol Res* Vol.27,No.3,(Mar 1994),pp.749–54,ISSN 1414-431X

Marrero, S.; Martínez, A. & González, S. (2006). [Correlation between diabetic foot degree and type of amputation in a Public Medical Assistance Center] *Informe médico.* Vol.8,No.4, (2006),pp.169-177, ISSN 1316 9688

Maslova, LV.; Kondrat'ev, BIu.; Maslov, LN. & Lishmanov, IuB. (1994). [The cardioprotective and antiadrenergic activity of an extract of Rhodiola rosea in stress]. *Eksp Klin Farmakol* Vol.57,No.6,(Nov-Dec 1994),pp.61–3, ISSN 0869-2092

Matsuda, T.; Kuroyanagi, M. & Sugiyama, S. (1994). Cell differentiation-inducing diterpenes from *Andrographis paniculata* Nees. *Chem Pharm Bull* (Tokyo) Vol.42,No.6(Jun 1994), pp.1216–25, ISSN 0009-2363

Mei, QB.; Tao, JY. & Cui, B. (1991). Advances in the pharmacological studies of radix *Angelica sinensis* (Oliv.) Diels (Chinese danggui). *Chin Med J* Vol.104,No.9(Sept 1991),pp.776–81, ISSN 0366-6999

Miyajima, S.; Shirai, A.; Yamamoto, S.; Okada, N. & Matsushita, T.(2005). Risk factors for major limb amputations in diabetic foot gangrene patients. *Diabetes Res Clin Pract* Vol.71,No.3,(Mar 2006),pp.272-9, ISSN 0168-8227

Moon, DO.; Choi, YH.; Kim, ND.; Park, YM. & Kim, GY.(2007). Anti-inflammatory effects of beta-lapachone in lipo polysaccharide estimulated BV2 microglia. *Int Immunopharmacol* Vol.7, No.4,(Apr 2007),pp.506-14, ISSN 1567-5769

Moss, SE.; Klein, R. & Klein, B. (1996). Long-term incidence of lower-extremity amputations in a diabetic population. *Arch Fam Med* Vol.5,No.7,(Jul-Aug 1996),pp.391–398, ISSN 1063-3987

Naik, Gh.; Priyadarsini, KI.; Satav, JG.; Banavalikar, MM.; Sohoni, DP.; Biyani, MK. & Mohan, H. (2003). Comparative antioxidant activity of individual herbal components used in Ayurvedic medicine. *Phytochemistry* Vol.63,No.1,(May 2003),pp.97–104, ISSN 0031-9422

Neufeldt V, Guralnik D (eds). (1988) Webster's New World Dictionary. Simon & Schuster, New York, USA

Nyamu, PN.; Otieno, CF.; Amayo, EO. & McLigeyo, SO. (2003). Risk factors and prevalence of diabetic foot ulcers at Kenyatta National Hospital, Nairobi. *East Afr Med J* Vol.80,No.1(Jan 2003),pp36-43, ISSN 0012-835X

Odama, N.; Murata, Y. & Nanba, H. (2004). Administration of a polysaccharide from *Grifola frondosa* stimulates immune function of normal mice. *J Med Food* Vol.7,No.2,(2004),pp.141–5, ISSN 1096-620X

Ohyama, K.; Akaike, T. & Hirobe, C. (2003). Cytotoxicity and apoptotic inducibility of *Vitex agnus-castus* fruit extract in cultured human normal and cáncer cells and effect on growth. *Biol Pharm Bull* Vol.26,No.1,(Jan 2003),pp.10–8, ISSN 0918-6158

Olalde, JA.; Magarici, M.; Amendola, F.; del Castillo, O.; Gonzalez, S. & Muhammad, A. (2008) Clinical outcomes of diabetic foot management with Circulat. *Phytother Res* Vol.22,No.10,(Oct 2008),pp.1292-8, ISSN: 1099-1573

Olalde Rangel, JA.; Magarici, M.; Amendola, F. & del Castillo, O. (2005). The Systemic Theory of Living Systems. Part IV: Systemic Medicine-The Praxis. Vol.2,No.4,(Dec 2005),pp. 429-439, ISSN 1741-4288

Olalde Rangel, JA. (2005). The Systemic Theory of Living Systems and Relevance to CAM: the Theory (Part III). *Evid Based Complement Alternat Med* Vol.2,No.3,(Sept 2005),pp.267-275, ISSN 1741-4288

Olalde Rangel, JA. (2005). The Systemic Theory of Living Systems and Relevance to CAM: The Theory (PartII). *Evid Based Complement Alternat Med* Vol.2,No.2,(Jun 2005),pp.129-137, ISSN 1741-4288

Olalde Rangel, JA. (2005). The Systemic Theory of Living Systems and Relevance to CAM: Part I: The Theory.*Evid Based Complement Alternat Med* Vol.2,No.1(Mar 2005),pp.13-18, ISSN 1741-4288

Owens, J. & Van de Castle, R. (2004). Gas Discharge Visualization Technique: Introduction to the concept of Energy Fields. In: Measuring Energy Fields, K. Korotkov, (Ed.), 11-22, Backbone Publishing, ISBN 097420191,Fair Lawn, USA

Palsdottir, A.; Cross, SJ.; Edwards, JH. & Carrol, MC. (1983). Correlation between a DNA restriction fragment length polymorphism and C4A6 protein. *Nature* Vol.306,No.5943,(Dec 1983),pp.615-616, ISSN 0028-0836

Park, EK.; Choo, MK.; Han, MJ. & Kim, DH. (2004). Ginsenoside Rh1 possesses antiallergic and anti-inflammatory activities. *Int Arch Allergy Immunol* Vol.133,No.2,(Feb 2004),pp.113-20, ISSN 1018-2438

Park, SH.; Lee, SG.; Kang, SK. & Chung, SH. (2006). *Acanthopanax senticosus* reverses fatty liver disease and hyperglycemia in ob/ob mice. *Arch Pharm Res* Vol.29,No.9,(Sept 2006),pp.768-76, ISSN 0253-6269

Pena, JC. (2002). [The concept of illness and kidney diseases in Nahuatl medicine. Synthesis of Mesoamerican pre-Columbian medicine]. *Rev Invest Clin* Vol.54,No.5,(Sep-Oct 2002),pp.474-81,ISSN 0034-8376

Pepe, C.; Rozza, A. & Veronesi, G. (1999). The evaluation by video capillaroscopy of the efficacity of a *Gingko biloba* extract with l-arginine and magnesium in the treatment of trophic lesions in patients with stage-IVchronic obliterating arteriopathy. *Minerva Cardioangiol* Vol.47,No.6,(Jun 1999),pp.223-30, ISSN 0026-4725

Pereira, EM.; Machado T, de B.; Leal, IC.; Jesus ,DM.; Damaso, CR.; Pinto, AV.; Giambiagi-deMarval, M.; Kuster, RM. Santos, & KR.(2006).*Tabebuia avellanedae* naphthoquinones: activity against methicillin-resistant staphylococcal strains, cytotoxic activity and in vivo dermal irritability analysis. *Ann Clin Microbiol Antimicrob* Vol.22(Mar 2006),pp.5, ISSN 1476-0711

Pinello, KC.; Fonseca, Ede S.; Akisue, G.; Silva, AP.; Salgado Oloris, SC.; Sakai, M.; Matsuzaki, P.; Nagamine, MK.; Palermo Neto, J. & Dagli, ML. (2005). Effects of *Pfaffia paniculata* (Brazilian ginseng) extract on macrophage activity. *Life Sci* Vol.78,No.12,(Feb 2006),pp.1287-92 ISSN: 0024-3205

Piscoya, J.; Rodriguez, Z.; Bustamante, SA.; Okuhama, NN.; Miller, MJ. & Sandoval, M .(2001). Efficacy and safety of freeze-dried cat's claw in osteo-arthritis of the knee: mechanisms of action of species *Uncaria guianensis*. *Inflamm Res* Vol.50,No.9,(Sept 2001),pp.442-8,ISSN 1023-3830

Planchon, SM.; Wuerzberger, S.; Frydman, B.; Witiak, DT.; Hutson, P.; Church DR.; Wilding, G. & Boothman, DA. (1995). b-Lapachone-mediated apoptosis in human promyelocytic leuke-mia (HL-60) and human prostate cancer cells: a p53-independent response. *Cancer Res* Vol.55,No.17(Sept 1995),pp.3706–11, ISSN 0008-5472

Plotnikov, MB.; Aliev, OI.; Vasil'ev, AS.; Maslov, MIu.; Dmitruk, SE. & Krasnov, EA. (2001). [Effect of *Rhaponticum carthamoides* extract on hemorheological properties of blood in rats with arterial hypertension]. *Eksp Klin Farmakol* Vol.64,No.6,(Nov-Dec 2001),pp.45-7, ISSN 0869-2092

Popiela, T.; Kulig, J.; Hanisch, J. & Bock, PR. (2001). Influence of a complementary treatment with oral enzymes on patients with colorectal cancers—an epidemiological retrolective cohort study. *Cancer Chemother Pharmacol* Vol.47,Suppl.1,(Jul 2001),pp.S55–63, ISSN 0344-5704

Popp, FA. (2003). Properties of biophotons and their theoretical implications. *Indian J Exp Biol* Vol.41,No.5, (May 2003),pp.391–402, ISSN 0019-5189

Prigogine, I. (1984). Order Out of Chaos. Bantam Books, ISBN 0553340824, New York, USA

Puri, A.; Saxena, R.;Saxena, RP.; Saxena, KC.; Srivastava, V. & Tandon, JS. (1993). Immunostimulant agents from *Andrographis paniculata. J Nat Prod* Vol.56,No.7,(Jul 1993),pp.95–9, ISSN 0163-3864

Randolph, RK.; Gellenbeck, K.; Stonebrook, K.; Brovelli, E.; Qian, Y.; Bankaitis-Davis, D. & Cheronis, J. (2003). Regulation of human immune gene Expression as influenced by a commercial blended *Echinacea* product: preliminary studies. *Exp Biol Med* (Maywood) Vol.228,No.9,(Oct 2003),pp.1051–6, ISSN 1535-3702

Raso, GM.; Pacilio, M.; Di Carlo, G.; Esposito, E.; Pinto, L. & Meli, R.(2002). In-vivo and in-vitro anti-inflammatory effect of *Echinacea purpurea* and *Hypericum perforatum. J Pharm Pharmacol Vol.*54,No.10,(Oct 2002),pp.1379-83, ISSN 0022-3573

Ratzmann, KP.; Drzimalla, E. & Raskovic, M. (1994). [The "diabetic foot" syndrome. Association with other complications and the incidence of amputation] *Med Klin (Munich)* Vol.89,No.9 (Sept 1994),pp.469-72, ISSN 0723-5003

Rayman, G.; Krishnan, ST. & Baker, NR. (2004). Are we underestimating diabetes-related lower-extremity amputation rates? Results and benefits of the first prospective study. *Diabetes Care* Vol.27,No.8,(Aug 2004),pp.1892-6,ISSN 0149-5992

Reay, JL.; Kennedy, DO. & Scholey, AB. (2005). Single doses of *Panax ginseng* (G115) reduce blood glucose levels and improve cognitive performance during sustained mental activity. *J Psychopharmacol* Vol.19,No.4(Jul 2004),pp.357-65, ISSN 0269-8811

Redman, DA. (2000). *Ruscus aculeatus* (butcher's broom) as a potential treatment for orthostatic hypotension, with a case report. *J Altern Complement Med* Vol.6,No.6,(Dec 2000),pp.539-49,ISSN 1075-5535

Rehman, J.; Dillow, JM.; Carter, SM.; Chou, J.; Le, B. & Maisel, AS. (1999). Increased production of antigen-specific immunoglobulins G and M following in vivo treatment with the medicinal plants *Echinacea angustifolia* and *Hydrastis canadensis. Immunol Lett* Vol.68,No.2-3(Jun 1999),pp.391–5, ISSN 0165-2478

Rigelsky, JM. & Sweet, BV. (2002).Hawthorn: pharmacology and therapeutic uses. *Am J Health Syst Pharm* Vol.59,No.5 (Mar 2002),pp.417–22, ISSN: 1079-2082

Risco, E.; Ghia, F.; Vila, R.; Iglesias, J.; Alvarez, E. & Canigueral, S. (2003). Immunomodulatory activity and chemical characterisation of sangre de drago (dragon's blood) from *Croton lechleri. Planta Med* Vol.69,No.9,(Sept 2003),pp.785–94, ISSN 0032-0943

Rotshteyn, Y. & Zito, SW. (2004). Application of modified *in vitro* screening procedure for identifying herbals possessing sulfonylurea-like activity. *J Ethnopharmacol* Vol.93,No.2-3,(Aug 2004),pp.337–44, ISSN 0378-8741

Ruffa, MJ.; Ferraro, G.; Wagner, ML.; Calcagno, ML.; Campos, RH. & Cavallaro, L. (2002). Cytotoxic effect of Argentine medicinal plant extracts on human hepatocellular carcinoma cell line. *J Ethnopharmacol* Vol. 79,No.3(Mar 2002),pp.335–9, ISSN 0378-8741

Santa Maria-Margalef, A.; Paciucci Barzanti, R. & Reventos Puigjaner, J. (2003). Antimitogenic effect of *Pygeum africanum* extracts on human prostatic cancer cell lines and explants from benign prostatic hyperplasia. *Arch Esp Urol Vol.*56,No.4,(May 2003),pp.369–78, ISSN 0004-0614

Sasagawa, M.; Cech, NB.; Gray, DE.; Elmer, GW. & Wenner, CA. (2006). *Echinacea* alkylamides inhibit interleukin-2 production by Jurkat T cells. *Int Immunopharmacol* Vol.6,No.7,(Jul 2006),pp.1214-21,ISSN 1567-5769

Savickiene, N.; Dagilyte, A. & Lukosius, A. (2002). Importance of biologically active components and plants in the pre-vention of complications of diabetes mellitus. *Medicina* (Kaunas) Vol.38,No.10(2002),pp.970–5, ISSN1010-660X

Scazzocchio, F.; Cometa, MF.; Tomassini, L. & Palmery, M. (2001). Antibacterial activity of *Hydrastis canadensis* extract and its major isolated alkaloids. *Planta Med* Vol.67,No.6,(Aug 2001),pp.561-4, ISSN 0032-0943

Selye, H. (1976). Stress of Life. McGraw-Hill, New York, USA

Shannon, CE. & Weaver, W. (1999).The Mathematical Theory of Communication, University of Illinois Press, ISBN 0-387-95457-0, Champaign, USA

Shao, BM.; Xu, W. & Dai, H. (2004). A study on the immune receptors for polysaccharides from the roots of *Astragalus membranaceus*, a Chinese medicinal herb. *Biochem Biophys Res Commun* Vol.320,No.4,(Aug 2004),pp.1103–11, ISSN 0006-291X

Shealy, CN. (1999). Natural Progesterone. Safe and Natural Hormone Replacement, Keats Publishing, ISBN 10-0879838892, Los Angeles,USA

Sheng, Y.; Pero, RW. & Amiri, A. (1998). Induction of apoptosis and inhibition of proliferation in human tumor cells treated with extracts of *Uncaria tomentosa*. *Anticancer Res* Vol.18,No.5A, (Sept-Oct 1998), pp.3363–8, ISSN 0250-7005

Schroedinger, E. (1992).What is Life? Cambridge University Press, Cambridge, USA

Siqueira, IR.; Fochesatto, C.; da Silva, AL.; Nunes, DS.; Battastini, AM.; Netto, CA. & Elisabetsky, E. (2003). *Ptychopetalum olacoides*, a traditional Amazonian "nerve tonic", possesses anticholinesterase activity. *Pharmacol Biochem Behav* Vol.75, No.3,(Jun 2003),pp.645–50, ISSN 0091-3057

Slawinska, D. & Slawinski, J. (1987). Ultraweak photon emission in model reactions of the *in vitro* formation of eumelanins and pheomelanins. *Pigment Cell Res* Vol.1,No.3,(1987),pp.171–5, ISSN 0893-5785

Smolina, TP.; Solov'eva, TF. & Besednova, NN. (2001). [Immunotropic activity of panaxans—bioglycans isolated from *ginseng*] *Antibiot Khimioter* Vol.46,No.7, (2001),pp.19-22, ISSN 0235-2990

Spasov, AA.; Wikman, GK.; Mandrikov, VB.; Mironova, IA & Neumoin, VV. (2000). A double-blind, placebo controlled pilot study of the stimulating and adaptogenic effect of *Rhodiola rosea* SHR-5 extract on the fatigue of students caused by stress during an examination period with a repeated low-dose regimen. *Phytomedicine* Vol.7,No.2,(Apr 2000),pp.85–9, ISSN 0944-7113

Stonier T. (1996). Information as a basic property of the universe. *Biosystems* Vol.38, No.2-3,(1996),pp.135–40, ISSN: 0303-2647

Sugimura, H. (1989). Effects of aqueous extracts from *Eleutherococcus* on the oxidative enzyme activities in mouse skeletal muscle. *Annual Proceedings of the Gifu Pharmaceutical University* Vol.38(1989)pp.38-48.

Sun, T. & Zhu, Y. (1999). The effect of PSP on immune function and living quality in patients receiving chemotherapy for gynecological malignancies. In: *Advanced Research in PSP*, Q. Yang (Ed.), 308–9, Hong Kong Association for Health Care Ltd, Hong Kong

Sun, Z.; Yang, Q. & Fei, H. (1999). The ameliorative effect of PSP on the toxic and side reactions of chemo and radiotherapy of cancers. In: *Advanced Research in PSP*, Q. Yang (Ed.), 304–7, Hong Kong Association for Health Care Ltd, Hong Kong

Takeda, K. and Okomura, K.(2004) CAM and NK cells. *Evid Based Complement Alternat Med* Vol.1,No.1,(Jun 2004), pp.17–27, ISSN 1741-4288

Takeda, M.; Tanno, Y.; Kobayashi, M.; Usa, M.; Ohuchi, N.; Satomi, S. & Inaba, H. (1998). A novel method of assessing carcinoma cell proliferation by biophoton emission. *Cancer Lett* Vol.127, No.1,(May 1998),pp.155–60, ISSN: 0304-3835

Tam, WY.; Chook, P.; Qiao, M.; Chan, LT.; Chan, TY.; Poon, YK.; Fung, KP.; Leung, PC. & Woo, KS. (2009). The efficacy and tolerability of adjunctive alternative herbal medicine [*Salvia miltiorrhiza* and *Pueraria lobata*] on vascular function and structure in coronary patients. *J Altern Complement Med* Vol.15,No.4 (April 2009),pp.415-21, ISSN 1557-7708

Tashmukhamedova, MA.; Almatov, KT.; Syrov, VN.; Sultanov, MB. & Abidov, AA. (1986). Comparative study of the effect of ecdysterone, turkesterone and nerobol on the function of rat liver mitochondria in experimental diabetes. *VoprMed Khim* Vol.32,No.5,(Sept-Oct 1986),pp.24-8, ISSN 0042-8809

Terasawa,K.(2004).Evidence-based reconstruction of Kampo medicine:part I -is Kampo CAM? *Evid Based Complement Alternat Med* Vol.1, No.1(Jun 2004),pp.11–6, ISSN 1741-4288

Thadani,U. (2004).Current medical management of chronic stable angina. *J Cardiovasc Pharmacol Ther* Vol.9,Suppl.1 (Sept 2004),pp.S11–29, ISSN 1074-2484

Thadani,U. (2003).The pursuit of optimum outcomes in stable angina. *Am J Cardiovasc Drugs* Vol.3,Suppl.1, (2003),pp.S11–20

Thadani,U. (1999).Management of stable angina pectoris. *Curr Opin Cardiol* Vol.14,No.4(Jul 1999),pp.349–358, ISSN 0268-4705

Thyagarajan, A.; Zhu, J. & Sliva, D.(2007). Combined effect of green tea and *Ganoderma lucidum* on invasive behavior of breast cancer cells. *Int J Oncol* Vol.30,No.4,(Apr 2007),pp.963-9, ISSN 1019-6439

Tilbary, RN. & Quickenden, TI. (1988). Spectral and time dependence studies of the ultraweak bioluminescence emitted by the bacterium *Escherichia coli. Photochem Photobiol* Vol.47,No.1,(1988),pp.145–50, ISSN 0031-8655

Tin-Hay, E.; Poh, KK.; Lim, YT.; Fatt-Hoe, A.; Lee, CH.; Low, AF.; Lee, CH.; Teo, SG.; Lim, J.; Lim, IH. & Tan, HC.(2009). Clinical predictors of stent thrombosis in the "real world" drug-eluting stent era. *Int J Cardiol* Vol.145,No.3,(Dec 2010),pp.422-25, ISSN 1874-1754

Trautner, C. Haastert, B.; Spraul, M.; Giani, G.& Berger, M.(2001). Unchanged incidence of lower-limb amputations in a German City, 1990-1998. *Diabetes Care* Vol.24,No.5,(May 2001),pp.855-9, ISSN 0149-5992

Tripathi,YB.; Singh, BK.; Pandey, RS. & Kumar, M. (2005). BHUx: A Patent Polyherbal Formulation to Prevent Atherosclerosis. *Evid Based Complement Alternat Med* Vol.2,No.2,(Jun 2005),pp.217-221, ISSN 1741-4288

Trushin,M.(2003).Studies on distant regulation of bacterial growth and light emission. *Microbiology* Vol.149,Part2(Feb 2003),pp.363–8, ISSN 1350-0872

Vaisberg, AJ.; Milla, M.; Planas, MC.; Cordova, JL.; de Agusti, ER.; Ferreyra, R.; Mustiga, MC.; Carlin, L. & Hammond, GB. (1989).Taspine is the cicatrizant principle in Sangre de Grado extracted from *Croton lechleri*. *Planta Med* Vol.55,No.2,(Apr 1989),pp.140-3, ISSN 0032-0943

Vandenbroek, I. Van Damme, P. & Van Puyvelde,L.; Arrazola, S.& De Kimpe, N. (2004). A comparison of traditional healer's medicinal plant knowledge in the Bolivian Andes and Amazon. *Soc Sci Med* Vol.59,No.4,(Aug 2004),pp.837–49, ISSN 0277 9536

Voeikov, VL. (2003).Mitogenic radiation, biophotons, and non-linear oxidative processes in aqueous media, In: *Integrative Biophysics Biophotonics,* FA. Popp, L. Beloussov, (Ed(s)), 331–359, Kluwer Academic Publishers, ISBN 978-140-2011-39-9, Dordrecht, The Netherlands

Volaco A, Chantelau E & Richter, B. (2004). Outcome of critical foot ischaemia in longstanding diabetic patients: a retrospective cohort study in a specialised tertiary care centre. *Vasa* Vol. 33,No.1,(2004),pp.36-41. ISSN 0301-1526

von Stockar, U. & Liu, J. (1999). Does microbial life always feed on negative entropy? Thermodynamic analysis of microbial growth. *Biochim Biophys Acta* Vol.1412,No.3,(Aug 1999),pp.191–211, ISSN 0006-3002

Vuksan, V.; Sievenpiper, JL.; Koo, VY.; Francis, T.; Beljan-Zdravkovic, U.; Xu, Z.& Vidgen, E.(2000). American ginseng (*Panax quinquefolius L*) reduces post-prandial glycemia in nondiabetic subjects and subjects with type 2 diabetes mellitus. *Arch Intern Med* Vol.160,No.7,(Apr 200),pp.1009-13,ISSN 0003-9926

Wago, H. & Deng, H. (2004).Chinese medicine and immunity, In: Complementary and Alternative Approaches to Biomedicine, E. L. Cooper, N. Yamaguchi, (Ed(s)), 167–79, KluwerAcademic/Plenum Publishers, ISBN 978-030-6482-88-5, New York,USA

Wang, BX.; Zhou, QL.; Yang, M.; Wang, Y.; Cui, ZW.; Liu, YQ. & Ikejima, T. (2003). Hypoglycemic mechanism of *ginseng* glycopeptide. *Acta Pharmacol Sin* Vol.24, No.1 (2003), pp.61-6, ISSN 1745-7254

Wang, RT.; Shan, BE. & Li, QX. (2002). Extracorporeal experimental study on immuno-modulatory activity of *Astragalus memhranaceus* extracts. *Zhongguo Zhong Xi Yi Jie He Za Zhi*, Vol. 22, No. 6, *(Jun 2002),*pp. 453–6, ISSN 0254-6272

Wasser, SP. & Weis, AL. (1999). Therapeutic effects of substances occurring in higher basidiomycetes mushrooms: a modern perspective. *Crit Rev Immunol* Vol.19 (1999), pp.65–96, ISSN 1040-8401

Wiener, N. (1954).*The Human Use of Human Beings*. Houghton-Miffin, ISBN: 0306803208, Boston

Winell, K.; Niemi, M. & Lepantalo, M. (2006). The national hospital discharge register data on lower limb amputations. *Eur J Vasc Endovasc Surg* Vol.32, No.1 (July 2006), pp.66-70, ISSN 1545-1550

World Health Organization. (2009) In: Cardiovascular disease: prevention and control. Available from http://www.who.int/dietphysicalactivity/ publications/facts/cvd/en/. 2009

World Health Organization. 2011. In: WHO Fact sheet N° 312. Availabe *http://www.who.int/mediacentre/factsheets/fs312/en/*

Wu, Y.; Wang, X. & Li, M. (1998). Effect of *Acanthopanacis senticosus* on exercise performance under constant endurance load for elderly. *Wei Sheng Yan Jiu* No.27,(1998), pp.421-4, ISSN 1000-8020

Yamada H. (2004). New scientific approach for natural medicines. In: *Complementary and Alternative Approaches to Biomedicine*, E.L. Cooper, N. Yamaguchi (Ed(s)), 27-33, Plenum Publishers, ISBN 978-030-6482-88-5, New York, USA

Yamaguchi, A.; Tanaka, M.; Naito, K.; Kimura, C.; Kobinata, T.; Okamura, H.; Ino, T. & Adachi, H. (2009).The efficacy of intravenous milrinone in left ventricular restoration. *Ann Thorac Cardiovasc Surg* Vol.8,No.15(August 2009),pp.233-8. ISSN 1341-1098

Yang, M.; Wang, BX. & Jin, YL. (1990). Effects of ginseng polysaccharides on reducing blood glucose and liver glycogen. *Zhongguo Yao Li Xue Bao*, No.11 (1990), pp.520-4, ISSN 0253-9756

Yang, T.; Jia, M.; Meng, J.; Wu, H. & Mei, Q. (2006). Immunomodulatory activity of polysaccharide isolated from *Angelica sinensis*. *Int J Biol Macromol* Vol.39, No. 4-5, (Nov 2006), pp.179-84, ISSN 1478-9868

Yin, ZZ.; Zhang, LY. & Xu, LN. (1980). The effect of dang-gui (*Angelica sinensis*) and its ingredient ferulic acid on rat platelet aggregation and release of 5-HT. *Yao Xue Xue Bao* Vol. 15, No.6, (Jun 1980) pp:321-6, ISSN 0513-4870

Young, HY.; Luo, YL.; Cheng, HY.; Hsieh, WC.; Liao, JC. & Peng, WH. (2005). Analgesic and anti-inflammatory activities of [6]-gingerol. *J Ethnopharmacol* Vol.96,No.1-2,(Jan 2005), pp.207-10, ISSN 1872-7573

Zaragoza, F.; Iglesias, I. & Benedi, J. (1985). Comparative study of the antiaggregation effects of anthocyanosides and other agents. *Arch Farmacol Toxicol* Vol.11,No.3,(Dec 1985), pp:183-8, ISSN 1578-5580

Zhang, HN. & Lin, ZB. (2004). Hypoglycemic effect of *Ganoderma lucidum* polysaccharides. *Acta Pharmacol Sin* Vol.25,No.2, (Feb 2004) pp.191-5, ISSN 1745-7254

Zhang, L.; Wang, Y.; Wang, LZ. & Gao, XM. (2004). Immunopotentiating effect of a 'Yang'-promoting formula of traditional Chinese medicine on aged female BALB/c mice. *Phytother Res* Vol.18, No.10, (Nov 2004), pp.857-61, ISSN 0951-418X

Zhang, Y.; Mills, GL. & Nair, G. (2002). Cyclooxygenase inhibitory and antioxidant compounds from the mycelia of the edible mushroom *Grifola frondosa*. *J Agric Food Chem* Vol.50,No.26,(Dec 2002),pp.7581-5, ISSN 1520-5118

Zhao, J.; Huang, X.; Tang, W.; Ren, P.; Xing, Z.; Tian, X.; Zhu, Z. & Wang, Y. (2007). Effect of oriental herbal prescription Guan-Xin-Er-Hao on coronary flow in healthy volunteers and antiapoptosis on myocardial ischemia-reperfusion in rat models. *Phytother Res* Vol.21,No.10,(Oct 2007), pp. 926-31, ISSN 0951-418X

Zhou, L.; Yang, Y.; Wang, X.; Liu, S.; Shang, W.; Yuan, G.; Li, F.; Tang, J.; Chen, M. & Chen, J. (2007). Berberine stimulates glucose transport through a mechanism distinct from insulin. *Metabolism* Vol.56,No.3,(2007):405-12,ISSN 0026-0495

Zhu, XL.; Chen, AF. & Lin, ZB. (2007). *Ganoderma lucidum* polysaccharides enhance the function of immunological effector cells in immunosuppressed mice. *J Ethnopharmacol* Vol.111, No.2, (May 2007), pp.219-26, ISSN 0378-8741

20

Effectiveness of Fenugreek for Lowering Hemoglobin (HbA1c) in Patients with Self-Management of Type 2 Diabetes: A Randomized Controlled Trial

Rashid Ansari[1] and Saiqaa Ansari[2]
[1]*School of Public Health, University of New England*
[2]*School of Population Health, University of Queensland*
Australia

1. Introduction

The incidence of type 2 diabetes is increasing worldwide, resulting in large measure from the increasing prevalence of obesity (Yale, 2000). Diabetes mellitus is a pandemic disease and is one of the main threats to human health (Narayan, 2005). In 2003, 194 million people worldwide, ranging in age from 20 to 79 years, had diabetes. It is projected that this number will be increased by 72% to 333 million by 2025, and nearly 80% of these cases will be in the poorer industrialized countries (IDF, 2003). According to a 2005 US Government estimate, approximately 21 million people in the United States have diabetes (Gerich, 2005). In 2002, diabetes was the sixth leading cause of death and had an estimated total cost of $132 billion (Hogan et al. 2003). Type 2 diabetes is a disease characterized by a dual defect: 1) by insulin resistance which prevents cells from using insulin properly, and 2) degrees of reduced pancreatic insulin secretion.

In the local context, according to World Health Organisation (WHO, 2004), prevalence of Type 2 diabetes in Pakistan for the year 2000 was 5.2 million and for 2030 it would be around 13.8 million. A quarter of the population of Pakistan would be classified as overweight or obese with the use of Indo-Asian-specific BMI cutoff values. Jafar et al (2006) have reported that prevalence of overweight was 25% and obesity was 10% in a large population-based sample of people over the age of 15 years in Pakistan. On the age-specific prevalence of overweight and obesity, they found that more than 40% of women and 30% of men aged 35–54 years were classified as overweight or obese.

It has been suggested in a variety of observational and epidemiological studies that physical activity may play a significant role in the prevention of type 2 diabetes mellitus. The relationships between physical activity and overweight are only beginning to be understood for the adult population, sedentary behaviours, particularly watching television (TV) and videos, surfing the internet have been found to be related to higher body mass index (BMI) for adult's population (Struber, 2004). The literature linking physical activity levels with risk of overweight in adults is not consistent but physical activity is an important component of effective obesity treatments (Saelens, 2003).

The main health promotion intervention here is the public health education which highlights the importance of physical activity for the prevention of type 2 diabetes in the middle-aged population of sub-continent and particularly Pakistan, which is experiencing a rapid and substantial decline of physical activity levels as a result of poor eating habits, unhealthy food supply, expansion of television, computerization, and mechanization, more prevalent car ownership and sedentary behaviour. In parallel with decreasing levels of physical activity, the prevalence of overweight and obesity has increased significantly in Pakistan and as a consequence, diabetes mellitus has become a major public health issue.

Therefore, promoting an active lifestyle or regular exercise has become the highest public health priority in that country to overcome the onslaught of type 2 diabetes. Also, the search for dietary adjuncts along with usual medical care to treat this life altering disease has become more important and dietary supplements that can modulate glucose homeostasis and potentially improve lipid parameters would be desirable. Fenugreek (Trigonella foenum-graecum Linn) is a dietary supplement that may hold promise in this regard and is one of the oldest medicinal plants, originating in India and Northern Africa and dating back to ancient Egyptian times (Jensen, 1992).

In Pakistan and India, fenugreek is commonly consumed as a condiment (Yoshikawa et al. 1997) and used medicinally as a lactation stimulant (Patil et al. 1997). Fenugreek seeds also lower serum triglycerides, total cholesterol (TC), and low-density lipoprotein cholesterol (LDL-C) (Al-Habori and Raman, 1998). The lipid-lowering effect of fenugreek might also be attributed to its estrogenic constituent, indirectly increasing thyroid hormones (Basch, 2003). The plant protein in fenugreek is 26%, so it might exert a lipid lowering effect (Sharma, 1986). Since a high proportion of diabetic patients in sub-continent suffer from malnutrition, the use of fenugreek which is rich in protein and fiber (48%), has a distinct advantage in these patients (Sharma, 1986).

This chapter addresses the effectiveness of fenugreek for lowering hemoglobin (HbA1c) in this randomized controlled trial and determines whether the intervention of taking fenugreek in combination of usual medical care lowers HbA1c in patients with type 2 diabetes. Effectiveness trials such as this are critical in determining if the interventions are effective in the practical world in which patients live. This randomized control trial addresses the research question "**Is Fenugreek treatment with medical care for patients with type 2 diabetes more effective than usual medical care and can it help to lower the haemoglobin in patients with poorly controlled type 2 diabetes"?** and test the hypothesis in relation to type 2 diabetic patients with usual medical care and usual medical care with self-management of fenugreek supplement and evaluates the effectiveness of the fenugreek treatment in comparison with the usual medical care in clinical settings.

2. Characteristics of type 2 diabetes

Type 2 diabetes is associated with certain ethnic groups, obesity, family history of diabetes, and physical inactivity, among other factors. Diabetes is a metabolic disease characterized by elevated concentrations of blood glucose for prolonged periods of time, i.e., hyperglycemia (Gerich, 2005). Chronic, untreated hyperglycemia can lead to serious complications that include cardiovascular diseases, blindness, kidney failure, and stroke. Furthermore, very low values of blood glucose (hypoglycemia) for even a short duration can result in loss of consciousness and coma. The figure 1 shows the complications of type 2 diabetes which is a syndrome characterized by insulin deficiency, insulin resistance, and increased hepatic glucose production. These metabolic abnormalities are treated by use of various medications which are designed to correct one or more of these metabolic abnormalities (Saltiel & Olefsky, 2001).

Type 2 diabetes is most common in adults, although younger people are also developing this type of disease. It starts with a slow onset with thirst, frequent urination, weight loss developing over weeks to months. It is also considered to run in families but it may happen with a person without a family history of diabetes as well. Most of the people who get this disease are overweight and obese. The treatment for type 2 diabetes differs at various stages of the condition. In its early stages, many people with type 2 diabetes can control their blood glucose levels by losing weight, eating properly and exercising. Many may subsequently need oral medication, and some people with type 2 diabetes may eventually need insulin shots to control their diabetes and avoid the disease's serious complications (Saltiel & Olefsky, 2001).
Even though there is no cure for diabetes, proper treatment and glucose control enable people with type 2 diabetes to live normal, productive lives. A major advance for people at risk of developing type 2 diabetes - such as family members of those with the condition - occurred recently when it was shown that diet and exercise can prevent or delay type 2 diabetes. People at high risk, who already had early signs of impaired glucose tolerance, significantly reduced their risk by losing only 5-7 percent of their body weight and performing moderate physical activity for 30 minutes/day.

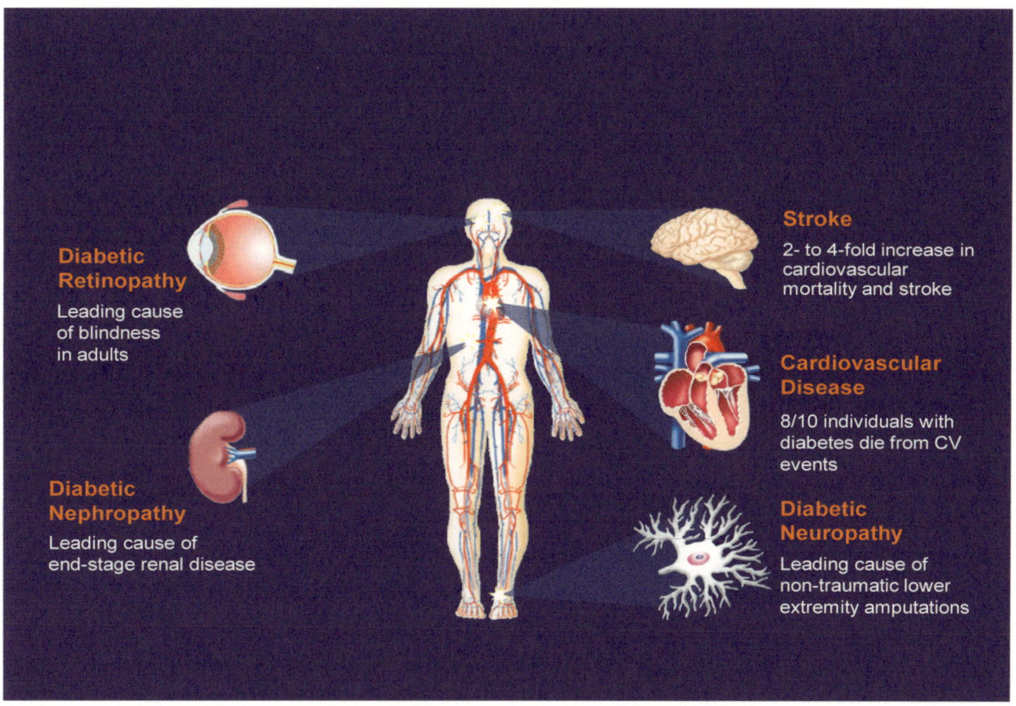

Fig. 1. Complications of type 2 diabetes - Source: Saltiel & Olefsky (2001)

The figure 1 shows the complications of type 2 diabetes from microvascular and macrovascular diseases and can have a devastating effect on quality of life and impose a heavy burden on healthcare systems.
Diabetic retinopathy *is* present in 21% of people in the world at the time type 2 diabetes is diagnosed (DSG, 1990), more than 60% have diabetes retinopathy during the first two decades of the disease and diabetic retinopathy is the leading cause of new blindness among

adults aged 20–74 years (Fong et al. 2003). Pakistan is ranked 6th among countries with the highest burden of diabetes (Wild et al. 2004), however, population-based data on the prevalence of diabetic retinopathy in Pakistan and on the visual impairment due to diabetic retinopathy is lacking and only the hospital-based data is available (Kayani et al. 2003).

Diabetic nephropathy is present in 18% of people diagnosed with diabetes (DSG, 1993) and is a leading cause of end-stage renal disease (Molitch et al. 2003)

Stroke: diabetes is associated with a 2- to 4-fold increase in cardiovascular mortality and stroke (Kannel et al. 1990).

Cardiovascular disease: 75% of individuals with type 2 diabetes die from cardiovascular causes (Gray & Yudkin, 1997).

Diabetic neuropathy *is* present in 12% of people at diagnosis (DSG, 1990) and diabetic neuropathy affects approximately 70% of people with diabetes and is a leading cause of non-traumatic lower extremity amputations (Mayfield et al. 2003). Therefore, early detection and treatment of diabetes is essential in order to reduce the impact of its serious complications.

2.1 Development of type 2 diabetes

Development of type 2 diabetes is the result of multifactorial influences that include lifestyle, environment and genetics. The disease arises when insulin resistance-induced compensatory insulin secretion is exhausted. A high-caloric diet coupled with a sedentary lifestyle is one of the major contributing factors in the development of the insulin resistance and pancreatic β-cell dysfunction as shown in Figure 2. However, a predisposing genetic background has long been suspected in playing a contributing role in the development of type 2 diabetes. By using whole-genome linkage analysis the entire genome of affected family members can be scanned and the family members monitored over several generations (Saltiel & Olefsky, 1996)

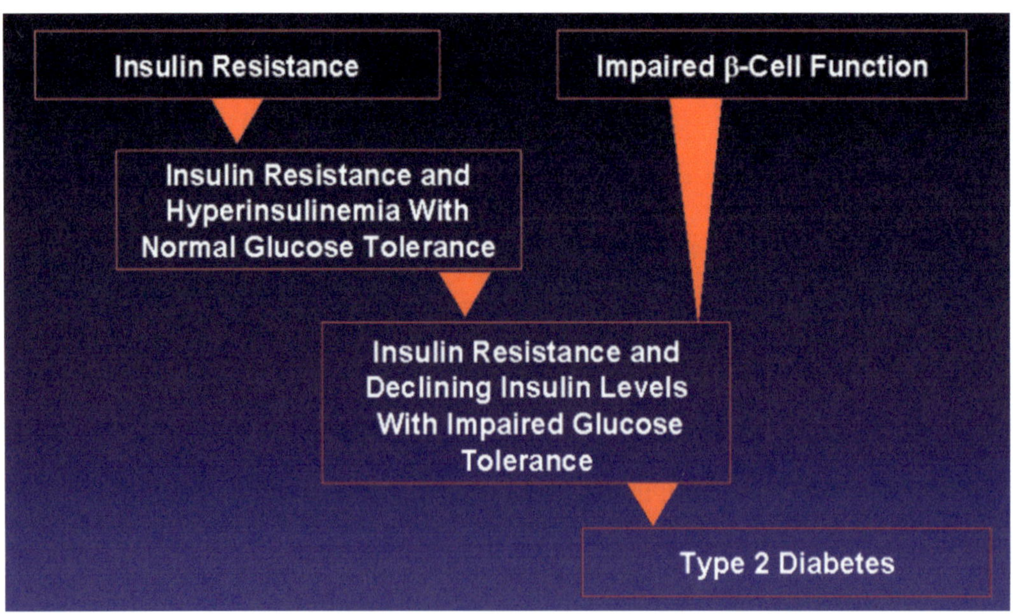

Fig. 2. Development of type 2 diabetes: Adapted from Saltiel & Olefsky (1996)

Although the metabolic syndrome is not exclusively associated with type 2 diabetes and the associated insulin resistance, the increasing prevalence of obesity and associated development of type 2 diabetes places insulin resistance as a major contributor to the syndrome. The metabolic syndrome is defined as a clustering of atherosclerotic cardiovascular disease risk factors that include visceral adiposity (obesity), insulin resistance, low levels of HDLs and a systemic proinflammatory state. There are key components to the metabolic syndrome which include in addition to insulin resistance (the hallmark feature of the syndrome), hypertension, dyslipidemia, chronic inflammation, impaired fibrinolysis, procoagulation and most telling central obesity.

3. Randomized controlled trials with fenugreek

The multiple trials in the past have shown conflicting results of the effect of fenugreek on the patients of type 2 diabetes. These studies showed some positive results on fasting serum glucose but did not examine hemoglobin (HbA1c) levels. Gupta et al (2001) reported the results of a small randomized, controlled, double-blind trial to evaluate the effects of fenugreek seeds on glycemic control. The authors reported that there were no significant differences between groups in mean glucose tolerance test values at the study's end. This study suggested that fenugreek seed extract and diet/exercise may be equally effective strategies for attaining glycemic control in type 2 diabetes. However, the trial may have been too small or brief to detect significant mean differences between groups.

Raghuram et al (1994) reported the results of a randomized, controlled, crossover trial of fenugreek seeds in 10 patients with type 2 diabetes. In the fenugreek-treated patients, statistically significant mean improvements were reported for glucose-tolerance test scores and serum-clearance rates of glucose. The absolute difference in glucose between the two groups was not mentioned. Sharma and Raghuram (1990) conducted two randomized, controlled, crossover studies in patients with type 2 diabetes. Significant mean improvements in fasting blood-glucose levels and glucose-tolerance test results were described in the fenugreek-treated patients.

Moosa et al (2006) conducted study to evaluate the effect of fenugreek on serum lipid profile in hypercholesteremic type 2 diabetic patients and concluded that fenugreek seeds powder significantly reduced serum total cholesterol, triglyceride and LDL-cholesterol but serum HDL-cholesterol level elevation was not significant. Neeraja and Rajyalakshmi (1996) presented a case series including six men with type 2 diabetes and six without diabetes. The cases suggested fenugreek reduced postprandial hyperglycemia primarily in subjects with diabetes, but less so in subjects without diabetes.

The results from several additional case series (Madar et al. 1988; Sharma, 1986; Sharma et al. 1996) also reported that fenugreek seeds may improve glycemic control in type 2 diabetes. The studies conducted to date have been methodologically weak, lacking adequate descriptions of blinding, randomization, baseline patient characteristics, statistical analysis, and standardization data for the therapy used. Demonstrating the efficacy of fenugreek has also been confounded by inconsistencies in the preparations, dosing regimens, and outcome measures used in the trials. Moreover, none of the investigations have been conducted over the longer period (Basch, 2003). The following table 1 gives the summary of Randomized Controlled Trials evaluating fenugreek use in diabetic patients.

Authors	Study Type	Condition	Sample size	Results
Gupta (2001)	Randomized Controlled Trials (Double-blinded)	Type 2 diabetes (hyperlipidemia)	N =25	Improved fasting glucose with fenugreek seeds and diet/exercise.
Raghuram (1994)	Randomized Controlled Trials (crossover study)	Type 2 diabetes	N =10	Improved peripheral glucose utilization with fenugreek seed supplementation
Sharma (1990)	Randomized Controlled Trials (crossover study	Type 2 diabetes	N =25	Improvement in reported diabetic symptoms
Neeraja (1996)	Case series with matched controls	Type 2 diabetes	N =12	Improvement of acute glycemic response with raw fenugreek seed powder
Moosa et al (2006)	Randomized Controlled Trials	Type 2 diabetes (hyperlipidemia)	N =30	Reduced serum total cholesterol with the use of fenugreek

Table 1. Summary of Randomized Controlled Trials evaluating the use of fenugreek in diabetes

4. Method of patient selection

The patients were recruited from the diabetic medical centre in rural area of Peshawar conducting the study of management of type 2 diabetes among the population aged 30-65 years. The patients were eligible and subjected to further screening if their records were found in the clinic database as patients with diabetes and had HbA1c >= 7.0% on a laboratory blood test during the last 6 months. Patients having coexisting liver, kidney or thyroid disorder were not included in the study. Also, the patients with allergy to fenugreek were excluded from the study.

The Word Health Organization (WHO, 2006) diabetes criteria were followed in the selection of the patients with diabetes as indicated in Table 2.

Condition	2 hour glucose	Fasting glucose
	mmol/l(mg/dl)	mmol/l(mg/dl)
Normal	<7.8 (<140)	<6.1 (<110)
Impaired fasting glycaemia	<7.8 (<140)	≥ 6.1(≥110) & <7.0(<126)
Impaired glucose tolerance	≥7.8 (≥140)	<7.0 (<126)
Diabetes mellitus	≥11.1 (≥200)	≥7.0 (≥126)

Table 2. World Health Organization (WHO, 2006). Diabetes Criteria for patients

The well known standard screening test for diabetes, the fasting plasma glucose (FPG), is also a component of diagnostic testing. The FPG test and the 75-g oral glucose tolerance test (OGTT) are both suitable tests for diabetes; however, the FPG test is preferred in clinical settings because it is easier and faster to perform, more convenient and acceptable to patients, and less expensive. This test was carried out and an FPG ≥126 mg/dl (7.0 mmol/l) considered being an indication for retesting, which was repeated on a different day to confirm a diagnosis. If the FPG is <126 mg/dl (7.0 mmol/l) and there is a high suspicion for diabetes, an OGTT was performed. A 2-h postload value in the OGTT ≥200 mg/dl (11.1 mmol/l) is a positive test for diabetes and was confirmed on an alternate day.

When it was found necessary, plasma glucose testing was also performed on individuals who have taken food or drink shortly before testing. Such tests are referred to as casual plasma glucose measurements and are given without regard to time of last meal. A casual plasma glucose level ≥200 mg/dl (11.1 mmol/l) with symptoms of diabetes is considered diagnostic of diabetes. A confirmatory FPG test or OGTT was also completed on such patients on a different day if the clinical condition of the patient permits.

Laboratory measurement of plasma glucose concentration is performed on venous samples with enzymatic assay techniques, and the above-mentioned values are based on the use of such methods. The A1C test values remain a valuable tool for monitoring glycemia, but it is not currently recommended for the screening or diagnosis of diabetes. Pencil and paper tests, such as the American Diabetes Association's risk test, may be useful for educational purposes but do not perform well as stand-alone tests. Capillary blood glucose testing using a reflectance blood glucose meter has also been used but because of the imprecision of this method, it is better used for self-monitoring rather than as a screening tool.

5. Determination of study sample size

The study sample size was determined based on the assumption of the estimation of Standard Deviation (SD). Therefore, the study design was selected to detect an effect size of 0.5 SD lowering of HbA1c. It was assumed that 15% patients might be lost to follow-up in control group over the period of three months and only 5 % patients will be lost to follow-up in intervention group. This assumption was based on the popularity of fenugreek seeds used by diabetic patients in sub-continent to manage their glycemic control. Taking into consideration all these factors, the following parameters were considered: α = Level of significance test = 0.05, Power = 0.8, m= the follow-up period 90 days (3 months), Standard Deviation (SD) = 0.5, the sample size was calculated for each group to detect an effect size of 0.5 SD. The sample size (N) for each group was =105; therefore, the total, N=210 patients were recruited to participate in both the groups.

6. Study population and randomization

Initially 325 patients with type 2 diabetes were invited to pre-randomized interview, out of which only 210 patients were included in the actual trial. Out of the 325 patients, 93 patients did not meet the inclusion criteria and 22 patients refused to participate in the trial. Finally, two hundred and ten (210) patients agreed to participate and signed informed consent documents at the clinic where they used to visit for their usual medical care for diabetes. Therefore, 102 patients were randomized to intervention group (fenugreek supplements) and 108 to the control group (usual medical care). Figure 3 shows their progress during the randomized controlled trial.

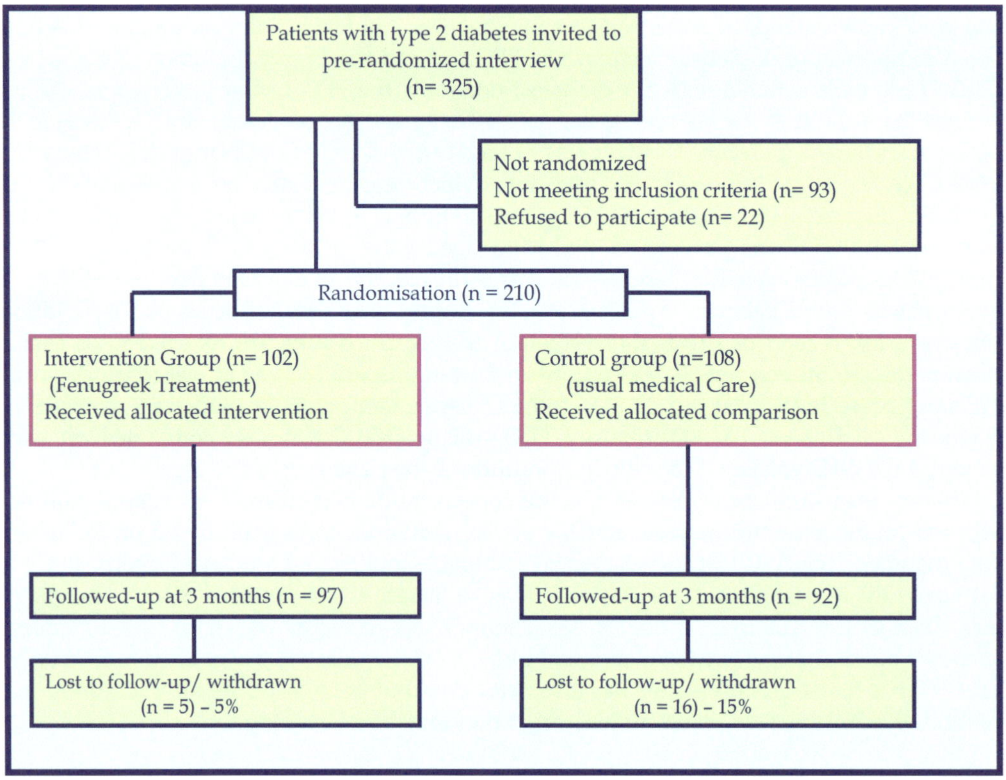

Fig. 3. Flow chart describing Randomized Controlled Trial of fenugreek treatment:

The sequence of allocation to treatments (a randomized list) was generated using the random number function in Excel worksheet. The baseline assessment was carried out prior to group allocation by an investigator/coordinator blind to the allocation sequence. The participants were issued a sealed envelope containing their group allocation. The randomization code was developed using a computer random number generator in a block size of eight patients. That helped to allocate patients to the intervention and control groups equally in each block - that is each patient would have an equal chance of allocation to either group. Once the randomization phase was completed, all patients were instructed to follow-up the usual medical care for their diabetes for the duration of the 90 days trial. The patients were allowed to adjust their usual medications as recommended by their doctors. In addition, each patient was asked to go for blood test for HbA1c on day 1 and then return to give blood sample after 90 days. In addition, participants were advised not to take any other new treatments for the management of type 2 diabetes during the trial periods.

The control group in randomized controlled trial received medical care from a physician-coordinated team. This team included physicians, nurses, dietitians, and mental health professionals with expertise and a special interest in diabetes. It is essential in this collaborative and integrated team approach that individuals with diabetes assume an active role in their care. The management plan in that group was based on individualized therapeutic alliance among the patient and family, the physician, and other members of the health care team. This plan has recognized diabetes self-management education as an integral component of care and in developing the plan, consideration was given to the patient's age, work schedule and conditions, physical activity, eating patterns, social situation and personality, cultural factors, and presence of complications of diabetes or other medical conditions. Treatment goals were set together with the patient, family, and health care team. Patient self-management was emphasized, and the plan emphasized the involvement of the patient in problem-solving as much as possible. A variety of strategies and techniques were employed to provide adequate education and development of problem-solving skills in the various aspects of diabetes management. During the implementation of the management plan it was assured that each aspect of diabetes management was understood and agreed on by the patient and the care providers and that the goals and treatment plan were reasonable.

Those patients randomized to take fenugreek (intervention group) received 100 gms fenugreek seeds powder from the pharmacy in the clinic. They were instructed to take 50 gms doses twice a day at lunch and dinner time in addition to their normal medications for diabetes. Those patients randomized to usual medical care (control group) were instructed to take their normal medicines and follow-up with their doctor as per their normal schedule. All participants were contacted again after 90 days (3-months) to give their blood sample for HbA1c testing. At that time, a questionnaire was sent via e-mail to participants in both intervention and control groups to assess the progress of the fenugreek treatment and clinical care without fenugreek.

The clinical and demographic characteristics of the patients in the two groups were well balanced at randomization. A demographic measure included age, gender, weight, ethnicity, religion, marital status, previous episodes of glycemic control, previous and current treatments of type 2 diabetes. The table 3 gives baseline characteristics of intervention and control groups in RCT trial.

Characteristics	**Intervention Group (n = 97)**	**Control Group (n = 92)**	**P-value**
Age (years)	Mean (62.5) ± SD (10.5)	Mean (59.5) ± SD (8.5)	0.78
Sex Male Female	 56% (n = 54) 44% (n = 43)	 58% (n = 53) 42% (n = 39)	
Body Mass Index (Kg/m2)	Mean (30.8) ± SD (6.5)	Mean (31.6) ± SD (6.5)	0.40
Fenugreek Intake Normal High	 98% (n=95) 2% (n = 2)	 - -	
Baseline Hemoglobin (HbA1c) %	Mean (8.5) ± SD (1.6)	Mean (8.4) ± SD (1.5)	0.59
Diabetes Medications	Mean (1.75) ± SD (0.8)	Mean (1.82) ± SD (0.8)	0.15

Table 3. Baseline characteristics of intervention and control groups in RCT trial

7. Type 2 diabetes treatments

7.1 Diabetes treatment with medications

The treatment options of type 2 diabetes is shown in figure 4 suggesting the specific areas of actions using medications which influence the various organs of the body to correct the metabolic abnormalities such as reducing the liver glucose production, slowing down absorption of sugars from the gut and reducing the insulin resistance. There are currently six distinct classes of hypoglycemic agents available to treat type 2 diabetes. These agents are Sulfonylurea (gliclazide, glipizide etc) - increase insulin secretion; Meglitinide (repaglinide) - increase insulin secretion; Biguanides (metformin) - reduce glucose production; Alpha-glycosidase (acrobase) - slow down absorption of sugar from the gut; Thiazolidendiones (pioglitazone) - reduce insulin resistance and Incretins - increase insulin secretion.

The patients in both the groups in RCT trials received medications recommended by their physicians. The most common combinations among both the groups were Meglitinide (repaglinide) with Thiazolidendiones and Sulfonylurea with Biguanides. However, the intervention group was given fenugreek as an additional supplement. The table 4 shows the hypoglycemic medications used by the patients during fenugreek RCT trial for 90 days.

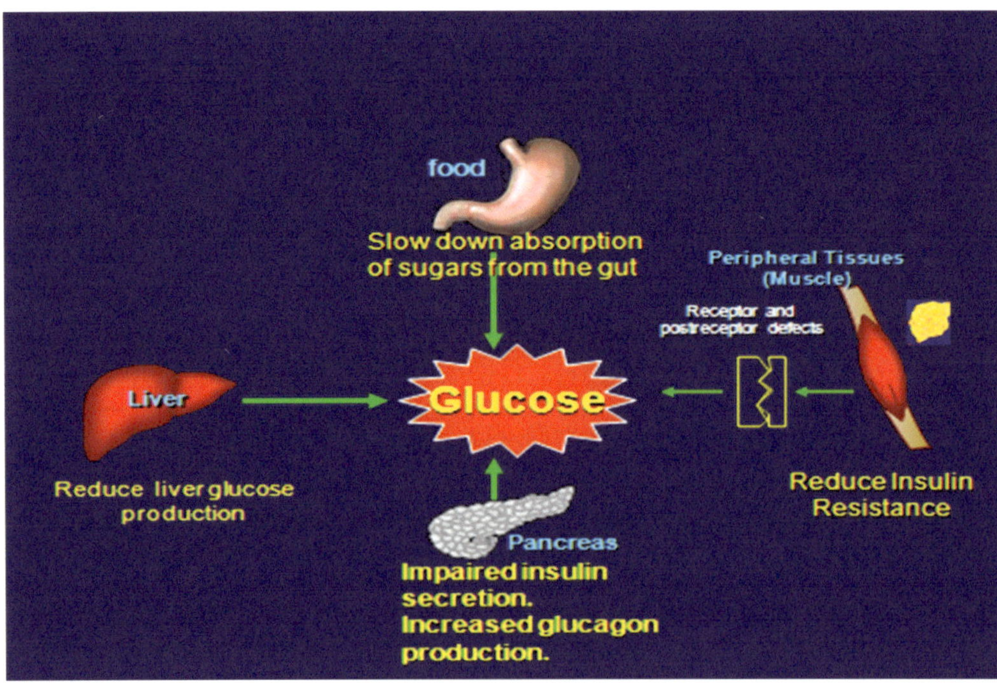

Fig. 4. Treatment options for type 2 diabetes - Source: Saltiel & Olefsky (2001)

Medication	Doses	Action
Sulfonylurea (Gliclazide)	30-120 mg/day	Increase insulin secretion
Meglitinide (Repaglinide)	0.5-4 mg/meal	Increase insulin secretion
Biguanides (Metformin)	25-3000 mg/day	Decrease hepatic glucose secretion
Thiazolidendione (Glitazone)	15-30 mg/day	Increase the insulin receptor number
Fenugreek (only for patients in intervention group)	100 gm/day	Help to lower HbA1c

Table 4. Hypoglycemic medications used by patients in fenugreek RCT trial

7.1.1 Details of hypoglycaemic medications used in RCT trial

The diabetes medications mentioned in table 4 work in different ways but the main function of all these medications include lowering blood sugar levels; help improve the body's use of glucose, decrease the symptoms of high blood sugar, help keeping patients with diabetes functioning normally and may prevent the complications, organ-damaging effects and premature deaths diabetes can cause. Since the drugs work in different ways, these are sometimes used in combination to enhance the effectiveness of treatment. In this RCT trial Sulfonylurea was used in combination with Biguanide (metformin) and Meglitinide was used in combination with Thiazolidinedione. However, fenugreek supplementation was only given to the patients in intervention group. The advantages and disadvantages of these medications used in RCT trial are given in Table 5 and the details of their mode of actions are summarized as follows:

Sulfonylurea: The sulfonylurea (Gliclazide) is an oral hypoglycemic drug and referred to as endogenous insulin secretagogues because the drug induces the pancreatic release of endogenous insulin. The fact that this drug induces pronounced hypoglycemia, treatment is initiated with the lowest possible dose and carefully monitored until the dose is found to control glucose level at 110-140mg/dL. The main function of Sulfonylurea is to bind and inhibit the pancreatic ATP-dependent potassium channel that is normally involved in glucose-mediated insulin secretion. Sulfonylurea has no significant effects on circulating triglycerides, lipoproteins or cholesterol.

Meglitinide: The meglitinide (repaglinide) is a non-sulfonylurea insulin secretagogues that is both fast acting and of short duration. Like the sulfonylurea, meglitinide therapy results in significant reduction in fasting glucose as well as HbA1c. The mechanism of action of the meglitinide is initiated by binding to a receptor on the pancreatic β-cell that is distinct from the receptors for the sulfonylurea. However, meglitinide do exerts effects on potassium conductance. Like the sulfonylurea, the meglitinide have no direct effects on the circulating levels of plasma lipids.

Biguanide: The biguanide (metformin) is a class of drugs that function to lower serum glucose levels by enhancing insulin-mediated suppression of hepatic glucose production and enhancing insulin-stimulated glucose uptake by skeletal muscle. Metformin is a member of this class and is currently the most widely prescribed insulin-sensitizing drug in current clinical use. Metformin administration does not lead to increased insulin release from the pancreas and as such the risk of hypoglycemia is minimal. Because the major site of action for metformin is the liver its use can be contraindicated in patients with liver dysfunction. The drug is ideal for obese patients and for younger type 2 diabetics.

Thiazolidinedione: The thiazolidinedione (pioglitazone) has proven useful in treating the hyperglycemia associated with insulin-resistance in both type 2 diabetes and non-diabetic conditions. The net effect of the thiazolidinedione is a potentiation of the actions of insulin in liver, adipose tissue and skeletal muscle, increased peripheral glucose disposal and a decrease in glucose output by the liver.

Medications	Advantages	Disadvantages
Sulfonylurea (Gliclazide)	Fast onset of action No effect on blood pressure No effect on LDL cholesterol Convenient dosing Low cost	Weight gain reported Risk of hypoglycemia
Meglitinide (Repaglinide)	No bad effect on cholesterol Rapid onset of action	Risk of hypoglycemia Weight gain reported Inconvenient dosing High cost
Biguanides (Metformin)	Low risk of hypoglycemia Not linked to weight gain Good effect on LDL cholesterol No ill effect on blood pressure Low cost	High risk of GI side effects (nausea and diarrhea) Risk of lactic acid build-up Less convenient dosing
Thiazolidendione (Glitazone)	Low risk of hypoglycemia Increase in HDL cholesterol Linked to decreased triglycerides Convenient dosing	Higher risk of heart failure Linked to weight gain Linked to risk of edema Linked to risk of anemia Slower onset of action Increase in LDL cholesterol

Table 5. Advantages and disadvantages of medications used by patients in fenugreek RCT trial

7.2 Diabetes treatment with diet and exercise

The normal diabetes treatment addresses the issues related to unhealthy lifestyles, such as lack of physical activity and excessive eating, which are the main causes to initiate and propagate the majority of type 2 diabetes (Michael, 2007). Studies have demonstrated strong relationship between excess weight and the risk of developing type 2 diabetes, hypertension, and hyperlipidemia. Therefore, the objective of physicians is to motivate patients to lose weight and exercise to improve the control of diabetes and slow down or even reverse the natural course of the disease (Michael, 2007).

However, it is difficult to overstate the importance of the relationship between lifestyle and the risk of developing type 2 diabetes. It has been demonstrated in recent studies that both women and men who have a BMI >35 kg/m^2 had a 20-fold increase in their risk of developing diabetes compared to people with a BMI of 18.5 - 24.9 kg/m^2 (Mokdad et al. 2001; Field et al. 2001). There are prospective studies which have demonstrated that lifestyle modification in the form of diet and regular moderate exercise sharply decrease the likelihood of developing type 2 diabetes in high-risk individuals who have impaired glucose tolerance or impaired fasting glucose. The effectiveness of this intervention superseded that of metformin therapy (Knowler et al. 2002). In this RCT trial, physicians compiled the flow scheme shown in Figure 5 which represents the method of treatment of type 2 diabetes by the combination of diet, exercise and medication for diabetes monitoring and control. It has been divided into two segments: for obese and normal weight patients and the combination of medication for both the groups of patients. The supplement of fenugreek was given to the patients belonging to intervention group.

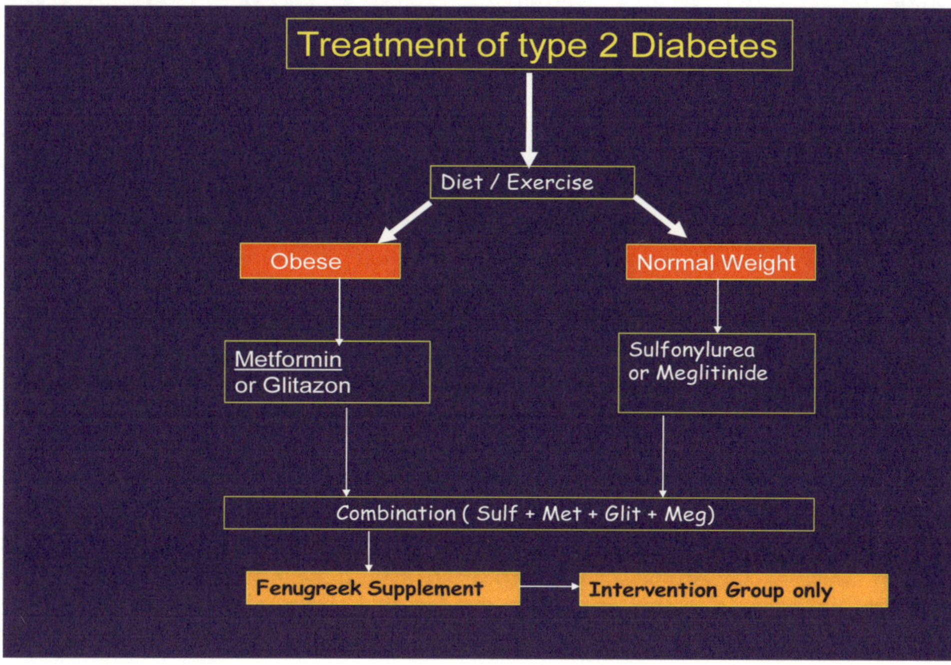

Fig. 5. Treatment of type 2 diabetes with the combination of diet, exercise and medications.

7.2.1 Dietary consideration for patients (intervention and control group)

It has been recommended that carbohydrate and monosaturated fat consumption for the patients with type 2 diabetes should comprise 60-70% of total calories. However, there is some concern that increased unsaturated fat consumption may promote weight gain in obese patients with type 2 diabetes and therefore may cause in reduction of insulin sensitivity (Bantle et al. 1993). The "glycemic index" is an attempt to compare the glycemic effects of various foods to a standard, such as white bread. Although several authors have proposed its clinical usefulness in controlling postprandial hyperglycemia, prospective studies have not demonstrated a clear improvement in hemoglobin (HbA1c) in patients using low-glycemic index diets (Michael, 2007).

The physicians in this trial have recommended the best mix of carbohydrate, protein, and fat that was adjusted to meet the metabolic goals and individual preference of the patients with diabetes in both the intervention and control groups. It has been recommended for individuals with diabetes, that the use of the glycemic index and glycemic load may provide a modest additional benefit for glycemic control over that observed when total carbohydrate is considered alone (ADA, 2011). Monitoring carbohydrate, whether by carbohydrate counting, choices, or experience-based estimation, remain a key strategy in achieving glycemic control. In addition, saturated fat intake should be less than 7% of total calories and the intake of trans fat should also be minimized.

7.2.2 Physical activity consideration for patients (intervention and control group)

Physical activity is a key component of lifestyle modification that can help individuals prevent or control type 2 diabetes. It is considered that diet is probably more important in the initial phases of weight loss, incorporating exercise as part of a weight loss regimen helps maintain weight and prevent weight regain (Klein et al. 2004). In this trial, the message was given to both the groups that as little as 30 minutes of moderate physical activity daily may offer greater benefits to these patients in managing their diabetes. It has also been reported that in patients with type 2 diabetes, structured regimens of physical activity for 8 weeks or longer improved HbA1c independent of changes in body mass (Sigal et al. 2006).

The evidence supports the contention that controlling blood glucose through modification of diet and lifestyle should be mainstay of diabetes therapy. It was found in this RCT that despite being one of the most time-consuming discussions with the patients in both the groups, this is probably the most important patient-physician discussion in regard to diabetes control and prevention of disease progression and complications.

8. Statistical analysis

We analysed the primary outcome by an un-paired sample t-test (mean difference between baseline and final HbA1c). The statistical analysis was carried out on an intention to treat basis and that was subject to the availability of data at follow up as well as at entry level for individual patients. The differences between mean changes were tested by unpaired t tests, and χ^2 tests (chi-squared test) were used to test for differences in proportions between the fenugreek treatment and clinical based treatment groups. For the χ^2 tests, the following formula was used.

$$\chi^2 = \Sigma \frac{(\text{observed} - \text{expected})^2}{\text{expected}}$$

In this study for example (using the data from Figure 3) - it shows that number of patients at three months follow-up who were allocated to intervention group to help lowering their glycemic control were 95 % as compared the patients in clinical care (85 %), so $\chi^2 = 5.73$, P=0.02). The association between the groups and outcome is considered statistically significant.

All the patients in intervention and control groups were provided glucometers to check their blood sugar three times in a day (Fasting sugar in the morning, at bed time and 2-hrs after meal) and record that on XL-worksheet prepared for them to enter the data. Then linear regression analysis was performed after three months between HbA1c and on the blood glucose results. The HbA1c and the self-glucose monitoring via a glucometer demonstrated a significant relationship (R = .90, P < 0.0001).

These findings are in agreement with the findings of Nathan et al. (2008) who reported that the linear regression analysis carried out by these authors between the HbA1c and blood glucose (BG) values provided the tightest correlations ($BG = 28.7 \times A1C - 46.7$, $R^2 = 0.84$, $P < 0.0001$), allowing calculation of an estimated average glucose for HbA1C values. The linear regression equations did not differ significantly across subgroups based on age, sex, diabetes type, race/ethnicity, or smoking status.

9. Results and discussions

The results of this randomized controlled trial support the hypothesis and research question that fenugreek supplement with usual medical care for type 2 diabetes is more effective than the usual medical care alone. The changes in HbA1c from baseline values in intervention and control groups after 3 months were calculated by unpaired sample t-test, the results are given in Table 6. At 3 months follow-up, the intervention group (fenugreek treatment) has shown significantly greater improvement and lowered HbA1c by 0.92% (95% CI, 0.34-1.50), p < 0.001 as compared with usual medical care alone lowering HbA1c by 0.42% (95% CI, 0.11-0.94), p = 0.12 in patents with poorly controlled diabetes.
The higher % age of lost to follow up throughout this trial (Figure 3) in those patients with usual medical care (15%) than in those treated by fenugreek (5%) suggests greater satisfaction with fenugreek supplement. The difference at 3 months follow up is the mean change for the intervention group minus the mean change for the control group. Therefore, the positive differences reflect more improvement in those treated by fenugreek supplement than in medical care alone.

RCT (Groups)	Baseline (HbA1c)	Final (HbA1c)	Difference	P-value
Treatment (n=97)	9.32 ± 2.2	8.4 ± 1.9	- 0.92 (95% CI, 0.34-1.50)	< .001
Control (n= 92)	9.10 ± 2.1	8.68 ± 1.6	- 0.42 (95% CI, 0.11- 0.94)	0.12

Table 6. Effect of Fenugreek on Hemoglobin (HbA1c) in type 2 diabetes

In patients with type 2 diabetes previous studies have shown an association between the degree of hyperglycemia and increased risk of microvascular complications (Klein, 1995), sensory neuropathy (Alder et al 1997), myocardial infarction (Klein, 1995; UKPDS,1998), stroke (Lehto et al. 1996), macrovascular mortality (Groeneveld et al. 1999) and all cause mortality (Wei et al. 1998; Knuiman et al. 1992). Generally, these studies measured glycemia as being high or low or assessed glycemia on a single occasion, whereas repeated measurements of glycemia over several moths or year would be more informative.
The existence of thresholds of glycemia—that is, concentrations above which the risk of complications markedly increases was studied in patients with type 2 diabetes by Stratton et al. (2000). The relative risk for myocardial infarction seems to increase with any increase in glycemia above the normal range (Fuller et al. 1983) as shown in figure 6 whereas the risk for microvascular disease is thought to occur only with more extreme concentrations of glycemia (Krolewski et al. 1995). The diabetes control and complications trial (DCCT) research group showed an association between glycemia and the progression of microvascular complications in patients with diabetes for hemoglobin HbA1C over the range of 6-11% after a mean of six years of follow up (DCCT, 1996).

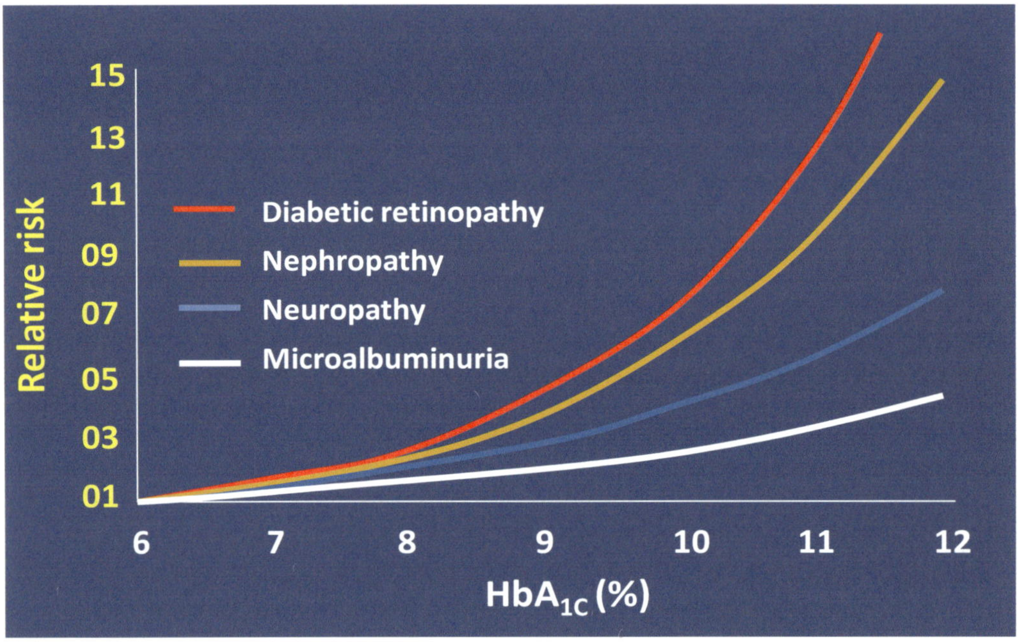

Source: Diabetic Control and Complications Trials (DCCT, 1996; Stratton et al. 2000)

Fig. 6. Relative risk of progression of diabetic complications by mean HbA1c

It has been reported by Stratton et al (2000) that the incidence of clinical complications was significantly associated with glycemia. That is each 1% reduction in updated mean HbA1c was associated with reductions in risk of 21% for any end point related to diabetes (95% confidence interval 17% to 24%, P<0.0001), 21% for deaths related to diabetes (15% to 27%, P<0.0001), 14% for myocardial infarction (8% to 21%, P<0.0001), and 37% for microvascular complications (33% to 41%, P<0.0001). The current fenugreek trial has demonstrated that there is a significant improvement after 3 months follow-up in the intervention group (fenugreek treatment) which has lowered HbA1c by 0.92% (95% CI, 0.34-1.50), p < 0.001 as compared to medical care alone lowering HbA1c by 0.42% (95% CI, 0.11-0.94), p = 0.12 in patents with poorly controlled diabetes. These finding are in agreement with the studies by Stratton et al (2000) that any reduction in HbA1c is likely to reduce the risk of complications, with the lowest risk being in those with HbA1c values in the normal range (< 6.0%).

10. Strength and weakness of the study

The strength of this trial is that it was an effectiveness trial that addressed the community clinical practice specific to the population in sub-continent and it has measured outcomes that are most significant to diabetes care providers. Previous trials have shown conflicting results about the efficacy of fenugreek to treat diabetes as summarized in Table 1 and none of the trials measured HbA1c as an outcome in their studies. There are several reasons of the success of this trial as compared to previous trials. The first reason is that this is the largest randomized fenugreek trial (n =210) to date in type 2 diabetes. The other reason is that we studied only patients with poorly controlled type 2 diabetes and finally, diabetics in sub-

continent may have different characteristics than those in other western countries due to their eating of different foods and drinking habits.
It is possible that the outcome measures associated with fenugreek treatment are subject to bias particularly when treatment was in progress or just afterwards. The main difference between usual medical care alone for the patients and usual medical care with fenugreek treatment occurred after 3 months period of trial. In order to reduce the bias, the questionnaire was sent to patients at home or via e-mail to minimize any chance that their answers might be affected by actual or perceived influence by medical practitioners at clinic. Also, the doctors did not know about those patients who were using fenugreek supplement and were blinded to the treatment allocation.

11. Contribution of the trial to public health

The main contribution of this study is to provide health professionals (diabetes care providers) and patients with type 2 diabetes an easily available, safe and cheap alternative (fenugreek seeds powder) to help them in the self-management and treatment of type 2 diabetes. The United Kingdom Prospective Diabetes Study (UKPDS) reported that a reduction of HbA1c from 7.9% to 7% lowers the risk of macro-vascular disease by 16%, retinopathy by 17% to 21% and nephropathy by 24% to 33% (UKPDS, 1998). Therefore, the results of this trial which have shown improvement in patients of diabetes by lowering HbA1c by 0.92% (95% CI, 0.34-1.50) might be expected to provide similar reductions in morbidity.

12. Future research

The use of fenugreek as a dietary supplement hold promise in future to be used in patients who manifest abnormalities of glucose monitoring and could benefit from a low-risk, inexpensive, food-based intervention aimed at normalizing their blood sugar levels and more specifically the HbA1c targets. However, the data collected to date on the benefits of fenugreek are sparse but may be used in future research for the development of well-designed, adequately powered, large scale randomized clinical trials for evaluating the effect of fenugreek seed powder on measures of insulin resistance, insulin secretion and better glucose control among the patients with type 2 diabetes.

13. Conclusion

In this randomized controlled trial, it has been shown that the levels of HbA1c reduced in the patients of poorly controlled type 2 diabetes who were taking 50 gms doses of fenugreek twice a day in addition to their normal medications for diabetes. These results of RCT support the hypothesis and the research question that fenugreek supplement with usual medical care for type 2 diabetes is more effective than the usual medical care alone. Therefore, it is recommended that fenugreek supplementation is safe and may be considered in patients with HBA1c > 7% as a potential means to lower the high levels of HbA1c.

14. Acknowledgement

The authors are highly thankful to Dr. Akif Ullah Khan, medical director of Ibn-Al-Nafees Medical Center, Peshawar- Pakistan for providing extensive help and support to carry out the RCT in his clinical settings in collaboration of his medical staff and helped to acquire the specific data of middle-aged population of Pakistan from the source www.pmrc.org.pk.The authors also extend their appreciation to Pakistan Medical Research Council for providing linkage to major national health studies, digital and electronic databases for educational and research purposes.

15. References

Adler AI, Boyko EJ, Ahroni AJ (1997), Risk factors for diabetic peripheral sensory neuropathy. Results of the Seattle prospective diabetic foot study. Diabetes Care; 20:1162-1167.

Al-Habori M, Raman A (1998). Antidiabetic and hypocholesterolaemic effects of fenugreek. Phytother Res; 12:233-242.

American Diabetes Association (2011). Standard of Medical care in Diabetes. Diabetes care, vol 34, Supplement 1 (S11-S61).

Bantle JP, Swanson JE, Thomas W et al (1993). Metabolic effects of dietary sucrose in type II diabetic subjects. *Diabetes Care* 16:1301–1305.

Basch, E, Ulbricht, C, Kuo, G et al (2003). Therapeutic applications of fenugreek. Alter Med rev; 8: 20-7.

DCCT Research Group (1996). The absence of a glycemic threshold for the development of long-term complications: the perspective of the diabetes control and complications trial. Diabetes; 45:1289-1298.

Diabetes Study Group (1990). UK Prospective Diabetes Studies, Diabetes Res; 13:1-11.

Diabetes study group (1993). Hypertension in Diabetes, J Hypertens; 11: 309-317.

Field AE, Coakley EH, Must A et al (2001). Impact of overweight on the risk of developing common chronic diseases during a 10-year period. *Arch Intern Med* 161:1581–1586.

Fong, DS, Aiello, L, Gardner, TW et al (2003). Diabetic Retinopathy, Diabetes Care; 26 (Suppl. 1): S99-S102.

Fuller JH, Shipley MJ, Rose G (1983). Mortality from coronary heart disease and stroke in relation to degree of glycaemia: the Whitehall study. BMJ; 287:867-870.

Gerich JE (2005). The importance of tight glycemic control. *Am J Med.* pp. 7–11.

Gray RP & Yudkin JS (1997). Cardiovascular disease in diabetes. In *Textbook of Diabetes* 2nd Edition, Blackwell Sciences.

Groeneveld Y, Petri H, Hermans J et al (1999). Relationship between blood glucose level and mortality in type 2 diabetes mellitus: a systematic review. Diabet Med; 116:2-13.

Gupta A, Gupta R, Lal B (2001). Effect of Trigonella foenum-graecum (fenugreek) seeds on glycaemic control and insulin resistance in type 2 diabetes mellitus: a double blind placebo controlled study. J Assoc Physicians India; 49:1057-1061.

Hogan P, Dall T, Nikolov P (2003). Economic costs of diabetes in the US in 2002. *Diabetes Care.* 26(3):917–932.

International Diabetes Federation (2003): Diabetes Atlas, 2nd ed. Brussels, IDF.

Jafar TH, Chaturvedi N, Pappas G (2006). Prevalence of overweight and obesity and their association with hypertension and diabetes mellitus in an Indo-Asian population. *CMAJ*; 175(9):1071-7.

Jensen, R (1992). Fenugreek overlooked but not forgotten. UCLA Lactation Alumni Newsletter; 1: 2-3.

Kannel WB, D'Agostino RB, Wilson PWF et al (1990. Diabetes, fibrinogen, and risk of cardiovascular disease: the Framingham experience. *Am Heart J.* 120:672–676.

Kayani, H, Rehan, N, Ullah, N (2003). Frequency of retinopathy among diabetes admitted in a teaching hospital of Lahore. J Ayub Med Coll, Abbottabad; 15(4): 53-6.

Klein R (1995) Hyperglycemia and microvascular and macrovascular disease in diabetes. Diabetes Care; 18:258-268.

Klein S, Sheard NF, Pi-Sunyer X et al (2004). Weight management through lifestyle modification for the prevention and management of type 2 diabetes: *Diabetes Care* 27:2067–2073.

Knowler WC, Barrett-Connor E, Fowler SE, et al (2002). Reduction in the incidence of type 2 diabetes with lifestyle intervention or metformin. N Engl J Med; 346:393–403.

Knuiman MW, Welborn TA, Whittall DE (1992). An analysis of excess mortality rates for persons with non-insulin-dependent diabetes mellitus in Western Australia using the Cox proportional hazards regression model. Am J Epidemiol; 135:638-648.

Krolewski AS, Laffel LM, Krolewski M et al (1995). Glycosylated hemoglobin and the risk of microalbuminuria in patients with insulin-dependent diabetes mellitus. N Engl J Med; 332:1251-1255.

Lehto S, Ronnemaa T, Pyörälä K (1996). Predictors of stroke in middle-aged patients with non-insulin-dependent diabetes. Stroke, 6; 27:63-68

Madar Z, Abel R, Samish S, Arad I (1988). Glucose-lowering effect of fenugreek in non-insulin dependent diabetics. Ear J Clin Nutr; 42:51-54.

Mayfield JA, Reiber, GE, Sanders, LJ et al *(2003).* Preventive Foot Care in people with Diabetes. *Diabetes Care* 2003; 26 (Suppl.1):S78–S79.

Michael, JE (2007). Diabetes Treatment: Diet and Exercise. Clinical Diabetes, vol. 25(3), 105-109.

Mokdad AH, Ford ES, Bowman BA et al (2003). Prevalence of obesity, diabetes, and obesity-related health risk factors, *JAMA* 289:76–79.

Molitch ME, de Fronze, RA, Franz, MJ et al (2003). Diabetic Nephropathy*, Diabetes Care*; 26 (Suppl. 1): S94–S98.

Moosa, ASM, Mamun, R, Asadi, AZS et al (2006). Hypolipidemic effects of fenugreek seed powder, Bangladesh J of Pharmacology, 1:64-67.

Narayan, K.M.V. (2005). The Diabetes Pandemic: Looking for the silver lining: Clinical diabetes. Volume 23, 2, p: 51-52.

Nathan D, Kuenen J, Borg R, et al (2008). Translating the A1c assay into estimated average glucose values. *Diabetes Care*: 31(8): 1473-1478

Neeraja A, Rajyalakshmi P (1996). Hypoglycemic effect of processed fenugreek seeds in humans. J Food Sci Technol; 33:427-430.

Patil SP, Niphadkar PV, Bapat MM (1997). Allergy to fenugreek (Trigonella foenum graecum). Ann Allergy Asthma Immunol; 78:297-300.

Raghuram TC, Sharma RD, Sivakumar B, et al (1994). Effect of fenugreek seeds on intravenous glucose disposition in non-insulin dependent diabetic patients. Phytother Res; 8:83-86.

Saelens, BE (2003). Helping individuals reduce sedentary behavior. In: Andersen RE, ed. *Obesity: Etiology, Assessment, Treatment, and Prevention.* Champaign, IL: Human Kinetics; 217 -238.

Saltiel, AR, Olefsky, JM (2001). Diabetes. Am Fam Physician; 63: 1747-56.

Sharma RD (1986). Effect of fenugreek seeds and leaves on blood glucose and serum insulin response in human subjects. Nutr Res; 6:1353-64.

Sharma RD (1986). Effect of fenugreek seeds and leaves on blood glucose and serum insulin responses in human subjects. Nutr Res; 6:1353-1364.

Sharma RD, Raghuram TC (1990). Hypoglycaemic effect of fenugreek seeds in non-insulin dependent diabetic subjects. Nutr Res; 10:731-739.

Sharma RD, Sarkar A, Hazra DK, et al (1996). Use of fenugreek seed powder in the management of non-insulin dependent diabetes mellitus. Nutr Res; 16:1331-1339.

Sigal RJ, Kenny GP, Wasserman DH et al (2006). Physical activity/exercise and type 2 diabetes: a consensus statement from the American Diabetes Association. *Diabetes Care* 29:1433–1438.

Stratton, IM, Adler, AI, Neil, HAW et al (2000). Association of glycemic with macrovascular and microvascular complications of type 2 diabetes: Prospective observational studies. BMJ 321: 405-412.

Struber, J (2004). Considering physical inactivity in relation to obesity. The Internet Journal of Allied Health Sciences and Practice; January, Vol 2 Nr 1.

UKPDS (1998). Intensive blood glucose control with sulphonylureas or insulin compared with conventional treatment and risk of complications in patients with type 2 diabetes. UK Prospective diabetes study (UKPDS) Group. Lancet; 352: 837-53.

Wei M, Gaskill SP, Haffner SM (1998). Effects of diabetes and level of glycaemia on all-cause and cardiovascular mortality. Diabetes Care; 21:1167-1172

WHO (2004). Expert Consultation: Appropriate body-mass index for Asian populations and its implications for policy and intervention. *Lancet*; 363:157-63.

Wild, S, Roglic, G, Green, A et al (2004). Global prevalence of diabetes: estimates for the year 2000 and projections for 2030. Diabetes care; 27(5):1047-53.

Yale JF (2000). Prevention of type 2 diabetes. Int J Clin Pract Suppl; 113:35-39.

Yoshikawa M, Murakami T, Komatsu H, et al (1997). Medicinal foodstuffs. IV. Fenugreek seed. (1): structures of trigoneosides Ia, Ib, IIa, IIb, IIIa, and IIIb, new furostanol saponins from the seeds of Indian Trigonella foenum-graecum L. Chem Pharm Bull (Tokyo); 45:81-87.